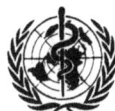

WORLD HEALTH ORGANIZATION

INTERNATIONAL AGENCY FOR RESEARCH ON CANCER

IARC MONOGRAPHS

ON THE

EVALUATION OF CARCINOGENIC

RISKS TO HUMANS

Some Thyrotropic Agents

VOLUME 79

This publication represents the views and expert opinions
of an IARC Working Group on the
Evaluation of Carcinogenic Risks to Humans,
which met in Lyon,

10–17 October 2000

2001

IARC MONOGRAPHS

In 1969, the International Agency for Research on Cancer (IARC) initiated a programme on the evaluation of the carcinogenic risk of chemicals to humans involving the production of critically evaluated monographs on individual chemicals. The programme was subsequently expanded to include evaluations of carcinogenic risks associated with exposures to complex mixtures, life-style factors and biological and physical agents, as well as those in specific occupations.

The objective of the programme is to elaborate and publish in the form of monographs critical reviews of data on carcinogenicity for agents to which humans are known to be exposed and on specific exposure situations; to evaluate these data in terms of human risk with the help of international working groups of experts in chemical carcinogenesis and related fields; and to indicate where additional research efforts are needed.

The lists of IARC evaluations are regularly updated and are available on Internet: http://monographs.iarc.fr/

This project was supported by Cooperative Agreement 5 UO1 CA33193 awarded by the United States National Cancer Institute, Department of Health and Human Services. Additional support has been provided since 1986 by the European Commission, since 1993 by the United States National Institute of Environmental Health Sciences and since 1995 by the United States Environmental Protection Agency through Cooperative Agreement Assistance CR 824264.

IARC Library Cataloguing in Publication Data

Some thyrotropic agents /
    IARC Working Group on the Evaluation of Carcinogenic Risks to Humans
    (2001 : Lyon, France)

    (IARC monographs on the evaluation of carcinogenic risks to humans ; 79)

    1. Carcinogens – congresses   2. Thyroid Carcinogens – congresses   I. IARC Working
    Group on the Evaluation of Carcinogenic Risks to Humans   II. Series

    ISBN 92 832 1279 7   (NLM Classification: W1)
    ISSN 1017-1606

PRINTED IN FRANCE

CONTENTS

NOTE TO THE READER

The term 'carcinogenic risk' in the *IARC Monographs* series is taken to mean the probability that exposure to an agent will lead to cancer in humans.

Inclusion of an agent in the *Monographs* does not imply that it is a carcinogen, only that the published data have been examined. Equally, the fact that an agent has not yet been evaluated in a monograph does not mean that it is not carcinogenic.

The evaluations of carcinogenic risk are made by international working groups of independent scientists and are qualitative in nature. No recommendation is given for regulation or legislation.

Anyone who is aware of published data that may alter the evaluation of the carcinogenic risk of an agent to humans is encouraged to make this information available to the Unit of Carcinogen Identification and Evaluation, International Agency for Research on Cancer, 150 cours Albert Thomas, 69372 Lyon Cedex 08, France, in order that the agent may be considered for re-evaluation by a future Working Group.

Although every effort is made to prepare the monographs as accurately as possible, mistakes may occur. Readers are requested to communicate any errors to the Unit of Carcinogen Identification and Evaluation, so that corrections can be reported in future volumes.

IARC WORKING GROUP ON THE EVALUATION OF CARCINOGENIC RISKS TO HUMANS: SOME THYROTROPIC AGENTS

Lyon, 10–17 October 2000

LIST OF PARTICIPANTS

Members[1]

C.C. Capen, Department of Veterinary Biosciences, College of Veterinary Medicine, Ohio State University, 1925 Coffey Road, Columbus, OH 43210-1093, USA (*Chairman*)

D.S. Cooper, Division of Endocrinology and Metabolism, Sinai Hospital, Medical Services, 2435 W. Belvedere Avenue, Suite 56, Baltimore, MD 21215, USA

B.A. Diwan, Carcinogenesis Study Section, National Cancer Institute, Frederick Cancer Research and Development Center, Building 358, Frederick, MD 21702-1201, USA

E. Dybing, Department of Environmental Medicine, National Institute of Public Health, PO Box 4404 Torshov, 0403 Oslo, Norway (*Vice-Chairman*)

C.L. Galli, Pharmacological Sciences Department, University of Milan, Via Balzaretti 9, 20133 Milan, Italy

G.C. Hard, American Health Foundation, 1 Dana Road, Valhalla, NY 10595, USA

T. Kauppinen, Finnish Institute of Occupational Health, Topeliuksenkatu 41 aA, 00250 Helsinki, Finland

R.J. Kavlock, Reproductive Toxicology Division, National Health and Environmental Effects Research Laboratory, Environmental Protection Agency, MD-71, Research Triangle Park, NC 27711, USA

C.D. Klaassen, Department of Pharmacology, Toxicology and Therapeutics, University of Kansas Medical Center, 3901 Rainbow Boulevard, Kansas City, KS 66160-7471, USA

R.M. McClain, 10 Powder Horn Terrace, Randolph, NJ 07869, USA

D. McGregor, 102 rue Duguesclin, 69006 Lyon, France

E. Negri, Laboratory of General Epidemiology, Mario Negri Institute of Pharmacological Research, via Eritrea 62, 20157 Milan, Italy

S. Olin, Risk Science Institute, International Life Sciences Institute, One Thomas Circle, 9th Floor, Washington DC 20005-5802, USA

---

[1] Unable to attend: J.E. Klaunig, Division of Toxicology, Department of Pharmacology and Toxicology, Indiana University School of Medicine, 635 Barnill Drive, MS 1021, Indianapolis, IN 46202-5120, USA

J.H. Olsen, Danish Cancer Society, Institute of Cancer Epidemiology, Box 839, 2100 Copenhagen Ø, Denmark

G.R. Rao, National Toxicology Program, National Institute of Environmental Health Sciences, PO Box 12233, MD B3-08, Research Triangle Park, NC 27709, USA

P.B. Ryan, Rollins School of Public Health, Emory University, 1518 Clifton Road NE, Atlanta, GA 30322, USA

T. Sanner, Department for Environmental and Occupational Cancer, The Norwegian Radium Hospital, Montebello, 0310 Oslo, Norway

E.K. Silbergeld, Program in Human Health and the Environment, University of Maryland, 10 South Pine Street MSTF 9-34, Baltimore, MD 21201, USA

F.M. Sullivan, Harrington House, 8 Harrington Road, Brighton, East Sussex BN1 6RE, United Kingdom

H. Watanabe, Department of Environment and Mutation, Research Institute for Radiation Biology and Medicine, Hiroshima University, 1-2-3 Kasumi, Minami-ku, Hiroshima 734, Japan

J. Whysner, Toxicology and Risk Assessment Program, American Health Foundation, 1 Dana Road, Valhalla, NY 10595-1599, USA

E. Zeiger, National Institute for Environmental Health Sciences, EC-14, PO Box 12233, Research Triangle Park, NC 27709, USA

Representatives/Observers

International Programme on Chemical Safety

J.L. Herrman, International Programme on Chemical Safety, World Health Organization, 1211 Geneva 27, Switzerland

NIEHS/National Toxicology Program

S. Lange, National Institute of Environmental Health Sciences, National Toxicology Program, A3-01, PO Box 12233, Research Triangle Park, NC 27709, USA

M. Shelby, National Institute of Environmental Health Sciences, National Toxicology Program, PO Box 12233, Research Triangle Park, NC 27709, USA

Technical Resources International Incorporated

T. Junghans, Technical Resources International Inc., 6500 Rock Spring Drive, Suite 650, Bethesda, MD 20817, USA

IARC Secretariat

R.A. Baan, Unit of Carcinogen Identification and Evaluation
M. Bird, Visiting Scientist in the Unit of Carcinogen Identification and Evaluation
R. Corvi, Unit of Genetic Cancer Susceptibility
S. Franceschi, Unit of Field and Intervention Studies
M. Friesen, Unit of Nutrition and Cancer
Y. Grosse, Unit of Carcinogen Identification and Evaluation

E. Heseltine (*Editor*)
V. Krutovskikh, Unit of Gene–Environment Interactions
W. Lee, Unit of Environmental Cancer Epidemiology
C. Malaveille, Unit of Endogenous Cancer Risk Factors
C. Partensky, Unit of Carcinogen Identification and Evaluation
J. Rice, Unit of Carcinogen Identification and Evaluation (*Head of Programme*)
E. Suonio, Unit of Carcinogen Identification and Evaluation
J. Wilbourn, Unit of Carcinogen Identification and Evaluation[1] *(Responsible Officer)*

Technical assistance
S. Egraz
M. Lézère
A. Meneghel
D. Mietton
J. Mitchell
E. Perez
S. Reynaud

---

[1] Until 31 December 2000

PREAMBLE

IARC MONOGRAPHS PROGRAMME ON THE EVALUATION OF CARCINOGENIC RISKS TO HUMANS

PREAMBLE

1. BACKGROUND

In 1969, the International Agency for Research on Cancer (IARC) initiated a programme to evaluate the carcinogenic risk of chemicals to humans and to produce monographs on individual chemicals. The *Monographs* programme has since been expanded to include consideration of exposures to complex mixtures of chemicals (which occur, for example, in some occupations and as a result of human habits) and of exposures to other agents, such as radiation and viruses. With Supplement 6 (IARC, 1987a), the title of the series was modified from *IARC Monographs on the Evaluation of the Carcinogenic Risk of Chemicals to Humans* to *IARC Monographs on the Evaluation of Carcinogenic Risks to Humans*, in order to reflect the widened scope of the programme.

The criteria established in 1971 to evaluate carcinogenic risk to humans were adopted by the working groups whose deliberations resulted in the first 16 volumes of the *IARC Monographs series*. Those criteria were subsequently updated by further ad-hoc working groups (IARC, 1977, 1978, 1979, 1982, 1983, 1987b, 1988, 1991a; Vainio *et al.*, 1992).

2. OBJECTIVE AND SCOPE

The objective of the programme is to prepare, with the help of international working groups of experts, and to publish in the form of monographs, critical reviews and evaluations of evidence on the carcinogenicity of a wide range of human exposures. The *Monographs* may also indicate where additional research efforts are needed.

The *Monographs* represent the first step in carcinogenic risk assessment, which involves examination of all relevant information in order to assess the strength of the available evidence that certain exposures could alter the incidence of cancer in humans. The second step is quantitative risk estimation. Detailed, quantitative evaluations of epidemiological data may be made in the *Monographs*, but without extrapolation beyond the range of the data available. Quantitative extrapolation from experimental data to the human situation is not undertaken.

The term 'carcinogen' is used in these monographs to denote an exposure that is capable of increasing the incidence of malignant neoplasms; the induction of benign neoplasms may in some circumstances (see p. 19) contribute to the judgement that the exposure is carcinogenic. The terms 'neoplasm' and 'tumour' are used interchangeably.

Some epidemiological and experimental studies indicate that different agents may act at different stages in the carcinogenic process, and several mechanisms may be involved. The aim of the *Monographs* has been, from their inception, to evaluate evidence of carcinogenicity at any stage in the carcinogenesis process, independently of the underlying mechanisms. Information on mechanisms may, however, be used in making the overall evaluation (IARC, 1991a; Vainio *et al.*, 1992; see also pp. 25–27).

The *Monographs* may assist national and international authorities in making risk assessments and in formulating decisions concerning any necessary preventive measures. The evaluations of IARC working groups are scientific, qualitative judgements about the evidence for or against carcinogenicity provided by the available data. These evaluations represent only one part of the body of information on which regulatory measures may be based. Other components of regulatory decisions vary from one situation to another and from country to country, responding to different socioeconomic and national priorities. **Therefore, no recommendation is given with regard to regulation or legislation, which are the responsibility of individual governments and/or other international organizations.**

The *IARC Monographs* are recognized as an authoritative source of information on the carcinogenicity of a wide range of human exposures. A survey of users in 1988 indicated that the *Monographs* are consulted by various agencies in 57 countries. About 2500 copies of each volume are printed, for distribution to governments, regulatory bodies and interested scientists. The Monographs are also available from IARC*Press* in Lyon and via the Distribution and Sales Service of the World Health Organization in Geneva.

3.   SELECTION OF TOPICS FOR MONOGRAPHS

Topics are selected on the basis of two main criteria: (a) there is evidence of human exposure, and (b) there is some evidence or suspicion of carcinogenicity. The term 'agent' is used to include individual chemical compounds, groups of related chemical compounds, physical agents (such as radiation) and biological factors (such as viruses). Exposures to mixtures of agents may occur in occupational exposures and as a result of personal and cultural habits (like smoking and dietary practices). Chemical analogues and compounds with biological or physical characteristics similar to those of suspected carcinogens may also be considered, even in the absence of data on a possible carcinogenic effect in humans or experimental animals.

The scientific literature is surveyed for published data relevant to an assessment of carcinogenicity. The IARC information bulletins on agents being tested for carcinogenicity (IARC, 1973–1996) and directories of on-going research in cancer epidemiology (IARC, 1976–1996) often indicate exposures that may be scheduled for future meetings. Ad-hoc working groups convened by IARC in 1984, 1989, 1991, 1993 and 1998 gave recommendations as to which agents should be evaluated in the IARC Monographs series (IARC, 1984, 1989, 1991b, 1993, 1998a,b).

As significant new data on subjects on which monographs have already been prepared become available, re-evaluations are made at subsequent meetings, and revised monographs are published.

4. DATA FOR MONOGRAPHS

The *Monographs* do not necessarily cite all the literature concerning the subject of an evaluation. Only those data considered by the Working Group to be relevant to making the evaluation are included.

With regard to biological and epidemiological data, only reports that have been published or accepted for publication in the openly available scientific literature are reviewed by the working groups. In certain instances, government agency reports that have undergone peer review and are widely available are considered. Exceptions may be made on an ad-hoc basis to include unpublished reports that are in their final form and publicly available, if their inclusion is considered pertinent to making a final evaluation (see pp. 25–27). In the sections on chemical and physical properties, on analysis, on production and use and on occurrence, unpublished sources of information may be used.

5. THE WORKING GROUP

Reviews and evaluations are formulated by a working group of experts. The tasks of the group are: (i) to ascertain that all appropriate data have been collected; (ii) to select the data relevant for the evaluation on the basis of scientific merit; (iii) to prepare accurate summaries of the data to enable the reader to follow the reasoning of the Working Group; (iv) to evaluate the results of epidemiological and experimental studies on cancer; (v) to evaluate data relevant to the understanding of mechanism of action; and (vi) to make an overall evaluation of the carcinogenicity of the exposure to humans.

Working Group participants who contributed to the considerations and evaluations within a particular volume are listed, with their addresses, at the beginning of each publication. Each participant who is a member of a working group serves as an individual scientist and not as a representative of any organization, government or industry. In addition, nominees of national and international agencies and industrial associations may be invited as observers.

6. WORKING PROCEDURES

Approximately one year in advance of a meeting of a working group, the topics of the monographs are announced and participants are selected by IARC staff in consultation with other experts. Subsequently, relevant biological and epidemiological data are collected by the Carcinogen Identification and Evaluation Unit of IARC from recognized sources of information on carcinogenesis, including data storage and retrieval systems such as MEDLINE and TOXLINE.

For chemicals and some complex mixtures, the major collection of data and the preparation of first drafts of the sections on chemical and physical properties, on analysis, on production and use and on occurrence are carried out under a separate contract funded by the United States National Cancer Institute. Representatives from industrial associations may assist in the preparation of sections on production and use. Information on production and trade is obtained from governmental and trade publications and, in some cases, by direct contact with industries. Separate production data on some agents may not be available because their publication could disclose confidential information. Information on uses may be obtained from published sources but is often complemented by direct contact with manufacturers. Efforts are made to supplement this information with data from other national and international sources.

Six months before the meeting, the material obtained is sent to meeting participants, or is used by IARC staff, to prepare sections for the first drafts of monographs. The first drafts are compiled by IARC staff and sent before the meeting to all participants of the Working Group for review.

The Working Group meets in Lyon for seven to eight days to discuss and finalize the texts of the monographs and to formulate the evaluations. After the meeting, the master copy of each monograph is verified by consulting the original literature, edited and prepared for publication. The aim is to publish monographs within six months of the Working Group meeting.

The available studies are summarized by the Working Group, with particular regard to the qualitative aspects discussed below. In general, numerical findings are indicated as they appear in the original report; units are converted when necessary for easier comparison. The Working Group may conduct additional analyses of the published data and use them in their assessment of the evidence; the results of such supplementary analyses are given in square brackets. When an important aspect of a study, directly impinging on its interpretation, should be brought to the attention of the reader, a comment is given in square brackets.

7.   EXPOSURE DATA

Sections that indicate the extent of past and present human exposure, the sources of exposure, the people most likely to be exposed and the factors that contribute to the exposure are included at the beginning of each monograph.

Most monographs on individual chemicals, groups of chemicals or complex mixtures include sections on chemical and physical data, on analysis, on production and use and on occurrence. In monographs on, for example, physical agents, occupational exposures and cultural habits, other sections may be included, such as: historical perspectives, description of an industry or habit, chemistry of the complex mixture or taxonomy. Monographs on biological agents have sections on structure and biology, methods of detection, epidemiology of infection and clinical disease other than cancer.

For chemical exposures, the Chemical Abstracts Services Registry Number, the latest Chemical Abstracts Primary Name and the IUPAC Systematic Name are recorded; other synonyms are given, but the list is not necessarily comprehensive. For biological agents, taxonomy and structure are described, and the degree of variability is given, when applicable.

Information on chemical and physical properties and, in particular, data relevant to identification, occurrence and biological activity are included. For biological agents, mode of replication, life cycle, target cells, persistence and latency and host response are given. A description of technical products of chemicals includes trade names, relevant specifications and available information on composition and impurities. Some of the trade names given may be those of mixtures in which the agent being evaluated is only one of the ingredients.

The purpose of the section on analysis or detection is to give the reader an overview of current methods, with emphasis on those widely used for regulatory purposes. Methods for monitoring human exposure are also given, when available. No critical evaluation or recommendation of any of the methods is meant or implied. The IARC published a series of volumes, *Environmental Carcinogens: Methods of Analysis and Exposure Measurement* (IARC, 1978–93), that describe validated methods for analysing a wide variety of chemicals and mixtures. For biological agents, methods of detection and exposure assessment are described, including their sensitivity, specificity and reproducibility.

The dates of first synthesis and of first commercial production of a chemical or mixture are provided; for agents which do not occur naturally, this information may allow a reasonable estimate to be made of the date before which no human exposure to the agent could have occurred. The dates of first reported occurrence of an exposure are also provided. In addition, methods of synthesis used in past and present commercial production and different methods of production which may give rise to different impurities are described.

Data on production, international trade and uses are obtained for representative regions, which usually include Europe, Japan and the United States of America. It should not, however, be inferred that those areas or nations are necessarily the sole or major sources or users of the agent. Some identified uses may not be current or major applications, and the coverage is not necessarily comprehensive. In the case of drugs, mention of their therapeutic uses does not necessarily represent current practice, nor does it imply judgement as to their therapeutic efficacy.

Information on the occurrence of an agent or mixture in the environment is obtained from data derived from the monitoring and surveillance of levels in occupational environments, air, water, soil, foods and animal and human tissues. When available, data on the generation, persistence and bioaccumulation of the agent are also included. In the case of mixtures, industries, occupations or processes, information is given about all agents present. For processes, industries and occupations, a historical description is also given, noting variations in chemical composition, physical properties and levels of occupational exposure with time and place. For biological agents, the epidemiology of infection is described.

Statements concerning regulations and guidelines (e.g., pesticide registrations, maximal levels permitted in foods, occupational exposure limits) are included for some countries as indications of potential exposures, but they may not reflect the most recent situation, since such limits are continuously reviewed and modified. The absence of information on regulatory status for a country should not be taken to imply that that country does not have regulations with regard to the exposure. For biological agents, legislation and control, including vaccines and therapy, are described.

8.   STUDIES OF CANCER IN HUMANS

(a)   Types of studies considered

Three types of epidemiological studies of cancer contribute to the assessment of carcinogenicity in humans—cohort studies, case–control studies and correlation (or ecological) studies. Rarely, results from randomized trials may be available. Case series and case reports of cancer in humans may also be reviewed.

Cohort and case–control studies relate the exposures under study to the occurrence of cancer in individuals and provide an estimate of relative risk (ratio of incidence or mortality in those exposed to incidence or mortality in those not exposed) as the main measure of association.

In correlation studies, the units of investigation are usually whole populations (e.g. in particular geographical areas or at particular times), and cancer frequency is related to a summary measure of the exposure of the population to the agent, mixture or exposure circumstance under study. Because individual exposure is not documented, however, a causal relationship is less easy to infer from correlation studies than from cohort and case–control studies. Case reports generally arise from a suspicion, based on clinical experience, that the concurrence of two events—that is, a particular exposure and occurrence of a cancer—has happened rather more frequently than would be expected by chance. Case reports usually lack complete ascertainment of cases in any population, definition or enumeration of the population at risk and estimation of the expected number of cases in the absence of exposure. The uncertainties surrounding interpretation of case reports and correlation studies make them inadequate, except in rare instances, to form the sole basis for inferring a causal relationship. When taken together with case–control and cohort studies, however, relevant case reports or correlation studies may add materially to the judgement that a causal relationship is present.

Epidemiological studies of benign neoplasms, presumed preneoplastic lesions and other end-points thought to be relevant to cancer are also reviewed by working groups. They may, in some instances, strengthen inferences drawn from studies of cancer itself.

(b)   Quality of studies considered

The Monographs are not intended to summarize all published studies. Those that are judged to be inadequate or irrelevant to the evaluation are generally omitted. They may be mentioned briefly, particularly when the information is considered to be a useful supplement to that in other reports or when they provide the only data available. Their inclusion does not imply acceptance of the adequacy of the study design or of the analysis and interpretation of the results, and limitations are clearly outlined in square brackets at the end of the study description.

It is necessary to take into account the possible roles of bias, confounding and chance in the interpretation of epidemiological studies. By 'bias' is meant the operation of factors in study design or execution that lead erroneously to a stronger or weaker association than in fact exists between disease and an agent, mixture or exposure circumstance. By 'confounding' is meant a situation in which the relationship with disease is made to appear stronger or weaker than it truly is as a result of an association between the apparent causal factor and another factor that is associated with either an increase or decrease in the incidence of the disease. In evaluating the extent to which these factors have been minimized in an individual study, working groups consider a number of aspects of design and analysis as described in the report of the study. Most of these considerations apply equally to case–control, cohort and correlation studies. Lack of clarity of any of these aspects in the reporting of a study can decrease its credibility and the weight given to it in the final evaluation of the exposure.

Firstly, the study population, disease (or diseases) and exposure should have been well defined by the authors. Cases of disease in the study population should have been identified in a way that was independent of the exposure of interest, and exposure should have been assessed in a way that was not related to disease status.

Secondly, the authors should have taken account in the study design and analysis of other variables that can influence the risk of disease and may have been related to the exposure of interest. Potential confounding by such variables should have been dealt with either in the design of the study, such as by matching, or in the analysis, by statistical adjustment. In cohort studies, comparisons with local rates of disease may be more appropriate than those with national rates. Internal comparisons of disease frequency among individuals at different levels of exposure should also have been made in the study.

Thirdly, the authors should have reported the basic data on which the conclusions are founded, even if sophisticated statistical analyses were employed. At the very least, they should have given the numbers of exposed and unexposed cases and controls in a case–control study and the numbers of cases observed and expected in a cohort study. Further tabulations by time since exposure began and other temporal factors are also important. In a cohort study, data on all cancer sites and all causes of death should have been given, to reveal the possibility of reporting bias. In a case–control study, the effects of investigated factors other than the exposure of interest should have been reported.

Finally, the statistical methods used to obtain estimates of relative risk, absolute rates of cancer, confidence intervals and significance tests, and to adjust for confounding should have been clearly stated by the authors. The methods used should preferably have been the generally accepted techniques that have been refined since the mid-1970s. These methods have been reviewed for case–control studies (Breslow & Day, 1980) and for cohort studies (Breslow & Day, 1987).

(c)   Inferences about mechanism of action

Detailed analyses of both relative and absolute risks in relation to temporal variables, such as age at first exposure, time since first exposure, duration of exposure, cumulative exposure and time since exposure ceased, are reviewed and summarized when available. The analysis of temporal relationships can be useful in formulating models of carcinogenesis. In particular, such analyses may suggest whether a carcinogen acts early or late in the process of carcinogenesis, although at best they allow only indirect inferences about the mechanism of action. Special attention is given to measurements of biological markers of carcinogen exposure or action, such as DNA or protein adducts, as well as markers of early steps in the carcinogenic process, such as proto-oncogene mutation, when these are incorporated into epidemiological studies focused on cancer incidence or mortality. Such measurements may allow inferences to be made about putative mechanisms of action (IARC, 1991a; Vainio *et al.*, 1992).

(d)   Criteria for causality

After the individual epidemiological studies of cancer have been summarized and the quality assessed, a judgement is made concerning the strength of evidence that the agent, mixture or exposure circumstance in question is carcinogenic for humans. In making its judgement, the Working Group considers several criteria for causality. A strong association (a large relative risk) is more likely to indicate causality than a weak association, although it is recognized that relative risks of small magnitude do not imply lack of causality and may be important if the disease is common. Associations that are replicated in several studies of the same design or using different epidemiological approaches or under different circumstances of exposure are more likely to represent a causal relationship than isolated observations from single studies. If there are inconsistent results among investigations, possible reasons are sought (such as differences in amount of exposure), and results of studies judged to be of high quality are given more weight than those of studies judged to be methodologically less sound. When suspicion of carcinogenicity arises largely from a single study, these data are not combined with those from later studies in any subsequent reassessment of the strength of the evidence.

If the risk of the disease in question increases with the amount of exposure, this is considered to be a strong indication of causality, although absence of a graded response is not necessarily evidence against a causal relationship. Demonstration of a decline in risk after cessation of or reduction in exposure in individuals or in whole populations also supports a causal interpretation of the findings.

Although a carcinogen may act upon more than one target, the specificity of an association (an increased occurrence of cancer at one anatomical site or of one morphological type) adds plausibility to a causal relationship, particularly when excess cancer occurrence is limited to one morphological type within the same organ.

Although rarely available, results from randomized trials showing different rates among exposed and unexposed individuals provide particularly strong evidence for causality.

When several epidemiological studies show little or no indication of an association between an exposure and cancer, the judgement may be made that, in the aggregate, they show evidence of lack of carcinogenicity. Such a judgement requires first of all that the studies giving rise to it meet, to a sufficient degree, the standards of design and analysis described above. Specifically, the possibility that bias, confounding or misclassification of exposure or outcome could explain the observed results should be considered and excluded with reasonable certainty. In addition, all studies that are judged to be methodologically sound should be consistent with a relative risk of unity for any observed level of exposure and, when considered together, should provide a pooled estimate of relative risk which is at or near unity and has a narrow confidence interval, due to sufficient population size. Moreover, no individual study nor the pooled results of all the studies should show any consistent tendency for the relative risk of cancer to increase with increasing level of exposure. It is important to note that evidence of lack of carcinogenicity obtained in this way from several epidemiological studies can apply only to the type(s) of cancer studied and to dose levels and intervals between first exposure and observation of disease that are the same as or less than those observed in all the studies. Experience with human cancer indicates that, in some cases, the period from first exposure to the development of clinical cancer is seldom less than 20 years; latent periods substantially shorter than 30 years cannot provide evidence for lack of carcinogenicity.

9.   STUDIES OF CANCER IN EXPERIMENTAL ANIMALS

All known human carcinogens that have been studied adequately in experimental animals have produced positive results in one or more animal species (Wilbourn *et al.*, 1986; Tomatis *et al.*, 1989). For several agents (aflatoxins, 4-aminobiphenyl, azathioprine, betel quid with tobacco, bischloromethyl ether and chloromethyl methyl ether (technical grade), chlorambucil, chlornaphazine, ciclosporin, coal-tar pitches, coal-tars, combined oral contraceptives, cyclophosphamide, diethylstilboestrol, melphalan, 8-methoxypsoralen plus ultraviolet A radiation, mustard gas, myleran, 2-naphthylamine, nonsteroidal estrogens, estrogen replacement therapy/steroidal estrogens, solar radiation, thiotepa and vinyl chloride), carcinogenicity in experimental animals was established or highly suspected before epidemiological studies confirmed their carcinogenicity in humans (Vainio *et al.*, 1995). Although this association cannot establish that all agents and mixtures that cause cancer in experimental animals also cause cancer in humans, nevertheless, **in the absence of adequate data on humans, it is biologically plausible and prudent to regard agents and mixtures for which there is *sufficient evidence* (see p. 24) of carcinogenicity in experimental animals as if they presented a carcinogenic risk to humans.** The possibility that a given agent may cause cancer through a species-specific mechanism which does not operate in humans (see p. 27) should also be taken into consideration.

The nature and extent of impurities or contaminants present in the chemical or mixture being evaluated are given when available. Animal strain, sex, numbers per group, age at start of treatment and survival are reported.

Other types of studies summarized include: experiments in which the agent or mixture was administered in conjunction with known carcinogens or factors that modify carcinogenic effects; studies in which the end-point was not cancer but a defined precancerous lesion; and experiments on the carcinogenicity of known metabolites and derivatives.

For experimental studies of mixtures, consideration is given to the possibility of changes in the physicochemical properties of the test substance during collection, storage, extraction, concentration and delivery. Chemical and toxicological interactions of the components of mixtures may result in nonlinear dose–response relationships.

An assessment is made as to the relevance to human exposure of samples tested in experimental animals, which may involve consideration of: (i) physical and chemical characteristics, (ii) constituent substances that indicate the presence of a class of substances, (iii) the results of tests for genetic and related effects, including studies on DNA adduct formation, proto-oncogene mutation and expression and suppressor gene inactivation. The relevance of results obtained, for example, with animal viruses analogous to the virus being evaluated in the monograph must also be considered. They may provide biological and mechanistic information relevant to the understanding of the process of carcinogenesis in humans and may strengthen the plausibility of a conclusion that the biological agent under evaluation is carcinogenic in humans.

(a)   Qualitative aspects

An assessment of carcinogenicity involves several considerations of qualitative importance, including (i) the experimental conditions under which the test was performed, including route and schedule of exposure, species, strain, sex, age, duration of follow-up; (ii) the consistency of the results, for example, across species and target organ(s); (iii) the spectrum of neoplastic response, from preneoplastic lesions and benign tumours to malignant neoplasms; and (iv) the possible role of modifying factors.

As mentioned earlier (p. 11), the *Monographs* are not intended to summarize all published studies. Those studies in experimental animals that are inadequate (e.g., too short a duration, too few animals, poor survival; see below) or are judged irrelevant to the evaluation are generally omitted. Guidelines for conducting adequate long-term carcinogenicity experiments have been outlined (e.g. Montesano *et al.*, 1986).

Considerations of importance to the Working Group in the interpretation and evaluation of a particular study include: (i) how clearly the agent was defined and, in the case of mixtures, how adequately the sample characterization was reported; (ii) whether the dose was adequately monitored, particularly in inhalation experiments; (iii) whether the doses and duration of treatment were appropriate and whether the survival of treated animals was similar to that of controls; (iv) whether there were adequate numbers of animals per group; (v) whether animals of each sex were used; (vi) whether animals were allocated randomly to groups; (vii) whether the duration of observation was adequate; and (viii) whether the data were adequately reported. If available, recent data on the incidence of specific tumours in historical controls, as well as in concurrent controls, should be taken into account in the evaluation of tumour response.

When benign tumours occur together with and originate from the same cell type in an organ or tissue as malignant tumours in a particular study and appear to represent a stage in the progression to malignancy, it may be valid to combine them in assessing tumour incidence (Huff *et al.*, 1989). The occurrence of lesions presumed to be pre-neoplastic may in certain instances aid in assessing the biological plausibility of any neoplastic response observed. If an agent or mixture induces only benign neoplasms that appear to be end-points that do not readily progress to malignancy, it should nevertheless be suspected of being a carcinogen and requires further investigation.

(b)   *Quantitative aspects*

The probability that tumours will occur may depend on the species, sex, strain and age of the animal, the dose of the carcinogen and the route and length of exposure. Evidence of an increased incidence of neoplasms with increased level of exposure strengthens the inference of a causal association between the exposure and the development of neoplasms.

The form of the dose–response relationship can vary widely, depending on the particular agent under study and the target organ. Both DNA damage and increased cell division are important aspects of carcinogenesis, and cell proliferation is a strong determinant of dose–response relationships for some carcinogens (Cohen & Ellwein, 1990). Since many chemicals require metabolic activation before being converted into their reactive intermediates, both metabolic and pharmacokinetic aspects are important in determining the dose–response pattern. Saturation of steps such as absorption, activation, inactivation and elimination may produce nonlinearity in the dose–response relationship, as could saturation of processes such as DNA repair (Hoel *et al.*, 1983; Gart *et al.*, 1986).

(c)   *Statistical analysis of long-term experiments in animals*

Factors considered by the Working Group include the adequacy of the information given for each treatment group: (i) the number of animals studied and the number examined histologically, (ii) the number of animals with a given tumour type and (iii) length of survival. The statistical methods used should be clearly stated and should be the generally accepted techniques refined for this purpose (Peto *et al.*, 1980; Gart *et al.*, 1986). When there is no difference in survival between control and treatment groups, the Working Group usually compares the proportions of animals developing each tumour type in each of the groups. Otherwise, consideration is given as to whether or not appropriate adjustments have been made for differences in survival. These adjustments can include: comparisons of the proportions of tumour-bearing animals among the effective number of animals (alive at the time the first tumour is discovered), in the case where most differences in survival occur before tumours appear; life-table methods, when tumours are visible or when they may be considered 'fatal' because mortality rapidly follows tumour development; and the Mantel-Haenszel test or logistic regression, when occult tumours do not affect the animals' risk of dying but are 'incidental' findings at autopsy.

In practice, classifying tumours as fatal or incidental may be difficult. Several survival-adjusted methods have been developed that do not require this distinction (Gart *et al.*, 1986), although they have not been fully evaluated.

10.   OTHER DATA RELEVANT TO AN EVALUATION OF CARCINOGENICITY AND ITS MECHANISMS

In coming to an overall evaluation of carcinogenicity in humans (see pp. 25–27), the Working Group also considers related data. The nature of the information selected for the summary depends on the agent being considered.

For chemicals and complex mixtures of chemicals such as those in some occupational situations or involving cultural habits (e.g. tobacco smoking), the other data considered to be relevant are divided into those on absorption, distribution, metabolism and excretion; toxic effects; reproductive and developmental effects; and genetic and related effects.

Concise information is given on absorption, distribution (including placental transfer) and excretion in both humans and experimental animals. Kinetic factors that may affect the dose–response relationship, such as saturation of uptake, protein binding, metabolic activation, detoxification and DNA repair processes, are mentioned. Studies that indicate the metabolic fate of the agent in humans and in experimental animals are summarized briefly, and comparisons of data on humans and on animals are made when possible. Comparative information on the relationship between exposure and the dose that reaches the target site may be of particular importance for extrapolation between species. Data are given on acute and chronic toxic effects (other than cancer), such as organ toxicity, increased cell proliferation, immunotoxicity and endocrine effects. The presence and toxicological significance of cellular receptors is described. Effects on reproduction, teratogenicity, fetotoxicity and embryotoxicity are also summarized briefly.

Tests of genetic and related effects are described in view of the relevance of gene mutation and chromosomal damage to carcinogenesis (Vainio *et al.*, 1992; McGregor *et al.*, 1999). The adequacy of the reporting of sample characterization is considered and, where necessary, commented upon; with regard to complex mixtures, such comments are similar to those described for animal carcinogenicity tests on p. 18. The available data are interpreted critically by phylogenetic group according to the end-points detected, which may include DNA damage, gene mutation, sister chromatid exchange, micronucleus formation, chromosomal aberrations, aneuploidy and cell transformation. The concentrations employed are given, and mention is made of whether use of an exogenous metabolic system *in vitro* affected the test result. These data are given as listings of test systems, data and references. The Genetic and Related Effects data presented in the *Monographs* are also available in the form of Graphic Activity Profiles (GAP) prepared in collaboration with the United States Environmental Protection Agency (EPA) (see also

Waters *et al.*, 1987) using software for personal computers that are Microsoft Windows® compatible. The EPA/IARC GAP software and database may be downloaded free of charge from *www.epa.gov/gapdb*.

Positive results in tests using prokaryotes, lower eukaryotes, plants, insects and cultured mammalian cells suggest that genetic and related effects could occur in mammals. Results from such tests may also give information about the types of genetic effect produced and about the involvement of metabolic activation. Some end-points described are clearly genetic in nature (e.g., gene mutations and chromosomal aberrations), while others are to a greater or lesser degree associated with genetic effects (e.g. unscheduled DNA synthesis). In-vitro tests for tumour-promoting activity and for cell transformation may be sensitive to changes that are not necessarily the result of genetic alterations but that may have specific relevance to the process of carcinogenesis. A critical appraisal of these tests has been published (Montesano *et al.*, 1986).

Genetic or other activity manifest in experimental mammals and humans is regarded as being of greater relevance than that in other organisms. The demonstration that an agent or mixture can induce gene and chromosomal mutations in whole mammals indicates that it may have carcinogenic activity, although this activity may not be detectably expressed in any or all species. Relative potency in tests for mutagenicity and related effects is not a reliable indicator of carcinogenic potency. Negative results in tests for mutagenicity in selected tissues from animals treated *in vivo* provide less weight, partly because they do not exclude the possibility of an effect in tissues other than those examined. Moreover, negative results in short-term tests with genetic end-points cannot be considered to provide evidence to rule out carcinogenicity of agents or mixtures that act through other mechanisms (e.g. receptor-mediated effects, cellular toxicity with regenerative proliferation, peroxisome proliferation) (Vainio *et al.*, 1992). Factors that may lead to misleading results in short-term tests have been discussed in detail elsewhere (Montesano *et al.*, 1986).

When available, data relevant to mechanisms of carcinogenesis that do not involve structural changes at the level of the gene are also described.

The adequacy of epidemiological studies of reproductive outcome and genetic and related effects in humans is evaluated by the same criteria as are applied to epidemiological studies of cancer.

Structure–activity relationships that may be relevant to an evaluation of the carcinogenicity of an agent are also described.

For biological agents—viruses, bacteria and parasites—other data relevant to carcinogenicity include descriptions of the pathology of infection, molecular biology (integration and expression of viruses, and any genetic alterations seen in human tumours) and other observations, which might include cellular and tissue responses to infection, immune response and the presence of tumour markers.

11.   SUMMARY OF DATA REPORTED

In this section, the relevant epidemiological and experimental data are summarized. Only reports, other than in abstract form, that meet the criteria outlined on p. 11 are considered for evaluating carcinogenicity. Inadequate studies are generally not summarized: such studies are usually identified by a square-bracketed comment in the preceding text.

(a)   Exposure

Human exposure to chemicals and complex mixtures is summarized on the basis of elements such as production, use, occurrence in the environment and determinations in human tissues and body fluids. Quantitative data are given when available. Exposure to biological agents is described in terms of transmission and prevalence of infection.

(b)   Carcinogenicity in humans

Results of epidemiological studies that are considered to be pertinent to an assessment of human carcinogenicity are summarized. When relevant, case reports and correlation studies are also summarized.

(c)   Carcinogenicity in experimental animals

Data relevant to an evaluation of carcinogenicity in animals are summarized. For each animal species and route of administration, it is stated whether an increased incidence of neoplasms or preneoplastic lesions was observed, and the tumour sites are indicated. If the agent or mixture produced tumours after prenatal exposure or in single-dose experiments, this is also indicated. Negative findings are also summarized. Dose–response and other quantitative data may be given when available.

(d)   Other data relevant to an evaluation of carcinogenicity and its mechanisms

Data on biological effects in humans that are of particular relevance are summarized. These may include toxicological, kinetic and metabolic considerations and evidence of DNA binding, persistence of DNA lesions or genetic damage in exposed humans. Toxicological information, such as that on cytotoxicity and regeneration, receptor binding and hormonal and immunological effects, and data on kinetics and metabolism in experimental animals are given when considered relevant to the possible mechanism of the carcinogenic action of the agent. The results of tests for genetic and related effects are summarized for whole mammals, cultured mammalian cells and nonmammalian systems.

When available, comparisons of such data for humans and for animals, and particularly animals that have developed cancer, are described.

Structure–activity relationships are mentioned when relevant.

For the agent, mixture or exposure circumstance being evaluated, the available data on end-points or other phenomena relevant to mechanisms of carcinogenesis from studies in humans, experimental animals and tissue and cell test systems are summarized within one or more of the following descriptive dimensions:

(i) Evidence of genotoxicity (structural changes at the level of the gene): for example, structure–activity considerations, adduct formation, mutagenicity (effect on specific genes), chromosomal mutation/aneuploidy

(ii) Evidence of effects on the expression of relevant genes (functional changes at the intracellular level): for example, alterations to the structure or quantity of the product of a proto-oncogene or tumour-suppressor gene, alterations to metabolic activation/inactivation/DNA repair

(iii) Evidence of relevant effects on cell behaviour (morphological or behavioural changes at the cellular or tissue level): for example, induction of mitogenesis, compensatory cell proliferation, preneoplasia and hyperplasia, survival of premalignant or malignant cells (immortalization, immunosuppression), effects on metastatic potential

(iv) Evidence from dose and time relationships of carcinogenic effects and interactions between agents: for example, early/late stage, as inferred from epidemiological studies; initiation/promotion/progression/malignant conversion, as defined in animal carcinogenicity experiments; toxicokinetics

These dimensions are not mutually exclusive, and an agent may fall within more than one of them. Thus, for example, the action of an agent on the expression of relevant genes could be summarized under both the first and second dimensions, even if it were known with reasonable certainty that those effects resulted from genotoxicity.

12.   EVALUATION

Evaluations of the strength of the evidence for carcinogenicity arising from human and experimental animal data are made, using standard terms.

It is recognized that the criteria for these evaluations, described below, cannot encompass all of the factors that may be relevant to an evaluation of carcinogenicity. In considering all of the relevant scientific data, the Working Group may assign the agent, mixture or exposure circumstance to a higher or lower category than a strict interpretation of these criteria would indicate.

(a)   Degrees of evidence for carcinogenicity in humans and in experimental animals and supporting evidence

These categories refer only to the strength of the evidence that an exposure is carcinogenic and not to the extent of its carcinogenic activity (potency) nor to the mechanisms involved. A classification may change as new information becomes available.

An evaluation of degree of evidence, whether for a single agent or a mixture, is limited to the materials tested, as defined physically, chemically or biologically. When the agents evaluated are considered by the Working Group to be sufficiently closely related, they may be grouped together for the purpose of a single evaluation of degree of evidence.

(i)   Carcinogenicity in humans

The applicability of an evaluation of the carcinogenicity of a mixture, process, occupation or industry on the basis of evidence from epidemiological studies depends on the variability over time and place of the mixtures, processes, occupations and industries. The Working Group seeks to identify the specific exposure, process or activity which is considered most likely to be responsible for any excess risk. The evaluation is focused as narrowly as the available data on exposure and other aspects permit.

The evidence relevant to carcinogenicity from studies in humans is classified into one of the following categories:

Sufficient evidence of carcinogenicity: The Working Group considers that a causal relationship has been established between exposure to the agent, mixture or exposure circumstance and human cancer. That is, a positive relationship has been observed between the exposure and cancer in studies in which chance, bias and confounding could be ruled out with reasonable confidence.

Limited evidence of carcinogenicity: A positive association has been observed between exposure to the agent, mixture or exposure circumstance and cancer for which a causal interpretation is considered by the Working Group to be credible, but chance, bias or confounding could not be ruled out with reasonable confidence.

Inadequate evidence of carcinogenicity: The available studies are of insufficient quality, consistency or statistical power to permit a conclusion regarding the presence or absence of a causal association between exposure and cancer, or no data on cancer in humans are available.

Evidence suggesting lack of carcinogenicity: There are several adequate studies covering the full range of levels of exposure that human beings are known to encounter, which are mutually consistent in not showing a positive association between exposure to the agent, mixture or exposure circumstance and any studied cancer at any observed level of exposure. A conclusion of 'evidence suggesting lack of carcinogenicity' is inevitably limited to the cancer sites, conditions and levels of exposure and length of observation covered by the available studies. In addition, the possibility of a very small risk at the levels of exposure studied can never be excluded.

In some instances, the above categories may be used to classify the degree of evidence related to carcinogenicity in specific organs or tissues.

(ii)   *Carcinogenicity in experimental animals*

The evidence relevant to carcinogenicity in experimental animals is classified into one of the following categories:

Sufficient evidence of carcinogenicity: The Working Group considers that a causal relationship has been established between the agent or mixture and an increased incidence of malignant neoplasms or of an appropriate combination of benign and malignant neoplasms in (a) two or more species of animals or (b) in two or more independent studies in one species carried out at different times or in different laboratories or under different protocols.

Exceptionally, a single study in one species might be considered to provide sufficient evidence of carcinogenicity when malignant neoplasms occur to an unusual degree with regard to incidence, site, type of tumour or age at onset.

Limited evidence of carcinogenicity: The data suggest a carcinogenic effect but are limited for making a definitive evaluation because, e.g. (a) the evidence of carcinogenicity is restricted to a single experiment; or (b) there are unresolved questions regarding the adequacy of the design, conduct or interpretation of the study; or (c) the agent or mixture increases the incidence only of benign neoplasms or lesions of uncertain neoplastic potential, or of certain neoplasms which may occur spontaneously in high incidences in certain strains.

Inadequate evidence of carcinogenicity: The studies cannot be interpreted as showing either the presence or absence of a carcinogenic effect because of major qualitative or quantitative limitations, or no data on cancer in experimental animals are available.

Evidence suggesting lack of carcinogenicity: Adequate studies involving at least two species are available which show that, within the limits of the tests used, the agent or mixture is not carcinogenic. A conclusion of evidence suggesting lack of carcinogenicity is inevitably limited to the species, tumour sites and levels of exposure studied.

(b)   *Other data relevant to the evaluation of carcinogenicity and its mechanisms*

Other evidence judged to be relevant to an evaluation of carcinogenicity and of sufficient importance to affect the overall evaluation is then described. This may include data on preneoplastic lesions, tumour pathology, genetic and related effects, structure–activity relationships, metabolism and pharmacokinetics, physicochemical parameters and analogous biological agents.

Data relevant to mechanisms of the carcinogenic action are also evaluated. The strength of the evidence that any carcinogenic effect observed is due to a particular mechanism is assessed, using terms such as weak, moderate or strong. Then, the Working Group assesses if that particular mechanism is likely to be operative in humans. The strongest indications that a particular mechanism operates in humans come from data on humans or biological specimens obtained from exposed humans. The data may be considered to be especially relevant if they show that the agent in question has caused changes in exposed humans that are on the causal pathway to carcinogenesis. Such data may, however, never become available, because it is at least conceivable that certain compounds may be kept from human use solely on the basis of evidence of their toxicity and/or carcinogenicity in experimental systems.

For complex exposures, including occupational and industrial exposures, the chemical composition and the potential contribution of carcinogens known to be present are considered by the Working Group in its overall evaluation of human carcinogenicity. The Working Group also determines the extent to which the materials tested in experimental systems are related to those to which humans are exposed.

(c)   *Overall evaluation*

Finally, the body of evidence is considered as a whole, in order to reach an overall evaluation of the carcinogenicity to humans of an agent, mixture or circumstance of exposure.

An evaluation may be made for a group of chemical compounds that have been eva-luated by the Working Group. In addition, when supporting data indicate that other, related compounds for which there is no direct evidence of capacity to induce cancer in humans or in animals may also be carcinogenic, a statement describing the rationale for this conclusion is added to the evaluation narrative; an additional evaluation may be made for this broader group of compounds if the strength of the evidence warrants it.

The agent, mixture or exposure circumstance is described according to the wording of one of the following categories, and the designated group is given. The categorization of an agent, mixture or exposure circumstance is a matter of scientific judgement, reflec-ting the strength of the evidence derived from studies in humans and in experimental animals and from other relevant data.

Group 1 —The agent (mixture) is carcinogenic to humans.
The exposure circumstance entails exposures that are carcinogenic to humans.

This category is used when there is *sufficient evidence* of carcinogenicity in humans. Exceptionally, an agent (mixture) may be placed in this category when evidence of carci-nogenicity in humans is less than sufficient but there is *sufficient evidence* of carcino-genicity in experimental animals and strong evidence in exposed humans that the agent (mixture) acts through a relevant mechanism of carcinogenicity.

Group 2

This category includes agents, mixtures and exposure circumstances for which, at one extreme, the degree of evidence of carcinogenicity in humans is almost sufficient, as well as those for which, at the other extreme, there are no human data but for which there is evidence of carcinogenicity in experimental animals. Agents, mixtures and exposure circumstances are assigned to either group 2A (probably carcinogenic to humans) or group 2B (possibly carcinogenic to humans) on the basis of epidemiological and experi-mental evidence of carcinogenicity and other relevant data.

Group 2A—The agent (mixture) is probably carcinogenic to humans.
The exposure circumstance entails exposures that are probably carcinogenic to humans.

This category is used when there is *limited evidence* of carcinogenicity in humans and *sufficient evidence* of carcinogenicity in experimental animals. In some cases, an agent (mixture) may be classified in this category when there is *inadequate evidence* of carcinogenicity in humans, *sufficient evidence* of carcinogenicity in experimental animals and strong evidence that the carcinogenesis is mediated by a mechanism that also operates in humans. Exceptionally, an agent, mixture or exposure circumstance may be classified in this category solely on the basis of *limited evidence* of carcinogenicity in humans.

Group 2B—The agent (mixture) is possibly carcinogenic to humans.
The exposure circumstance entails exposures that are possibly carcinogenic to humans.

This category is used for agents, mixtures and exposure circumstances for which there is *limited evidence* of carcinogenicity in humans and less than *sufficient evidence* of carcinogenicity in experimental animals. It may also be used when there is *inadequate evidence* of carcinogenicity in humans but there is *sufficient evidence* of carcinogenicity in experimental animals. In some instances, an agent, mixture or exposure circumstance for which there is *inadequate evidence* of carcinogenicity in humans but *limited evidence* of carcinogenicity in experimental animals together with supporting evidence from other relevant data may be placed in this group.

Group 3—The agent (mixture or exposure circumstance) is not classifiable as to its carcinogenicity to humans.

This category is used most commonly for agents, mixtures and exposure circumstances for which the *evidence of carcinogenicity* is *inadequate* in humans and *inadequate* or *limited* in experimental animals.

Exceptionally, agents (mixtures) for which the *evidence of carcinogenicity* is *inadequate* in humans but *sufficient* in experimental animals may be placed in this category when there is strong evidence that the mechanism of carcinogenicity in experimental animals does not operate in humans.

Agents, mixtures and exposure circumstances that do not fall into any other group are also placed in this category.

Group 4—The agent (mixture) is probably not carcinogenic to humans.

This category is used for agents or mixtures for which there is *evidence suggesting lack of carcinogenicity* in humans and in experimental animals. In some instances, agents or mixtures for which there is *inadequate evidence* of carcinogenicity in humans but *evidence suggesting lack of carcinogenicity* in experimental animals, consistently and strongly supported by a broad range of other relevant data, may be classified in this group.

References

Breslow, N.E. & Day, N.E. (1980) *Statistical Methods in Cancer Research*, Vol. 1, *The Analysis of Case–Control Studies* (IARC Scientific Publications No. 32), Lyon, IARC*Press*

Breslow, N.E. & Day, N.E. (1987) *Statistical Methods in Cancer Research*, Vol. 2, *The Design and Analysis of Cohort Studies* (IARC Scientific Publications No. 82), Lyon, IARC*Press*

Cohen, S.M. & Ellwein, L.B. (1990) Cell proliferation in carcinogenesis. *Science*, **249**, 1007–1011

Gart, J.J., Krewski, D., Lee, P.N., Tarone, R.E. & Wahrendorf, J. (1986) *Statistical Methods in Cancer Research*, Vol. 3, *The Design and Analysis of Long-term Animal Experiments* (IARC Scientific Publications No. 79), Lyon, IARC*Press*

Hoel, D.G., Kaplan, N.L. & Anderson, M.W. (1983) Implication of nonlinear kinetics on risk estimation in carcinogenesis. *Science*, **219**, 1032–1037

Huff, J.E., Eustis, S.L. & Haseman, J.K. (1989) Occurrence and relevance of chemically induced benign neoplasms in long-term carcinogenicity studies. *Cancer Metastasis Rev.*, **8**, 1–21

IARC (1973–1996) *Information Bulletin on the Survey of Chemicals Being Tested for Carcinogenicity/Directory of Agents Being Tested for Carcinogenicity*, Numbers 1–17, Lyon, IARC*Press*

IARC (1976–1996), Lyon, IARC*Press*

> *Directory of On-going Research in Cancer Epidemiology 1976.* Edited by C.S. Muir & G. Wagner

> *Directory of On-going Research in Cancer Epidemiology 1977* (IARC Scientific Publications No. 17). Edited by C.S. Muir & G. Wagner

> *Directory of On-going Research in Cancer Epidemiology 1978* (IARC Scientific Publications No. 26). Edited by C.S. Muir & G. Wagner

> *Directory of On-going Research in Cancer Epidemiology 1979* (IARC Scientific Publications No. 28). Edited by C.S. Muir & G. Wagner

> *Directory of On-going Research in Cancer Epidemiology 1980* (IARC Scientific Publications No. 35). Edited by C.S. Muir & G. Wagner

> *Directory of On-going Research in Cancer Epidemiology 1981* (IARC Scientific Publications No. 38). Edited by C.S. Muir & G. Wagner

> *Directory of On-going Research in Cancer Epidemiology 1982* (IARC Scientific Publications No. 46). Edited by C.S. Muir & G. Wagner

> *Directory of On-going Research in Cancer Epidemiology 1983* (IARC Scientific Publications No. 50). Edited by C.S. Muir & G. Wagner

> *Directory of On-going Research in Cancer Epidemiology 1984* (IARC Scientific Publications No. 62). Edited by C.S. Muir & G. Wagner

> *Directory of On-going Research in Cancer Epidemiology 1985* (IARC Scientific Publications No. 69). Edited by C.S. Muir & G. Wagner

> *Directory of On-going Research in Cancer Epidemiology 1986* (IARC Scientific Publications No. 80). Edited by C.S. Muir & G. Wagner

> *Directory of On-going Research in Cancer Epidemiology 1987* (IARC Scientific Publications No. 86). Edited by D.M. Parkin & J. Wahrendorf

> *Directory of On-going Research in Cancer Epidemiology 1988* (IARC Scientific Publications No. 93). Edited by M. Coleman & J. Wahrendorf

> *Directory of On-going Research in Cancer Epidemiology 1989/90* (IARC Scientific Publications No. 101). Edited by M. Coleman & J. Wahrendorf

> *Directory of On-going Research in Cancer Epidemiology 1991* (IARC Scientific Publications No.110). Edited by M. Coleman & J. Wahrendorf

> *Directory of On-going Research in Cancer Epidemiology 1992* (IARC Scientific Publications No. 117). Edited by M. Coleman, J. Wahrendorf & E. Démaret

Directory of On-going Research in Cancer Epidemiology 1994 (IARC Scientific Publications No. 130). Edited by R. Sankaranarayanan, J. Wahrendorf & E. Démaret

Directory of On-going Research in Cancer Epidemiology 1996 (IARC Scientific Publications No. 137). Edited by R. Sankaranarayanan, J. Wahrendorf & E. Démaret

IARC (1977) *IARC Monographs Programme on the Evaluation of the Carcinogenic Risk of Chemicals to Humans*. Preamble (IARC intern. tech. Rep. No. 77/002)

IARC (1978) *Chemicals with* Sufficient Evidence *of Carcinogenicity in Experimental Animals—* IARC Monographs *Volumes 1–17* (IARC intern. tech. Rep. No. 78/003)

IARC (1978–1993) *Environmental Carcinogens. Methods of Analysis and Exposure Measurement*, Lyon, IARCPress

    Vol. 1. Analysis of Volatile Nitrosamines in Food (IARC Scientific Publications No. 18). Edited by R. Preussmann, M. Castegnaro, E.A. Walker & A.E. Wasserman (1978)

    Vol. 2. Methods for the Measurement of Vinyl Chloride in Poly(vinyl chloride), Air, Water and Foodstuffs (IARC Scientific Publications No. 22). Edited by D.C.M. Squirrell & W. Thain (1978)

    Vol. 3. Analysis of Polycyclic Aromatic Hydrocarbons in Environmental Samples (IARC Scientific Publications No. 29). Edited by M. Castegnaro, P. Bogovski, H. Kunte & E.A. Walker (1979)

    Vol. 4. Some Aromatic Amines and Azo Dyes in the General and Industrial Environment (IARC Scientific Publications No. 40). Edited by L. Fishbein, M. Castegnaro, I.K. O'Neill & H. Bartsch (1981)

    Vol. 5. Some Mycotoxins (IARC Scientific Publications No. 44). Edited by L. Stoloff, M. Castegnaro, P. Scott, I.K. O'Neill & H. Bartsch (1983)

    Vol. 6. N-Nitroso Compounds (IARC Scientific Publications No. 45). Edited by R. Preussmann, I.K. O'Neill, G. Eisenbrand, B. Spiegelhalder & H. Bartsch (1983)

    Vol. 7. Some Volatile Halogenated Hydrocarbons (IARC Scientific Publications No. 68). Edited by L. Fishbein & I.K. O'Neill (1985)

    Vol. 8. Some Metals: As, Be, Cd, Cr, Ni, Pb, Se, Zn (IARC Scientific Publications No. 71). Edited by I.K. O'Neill, P. Schuller & L. Fishbein (1986)

    Vol. 9. Passive Smoking (IARC Scientific Publications No. 81). Edited by I.K. O'Neill, K.D. Brunnemann, B. Dodet & D. Hoffmann (1987)

    *Vol. 10. Benzene and Alkylated Benzenes (*IARC Scientific Publications No. 85). Edited by L. Fishbein & I.K. O'Neill (1988)

    Vol. 11. Polychlorinated Dioxins and Dibenzofurans (IARC Scientific Publications No. 108). Edited by C. Rappe, H.R. Buser, B. Dodet & I.K. O'Neill (1991)

    Vol. 12. Indoor Air (IARC Scientific Publications No. 109). Edited by B. Seifert, H. van de Wiel, B. Dodet & I.K. O'Neill (1993)

IARC (1979) *Criteria to Select Chemicals for* IARC Monographs (IARC intern. tech. Rep. No. 79/003)

IARC (1982) *IARC Monographs on the Evaluation of the Carcinogenic Risk of Chemicals to Humans*, Supplement 4, *Chemicals, Industrial Processes and Industries Associated with Cancer in Humans* (IARC Monographs, Volumes 1 to 29), Lyon, IARCPress

IARC (1983) *Approaches to Classifying Chemical Carcinogens According to Mechanism of Action* (IARC intern. tech. Rep. No. 83/001)

IARC (1984) *Chemicals and Exposures to Complex Mixtures Recommended for Evaluation in IARC Monographs and Chemicals and Complex Mixtures Recommended for Long-term Carcinogenicity Testing* (IARC intern. tech. Rep. No. 84/002)

IARC (1987a) *IARC Monographs on the Evaluation of Carcinogenic Risks to Humans*, Supplement 6, *Genetic and Related Effects: An Updating of Selected* IARC Monographs *from Volumes 1 to 42*, Lyon, IARC*Press*

IARC (1987b) *IARC Monographs on the Evaluation of Carcinogenic Risks to Humans*, Supplement 7, *Overall Evaluations of Carcinogenicity: An Updating of* IARC Monographs *Volumes 1 to 42*, Lyon, IARC*Press*

IARC (1988) *Report of an IARC Working Group to Review the Approaches and Processes Used to Evaluate the Carcinogenicity of Mixtures and Groups of Chemicals* (IARC intern. tech. Rep. No. 88/002)

IARC (1989) *Chemicals, Groups of Chemicals, Mixtures and Exposure Circumstances to be Evaluated in Future IARC Monographs, Report of an ad hoc Working Group* (IARC intern. tech. Rep. No. 89/004)

IARC (1991a) *A Consensus Report of an IARC Monographs Working Group on the Use of Mechanisms of Carcinogenesis in Risk Identification* (IARC intern. tech. Rep. No. 91/002)

IARC (1991b) *Report of an ad-hoc* IARC Monographs *Advisory Group on Viruses and Other Biological Agents Such as Parasites* (IARC intern. tech. Rep. No. 91/001)

IARC (1993) *Chemicals, Groups of Chemicals, Complex Mixtures, Physical and Biological Agents and Exposure Circumstances to be Evaluated in Future* IARC Monographs, *Report of an ad-hoc Working Group* (IARC intern. Rep. No. 93/005)

IARC (1998a) *Report of an ad-hoc* IARC Monographs *Advisory Group on Physical Agents* (IARC Internal Report No. 98/002)

IARC (1998b) *Report of an ad-hoc* IARC Monographs *Advisory Group on Priorities for Future Evaluations* (IARC Internal Report No. 98/004)

McGregor, D.B., Rice, J.M. & Venitt, S., eds (1999) *The Use of Short and Medium-term Tests for Carcinogens and Data on Genetic Effects in Carcinogenic Hazard Evaluation* (IARC Scientific Publications No. 146), Lyon, IARC*Press*

Montesano, R., Bartsch, H., Vainio, H., Wilbourn, J. & Yamasaki, H., eds (1986) *Long-term and Short-term Assays for Carcinogenesis—A Critical Appraisal* (IARC Scientific Publications No. 83), Lyon, IARC*Press*

Peto, R., Pike, M.C., Day, N.E., Gray, R.G., Lee, P.N., Parish, S., Peto, J., Richards, S. & Wahrendorf, J. (1980) Guidelines for simple, sensitive significance tests for carcinogenic effects in long-term animal experiments. In: *IARC Monographs on the Evaluation of the Carcinogenic Risk of Chemicals to Humans*, Supplement 2, *Long-term and Short-term Screening Assays for Carcinogens: A Critical Appraisal*, Lyon, IARC*Press*, pp. 311–426

Tomatis, L., Aitio, A., Wilbourn, J. & Shuker, L. (1989) Human carcinogens so far identified. *Jpn. J. Cancer Res.*, **80**, 795–807

Vainio, H., Magee, P.N., McGregor, D.B. & McMichael, A.J., eds (1992) *Mechanisms of Carcinogenesis in Risk Identification* (IARC Scientific Publications No. 116), Lyon, IARC*Press*

Vainio, H., Wilbourn, J.D., Sasco, A.J., Partensky, C., Gaudin, N., Heseltine, E. & Eragne, I. (1995) Identification of human carcinogenic risk in IARC Monographs. *Bull. Cancer,* **82**, 339–348 (in French)

Waters, M.D., Stack, H.F., Brady, A.L., Lohman, P.H.M., Haroun, L. & Vainio, H. (1987) Appendix 1. Activity profiles for genetic and related tests. In: *IARC Monographs on the Evaluation of Carcinogenic Risks to Humans*, Suppl. 6, *Genetic and Related Effects: An Updating of Selected IARC Monographs from Volumes 1 to 42*, Lyon, IARC*Press*, pp. 687–696

Wilbourn, J., Haroun, L., Heseltine, E., Kaldor, J., Partensky, C. & Vainio, H. (1986) Response of experimental animals to human carcinogens: an analysis based upon the IARC Monographs Programme. *Carcinogenesis*, **7**, 1853–1863

GENERAL REMARKS ON THE SUBSTANCES CONSIDERED

This seventy-ninth volume of *IARC Monographs* contains evaluations of the carcinogenic risk to humans of 19 chemicals that have produced thyroid tumours in rodents. Unless otherwise stated, the term 'thyroid tumour', as used in this volume, refers to neoplasms of thyroid follicular cell origin.

These substances have diverse uses. A number are used as drugs, including so-called 'anti-thyroid' agents (methimazole, methylthiouracil, propylthiouracil and thiouracil), sedatives (doxylamine succinate and phenobarbital), antifungal agents (griseofulvin), diuretics (spironolactone) and antibacterial agents (sulfamethazine and sulfamethoxazole). The others are or have been used in agriculture as pesticides (amitrole, chlordane, heptachlor, hexachlorobenzene and toxaphene), in foods or cosmetics (kojic acid), in hair dyes (2,4-diaminoanisole) and as industrial chemicals (*N*,*N*'-diethylthiourea, ethylenethiourea, and thiourea). Many of these agents have been evaluated previously in *IARC Monographs*, but some (*N*,*N*'-diethylthiourea, doxylamine succinate, kojic acid, methimazole and sulfamethazine) are evaluated for the first time.

Since the previous evaluations of these agents in the *Monographs* series, new data, particularly on mechanisms, have become available. Such data now play an important role in making overall evaluations of carcinogenicity to humans (Vainio *et al.*, 1992). A number of guidelines have been developed for the use of information on the mechanisms of induction of tumours of the kidney, urinary bladder and thyroid gland in rodents in making IARC evaluations (Capen *et al.*, 1999), and these guidelines were used in the present volume.

Use of anti-thyroid drugs in humans

Thioureylene anti-thyroid drugs belong to the family of thionamides, which are heterocyclic thiourea derivatives that potently inhibit thyroid hormone synthesis. They were developed in the mid-1940s to early 1950s on the basis of observations that thiourea and thiocarbamide are goitrogenic in animals. Thiouracil was the first 'anti-thyroid drug' to be used clinically, but its use was short-lived because of toxicity and because other, more active drugs (i.e. propylthiouracil, methylthiouracil and methimazole) were soon developed (Astwood & VaanderLaan, 1945; Stanley & Astwood, 1949). In addition to propylthiouracil and methimazole, the 3-carbethoxy derivative of methimazole, carbimazole, is widely used in Europe and Asia. Carbimazole is metabolized *in vivo* to methimazole, which exerts the anti-thyroid effects. It has been estimated that 0.1–0.3% of the population in a number of developed countries is taking antithyroid drugs at any given time (Anon., 1988).

The mechanism of action of thioureylene anti-thyroid drugs is still not completely understood. The drugs are actively concentrated by the thyroid gland. They act to block the formation of thyroid hormone by inhibiting two key steps in intrathyroidal hormone synthesis: (i) incorporation of oxidized iodine into tyrosine residues in thyroglobulin to form iodotyrosines (the so-called 'organification' step), and (ii) the 'coupling reaction', wherein iodotyrosine residues within the thyroglobulin molecule couple to form the iodothyronines, thyroxine (T4) and triiodothyronine (T3) (Taurog, 1976) (see Figure 1). The organification step is catalysed by the haem-containing glycoprotein enzyme thyroid peroxidase (TPO), which provides a haem-bound oxidized iodine moiety (TPO-I$^+$). Although antithyroid drugs are potent inhibitors of TPO *in vitro*, their mechanism of action *in vivo* is more complex. It now appears that, within the thyroid gland, the drugs themselves serve as TPO substrates. Upon entry into the thyroid, they are iodinated and thus act as TPO competitors by diverting the oxidized iodine species (TPO-I$^+$) away from the organification process (Davidson *et al.*, 1978; Engler *et al.*, 1982). The inhibitory effects of antithyroid drugs on the coupling process are less well characterized but also probably involve interference with TPO (Cooper, 2000).

Anti-thyroid drugs may have other, less well-documented intrathyroidal effects. There is evidence that they can interfere with thyroglobulin synthesis (Monaco *et al.*, 1980) and possibly with the thyroglobulin structure (Papapetrou *et al.*, 1975), but the clinical significance of these observations is uncertain. The drugs have no effect on iodine trapping by the thyroid, nor do they interfere with thyroid hormone secretion by the gland.

In addition to these intrathyroidal effects that relate to thyroid hormone synthesis, the drugs also have potentially clinically important extrathyroidal effects. The first is the inhibition by propylthiouracil (but not methimazole) of 5'-deiodinase type I, the enzyme that catalyses the conversion of T4 to T3 in peripheral tissues. T3 is the biologically active form of thyroid hormone and, since 80% of daily T3 production arises from peripheral T4 deiodination rather than from direct glandular secretion, inhibition of this enzyme by propylthiouracil causes an immediate decrease in serum T3 concentrations (Cooper *et al.*, 1982). However, this effect probably does not confer a clinical advantage of propylthiouracil over methimazole, except in severe thyrotoxicosis ('thyroid storm'). The second extrathyroidal effect relates to possible effects on the immune system. Graves disease, the commonest cause of hyperthyroidism by far, is an autoimmune disease. Numerous in-vitro and in-vivo studies (summarized by Cooper, 1998) have suggested that the thionamide anti-thyroid drugs have immunosuppressive effects, and it is these effects that are thought to be responsible for the remissions that are seen in anywhere from 20 to 80% of patients after a 12–24-month course of drug therapy. However, it is also possible that anti-thyroid drugs simply control the hyperthyroid state

Figure 1. Thyronine, thyroid hormones and precursors

Thyronine

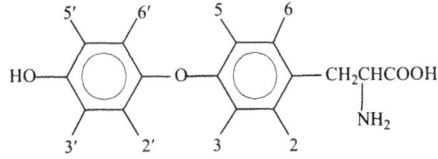

Thyroxine (= T_4)

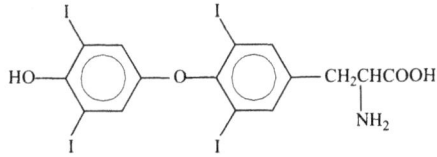

3,5,3'-Triiodothyronine (= T_3)

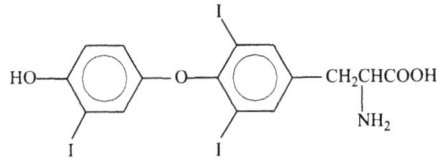

3,3',5'-Triiodothyronine (= rT_3)

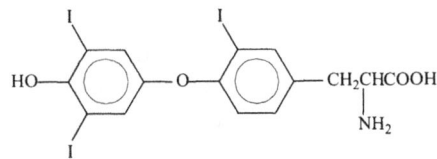

Diiodotyrosine

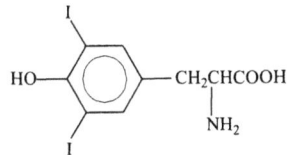

Iodotyrosine

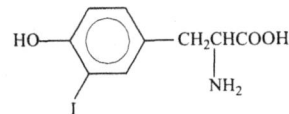

From Hardman *et al.* (1995)

by permitting the disordered immune system to return to normal after correction of thyroid hormone concentrations in the blood (Cooper, 1998).

At present, the only clinical use of the thionamide anti-thyroid drugs is in the treatment of hyperthyroidism caused by Graves disease, toxic thyroid nodules, toxic multinodular goitre and several other rare causes of hyperthyroidism. In patients with Graves disease, anti-thyroid drugs are used in two contexts. In some patients, they are given for several months to normalize thyroid function prior to definitive therapy with either radioiodine or surgery. In other patients, they are given for 1–2 years, in the hope that the patient will enter a period of remission.

Thyroid cancer in humans

In humans, thyroid cancer is relatively rare. The great majority of thyroid cancers arise from the epithelial elements of the gland, mostly from the follicular cells (Robbins *et al.*, 1984). Thyroid carcinomas fall into two broad groups: differentiated and undifferentiated (anaplastic). The former group is subdivided into two types, papillary and follicular. Medullary carcinoma derives from parafollicular cells (i.e. calcitonin-producing cells, or C-cells) and accounts for 5–15% of most series of thyroid carcinomas (Franceschi *et al.*, 1993). The etiology of this type is separate from those of other thyroid carcinomas, inheritance being an important determinant (Ron, 1996).

Thyroid carcinomas vary widely in the degree of malignancy, ranging from relatively benign to rapidly fatal. The difference depends almost entirely on the histological type. A 'pool' of individuals with occult thyroid carcinomas (mostly of the papillary type) is probably present in most populations, even among young people. Large differences in the estimated frequency of cancer at this site can therefore be due to variation in diagnostic intensity. Data on changing trends of incidence and mortality are thus subject to reservation, depending on the degree to which they have been influenced by changing diagnostic criteria and the precision of histopathological description.

Mortality rates from thyroid cancer have decreased in most developed countries, and the decreases have been especially marked in Austria, Iceland and Switzerland, where the rates were relatively elevated in the early 1990s (i.e. approximately 2/100 000 compared to < 1/100 000 nearly everywhere else). Mortality rates have also decreased in the United Kingdom and the USA. Upward trends in the incidence of thyroid cancer were recorded in most developed countries at least up to the 1970s or early 1980s, with stabilization thereafter (Franceschi *et al.*, 1993). Thyroid cancer shows a two- to threefold higher incidence in women than in men.

Thyroid function is regulated by pituitary (thyroid-stimulating hormone; TSH) and hypothalamic (thyrotropin-releasing hormone) mediators and by the glandular organic iodine content. The role of elevated TSH concentrations in the pathogenesis of thyroid cancer in humans is unclear, as epidemiological studies have shown excess incidences of thyroid cancer in both iodine-rich and iodine-deficient areas, and both iodine deficiency and iodine excess may enhance TSH secretion. Endemic goitre due to iodine excess has been demonstrated among fishermen in Japan (Suzuki *et al.*, 1965; Okamura *et al.*, 1987) and Norway (Jorgensen & Svindland, 1991) who eat large quantities of iodine-rich seaweed, and in persons living in areas in China where the iodine concentration in the drinking-water is very high (Li *et al.*, 1987) and where large quantities of iodine-rich salt or pickled vegetables (Zhu *et al.*, 1984) are ingested. Papillary carcinomas of the thyroid represent the vast majority of thyroid cancers in iodine-sufficient areas, whereas follicular and anaplastic carcinomas occur more frequently in iodine-deficient areas (Williams *et al.*, 1977).

Few epidemiological data are available on the relationship between thyroid cancer and TSH concentrations. Only one study provided information on TSH concentrations in serum during the preclinical phase of thyroid cancer. In this study, sera were available for 43 patients with thyroid cancer and 128 healthy controls, which had been collected on average 4 years earlier in a large Norwegian serum bank. No difference in TSH concentration was found, whereas higher concentrations of thyroid-binding globulin were measured in the sera of thyroid cancer patients than in those of controls. The increase in thyroid-binding globulin was interpreted as representing either secretion from a slowly growing, subclinical tumour or leakage from normal follicles (Thoresen *et al.*, 1988).

Only two case–control studies have provided data on the risk for thyroid cancer in relation to residence in areas endemic for goitre. In an Italian study, the relative risk for having resided in such an area was 1.3 for < 20 years of residence and 1.6 for 20 or more years (D'Avanzo *et al.*, 1995). In a study in Sweden, a trend towards an association was found with duration of residence in areas endemic for goitre (Galanti *et al.*, 1995).

The results are far more consistent with respect to the role of previous benign thyroid disease. In a re-analysis of the data from 12 case–control studies in Asia, Europe and the USA, involving a total of 2094 women and 425 men with cancer of the thyroid and 3248 female and 928 male controls, persons with a history of benign thyroid nodules or adenomas had a high risk for thyroid cancer (odds ratio, 30; 95% confidence interval [CI], 15–62 for women; 18 cases versus 0 controls in men). The pooled odds ratios associated with a history of goitre were 5.9 (95% CI, 4.2–8.1) for women and 38 (95% CI, 5.0–291) for men, whereas a history of hypothyroidism or hyperthyroidism was not significantly associated with risk. The excess risk associated with benign nodules or adenomas and goitre was greatest within 2–4 years before diagnosis of thyroid cancer, but an elevated odds ratio was present 10 years or more before diagnosis of cancer (Franceschi *et al.*, 1999).

Most thyroid disorders, including cancer, are several times more prevalent in women than in men, which indicates a possible role of female hormones (Franceschi *et al.*, 1993). In a pooled analysis of 14 case–control studies (2247 female cases of thyroid cancer and 3699 controls), however, parity and a history of spontaneous or induced abortions or infertility were not associated with risk. The odds ratio was above unity for women who had first given birth at a late age (1.1; 95% CI, 1.0–1.3 for a 5-year delay) (Negri *et al.*, 1999). The odds ratio was significantly increased for women who were currently using oral contraceptives (odds ratio, 1.5; 95% CI, 1.0–2.1) but declined with increasing time since cessation of use (La Vecchia *et al.*, 1999). The moderate excess risk among current users of oral contraceptives, if not due to increased surveillance for thyroid masses among such users, is similar to that described for breast cancer (Collaborative Group on Hormonal Factors in Breast Cancer, 1996) and would imply a role of female hormones in the promotion of thyroid cancer.

Ionizing radiation is the only well-defined risk factor for thyroid carcinoma. A pooled analysis of five cohort studies and two case–control investigations, cumulating over 3 000 000 person–years of follow-up and 700 thyroid cancers, showed that, for persons exposed to radiation before the age of 15 years, the dose–response relationship was best described by a linear equation, even down to very low doses (0.10 Gy) (Ron *et al.*, 1995). The epidemic of thyroid carcinoma in children exposed to radioiodines as a result of the Chernobyl nuclear reactor accident in 1986 was described in a previous monograph (IARC, 2001).

Epidemiological data on thyroid carcinoma unrelated to exposure to ionizing radiation are scanty. The few studies available generally did not address the specific compounds included in this volume. For example, one cohort study and two case–control studies were carried out among patients receiving anti-thyroid drugs, the identity of which was not specified. These reports are reviewed in each of the four monographs dealing with these drugs (methimazole, methylthiouracil, propylthiouracil and thiouracil). Some compounds (e.g. phenobarbital, chlordane and hexachlorobenzene) have been studied in relation to other cancers. Exposure to non-radioactive chemicals has not been shown to result in the development of thyroid carcinoma in humans.

Pathogenesis of thyroid neoplasms in humans

Studies on the pathogenesis of thyroid neoplasms in humans have tended to focus on structural changes in cancer-related genes in thyroid tumours, rather than on hormonal factors. Most of the work involved molecular studies of human tumours for which no cause was determined, but in some cases the development of a well-differentiated carcinoma has been strongly correlated with a history of exposure to external radiation or to iodine deficiency.

Chromosomal abnormalities have been identified in follicular and papillary thyroid adenomas and carcinomas and in medullary thyroid neoplasms (Gillenwater & Weber, 1997; Kroll *et al.*, 2000), as well as in mixed medullary-follicular carcinomas (Volante *et al.*, 1999). These chromosomal changes are associated with alterations in both oncogenes and tumour suppressor genes. Considerable research has focused on the *met, ras* and *ret* proto-oncogenes and on chimaeric oncogenes, such as the newly identified *PAX8-PPARγl* fusion oncogene (Kroll *et al.*, 2000). Later-stage mutational events in thyroid carcinogenesis may involve mutations in *p53*. Mutated oncogenes are found in 15–70% of thyroid carcinomas, depending on the tumour type (Gillenwater & Weber, 1997; Lazzereschi *et al.*, 1997).

Many of the genetic changes that have been identified in human thyroid tumours arise relatively early in tumorigenesis. They indicate the involvement of multiple genetic pathways, some of which are important to thyroid function, e.g. by altering the TSH receptor and its associated signal transducers (reviewed by Suarez, 2000). Constitutive activation of the TSH receptor signal cascade is responsible for the hyperfunctional state of 25–30% of thyroid follicular toxic adenomas and hyper-functioning tumours (Suarez, 2000).

Thyroid tumours in experimental animals

The background, naturally occurring or 'spontaneous' rate of thyroid follicular-cell tumours in rodents has been reported to be low (Huff, 1999). Among more than 1300 control male and female B6C3F$_1$ mice and Fischer 344 rats used in assays conducted within the National Toxicology Program in the USA, the frequency was about 2% in male and female mice and male rats and 1% in female rats (range, 0–8%).

In contrast to the general lack of evidence for a role of environmental carcinogens other than ionizing radiation in thyroid carcinogenesis in humans, a large number of chemicals, including genotoxic agents such as *N*-nitrosoalkylureas and *N*-nitrosamines, have produced thyroid tumours in rodents (see Dybing & Sanner, 1999; Huff, 1999; Wilbourn *et al.*, 1999). Some of these compounds have genotoxic effects and may also affect TSH; other chemicals that cause thyroid tumours in rats or mice have no detectable genotoxic activity. Such agents often also produce hepatocellular tumours, particularly in mice (see McClain & Rice, 1999). A significant number of pharma-ceutical drugs and agricultural chemicals introduced for general use since 1970 cause thyroid follicular cell tumours in rats or mice or both. However, as many of the bio-assays demonstrating this effect have not been published in the open scientific literature, data on tumours induced by many compounds that might have been chosen for evaluation in this volume were not available.

The lack of evidence for a role of chemicals in the causation of human thyroid neoplasms, in contrast to the frequent observation of thyroid tumours in bioassays for carcinogenicity in experimental animals, raises the question of whether, and in what way, thyroid tumours in laboratory animals predict a cancer hazard for humans (Capen, 1997).

Mechanisms of thyroid follicular-cell proliferation and neoplasia in animals

Little information is available about structural alterations in cancer-related genes in thyroid tumours from rats and mice, in contrast to human thyroid tumours.

There is overwhelming evidence that TSH-induced growth of thyroid epithelial cells plays a critical role in thyroid tumorigenesis in rodents (Thomas & Williams, 1999), whether induced by a carcinogenic chemical or not. Simply feeding an iodine-deficient diet to rats is sufficient to cause not only goitre but thyroid follicular cell adenoma and carcinoma as well (Ohshima & Ward, 1986). The induction of thyroid follicular cell tumours in rats and mice by agents judged to be nongenotoxic is probably primarily a response to dysregulation of the thyroid–pituitary axis of hormonal control of thyroid follicular cell proliferation and function. Prolonged stimulation of the thyroid by TSH, leading to diffuse follicular cell hyperplasia, is an important mechanism in thyroid carcinogenesis in these rodents. Such stimulation can result from decreased synthesis, increased secretion, altered transport and storage or altered metabolism of thyroid hormones (Hard, 1998; Capen et al., 1999).

After iodine is taken up in the follicular cell, it is oxidized by thyroid peroxidase and bound to tyrosyl residues of the thyroid-specific protein thyroglobulin. Mono-iodotyrosine and diiodotyrosine are coupled to form T3 and T4, which are released into the circulation where they are bound to plasma proteins (thyroid-binding globulin in humans and albumin in rats). More T4 than T3 is released from the thyroid, but T4 is deiodinated by 5′-monodeiodinase type I peripherally to produce T3 locally. The circulating concentrations of T4 are monitored by the thyrotropic cells of the pituitary, which are responsible for the production of TSH. In the pituitary, T4 is metabolized to T3 by 5′-deiodinase type II, and the T3 then binds to specific receptors in the cell nucleus. A decrease in T3 receptor occupancy results in stimulation of TSH synthesis and secretion.

Xenobiotics can affect thyroid homeostasis by:
- inhibition of iodine uptake by the thyroid (perchlorates, thiocyanates);
- inhibition of thyroid peroxidase and a decrease in iodine utilization (sulfonamides, propylthiouracil, methimazole, thiourea);
- inhibition of T4 or T3 release from the thyroid (lithium, excess iodide);
- increased metabolism of T4 in the liver (phenobarbital, spironolactone, chlordane); and
- inhibition of 5′-monodeiodinase, decreasing conversion of T4 to active T3 in peripheral tissues (propylthiouracil).

If disruption of thyroid function and consequent stimulation of TSH production by the pituitary is sufficiently intense and prolonged, proliferative changes in thyroid follicular epithelium will result, which, in rats and mice, may progress to tumours (Capen, 1997).

Application of mechanistic evidence in evaluations of chemicals that cause thyroid tumours in experimental animals

Criteria for the use of mechanistic data to assess the predictive value of thyroid follicular cell tumours in rodents for evaluating the carcinogenic hazard of chemicals to humans have been described (Capen et al., 1999). These criteria are as follows:

– Agents that lead to the development of thyroid neoplasia through an adaptive physiological mechanism belong to a different category from those that lead to neoplasia through genotoxic mechanisms or through mechanisms involving pathological responses with necrosis and repair.

– Agents that cause thyroid follicular-cell neoplasia in rodents solely through hormonal imbalance can be identified on the basis of the following criteria.

  • No genotoxic activity (agent and/or metabolite) was found in an overall evaluation of the results of tests *in vivo* and *in vitro*.

  • Hormone imbalance was demonstrated under the conditions of the assay for carcinogenicity.

  • The mechanism whereby the agent leads to hormone imbalance has been defined.

– When tumours are observed both in the thyroid and at other sites, they should be evaluated separately on the basis of the modes of action of the agent.

– Agents that induce thyroid follicular-cell tumours in rodents by interfering with thyroid hormone homeostasis can, with some exceptions, notably the sulfonamides, also interfere with thyroid hormone homeostasis in humans if given at a sufficient dose for a sufficient time. These agents can be assumed not to be carcinogenic in humans at concentrations that do not lead to alterations in thyroid hormone homeostasis.

The Working Group considered that some clarification of these criteria was desirable. Specifically, the 'conditions' of the carcinogenicity assay, referred to above, are meant to indicate that hormonal assays and morphological evaluation of the thyroid gland should be carried out in animals of the same species, and preferably the same strain, as were used in the bioassay in which thyroid tumours developed, but not necessarily as part of the bioassay itself. Animals used in hormonal assays should be treated by the same route and dose as animals in which tumours developed in bioassays for carcinogenicity.

Evidence for hormonal imbalance could include measurements of serum thyroid hormone and TSH and of morphological changes characteristic of increased TSH stimulation, including increased thyroid gland weight and diffuse follicular-cell hyperplasia and/or hypertrophy.

General statement regarding the determination of genotoxicity or non-genotoxicity of a substance

There is no general agreement about the numbers or types of tests that are needed to determine the genotoxicity or non-genotoxicity of a substance. It is generally agreed, however, that tests for gene mutation and for chromosomal damage are required (McGregor *et al.*, 1999). The tests for gene mutation most widely used involve bacteria (usually *Salmonella*) and mammalian cells *in vitro*, with and without exogenous metabolic activation. The assays for chromosomal damage include cytogenetic analysis *in vitro* or *in vivo* and tests for micronucleus formation *in vitro* and *in vivo*. As a rule, a substance that reproducibly induces gene mutation or chromosomal damage (measured as aberrations or micronuclei) is to be considered a genotoxic agent. It should be specified whether the evidence of genotoxicity is based on the results of in-vitro tests, in-vivo tests or both.

It is more difficult to find agreement on the tests and patterns of test results necessary to declare a substance non-genotoxic. In order to do so, a consistent pattern of negative results should have been found in bacteria and mammalian cells *in vitro* and in mammals *in vivo*.

For most of the agents reviewed in this *Monographs* volume, few data were available from adequate tests of genetic toxicity. The lack of adequate data on genotoxicity precluded application of the above criteria to a number of the substances considered in this volume.

References

Anon. (1988) Risk of agranulocytosis and aplastic anaemia in relation to use of antithyroid drugs. International Agranulocytosis and Aplastic Anaemia Study. *Br. med. J.*, **297**, 262–265

Astwood, E.B. & VaanderLaan, W.P. (1945) Thiouracil derivatives of greater activity for the treatment of hyperthyroidism. *J. clin. Endocrinol.*, **5**, 424–430

Capen, C.C. (1997) Mechanistic data and risk assessment of selected toxic end points of the thyroid gland. *Toxicol. Pathol.*, **25**, 39–48

Capen, C.C., Dybing, E., Rice, J.M. & Wilbourn, J.D., eds (1999) *Species Differences in Thyroid, Kidney and Urinary Bladder Carcinogenesis* (IARC Scientific Publications No. 147), Lyon, IARC*Press*

Collaborative Group on Hormonal Factors in Breast Cancer (1996) Breast cancer and hormonal contraceptives: Collaborative reanalysis of individual data on 53 297 women with breast cancer and 100 239 women without breast cancer from 54 epidemiological studies. *Lancet*, **347**, 1713–1727

Cooper, D.S. (1998) Antithyroid drugs for the treatment of hyperthyroidism caused by Graves' disease. *Endocrinol. Metab. Clin. N. Am.*, **27**, 225–247

Cooper, D.S. (2000) Treatment of thyrotoxicosis. In: Bravermann, L.E. & Utiger, R.D., eds, *Werner & Ingbar's, The Thyroid. A Fundamental and Clinical Text*, 8th Ed., Philadelphia, Lippincott Williams & Wilkins, pp. 691–715

Cooper, D.S., Saxe, V.C., Meskill, M., Maloof, F. & Ridgway, E.C. (1982) Acute effects of propylthiouracil (PTU) on thyroidal iodide organification and peripheral deiodination: Correlation with serum PTU levels measured by radioimmunoassay. *J. clin. Endocrinol. Metab.*, **54**, 101–107

D'Avanzo, B., La Vecchia, C., Franceschi, S., Negri, E. & Talamini, R. (1995) History of thyroid diseases and subsequent thyroid cancer risk. *Cancer Epidemiol. Biomarkers Prev.*, **4**, 193–199

Davidson, B., Soodak, M., Neary, J.T., Strout, H.V., Kieffer, J.D., Mover, H. & Maloof, F. (1978) The irreversible inactivation of thyroid peroxidase by methylmercaptoimidazole, thiouracil, and propylthiouracil *in vitro* and its relationship to in vivo findings. *Endocrinology*, **103**, 871–882

Dybing, E. & Sanner, T. (1999) Species differences in chemical carcinogenesis of the thyroid gland, kidney and urinary bladder. In: Capen, C.C., Dybing, E., Rice, J.M. & Wilbourn, J.D., eds, *Species Differences in Thyroid, Kidney and Urinary Bladder Carcinogenesis* (IARC Scientific Publications No. 147), Lyon, IARC*Press*, pp. 15–32

Engler, H., Taurog, A. & Nakashima, T. (1982) Mechanism of inactivation of thyroid peroxidase by thioureylene drugs. *Biochem. Pharmacol.*, **31**, 3801–3806

Franceschi, S., Boyle, P., Maisonneuve, P., La Vecchia, C., Burt, A.D., Kerr, D.J. & McFarlane, G.J. (1993) The epidemiology of thyroid carcinoma. *Crit. Rev. Oncogenesis*, **4**, 25–52

Franceschi, S., Preston-Martin, S., Dal Maso, L., Negri, E., La Vecchia, C., Mack, W.J., McTiernan, A., Kolonel, L., Mark, S.D., Mabuchi, K., Jin, F., Wingren, G., Galanti, R., Hallquist, A., Glattre, E., Lund, E., Levi, F., Linos, D. & Ron, E. (1999) A pooled analysis of case–control studies of thyroid cancer. IV. Benign diseases. *Cancer Causes Control*, **10**, 583–595

Galanti, M.R., Sarén, P., Karlsson, A., Grimelius, L. & Ekbom, A. (1995) Is residence in areas of endemic goiter a risk factor for thyroid cancer? *Int. J. Cancer*, **61**, 615–621

Gillenwater, A.M. & Weber, R.S. (1997) Thyroid carcinoma. *Cancer Treat. Res.*, **90**, 149–169

Hard, G.C. (1998) Recent developments in the investigation of thyroid regulation and thyroid carcinogenesis. *Environ. Health Perspectives*, **106**, 427–436

Hardman, J.G., Limbird, L.E., Molinoff, P.B., Ruddon, R.W. & Gilman, A.G., eds (1995) *Goodman & Gilman's The Pharmacological Basis of Therapeutics*, 9th Ed., New York, McGraw-Hill, p. 1384

Huff, J. (1999) Chemicals associated with tumours of the kidney, urinary bladder and thyroid gland in laboratory rodents from 2000 NTP/NCI bioassays for carcinogenicity. In: Capen, C.C., Dybing, E., Rice, J.M. & Wilbourn, J.D., eds, *Species Differences in Thyroid, Kidney and Urinary Bladder Carcinogenesis* (IARC Scientific Publications No. 147), Lyon, IARC*Press*, pp. 211–225

IARC (2001) *IARC Monographs on the Evaluation of Carcinogenic Risks to Humans*, Vol. 78, *Ionizing Radiation, Part 2 — Some Internally Deposited Radionuclides*, Lyon, IARC*Press*

Jorgensen, H. & Svindland, O. (1991) Hyperthyreosis and hypothyreosis after use of iodine-containing natural products and iodine-containing vitamin and mineral supplements. *Tidsskr. Nor. Laegeforen.*, **111**, 3153–3155

Kroll, T.G., Sarraf, P., Pecciarini, L., Chen, C.J., Mueller, E., Spiegelman, B.M. & Fletcher, J.A. (2000) PAX8/PPARgamma1 fusion oncogene in human thyroid carcinoma. *Science*, **289**, 1357–1360

La Vecchia, C., Ron, E., Franceschi, S., Dal Maso, L., Mark, S.D., Chatenoud, L., Braga, C., Preston-Martin, S., McTiernan, A., Kolonel, L., Mabuchi, K., Jin, F., Wingren, G., Galanti, M.R., Hallquist, A., Lund, E., Levi, F., Linos, D. & Negri, E. (1999) A pooled analysis of case–control studies of thyroid cancer. III. Oral contraceptives, menopausal replacement therapy and other female hormones. *Cancer Causes Control*, **10**, 157–166

Lazzereschi, D., Mincione, G., Coppo, A., Ranieri, A., Turco, A., Buccheschi, G., Pelicano, S. & Colletta, G. (1997) Oncogenes and antioncogenes involved in human thyroid carcinogenesis. *J. exp. Clin. Cancer Res.*, **16**, 325–332

Li, M., Liu, D.R., Qu, C.Y., Zhang, P.Y., Qian, Q.D., Zhang, C.D., Jia, Q.Z., Wang, H.X., Eastman, C.J., Boyages, S.C., Collins, J.K., Jupp, J.J. & Maberly, G.F. (1987) Endemic goitre in central China caused by excessive iodine intake. *Lancet*, **ii**, 257–259

McClain, R.M. & Rice, J.M. (1999) A mechanistic relationship between thyroid follicular cell tumours and hepatocellular neoplasms in rodents. In: Capen, C.C., Dybing, E., Rice, J.M. & Wilbourn, J.D., eds, *Species Differences in Thyroid, Kidney and Urinary Bladder Carcinogenesis* (IARC Scientific Publications No. 147), Lyon, IARC*Press*, pp. 61–68

McGregor, D.B., Rice, J.M. & Venitt, S., eds (1999) *The Use of Short- and Medium-term Tests for Carcinogens and Data on Genetic Effects in Carcinogenic Hazard Evaluation* (IARC Scientific Publications No. 146), Lyon, IARC*Press*

Monaco, F., Santolamazza, C., De Ros, I. & Andreoli, A. (1980) Effects of propylthiouracil and methylmercaptoimidazole in thyroglobulin synthesis. *Acta endocrinol.*, **93**, 32–36

Negri, E., Dal Maso, L., Ron, E., La Vecchia, C., Mark, S.D., Preston-Martin, S., McTiernan, A., Kolonel, L., Yoshimoto, Y., Jin, F., Wingren, G., Rosaria Galanti, M., Hardell, L., Glattre, E., Lund, E., Levi, F., Linos, D., Braga, C. & Franceschi, S. (1999) A pooled analysis of case–control studies of thyroid cancer. II. Menstrual and reproductive factors. *Cancer Causes Control*, **10**, 143–155

Ohshima, M. & Ward, J.M. (1986) Dietary iodine deficiency as a tumor promoter and carcinogen in male F344/NCr rats. *Cancer Res.*, **46**, 877–883

Okamura, K., Nakashima, T., Ueda, K., Inoue, K., Omae, T. & Fujishima, M. (1987) Thyroid disorders in the general population of Hisayama, Japan, with special reference to prevalence and sex differences. *Int. J. Epidemiol.*, **16**, 545–549

Papapetrou, P.D., Mothon, S. & Alexander, W.D. (1975) Binding of the 35-S of 35-S-propylthiouracil by follicular thyroglobulin *in vivo* and *in vitro*. *Acta endocrinol.*, **79**, 248–258

Robbins, S.L., Cotram, R.S. & Kumar, V. (1984) *Pathologic Basis of Disease*, Philadelphia, W.B. Saunders, pp. 1201–1225

Ron, E. (1996) Thyroid cancer. In: Schottenfeld, D. & Fraumeni, J.F., Jr, eds, *Cancer Epidemiology and Prevention*, 2nd Ed., New York, Oxford University Press, pp. 1000–1021

Ron, E., Lubin, J.H., Shore, R.E., Mabuchi, K., Modan, B., Pottern, L.M., Schneider, A.B., Tucker, M.A. & Boice, J.D., Jr (1995) Thyroid cancer after exposure to external radiation: Pooled analysis of seven studies. *Radiat. Res.*, **141**, 259–277

Stanley, M.M. & Astwood, E.B. (1949) 1-Methyl-2-mercaptoimidazole: An antithyroid compound highly active in man. *Endocrinology*, **44**, 588–589

Suarez, H.G. (2000) Molecular basis of epithelial thyroid tumorigenesis. *C. R. Acad. Sci. III*, **323**, 519-528

Suzuki, H., Higuchi, T., Sawa, K., Ohtaki, S. & Horiuchi, Y. (1965) 'Endemic goitre' in Hokkaido, Japan. *Acta endocrinol.*, **50**, 161–176

Taurog, A. (1976) The mechanism of action of thioureylene antithyroid drugs. *Endocrinology*, **98**, 1031–1046

Thomas, G.A. & Williams, E.D. (1999) Thyroid stimulating hormone (TSH)-associated follicular hypertrophy and hyperplasia as a mechanism of thyroid carcinogenesis in mice and rats. In: Capen, C.C., Dybing, E., Rice, J.M. & Wilbourn, J.D., eds, *Species Differences in Thyroid, Kidney and Urinary Bladder Carcinogenesis* (IARC Scientific Publications No. 147), Lyon, IARC*Press*, pp. 45–59

Thoresen, S.Ø., Myking, O., Glattre, E., Rootwelt, K., Andersen, A. & Foss, O.P. (1988) Serum thyroglobulin as a preclinical tumour marker in subgroups of thyroid cancer. *Br. J. Cancer*, **57**, 105–108

Vainio, H., Magee, P., McGregor, D. & McMichael, A.J., eds (1992) *Mechanisms of Carcinogenesis in Risk Identification* (IARC Scientific Publications No. 116), Lyon, IARC*Press*

Volante, M., Papotti, M., Roth, J., Saremaslani, P., Speel, E.J., Lloyd, R.V., Carney, J.A., Heitz, P.U., Bussolati, G. & Komminoth, P. (1999) Mixed medullary–thyroid carcinoma. Molecular evidence for a dual origin of tumor components. *Am. J. Pathol.*, **155**, 1499–1509

Wilbourn, J.D., Partensky, C. & Rice, J.M. (1999) Agents that induce epithelial neoplasms of the urinary bladder, renal cortex and thyroid follicular lining in experimental animals and humans: Summary of data from *IARC Monographs* Volumes 1–69. In: Capen, C.C., Dybing, E., Rice, J.M. & Wilbourn, J.D., eds, *Species Differences in Thyroid, Kidney and Urinary Bladder Carcinogenesis* (IARC Scientific Publications No. 147), Lyon, IARC*Press*, pp. 191–209

Williams, E.D., Doniach, I., Bjarnason, O. & Michie, W. (1977) Thyroid cancer in an iodine rich area. A histopathological study. *Cancer*, **39**, 215–222

Zhu, X.Y., Lu, T.Z., Song, X.K., Li, X.T., Gao, S.M., Yang, H.M., Ma, T., Li, Y.Z. & Zhang, W.Q. (1984) Endemic goiter due to iodine rich salt and its pickled vegetables. *Chin. med. J.*, **97**, 545–548

THE MONOGRAPHS

DRUGS

ANTI-THYROID DRUGS

METHIMAZOLE

1. Exposure Data

1.1 Chemical and physical data

1.1.1 *Nomenclature*

Chem. Abstr. Serv. Reg. No.: 60-56-0
Deleted CAS Reg. Nos: 4708-61-6; 85916-84-3
Chem. Abstr. Name: 1,3-Dihydro-1-methyl-2*H*-imidazole-2-thione
IUPAC Systematic Names: 1-Methylimidazole-2-thiol; 1-methyl-4-imidazoline-2-thione
Synonyms: 2-Mercapto-1-methyl-1*H*-imidazole; 2-mercapto-1-methylimidazole; mercazolylum; 1-methyl-1,3-dihydroimidazole-2-thione; *N*-methylimidazolethiol; 1-methyl-2-imidazolethiol; 1-methyl-1*H*-imidazole-2-thiol; 1-methylimidazole-2(3*H*)-thione; 1-methyl-2-mercaptoimidazole; 1-methyl-2-mercapto-1*H*-imidazole; *N*-methyl-2-mercaptoimidazole; 1-methyl-2-thioimidazole; thiamazole

1.1.2 *Structural and molecular formulae and relative molecular mass*

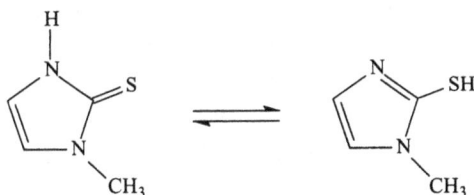

$C_4H_6N_2S$ Relative molecular mass: 114.17

1.1.3 *Chemical and physical properties of the pure substance*

(a) *Description*: White to pale-buff, crystalline powder (Aboul-Enein & Al-Badr, 1979)
(b) *Boiling-point*: 280 °C (decomposes) (Lide & Milne, 1996)
(c) *Melting-point*: 146 °C (Lide & Milne, 1996)

(d) *Spectroscopy data*: Infrared [prism (20239, 57116), grating (18391, 57116)], ultraviolet (6780), nuclear magnetic resonance [proton (6068, 30101), C-13 (2452)] and mass spectral data have been reported (Sadtler Research Laboratories, 1980; Lide & Milne, 1996).

(e) *Solubility*: Very soluble in water (200 g/L); soluble in chloroform and ethanol; slightly soluble in benzene, diethyl ether and ligroin (Gennaro, 1995; Lide & Milne, 1996)

1.1.4   *Technical products and impurities*

Methimazole is available as 5- and 10-mg scored tablets (Gennaro, 1995).

Trade names for methimazole include Basolan, Danantizol, Favistan, Frentirox, Mercazole, Metazole, Metibasol, Metothyrine, Strumazol, Tapazole, Thacapzol, Thiamethazole, Thycapzol, Thyrozol and Tirodril (Budavari, 2000; Royal Pharmaceutical Society of Great Britain, 2000; Swiss Pharmaceutical Society, 2000).

1.1.5   *Analysis*

Several international pharmacopoeias specify infrared absorption spectrophotometry with comparison to standards and colorimetry as the methods for identifying methimazole; titration with sodium hydroxide is used to assay its purity and for its content in pharmaceutical preparations (The Society of Japanese Pharmacopoeia, 1996; AOAC International, 1998; US Pharmacopeial Convention, 1999).

Methods have been reported for the analysis of methimazole in biological fluids (blood, milk, serum, urine), tissues, incubation material and dried animal feed. The methods include capillary zone electrophoresis with ultraviolet detection, micellar electrokinetic chromatography, thin-layer chromatography, high-performance thin-layer chromatography, high-performance liquid chromatography (HPLC) with atmospheric pressure chemical ionization–mass spectrometry, reversed-phase HPLC with ultraviolet detection and gas chromatography with negative-ion chemical ionization–mass spectrometry (Moretti *et al.*, 1986, 1988; Centrich Escarpenter & Rubio Hernández, 1990; Watson *et al.*, 1991; De Brabander *et al.*, 1992; Moretti *et al.*, 1993; Batjoens *et al.*, 1996; Blanchflower *et al.*, 1997; Le Bizec *et al.*, 1997; Buick *et al.*, 1998; Vargas *et al.*, 1998; Esteve-Romero *et al.*, 1999).

1.2   Production

Methimazole can be prepared by reacting aminoacetaldehyde diethyl acetal with methyl isothiocyanate or by reacting thiocyanic acid with *N*-substituted amino acetals (Aboul-Enein & Al-Badr, 1979; Budavari, 2000).

Information available in 2000 indicated that methimazole was manufactured by three companies in China, two companies in Germany and one company each in Japan, Slovakia and Switzerland (CIS Information Services, 2000a).

Information available in 2000 indicated that methimazole was used in the formulation of pharmaceuticals by five companies in Taiwan, four companies in Germany, three companies in Turkey, two companies each in the Islamic Republic of Iran and Italy and one company each in Argentina, Austria, Belgium, Brazil, Canada, Denmark, Greece, Israel, Mexico, the Netherlands, Peru, the Philippines, Poland, Portugal, the Republic of Korea, Spain, Sweden, Thailand, the Ukraine, the USA and Venezuela (CIS Information Services, 2000b).

1.3   Use

Methimazole is used to control the symptoms of hyperthyroidism associated with Graves disease and to maintain patients in a euthyroid state for several years, until spontaneous remission occurs (American Hospital Formulary Service, 2000).

Methimazole is an anti-thyroid drug, developed in 1949, that is widely used in the treatment of hyperthyroidism. The usual starting dose is 10–30 mg/day, given orally as a single daily dose. Doses as high as 120 mg/day (20 mg every 4 h) may be used in severe thyrotoxicosis ('thyroid storm') (Cooper, 1998). Studies have shown better compliance with methimazole than with propylthiouracil (see monograph in this volume), most likely due to the single daily dose of the former (Nicholas et al., 1995). The long duration of action of methimazole makes multiple dosing unnecessary in the vast majority of patients (Roti et al., 1989). There are no intravenous preparations of methimazole, but it has been administered rectally to seriously ill patients who cannot take oral medications. The dose of methimazole is not different for infants, children or the elderly (Cooper, 1998), and it is considered unnecessary to alter the dose for patients with hepatic or renal disease (Cooper, 2000; see also section 4).

Carbimazole, the 3-carbethoxy derivative of methimazole, is converted to methimazole in vivo. It is also in widespread use as an anti-thyroid agent in Europe and Japan. In the USA, propylthiouracil is used as the primary therapy for hyperthyroidism in pregnancy, but methimazole or carbimazole is used as the first treatment in many parts of the world (Masiukiewicz & Burrow, 1999). The doses used are similar to those for non-pregnant women, with an effort to minimize them when possible to avoid fetal hypothyroidism. Methimazole is considered to be safe for use at low doses by lactating women (Azizi, 1996; Azizi et al., 2000).

Anti-thyroid drugs, including methimazole, may be given for several weeks up to 1–2 years. After initiation of therapy, thyroid function improves slowly, returning to normal only by 6–12 weeks of treatment (Okamura et al., 1987). The time that it takes a patient to achieve a euthyroid state depends on a variety of clinical factors, including the severity of the hyperthyroidism at baseline, the size of the thyroid (correlated with intrathyroidal hormonal stores) and the dose of the anti-thyroid drug. Often, as thyroid function improves, the dose of antithyroid drug can be reduced. For example, mainte-nance doses of methimazole of 2.5–5 mg/day may be adequate to control thyroid function for an extended period. Low doses of anti-thyroid drugs are most successfully used in areas of the world with marginal iodine sufficiency, as high intrathyroidal iodine concentrations would be expected to offset the effects of the drugs (Azizi, 1985).

Methimazole and carbimazole are also used to treat feline hyperthyroidism (Prince, 2000). Methimazole has been used illegally in cattle as a fattening agent (Martínez-Frías et al., 1992).

Methimazole is also used in cyanide-free silver electroplating (Budavari, 2000).

1.4   Occurrence

1.4.1   *Occupational exposure*

According to the 1981–83 National Occupational Exposure Survey (National Insti-tute for Occupational Safety and Health, 2000) about 700 workers, including phar-macists, health aides and metal-plating machine operators, were potentially exposed to methimazole in the USA.

1.4.2   *Environmental occurrence*

No data were available to the Working Group.

1.5   Regulations and guidelines

Methimazole is listed in the pharmacopoeias of Italy, Japan, Poland, Taiwan and the USA (The Society of Japanese Pharmacopoeia, 1996; Wang et al., 1998; US Pharmaco-peial Convention, 1999; Royal Pharmaceutical Society of Great Britain, 2000) and is also registered for human use in the Netherlands, Portugal, Spain and Sweden (Instituto Nacional de Farmacia e do Medicamento, 2000; Medical Products Agency, 2000; Medicines Evaluation Board Agency, 2000; Spanish Medicines Agency, 2000).

2.   Studies of Cancer in Humans

No information was available specifically on methimazole.

2.1   Cohort studies

Dobyns et al. (1974) followed up 34 684 patients treated in England and the USA for hyperthyroidism between 1946 and 1964, 1238 of whom had been treated for at least 1 year with unspecified anti-thyroid drugs. No malignant thyroid neoplasm was found within 1 year of treatment. By 1968, more cases of thyroid neoplasm were found at follow-up among patients initially treated with anti-thyroid drugs (4 malignant tumours and 18 adenomas in 1238 patients) than among those initially treated with [131]I (19 malignant tumours and 41 adenomas in 21 714 patients) or (partial) thyroidectomy (4 malignant tumours and 14 adenomas in 11 732 patients). The authors suggested that more neoplasms were found in the drug-treated patients because subsequent thyroidectomy was more frequent in this group (30% of drug-treated patients, as compared with 0.5% of those initially treated with ^{131}I and 1.2% of those treated with primary thyroidectomy), which provided more opportunity for identification of neoplasms. [The Working Group noted that rates could not be calculated because person–years were not provided, and the ages of the groups were not given.]

Ron *et al.* (1998) updated the report of Dobyns *et al.* (1974) and followed-up 35 593 patients treated for hyperthyroidism between 1946 and 1964 in 25 clinics in the USA and one in the United Kingdom. By December 1990, about 19% had been lost to follow-up, and 50.5% of the study cohort had died. A total of 1374 patients (1094 women) had been treated with anti-thyroid drugs only, 10 439 (7999 women) with ^{131}I and drugs, 10 381 (8465 women) with thyroidectomy and drugs, 2661 (2235 women) with a combination of the three types of treatment and the remainder by other means. The drugs used during the study period were chiefly thiourea derivatives and iodine compounds. One year or more after the start of the study, the standardized mortality ratio (SMR) in comparison with the general population for the patients treated with anti-thyroid drugs only was 1.3 (95% confidence interval [CI], 1.1–1.6) for deaths from all cancers, which was chiefly due to significantly more deaths from oral cancer (4.2; 95% CI, 1.3–9.7; five cases) and brain tumours (3.7; 95% CI, 1.2–8.6; five cases). The excess risk for death from brain cancer persisted after exclusion of cases prevalent at the time of entry into the study. No deaths from thyroid carcinoma were recorded. The SMR for all cancers was approximately 1.0 in patients treated with ^{131}I or surgery (with or without anti-thyroid drugs), but the SMR for thyroid cancer was fourfold higher (3.9; 95% CI, 2.5–5.9; 24 cases observed) among patients who had been treated with ^{131}I with or without drugs. The authors noted that the group treated with drugs only was small; the type, quantity and dates of drug use were generally not available; and many patients had cancer before entry into the study, suggesting that some, but not all, of the excess could be attributed to the selection of patients with health problems for drug therapy. [The Working Group noted that the expected number of deaths from thyroid carcinomas was not reported, although it would almost certainly have been less than 1.0. Results were given for patients treated only with drugs but not for those given drugs with other treatment.]

2.2   Case–control studies

Ron *et al.* (1987) conducted a study of 159 cases of thyroid cancer and 285 population controls in Connecticut, USA, between 1978 and 1980. The use of anti-thyroid medications was not associated with an increased risk [relative risks not shown].

In a study carried out in northern Sweden between 1980 and 1989, 180 cases of thyroid cancer and 360 population controls were evaluated (Hallquist *et al.*, 1994). Use of anti-thyroid drugs (two cases and two controls) was associated with a relative risk of 2.0 (95% CI, 0.2–21).

3.   Studies of Cancer in Experimental Animals

Studies on the carcinogenicity of anti-thyroid chemicals, including methimazole, in experimental animals have been reviewed (Paynter *et al.*, 1988).

3.1   Oral administration

Mouse: Groups of 78 male and 104 female C3H mice, 2 months of age, received methimazole (pharmaceutical grade) in their drinking-water at a starting dose of 35 mg/L, increased gradually over 26 months to 500 mg/L, when the study was terminated. The control groups comprised 57 male and 81 female untreated mice. No statistically significant increase in the incidence of tumours was seen at any site. An increased incidence of hyperplasia of thyroid gland epithelium in treated mice was described, but the actual incidences were not provided (Jemec, 1970).

Groups of 40 male and 35 female C3H/FIB mice, 2 months of age, received methimazole [purity not specified] at a dose of 250 mg/L of demineralized water in conjunction with a low-iodine pelleted diet (iodine content, 90 μg/kg) for up to 22 months. [The Working Group noted that this concentration of iodine in the diet was 10–30 times lower than that in standard diets used in carcinogenicity studies.] The concentration of methimazole was increased to 500 mg/L when the mice were 4 months old. Groups of 50 male and 50 female mice fed the low-iodine diet served as untreated controls. In addition, groups of 80 male and 108 female mice received methimazole in the drinking-water in conjunction with a high-iodine diet (iodine content, 9–10 mg/kg), the starting dose being 35 mg/L of water, increased gradually over 26 months to 500 mg/L. [The Working Group noted that this concentration of iodine in the diet was 3–10 times that in standard diets used in carcinogenicity studies.] Groups of 236 male and 239 female mice fed the high-iodine diet served as untreated controls. A statistically significant increase ($p < 0.01$) in the incidence of thyroid follicular-cell adenomas was reported over four periods of observation in the methimazole-treated mice on a low-iodine diet, the incidence being 7/75, including 3/75 in which pulmonary metastases were found. In contrast, the incidences of adenomas in untreated controls on a low-iodine diet or a high-iodine diet and in the methimazole-treated group on a high-iodine diet were 1/150, 0/249 and 0/118, respectively (Jemec, 1977).

Rat: Groups of 25 male and 25 female rats (obtained from Harlan Industries, Cumberland, IN, USA), weighing 86–136 g [age not specified] were given diets containing methimazole (stated as pure) at concentrations of 5, 30 or 180 mg/kg of diet (equivalent to 0.25, 2.5 or 9.0 mg/kg bw per day) for 2 years. The control groups, consisting of 50 males and 50 females, received the diet without methimazole. Survival was poor in the group at the highest dose, the mortality rate being 50% in the first year (compared with < 10% in the other groups), and only 6% were still alive at 2 years, compared with 16–20% in the other groups. The incidence of thyroid follicular-cell tumours was increased at the two higher doses, the incidences for follicular adenoma in males and females combined being 1/55 (2%), 1/8 (13%), 31/55 (56%) and 17/32 (53%) at 0, 5, 30 and 180 mg/kg of diet, respectively [statistical significance not stated], the denominators representing the number of rats surviving when the first tumour was detected in each group. A treatment-related increase in the incidence of follicular adenocarcinoma was found in survivors, the incidences for males and females combined being 1/17 (6%), 5/42 (12%) and 5/24 (21%) at 0, 30 and 180 mg/kg of diet, respectively. The incidence of thyroid follicular hyperplasia was increased in both males and females receiving methimazole at 30 and 180 mg/kg of diet (Owen *et al.*, 1973). [The Working Group noted the inconsistency in the sizes of the groups with thyroid tumours, particularly those with adenomas at 30 mg/kg of diet.]

3.2   Administration with known carcinogens

Rat: In medium-term initiation–promotion bioassays, groups of 20 male Wistar rats were given *N*-nitrosoethyl-*N*-hydroxyethylamine as an initiating agent and either trisodium nitrilotriacetate, hydroquinone or potassium dibasic phosphate as the promoting agents, and the effects of methimazole on renal tumour induction were tested. Rats initiated with the nitrosamine underwent nephrectomy of the left kidney and were fed the renal tumour promoters, either alone or in combination with methimazole, in the diet for 20 weeks at concentrations of 1% for trisodium nitrilotriacetate, 2% for hydroquinone, 10% for potassium dibasic phosphate and 300 mg/kg of diet for methimazole. Although methimazole reduced the incidences of renal tubule hyperplasia in each group, it had no effect on the incidence of renal tumours (Konishi *et al.*, 1995).

4. Other Data Relevant to an Evaluation of Carcinogenicity and its Mechanisms

4.1   Absorption, distribution, metabolism and excretion

4.1.1   Humans

Jansson *et al.* (1985) studied the pharmacokinetics of methimazole in healthy, thyrotoxic and hypothyroid persons before and after therapeutic doses for the treatment of euthyroidism. The initial distribution half-time of methimazole was reported to be 0.10–0.23 h, with an elimination half-time of 4.9–5.7 h after intravenous adminis-tration. Almost complete oral absorption was observed, with an absolute bioavailability of 93% in fasting persons. There were only minor interindividual variations in the pharmacokinetics, with the exception of one hypothyroid patient who showed a rapid elimination half-time in both the hypothyroid and euthyroid states (2.6 and 2.4 h, respectively). Hengstmann and Hohn (1985) reported elimination half-times of 2–3 h in euthyroid subjects and ~6 h in hyperthyroid patients. The elimination rate was lower in the hyperthyroid patients than in euthyroid subjects and was not restored when normal thyroid function was achieved. Although renal insufficiency had no effect, patients with hepatic failure had a prolonged elimination half-time of methimazole, the prolongation being proportional to the degree of impairment (Jansson *et al.*, 1985). In hyperthyroid patients receiving carbimazole (1-methyl-2-thio-3-carbethoxyimidazole; see section 1) who then underwent thyroidectomy, the intrathyroidal concentration of methimazole was 518 ng/g of thyroid tissue 3–6 h after administration (Jansson *et al.*, 1983).

The concentrations of methimazole were measured in blood and milk from five lactating women after oral administration of 40 mg of carbimazole, which is rapidly and completely transformed to methimazole. After 1 h, the mean concentrations of methimazole had reached 253 µg/L in serum and 182 µg/L in milk. Methimazole was not bound to protein in the serum, and its concentration in serum was comparable to that in milk. The total amount of methimazole excreted in milk over 8 h was 34 µg (range, 29–47 µg) or about 0.14% of the dose administered (Johansen *et al.*, 1982).

In isolated, perfused, term human placentae, methimazole at doses of 1.5 and 15 µg/mL in either a protein-free perfusate (low dose only) or a perfusate containing 40 g/L bovine albumin readily crossed the placenta and reached equilibrium within 2 h. The transfer of methimazole was similar to that of propylthiouracil (see monograph in this volume; Mortimer *et al.*, 1997).

4.1.2   Experimental systems

In studies in which radiolabelled methimazole was administered to Sprague-Dawley rats intravenously, intraperitoneally or orally (the drug was reported to be completely absorbed after oral administration), about 5% was found to be bound to plasma proteins, and it seemed to be ubiquitously distributed to all tissues studied, although Pittman *et al.* (1971) reported that the thyroid and adrenal glands had the highest organ:plasma ratios. Approximately 10% of the administered radiolabel appeared in the bile, whereas 77–95% was excreted into the urine, with negligible amounts in the faeces, suggesting enterohepatic circulation. The half-time of urinary excretion of radiolabel was 5–7 h, regardless of the route of administration. Of the total radiolabel excreted in the urine, 14–21% was associated with unchanged drug. The major urinary and biliary metabolite was methimazole glucuronide (36–48%), and three other unidentified metabolites were found in the bile (Sitar & Thornhill, 1973; Skellern *et al.*, 1973; Skellern & Steer, 1981).

Lee and Neal (1978) demonstrated that incubation *in vitro* of methimazole with rat hepatic microsomes led to the formation of 3-methyl-2-thiohydantoin and *N*-methyl-imidazole. They also showed that radiolabelled methimazole bound to microsomal macromolecules and that this binding was stimulated by NADPH. The cytochrome P450 and flavin-containing monooxygenase systems of rat hepatic microsomes have been implicated in these reactions (see section 4.2.2).

4.1.3 *Comparison of animals and humans*

In humans and rodents, methimazole is readily absorbed and rapidly excreted with a half-time of 5 h. In rats, glucuronidation is the main metabolic pathway; less is known about the metabolism of methimazole in humans.

4.2 Toxic effects

4.2.1 *Humans*

(a) *Effects on thyroid function at therapeutic doses*

Methimazole is commonly used to treat hyperthyroidism. It inhibits intrathyroidal synthesis of thyroid hormones by interfering with thyroid peroxidase-mediated iodine utilization. As a result, the concentrations of thyroxine (T4) and triiodothyronine (T3) in serum are decreased (Cooper, 2000). In some studies, hyperthyroid patients became hypothyroid if the dose of methimazole was not monitored carefully. In one study, 100% of patients became hypothyroid within 12 weeks while taking 40 mg/day (Kallner *et al.*, 1996).

(b) *Other studies in humans*

Most of the toxic effects of methimazole are considered to be allergenic, including fever, skin rashes and arthralgia. Agranulocytosis is the most significant major side-effect, occurring in 4 of 13 patients investigated in one study. Cholestatic jaundice is a rare severe side-effect (Vitug & Goldman, 1985). The side-effects of methimazole appear to be dose-related (Cooper, 1999). In a study of the toxic effects of methimazole in hyperthyroid patients receiving high daily doses of 40–120 mg, the major effects were agranulocytosis, granulocytopenia and abnormal liver function in 3% of patients, whereas 13% showed minor effects such as arthralgia, skin rash and gastric intolerance (Romaldini *et al.*, 1991). Other reports also indicate that rashes and agranulocytosis are the major side-effects (Wiberg & Nuttall, 1972; Van der Klauw *et al.*, 1999). At high doses (up to 120 mg/day), the incidence (32%) and severity of side-effects were increased (Wiberg & Nuttall, 1972; Meyer-Gessner *et al.*, 1994).

Methimazole therapy induced changes in plasma lipid peroxidation and the antioxidant system in hyperthyroid and euthyroid patients. Lipid peroxide plasma concentrations were decreased while ascorbic acid and vitamin E levels were significantly increased in euthyroid patients in comparison with hyperthyroid patients. Plasma glutathione peroxidase activity was increased and glutathione transferase activity was significantly decreased after euthyroidism was sustained with methimazole therapy (Ademoglu *et al.*, 1998).

Thyroglobulin mRNA levels and accumulation of thyroglobulin in the culture medium were enhanced by addition of methimazole to the Fischer rat thyroid cell line 5. The effect on *Tg* gene expression was independent of thyroid-stimulating hormone (TSH) or insulin concentrations, and methimazole did not alter TSH-induced cAMP production. Both iodide and cycloheximide (a protein synthesis inhibitor) inhibited the stimulatory effects of methimazole on protein synthesis (Leer *et al.*, 1991).

4.2.2 *Experimental systems*

Male marmosets (*Callithrix jacchus*) were given methimazole at an oral dose of 10 or 30 mg/kg bw per day for 4 weeks. Marked hypertropy of follicular epithelial cells was observed, with a significant decrease in the plasma T4 concentration. Hypertrophied epithelial cells were filled with dilated rough endoplasmic reticulum and reabsorbed intracellular colloid, with vacuoles that were positive to anti-T4 immunostaining (Kurata *et al.*, 2000).

Hood *et al.* (1999) examined the effect in rats of various concentrations of methimazole in the diet. The concentrations of total and free T4 were reduced by more than 95% after 21 days of treatment with increasing dietary concentrations of 30, 100, 300 and 1000 ppm (mg/kg), and those of total and free T3 were reduced by 60%. Feeding rats with diets containing 30 ppm (mg/kg) methimazole for 21 days resulted in a 5.6-fold increase in TSH, a 14-fold increase in thyroid follicular-cell proliferation and a twofold increase in thyroid weight. The increases in thyroid weight and follicular-cell proliferation were significantly correlated with the increase in TSH.

Administration of methimazole at a concentration of 0.05% in the drinking-water for 32 days to male Sprague-Dawley rats decreased the serum concentrations of T3 (by 80%) and T4 (by 90%) and also decreased the rate of body-weight gain, colonic temperature, systolic blood pressure and heart rate when compared with vehicle-treated rats

(Bhargava *et al.*, 1988). Methimazole given in combination with DL-buthionine sulfoximine, an inhibitor of glutathione synthesis, caused centrilobular necrosis of hepatocytes and increased hepatic serum alanine aminotransferase activity in male ICR mice. Methimazole given to mice with normal levels of glutathione produced only a marginal increase in serum alanine aminotransferase activity and was not hepatoxic. Pretreatment with hepatic cytochrome P450 monooxygenase inhibitors prevented or at least greatly reduced the hepatotoxicity of methimazole in combination with DL-buthionine sulfoximine. Competitive substrates for flavin-containing monooxygenases also eliminated the hepatotoxicity of the two compounds in combination, indicating that methimazole is metabolized to an active hepatotoxicant by both cytochrome P450 monooxygenases and flavin-containing monooxygenases, and that inadequate rates of detoxication of the resulting metabolite(s) are responsible for the hepatotoxicity in glutathione-depleted mice (Mizutani *et al.*, 1999).

Methimazole was toxic to the olfactory system in Long-Evans rats given a single intraperitoneal dose of ≥ 25 mg/kg bw or an oral dose of ≥ 50 mg/kg bw. A 300-mg/kg bw intraperitoneal dose resulted in almost complete destruction of the olfactory epithelium (Genter *et al.*, 1995). Bergman and Brittebo (1999) reported that [^{3}H]methimazole given to NMRI mice by intravenous injection showed selective covalent binding to Bowman glands in the olfactory mucosa, bronchial epithelium in the lungs and centrilobular parts of the liver. Extensive lesions of the olfactory mucosa were observed after two consecutive intraperitoneal doses of methimazole, but these were efficiently repaired within 3 months. Pretreatment with T4 did not protect against toxicity, but pretreatment with metyrapone (a cytochrome P450 inhibitor) completely prevented methimazole-induced toxicity and covalent binding in the olfactory mucosa and bulb.

4.3 Reproductive and developmental effects

4.3.1 *Humans*

Pregnancy outcomes after use of methimazole during gestation have been reviewed. No differences in the rates of malformations were seen in the infants of hyperthyroid mothers who had and had not taken methimazole; however, 17 cases of aplasia cutis congenita were found in the offspring of women who had used methimazole. The authors estimated an expected incidence of 9.4 cases on the basis of the overall incidence of hyperthyroidism during pregnancy, the prevalence of methimazole use by hyperthyroid patients and the background incidence of the effect. They also reported that no signs of intellectual impairment were found in four studies involving 101 children whose mothers had undergone thioamide therapy (Mandel *et al.*, 1994). Other cases of aplasia cutis have been reported in infants whose mothers were treated with methimazole during pregnancy (Sargent *et al.*, 1994; Vogt *et al.*, 1995). Martínez-Frías *et al.* (1992) suggested that an increase in the incidence of aplasia cutis noted between 1980 and 1990 in the Spanish Collaborative Study of Congenital Malformations might have been due to illicit use of methimazole in animal feed, although no actual exposure was confirmed in this report. In contrast, no significant increase in the overall incidence of congenital malformations was noted in 36 women on methimazole therapy, and, in particular, no scalp defects were observed in the exposed infants (Wing *et al.*, 1994). Similarly, a review of nearly 50 000 pregnancies in the Netherlands found no association between exposure to methimazole and defects of the skin or scalp (Van Dijke *et al.*, 1987). An association between use of methimazole and choanal and oesophageal atresia has also been reported (summarized by Clementi *et al.*, 1999).

Thyroid status at delivery was evaluated in the infants of 43 women who had been treated with methimazole for Graves disease for at least 4 weeks during pregnancy and compared with that of the infants of 32 women with no history of thyroid problems. The doses ranged from 2.5 to 20 mg/day. No difference was found in the mean concentration of free T4 or TSH in the cord blood of infants in the two groups. A similar lack of effect was seen in 34 women treated with propylthiouracil (see monograph in this volume; Momotani *et al.*, 1997).

4.3.2   *Experimental systems*

Postnatal neurological development was evaluated in the offspring of groups of eight Sprague-Dawley rats given drinking-water containing methimazole at a concentration of 0 or 0.1 g/L from day 17 of gestation to postnatal day 10. The growth of offspring was reduced relative to that of controls after postnatal day 2, and they showed significant delays in acquisition of the surface-righting response (at 14 days *vs* 7 days in controls), auditory startle reflex (at 18 *vs* 12 days) and eye opening (at 17 *vs* 15 days). They also showed a significant reduction in locomotor activity in a 10-min open-field test at 21 days (Comer & Norton, 1982). In a study of the same design, 6-week-old, 4-month-old and 6-month-old rat offspring showed a pattern of relative decreases in locomotor activity in a residential maze, the result of a lack of habituation and a lack of a diurnal motor pattern. The treated offspring also had an asymmetric walking gait and alterations in exploratory patterns in a radial-arm maze. The two sexes were affected equally in all measures (Comer & Norton, 1985).

In groups of three Wistar rats given drinking-water containing methimazole at a concentration of 0 or 0.025% from day 8 of gestation, the total serum T3 and T4 concentrations were significantly reduced on day 18 of gestation, but fetal body weights were not affected nor were there any changes in the histological appearance of the testes. Treatment of offspring with 0 or 0.05% methimazole in the drinking-water from birth onwards significantly reduced the total serum concentrations of T3 and T4 at 21 and 50 days of age and reduced both body-weight gain and testis weight. [These rats were not old enough for the enlarged testes and enhanced sperm production observed in rats similarly treated with propylthiouracil (see monograph in this volume) to be seen]. Serum follicular-stimulating hormone and luteinizing hormone concentrations were reduced at 35 and 50 days of age. The hypothyroid rats showed delayed maturation of the testes, as seen by a decrease in the diameter of the seminiferous tubules and a reduction in the number of germ cells per cross-section. Sertoli cells also showed retarded development. With the exception of the reduction in total T4 concentration, the effects were reversible by concomitant administration of L-T3 (100 µg/kg bw every other day) (Francavilla *et al.*, 1991).

The teratogenic potential of methimazole was compared with that of ethylene-thiourea (see monograph in this volume) in rat embryo cultures. Exposure of 9.5-day-old Wistar rat embryos to methimazole at a concentration of 100 µmol/L for 48 h did not affect the morphology of the embryos, but at 500 µmol/L the mean apparent embryonic age and somite number were statistically significantly lower than those of controls. At higher concentrations (1, 2 and 5 mmol/L), the yolk-sac diameter and crown–rump length were also lower ($p < 0.05$) than those of controls. While some similarities in embryonic responses were noted, the failure of closure of the cranial region in many embryos exposed to methimazole was not seen in embryos exposed to ethylenethiourea, and other effects seen in ethylenethiourea-exposed embryos were not seen in those exposed to methimazole (Stanisstreet *et al.*, 1990).

The effect of methimazole-induced hypothyroidism during the neonatal period on testicular development was studied in Sprague-Dawley rats. Dams were given 0 or 0.025% methimazole in the drinking-water for 25 days from the day of parturition. Only male offspring were maintained in the litters [number of litters per group not specified]. Serum thyroid hormone concentrations were depressed at 25 days of age, but were normal by day 45. Body-weight gain was reduced early in life and remained 11% lower than that of controls at 90 days of age. At 90 days of age, the testis weights were increased by 18%, and daily sperm production was slightly increased. The effects were largely equivalent to those obtained after exposure to 0.004% propyl-thiouracil during the same neonatal period (Cooke *et al.*, 1993).

Postnatal development of Swiss Webster mice was examined after administration of 0 (10 dams) or 0.1 g/L (12 dams) methimazole in the drinking-water from day 16 of gestation through day 10 of lactation. There was no effect on litter size at birth. Body weights were reduced through young adulthood, after which the effect was no longer significant. Developmental milestones (incisor eruption, eye opening, vaginal opening, testis descent) were unaffected. Surface–righting time (tested on days 7–11), negative geotaxis (tested on days 6, 8 and 10) and swimming ontogeny (tested on days 4–20) were affected by exposure. There were no effects on rotarod performance on day 52 or on brain weights on day 120 (Rice *et al.*, 1987).

Neurological effects were studied in Fischer 344 rats exposed to methimazole in the drinking-water from gestational day 17 through lactational day 10 at a dose of 0, 0.01, 0.03 or 0.1 g/L, with approximately 12 litters per group. A number of indicators of neurological maturation, behaviour, thermoregulation, neurophysiology and morphology were measured at various ages. Pup weight (day 4), age at incisor eruption, thyroid histopathology (day 11), flash-evoked potential (day 14) and somatosensory-evoked potentials in the 60–120-Hz range (day 90) were significantly altered at all doses. Thermoregulation (day 12) was reduced and kidney weights increased (day 11) at concentrations ≥ 0.03 g/L. Body weight (day 12) and auditory brainstem responses (day 90) were affected at the highest concentration. Body weights on day 14 were normal in all treated groups (Albee *et al.*, 1989).

4.4   Effects on enzyme induction or inhibition and gene expression

No data were available to the Working Group.

4.5   Genetic and related effects

4.5.1   *Humans*

No data were available to the Working Group.

4.5.2   *Experimental systems* (see Table 1 for references)

Methimazole did not induce forward mutation in a fluctuation test with *Klebsiella pneumoniae*.

Methimazole induced chromosomal aberrations in a cell line derived from mouse mammary carcinoma and inhibited cell-to-cell communication in a primary culture of rat thyrocytes. Incubation of methimazole-treated thyrocytes from Sprague-Dawley rats with TSH did not affect the inhibitory effects of methimazole on gap-junctional intercellular communication.

No chromosomal aberrations were induced in bone-marrow cells, spermatogonia or primary spermatocytes of mice treated subcutaneously with methimazole for up to 5 days. The bone-marrow cells from these mice did not contain micronuclei. The frequency of sister chromatid exchange was increased in T lymphocytes of mice given 0.1% methimazole in the drinking-water for 2–6 weeks.

Subcutaneous injection of methimazole did not induce dominant lethal mutations in male mice.

4.6   Mechanistic considerations

Methimazole belongs to a class of drugs used in the treatment of hyperthyroidism, which act by interfering with the functioning of thyroid peroxidase. The mode of action in experimental animals is inhibition of thyroid peroxidase, which decreases thyroid hormone production and increases cell proliferation by increasing the secretion of TSH. This is the probable basis of the tumorigenic activity of methimazole for the thyroid in experimental animals.

Table 1. Genetic and related effects of methimazole

Test system	Result[a] Without exogenous metabolic system	Result[a] With exogenous metabolic system	Dose[b] (LED/HID)	Reference
Klebsiella pneumoniae, forward mutation	–	NT	5023	Voogd *et al.* (1979)
Chromosomal aberrations, C3H mouse mammary carcinoma cell line *in vitro*	+	NT	365	Kodama *et al.* (1980)
Inhibition of gap-junctional intercellular communication, primary thyrocyte cultures from Sprague-Dawley rats	+	NT	0.1	Asakawa *et al.* (1992)
Sister chromatid exchange, C57BL6 mouse T lymphocytes *in vivo*	+		0.1% in drinking-water, 2–6 weeks	Liu *et al.* (1995)
Chromosomal aberrations, Slc-ICR mouse bone-marrow cells, primary spermatocytes and spermatogonia *in vivo*	–		180 sc × 5	Hashimoto *et al.* (1987)
Micronucleus formation, Slc-ICR mouse bone-marrow cells *in vivo*	–		180 sc × 5	Hashimoto *et al.* (1987)
Dominant lethal mutation, male ICR mice *in vivo*	–		90 sc × 1	Akatsuka *et al.* (1979)

[a] +, positive; –, negative; NT, not tested
[b] LED, lowest effective dose; HID, highest ineffective dose; in-vitro tests, µg/mL; in-vivo tests, mg/kg bw per day; sc, subcutaneous

Methimazole was not adequately tested to support a conclusion regarding its classi-fication as a genotoxin or a non-genotoxin. It inhibited gap-junctional intercellular communication in primary rat hepatocytes *in vitro*.

5. Summary of Data Reported and Evaluation

5.1   Exposure data

Methimazole is an anti-thyroid drug, introduced in 1949, which is widely used in the treatment of hyperthyroidism. It has been used as a fattening agent in cattle, but this use has been banned.

5.2   Human carcinogenicity studies

No epidemiological data on use of methimazole and cancer were found. However, two analyses were published of one cohort study conducted in the United Kingdom and the USA of the cancer risk of patients, mainly women, with hyperthyroidism who had been treated with anti-thyroid drugs. The earlier analysis showed more malignant thyroid neoplasms in patients receiving these drugs than in those treated with surgery or ^{131}I, but the excess may have been due to closer surveillance of the patients given drugs owing to more frequent use of thyroidectomy. In the later analysis, patients with hyperthyroidism treated only with anti-thyroid drugs had a modest increase in the risk for death from cancer, due chiefly to oral cancer and cancer of the brain. Neither report provided information on the type, quantity or dates of anti-thyroid drug use.

Two case–control studies of cancer of the thyroid showed no significant asso-ciation with treatment with anti-thyroid medications.

5.3   Animal carcinogenicity data

Methimazole was tested by oral administration in two limited studies in mice and in one study in rats. In one study in mice, it increased the incidence of thyroid follicular-cell adenomas but only in conjunction with a low-iodine diet. It produced thyroid follicular-cell adenomas and carcinomas in the study in rats.

5.4   Other relevant data

In humans and rodents, methimazole is readily absorbed and rapidly excreted. In rats, glucuronidation is the major metabolic pathway; less is known about its meta-bolism in humans.

The mode of action of methimazole in the thyroid in experimental animals involves inhibition of thyroid peroxidase, which decreases thyroid hormone production and increases proliferation by increasing the secretion of thyroid-stimulating hormone. This is the probable basis for the tumorigenic activity of methimazole for the thyroid in experimental animals.

While the overall incidence of malformations in the infants of women given methimazole during pregnancy does not appear to be elevated, there is equivocal evidence for an association with the occurrence of aplasia cutis, a skin defect. Most of the studies in experimental animals focused on the consequences of hypothyroidism subsequent to perinatal or early postnatal exposure of rats to methimazole; effects on adult neurobehavioural and testicular function were found. Neurobehavioural effects have also been reported in mice exposed perinatally to methimazole.

Methimazole has not been adequately tested for its ability to induce gene mutations. It induced chromosomal aberrations in mammalian cells *in vitro*, but the results of studies of its ability to induce chromosomal damage *in vivo* were mainly negative.

5.5   Evaluation

There is *inadequate evidence* in humans for the carcinogenicity of methimazole.

There is *limited evidence* in experimental animals for the carcinogenicity of methimazole.

Overall evaluation

Methimazole is *not classifiable as to its carcinogenicity to humans (Group 3).*

6.   References

Aboul-Enein, H.Y. & Al-Badr, A.A. (1979) Methimazole. *Anal. Profiles Drug Subst.*, **8**, 351–370

Ademoglu, E., Gökkusu, C., Yarman, S. & Azizlerli, H. (1998) The effect of methimazole on the oxidant and antioxidant system in patients with hyperthyroidism. *Pharmacol. Res.*, **38**, 93–96

Akatsuka, K., Hashimoto, T., Takeuchi, K. & Ohhira, M. (1979) [Mutagenicity test of antithyroid agent, methimazole — Dominant lethal mutation test on male mice.] *J. toxicol. Sci.*, **4**, 127–138 (in Japanese)

Albee, R.R., Mattsson, J.L., Johnson, K.A., Kirk, H.D. & Breslin, W.J. (1989) Neurological consequences of congenital hypothyroidism in Fischer 344 rats. *Neurotoxicol. Teratol.*, **11**, 171–183

American Hospital Formulary Service (2000) *Methimazole*, Bethesda, MD, American Society of Health — System Pharmacists [AHFS First CD-ROM]

AOAC International (1998) AOAC Official Method 967.32. Methimazole in Drugs. In: *Official Methods of Analysis of AOAC International*, 15th Ed., Gaithersburg, MD [CD-ROM]

Asakawa, H., Yamasaki, Y., Hanafusa, T., Kono, N. & Tarui, S. (1992) Cell-to-cell communication in cultured rat thyroid monolayer cells is inhibited dose-dependently by methimazole. *Res. Commun. chem. Pathol. Pharmacol.*, **77**, 131–145

Azizi, F. (1985) Environmental iodine intake affects the response to methimazole in patients with diffuse toxic goiter. *J. clin. Endocrinol. Metab.*, **61**, 374–377

Azizi, F. (1996) Effect of methimazole treatment of maternal thyrotoxicosis on thyroid function in breast-feeding infants. *J. Pediatr.*, **128**, 855–858

Azizi, F., Khoshniat, M., Bahrainian, M. & Hedayati, M. (2000) Thyroid function and intellectual development of infants nursed by mothers taking methimazole. *J. clin. Endocrinol. Metab.*, **85**, 3233–3238

Batjoens, P., De Brabander, H.F. & De Wasch, K. (1996) Rapid and high-performance analysis of thyreostatic drug residues in urine using as chromatography–mass spectrometry. *J. Chromatogr., A.*, **750**, 127–132

Bergman, U. & Brittebo, E. (1999) Methimazole toxicity in rodents: Covalent binding in the olfactory mucosa and detection of glial fibrillary acidic protein in the olfactory bulb. *Toxicol. appl. Pharmacol.*, **155**, 190–200

Bhargava, H.N., Ramarao, P. & Gulati, A. (1988) Effect of methimazole-induced hypothyroidism on multiple opioid receptors in rat brain regions. *Pharmacology*, **37**, 356–364

Blanchflower, W.J., Hughes, P.J., Cannavan, A., McCoy, M.A. & Kennedy, D.G. (1997) Determination of thyreostats in thyroid and urine using high-performance liquid chromatography–atmospheric pressure chemical ionization mass spectrometry. *Analyst*, **122**, 967–972

Budavari, S., ed. (2000) *The Merck Index*, 12th Ed., Version 12:3, Whitehouse Station, NJ, Merck & Co. & Boca Raton, FL, Chapman & Hall/CRC [CD-ROM]

Buick, R.K., Barry, C., Traynor, I.M., McCaughey, W.J. & Elliott, C.T. (1998) Determination of thyreostat residues from bovine matrices using high-performance liquid chromatography. *J. Chromatogr. B. Biomed. Sci. Appl.*, **720**, 71–79

Centrich Escarpenter, F. & Rubio Hernández, D. (1990) [Analysis of thyrostatics in the thyroid glands by thin layer chromatography and HPLC–UV.] *An. Bromatol.*, **42**, 337–344 (in Spanish)

CIS Information Services (2000a) *Directory of World Chemical Producers (Version 2000.1)*, Dallas, TX [CD-ROM]

CIS Information Services (2000b) *Worldwide Bulk Drug Users Directory (Version 2000)*, Dallas, TX [CD-ROM]

Clementi, M., Di Gianantonio, E., Pelo, E., Mammi, I., Basile, R.T. & Tenconi, R. (1999) Methimazole embryopathy: Delineation of the phenotype. *Am. J. med. Genet.*, **83**, 43–46

Comer, C.P. & Norton, S. (1982) Effects of perinatal methimazole exposure on a developmental test battery for neurobehavioral toxicity in rats. *Toxicol. appl. Pharmacol.*, **63**, 133–141

Comer, C.P. & Norton, S. (1985) Behavioral consequences of perinatal hypothyroidism in postnatal and adult rats. *Pharmacol. Biochem. Behav.*, **22**, 605–611

Cooke, P.S., Kirby, J.D. & Porcelli, J. (1993) Increased testis growth and sperm production in adult rats following transient neonatal goitrogen treatment: Optimization of the propyl-thiouracil dose and effects of methimazole. *J. Reprod. Fertil.*, **97**, 493–499

Cooper, D.S. (1998) Antithyroid drugs for the treatment of hyperthyroidism caused by Graves' disease. *Endocrinol. Metab. Clin. N. Am.*, **27**, 225–247

Cooper, D.S. (1999) The side-effects of antithyroid drugs. *Endocrinologist*, **9**, 457–467

Cooper, D.S. (2000) The treatment of hyperthyroidism. In: Braverman, L.E. & Utiger, R.D., eds, *Werner & Ingbar's. The Thyroid. A Fundamental and Clinical Text*, 8th Ed., Philadelphia, PA, J.B. Lippincott, pp. 691–715

De Brabander, H.F., Batjoens, P. & Van Hoof, J. (1992) Determination of thyreostatic drugs by HPTLC with confirmation by GC-MS. *J. planar Chromatogr.-Mod. TLC*, **5**, 124–130

Dobyns, B.M., Sheline, G.E., Workman, J.B., Tompkins, E.A., McConahey, W.M. & Becker, D.V. (1974) Malignant and benign neoplasms of the thyroid in patients treated for hyper-thyroidism: A report of the Cooperative Thyrotoxicosis Therapy Follow-up Study. *J. clin. Endocrinol. Metab.*, **38**, 976–998

Esteve-Romero, J., Escrig-Tena, I., Simó-Alfonso, E.F. & Ramis-Ramos, G. (1999) Determi-nation of thyreostatics in animal feed by micellar electrokinetic chromatography. *Analyst*, **124**, 125–128

Francavilla, S., Cordeschi, G., Properzi, G., Di Cicco, L., Jannini, E.A., Palmero, S., Fugassa, E., Loras, B. & D'Armiento, M. (1991) Effect of thyroid hormone on the pre- and post-natal development of the rat testis. *J. Endocrinol.*, **129**, 35–42

Gennaro, A.R. (1995) *Remington: The Science and Practice of Pharmacy*, 19th Ed., Vol. II, Easton, PA, Mack Publishing Co., p. 1086

Genter, M.B., Deamer, N.J., Blake, B.L., Wesley, D.S. & Levi, P.E. (1995) Olfactory toxicity of methimazole: Dose–response and structure–activity studies and characterization of flavin-containing monooxygenase activity in the Long-Evans rat olfactory mucosa. *Toxicol. Pathol.*, **23**, 477–486

Hallquist, A., Hardell, L., Degerman, A. & Boquist, L. (1994) Thyroid cancer: Reproductive factors, previous diseases, drug intake, family history and diet. A case–control study. *Eur. J. Cancer Prev.*, **3**, 481–488

Hashimoto, T., Takeuchi, K., Ohno, S. & Komatsu, S. (1987) Mutagenicity tests of the antithyroid agent thiamazole. Cytogenetic studies on male mice. *J. toxicol. Sci.*, **12**, 23–32

Hengstmann, J.H. & Hohn, H. (1985) Pharmacokinetics of methimazole in humans. *Klin. Wochenschr.*, **63**, 1212–1217

Hood, A., Liu, Y.P., Gattone, V.H.II & Klaassen, C.D. (1999) Sensitivity of thyroid gland growth to thyroid stimulating hormone (TSH) in rats treated with antithyroid drugs. *Toxicol. Sci.*, **49**, 263–271

Instituto Nacional de Farmacia e do Medicamento (2000) Lisbon

Jansson, R., Dahlberg, P.A., Johansson, H. & Lindstrom, B. (1983) Intrathyroidal concen-trations of methimazole in patients with Graves' disease. *J. clin. Endocrinol. Metab.*, **57**, 129–132

Jansson, R., Lindström, B. & Dahlberg, P.A. (1985) Pharmacokinetic properties and bio-availability of methimazole. *Clin. Pharmacokinet.*, **10**, 443–450

Jemec, B. (1970) Studies of the goitrogenic and oncogenic effect of thycapzol on C_3H mice. *Acta pathol. microbiol. scand.*, **78**, 151–160

Jemec, B. (1977) Studies of the tumorigenic effect of two goitrogens. *Cancer*, **40**, 2188–2202

Johansen, K., Nyboe Andersen, A., Kampmann, J.P., Mølholm Hansen, J. & Mortensen, H.B. (1982) Excretion of methimazole in human milk. *Eur. J. clin. Pharmacol.*, **23**, 339–341

Kallner, G., Vitols, S. & Ljunggren, J.G. (1996) Comparison of standardized initial doses of two antithyroid drugs in the treatment of Graves' disease. *J. intern. Med.*, **239**, 525–529

Kodama, F., Fukushima, K. & Umeda, M. (1980) Chromosome aberrations induced by clinical medicines. *J. toxicol. Sci.*, **5**, 141–149

Konishi, N., Kitamura, M., Hayashi, I., Matsuda, H., Tao, M., Naitoh, H., Kitahori, Y. & Hiasa Y. (1995) Effect of methimazole on rat renal carcinogenesis induced by N-ethyl-N-hydroxyethylnitrosamine. *Toxicol. Pathol.*, **23**, 606–611

Kurata, Y., Wako, Y., Tanaka, K., Inoue, Y. & Makinodan, F. (2000) Thyroid hyperactivity induced by methimazole, spironolactone and phenobarbital in marmosets (*Callithrix jacchus*): Histopathology, plasma thyroid hormone levels and hepatic T_4 metabolism. *J. vet. Med. Sci.*, **62**, 607–614

Le Bizec, B., Monteau, F., Maume, D., Montrade, M.P., Gade, C. & Andre, F. (1997) Detection and identification of thyreostats in the thyroid gland by gas chromatography–mass spectrometry. *Anal. chim. Acta*, **340**, 201–208

Lee, P.W. & Neal, R.A. (1978) Metabolism of methimazole by rat liver cytochrome P-450-containing monoxygenases. *Drug Metab. Disposition*, **6**, 591–600

Leer, L.M., Cammenga, M. & De Vijlder, J.J.M. (1991) Methimazole and propylthiouracil increase thyroglobulin gene expression in FRTL-5 cells. *Mol. cell. Endocrinol.*, **82**, R25–R30

Lide, D.R. & Milne, G.W.A. (1996) *Properties of Organic Compounds*, Version 5.0, Boca Raton, FL, CRC Press [CD-ROM]

Liu, W.K., Tsui, K.W., Lai, K.W.H. & Xie, Y. (1995) Sister-chromatid exchanges in lymphocytes from methimazole-induced hypothyroid mice. *Mutat. Res.*, **326**, 193–197

Mandel, S.J., Brent, G.A. & Larsen, P.R. (1994) Review of antithyroid drug use during pregnancy and report of a case of aplasia cutis. *Thyroid*, **4**, 129–133

Martínez-Frías, M.L., Cereijo, A., Rodríguez-Pinilla, E. & Urioste, M. (1992) Methimazole in animal feed and congenital aplasia cutis [Letter to the Editor]. *Lancet*, **339**, 742–743

Masiukiewicz, U.S. & Burrow, G.N. (1999) Hyperthyroidism in pregnancy: Diagnosis and treatment. *Thyroid*, **9**, 647–652

Medical Products Agency (2000) Uppsala

Medicines Evaluation Board Agency (2000) The Hague

Meyer-Gessner, M., Benker, G., Lederbogen, S., Olbricht, T. & Reinwein, D. (1994) Antithyroid drug-induced agranulocytosis: Clinical experience with 10 patients in one institution and review of the literature. *J. endocrinol. Invest.*, **17**, 29–36

Mizutani, T., Murakami, M., Shirai, M., Tanaka, M. & Nakanishi, K. (1999) Metabolism-dependent hepatotoxicity of methimazole in mice depleted of glutathione. *J. appl. Toxicol.*, **19**, 193–198

Momotani, N., Noh, J.Y., Ishikawa, N. & Ito, K. (1997) Effects of propylthiouracil and methimazole on fetal thyroid status in mothers with Graves' hyperthyroidism. *Endocrinology*, **82**, 3633–3636

Moretti, G., Amici, M. & Cammarata, P. (1986) [Determination of methylthiouracil and analogous thyrostatics in animal tissues by HPTLC after solid-phase purification.] *Riv. Soc. Ital. Sci. Aliment.*, **15**, 35–39 (in Italian)

Moretti, G., Amici, M., Cammarata, P. & Fracassi, F. (1988) Identification of thyrostatic drug residues in animal thyroids by high-performance thin-layer chromatography and fluorescence reaction detection. *J. Chromatogr.*, **442**, 459–463

Moretti, G., Betto, R., Cammarata, P., Fracassi, F., Giambenedetti, M. & Borghese, A. (1993) Determination of thyreostatic residues in cattle plasma by high-performance liquid chromatography with ultraviolet detection. *J. Chromatogr. B. Biomed. Sci. Appl.*, **616**, 291–296

Mortimer, R.H., Cannell, G.R., Addison, R.S., Johnson, L.P., Roberts, M.S. & Bernus, I. (1997) Methimazole and propylthiouracil equally cross the perfused human term placental lobule. *J. clin. Endocrinol. Metab.*, **82**, 3099–3102

National Institute for Occupational Safety and Health (2000) *National Occupational Exposure Survey 1981–83*, Cincinnati, OH, Department of Health and Human Services, Public Health Service

Nicholas, W.C., Fischer, R.G., Stevenson, R.A. & Bass, J.D. (1995) Single daily dose of methimazole compared to every 8 hours propylthiouracil in the treatment of hyperthyroidism. *South. med. J.*, **88**, 973–976

Okamura, K., Ikenoue, H., Shiroozu, A., Sato, K., Yoshinari, M. & Fujishima, M. (1987) Reevaluation of the effects of methylmercaptoimidazole and propylthiouracil in patients with Graves' hyperthyroidism. *J. clin. Endocrinol. Metab.*, **65**, 719–723

Owen, N.V., Worth, H.M. & Kiplinger, G.F. (1973) The effects of long-term ingestion of methimazole on the thyroids of rats. *Food Cosmet. Toxicol.*, **11**, 649–653

Paynter, O.E., Burin, G.J., Jaeger, R.B. & Gregorio, C.A. (1988) Goitrogens and thyroid follicular cell neoplasia: Evidence for a threshold process. *Regul. Toxicol. Pharmacol.*, **8**, 102–119

Pittman, J., Beschi, R. & Smitherman, T. (1971) Methimazole: Its absorption and excretion in man and tissue distribution in rats. *J. clin. Endocrinol. Metab.*, **33**, 182–185

Prince, J. (2000) *Methimazole, the Use of Methimazole (Tepazole) in Dogs and Cats*, Rhinelander, WI, Foster & Smith [www.petinfocenter.com/pharmacy/methimazole.htm]

Rice, S.A., Millan, D.P. & West, J.A. (1987) The behavioral effects of perinatal methimazole administration in Swiss Webster mice. *Fundam. appl. Toxicol.*, **8**, 531–540

Romaldini, J.H., Werner, M.C., Bromberg, N. & Werner, R.S. (1991) Adverse effects related to antithyroid drugs and their dose regimen. *Exp. clin. Endocrinol.*, **97**, 261–264

Ron, E., Kleinerman, R.A., Boice, J.D., Jr, LiVolsi, V.A., Flannery, J.T. & Fraumeni, J.F., Jr (1987) A population-based control study of thyroid cancer. *J. natl Cancer Inst.*, **79**, 1–12

Ron, E., Doody, M.M., Becker, D.V., Brill, A.B., Curtis, R.E., Goldman, M.B., Harris, B.S.H., Hoffman, D.A., McConahey, W.M., Maxon, H.R., Preston-Martin, S., Warshauer, E., Wong, F.L. & Boice, J.D., Jr for the Cooperative Thyrotoxicosis Therapy Follow-up Study Group (1998) Cancer mortality following treatment for adult hyperthyroidism. *J. Am. med. Assoc.*, **280**, 347–355

Roti, E., Gardini, E., Minelli, R., Salvi, M., Robuschi, G. & Braverman, L.E. (1989) Methimazole and serum thyroid hormone concentrations in hyperthyroid patients: Effects of single and multiple daily doses. *Ann. intern. Med.*, **111**, 181–182

Royal Pharmaceutical Society of Great Britain (2000) *Martindale, The Extra Pharmacopoeia*, 13th Ed., London, The Pharmaceutical Press [MicroMedex Online]

Sadtler Research Laboratories (1980) *Sadtler Standard Spectra, 1980 Cumulative Molecular Formula Index*, Philadelphia, PA, p. 36

Sargent, K.A., Stopfer, J.E., Mallozzi, A.E., Khandelwal, M., Quashie, C. & Schneider, A.S. (1994) Apparent scalp–ear–nipple (Findlay) syndrome in a neonate exposed to methimazole *in utero* (Abstract). *Am. J. hum. Genetics*, **55**, A312

Sitar, D.S. & Thornhill, D.P. (1973) Methimazole: Absorption, metabolism and excretion in the albino rat. *J. Pharmacol. exp. Ther.*, **184**, 432–439

Skellern, G.C. & Steer, S.T. (1981) The metabolism of [2-^{14}C]methimazole in the rat. *Xenobiotica*, **11**, 627–634

Skellern, G.G., Stenlake, J.B. & Williams, W.D. (1973) The absorption, distribution, excretion and metabolism of [2-^{14}C]methimazole in rat. *Xenobiotica*, **3**, 121–132

Society of Japanese Pharmacopoeia (1996) *The Japanese Pharmacopoeia JP XIII*, 13th Ed., Tokyo, pp. 662–663

Spanish Medicines Agency (2000) Madrid

Stanisstreet, M., Herbert, L.C. & Pharoah, P.O.D. (1990) Effects of thyroid antagonists on rat embryos cultured in vitro. *Teratology*, **41**, 721–729

Swiss Pharmaceutical Society (2000) *Index Nominum. International Drug Directory*, 16th Ed., Stuttgart, Medpharm Scientific Publishers [MicroMedex Online]

US Pharmacopeial Convention (1999) *The 2000 US Pharmacopeia*, 24th rev./*The National Formulary*, 19th rev., Rockville, MD, pp. 1066–1067, 2278

Van der Klauw, M.M., Goudsmit, R., Halie, M.R., van't Veer, M.B., Herings, R.M.C., Wilson, J.H.P. & Stricker, B.H.C. (1999) A population-based case–cohort study of drug-associated agranulocytosis. *Arch. intern. Med.*, **159**, 369–374

Van Dijke, C.P., Heydendael, R.J. & De Kleine, M.J. (1987) Methimazole, carbimazole, and congenital skin defects. *Ann. intern. Med.*, **106**, 60–61

Vargas, G., Havel, J. & Frgalová, K. (1998) Capillary zone electrophoresis determination of thyreostatic drugs in urine. *J. capillary Electrophor.*, **5**, 9–12

Vitug, A.C. & Goldman, J.M. (1985) Hepatotoxicity from antithyroid drugs. *Horm. Res.*, **21**, 229–234

Vogt, T., Stolz, W. & Landthaler, M. (1995) Aplasia cutis congenita after exposure to methimazole: A causal relationship? *Br. J. Dermatol.*, **133**, 994–996

Voogd, C.E., van der Stel, J.J. & Jacobs, J.J.J.A.A. (1979) Mutagenic action of nitroimidazoles. IV. A comparison of the mutagenic action of several nitroimidazoles and some imidazoles. *Mutat. Res.*, **66**, 207–221

Wang, P.-W., Liu, R.-T., Tung, S.-C., Chien, W.-Y., Lu, Y.-C., Chen, C.-H., Kuo, M.-C., Hsieh, J.-R. & Wang, S.-T. (1998) Outcome of Graves' disease after antithyroid drug treatment in Taiwan. *J. Formos. Med. Assoc.*, **97**, 619–625

Watson, D.G., Bates, C.D., Skellern, G.G., Mairs, R. & Martin, S. (1991) Analysis of thiocarbamides by gas chromatography–negative-ion chemical-ionization mass spectrometry. *Rapid Commun. Mass Spectrom.*, **5**, 141–142

Wiberg, J.J. & Nuttall, F.Q. (1972) Methimazole toxicity from high doses. *Ann. intern. Med.*, **77**, 414–416

Wing, D.A., Millar, L.K., Koonings, P.P., Montoro, M.N. & Mestman, J.H. (1994) A comparison of propylthiouracil versus methimazole in the treatment of hyperthyroidism in pregnancy. *Am. J. Obstet. Gynecol.*, **170**, 90–95

METHYLTHIOURACIL

This substance was considered by previous working groups, in 1974 (IARC, 1974) and 1987 (IARC, 1987). Since that time, new data have become available, and these have been incorporated into the monograph and taken into consideration in the present evaluation.

1. Exposure Data

1.1   Chemical and physical data

1.1.1   *Nomenclature*

Chem. Abstr. Serv. Reg. No.: 56-04-2
Deleted CAS Reg. Nos: 1123-10-0; 31909-18-9; 91795-77-6
Chem. Abstr. Name: 2,3-Dihydro-6-methyl-2-thioxo-4(1*H*)-pyrimidinone
IUPAC Systematic Name: 6-Methyl-2-thiouracil
Synonyms: 4-Hydroxy-2-mercapto-6-methylpyrimidine; 4-hydroxy-6-methyl-2-mercaptopyrimidine; 2-mercapto-4-methyl-6-hydroxypyrimidine; 2-mercapto-6-methyl-4-pyrimidinol; 2-mercapto-6-methylpyrimidin-4-one; 6-methyl-2-mercapto-uracil; 4-methyl-2-thiouracil; MTU; 2-thio-6-methyluracil; 6-thio-4-methyluracil

1.1.2   *Structural and molecular formulae and relative molecular mass*

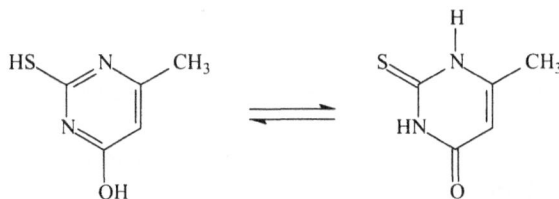

$C_5H_6N_2OS$ Relative molecular mass: 142.18

1.1.3   *Chemical and physical properties of the pure substance*

(a) *Description*: Crystalline solid (Budavari, 2000)
(b) *Boiling-point*: Sublimes (Lide & Milne, 1996)
(c) *Melting-point*: 330 °C (sublimes) (Lide & Milne, 1996)
(d) *Spectroscopy data*: Infrared [prism (8429), grating (24088)], ultraviolet (2236), nuclear magnetic resonance [proton (11278), C-13 (1639)] and mass spectral data have been reported (Sadtler Research Laboratories, 1980; Lide & Milne, 1996).
(e) *Solubility*: Insoluble in water; slightly soluble in benzene, diethyl ether, ethanol and methanol (Lide & Milne, 1996)

1.1.4   *Technical products and impurities*

Trade names for methylthiouracil include Alkiron, Antibason, Basecil, Basethyrin, Metacil, Methacil, Methiacil, Methicil, Methiocil, Muracil, Prostrumyl, Strumacil, Thimecil, Thiothymin, Thyreonorm, Thyreostat, Thyreostat I, Tiomeracil and Tiorale M.

1.1.5   *Analysis*

Methods have been reported for the analysis of methylthiouracil in biological fluids (blood, milk, serum, urine), tissues, dried animal feed and feed additives. The methods include capillary zone electrophoresis with ultraviolet detection, micellar electrokinetic chromatography, thin-layer chromatography, high-performance thin-layer chromatography, high-performance liquid chromatography (HPLC) with atmospheric pressure chemical ionization–mass spectrometry, reversed-phase HPLC with ultraviolet and electrochemical detection and gas chromatography with mass spectrometry (Saldaña Monllor *et al.*, 1980; Moretti *et al.*, 1986; Hooijerink & De Ruig, 1987; Moretti *et al.*, 1988; Centrich Escarpenter & Rubio Hernández, 1990; De Brabander *et al.*, 1992; Moretti *et al.*, 1993; Batjoens *et al.*, 1996; Krivánková *et al.*, 1996; Blanchflower *et al.*, 1997; Le Bizec *et al.*, 1997; Yu *et al.*, 1997; Buick *et al.*, 1998; Vargas *et al.*, 1998; Esteve-Romero *et al.*, 1999).

1.2   Production

Methylthiouracil can be made by condensation of ethyl acetoacetate with thiourea (IARC, 1974)

Information available in 2000 indicated that methylthiouracil was manufactured by two companies each in China and Germany and one company each in Austria, Italy and Japan (CIS Information Services, 2000a; Herbrand, 2000).

Information available in 2000 indicated that methylthiouracil was used in the formulation of pharmaceutical drugs by one company in Poland (CIS Information Services, 2000b).

1.3   Use

Methylthiouracil was introduced in the mid-1940s, at the same time as propyl-thiouracil, as a thionamide anti-thyroid drug for the treatment of hyperthyroidism. The usual dose is 200 mg/day in two to four equally spaced doses. Methylthiouracil is no longer in clinical use in most countries, although it may be used to a limited degree in some eastern European countries. It has not been registered for human use since 1958 in Sweden, 1986 in the United Kingdom and 1988 in the Netherlands (Medical Products Agency, 2000; Medicines Control Agency, 2000; Medicines Evaluation Board Agency, 2000). A MEDLINE search revealed no references to use of methylthiouracil since 1987 (Junik *et al.*, 1987). This may be related to the higher rate of adverse reactions than with propylthiouracil or methimazole (see monographs in this volume) (Van der Laan & Storrie, 1955).

1.4   Occurrence

1.4.1   *Occupational exposure*

No data were available to the Working Group.

1.4.2   *Environmental occurrence*

No data were available to the Working Group.

1.5   Regulations and guidelines

Methylthiouracil is listed in the current pharmacopoeias of Austria, Poland and Switzerland. It was previously listed in the pharmacopoeias of the former East Germany, Italy, Japan (1976), the United Kingdom (1973) and the USA (XXI) (Royal Pharmaceutical Society of Great Britain, 2000; Swiss Pharmaceutical Society, 2000). It was also formerly listed in the International Pharmacopoeia (II).

2.   Studies of Cancer in Humans

No information was available specifically on methylthiouracil.

2.1   Cohort studies

Dobyns *et al.* (1974) followed up 34 684 patients treated in England and the USA for hyperthyroidism between 1946 and 1964, 1238 of whom had been treated for at least 1 year with unspecified anti-thyroid drugs. No malignant thyroid neoplasm was found within 1 year of treatment. By 1968, more cases of thyroid neoplasm were found at follow-up among patients initially treated with anti-thyroid drugs (4 malignant tumours and 18 adenomas in 1238 patients) than among those initially treated with ^{131}I (19 malignant tumours and 41 adenomas in 21 714 patients) or (partial) thyroidectomy (4 malignant tumours and 14 adenomas in 11 732 patients). The authors suggested that more neoplasms were found in the drug-treated patients because subsequent thyroidec- tomy was more frequent in this group (30% of drug-treated patients, as compared with 0.5% of those initially treated with ^{131}I and 1.2% of those treated with primary thyroidectomy), which provided more opportunity for identification of neoplasms. [The Working Group noted that rates could not be calculated because person–years were not provided, and the ages of the groups were not given.]

Ron *et al.* (1998) updated the report of Dobyns *et al.* (1974) and followed-up 35 593 patients treated for hyperthyroidism between 1946 and 1964 in 25 clinics in the USA and one in the United Kingdom. By December 1990, about 19% had been lost to follow-up, and 50.5% of the study cohort had died. A total of 1374 patients (1094 women) had been treated with anti-thyroid drugs only, 10 439 (7999 women) with ^{131}I and drugs, 10 381 (8465 women) with thyroidectomy and drugs, 2661 (2235 women) with a combination of the three types of treatment and the remainder by other means. The drugs used during the study period were chiefly thiourea derivatives and iodine compounds. One year or more after the start of the study, the standardized mortality ratio (SMR) in comparison with the general population for the patients treated with anti-thyroid drugs only was 1.3 (95% confidence interval [CI], 1.1–1.6) for deaths from all cancers, which was chiefly due to significantly more deaths from oral cancer (4.2; 95% CI, 1.3–9.7; five cases) and brain tumours (3.7; 95% CI, 1.2–8.6; five cases). The excess risk for death from brain cancer persisted after exclusion of cases prevalent at the time of entry into the study. No deaths from thyroid carcinoma were recorded. The SMR for all cancers was approximately 1.0 in patients treated with ^{131}I or surgery (with or without anti-thyroid drugs), but the SMR for thyroid cancer was fourfold higher (3.9; 95% CI, 2.5–5.9; 24 cases observed) among patients who had been treated with ^{131}I with or without drugs. The authors noted that the group treated with drugs only was small; the type, quantity and dates of drug use were generally not available; and many patients had cancer before entry into the study, suggesting that some, but not all, of the excess could be attributed to the selection of patients with health problems for drug therapy. [The Working Group noted that the expected number of deaths from thyroid carcinomas was not reported, although it would almost certainly have been less than 1.0. Results were given separately for patients treated only with drugs and not for those given drugs with other treatment.]

2.2   Case–control studies

Ron *et al.* (1987) conducted a study of 159 cases of thyroid cancer and 285 population controls in Connecticut, USA, between 1978 and 1980. The use of anti-thyroid medications was not associated with an increased risk [relative risks not shown].

In a study carried out in northern Sweden between 1980 and 1989, 180 cases of thyroid cancer and 360 population controls were evaluated (Hallquist *et al.*, 1994). Use of anti-thyroid drugs (two cases and two controls) was associated with a relative risk of 2.0 (95% CI, 0.2–21).

3. Studies of Cancer in Experimental Animals

Methylthiouracil was evaluated in a previous monograph (IARC, 1974). Although there have been several new studies on the carcinogenicity of methylthiouracil in animals, no conventional bioassays have been reported. The summaries of the most relevant studies from the previous monograph are either repeated here or the studies are analysed in greater depth. Studies on the carcinogenicity of anti-thyroid chemicals, including methylthiouracil, in experimental animals have been reviewed (Doniach, 1970; Christov & Raichev, 1972a).

3.1   Oral administration

Mouse: In a study published since the previous evaluation, groups of 94 male and 82 female C3H/FIB mice, 2 months of age, were given methylthiouracil [purity not specified] in their drinking-water at a concentration of 0 or 1000 mg/L in conjunction with an iodine-rich diet (9–10 mg/kg). A group of 236 male and 239 female mice served as untreated controls on an iodine-rich diet. Another group of 42 males and 53 females of the same strain and age received methylthiouracil mixed into pelleted diet at a concentration of 2000 mg/kg, which was increased to 5000 mg/kg of diet when they were 4 months of age, in conjunction with an iodine-poor diet (90 µg/kg). Groups of 50 males and 50 females served as untreated controls on iodine-poor diet. Groups of animals were killed after 6–22 months of treatment. Methylthiouracil caused a statistically significant increase ($p < 0.01$) in the incidence of thyroid adenomas in mice on the iodine-poor diet (23/75, including 13/75 with pulmonary metastases). In contrast, the incidences of thyroid adenoma were 1/150 in control mice on the iodine-poor diet, 0/249 in control mice on the iodine-rich diet and 2/167 in methylthiouracil-treated mice on the iodine-rich diet. Methylthiouracil also produced hepatomas in 28/75 mice on the iodine-poor diet ($p < 0.01$), in 6/167 mice on the iodine-rich diet, in 2/150 control mice on the iodine-poor diet and in 6/249 control mice on the iodine-rich diet. All of these incidences refer to pooled males and females (Jemec, 1977).

Rat: Groups of female Long-Evans rats, approximately 9 months of age, were given methylthiouracil [route not specified clearly but presumed to be dietary] at a dose of 0 (31 rats at start) or 2.5 mg/rat per day (34 rats at start) in combination with a low-iodine diet (average, 100–150 µg/kg of diet) for 24–33 months. Administration of methylthiouracil resulted in thyroid hyperplasia in 22/24 rats, 'nodular thyroid changes' in 15/24 rats and thyroid carcinoma in 8/24 rats examined. In the group receiving the low-iodine diet only, 1/31 had thyroid hyperplasia, 3/31 had nodular changes and 0/31 had thyroid carcinoma (Field *et al.*, 1959). [The Working Group considered the nodular changes to be adenomas.]

In a study published since the previous evaluation, two groups of inbred Wistar/FIB rats (39 and 57 animals at start), 2 months of age, were given methylthiouracil [purity not specified] in their drinking-water at a concentration of 0 (control) or 0.1% [length of exposure not specified]. A third group (43 rats at start) was hypophysectomized, given methylthiouracil (0.1%) 5–6 days after the operation and killed 7–8 months later. The author reported that the average age at death did not differ significantly in the three groups. Thyroid tumours occurred in 16/57 intact rats given methylthiouracil, 0/39 of the controls and 0/32 hypophysectomized rats receiving methylthiouracil. Of the 16 tumour-bearing rats given methylthiouracil only, nine had thyroid adenomas and seven had carcinomas metastasizing to the lungs. As part of a second experiment, groups of Wistar/FIB rats [initial numbers and sex not specified], 2 months of age, were given methylthiouracil [purity not specified] in the drinking-water at a concentration of 0 (control) or 0.25% for 2 years. Methylthiouracil induced thyroid adenomas in 11/30 rats (five with pulmonary nodules), whereas none were seen in 33 controls (Jemec, 1980).

In another study published since the previous evaluation, groups of white random-bred rats, 3 months of age, were given methylthiouracil [purity not specified] in the drinking-water at a concentration of 0 or 0.1% until natural death or were killed when moribund. Methylthiouracil produced thyroid tumours in 39/58 treated rats (38 adenomas, one carcinoma; $p < 0.01$) and produced thyroid adenomas in 3/100 controls (Alexandrov *et al.*, 1989).

Hamster: Groups of hamsters, 3 months of age, were given methylthiouracil [purity not specified] in the drinking-water at a concentration of 0 (control) or 0.2%. Between four and 12 animals in each group were killed at regular intervals after 2–12 months of exposure. The first thyroid adenoma was recorded after 5 months of treatment with methylthiouracil; the total incidence of animals with thyroid adenomas by the end of the experiment was 20/77 treated hamsters and 0/37 controls (Christov & Raichev, 1972b).

3.2   Administration with known carcinogens

Rat: Groups of Debrecen or CB albino rats of each sex [initial numbers unspecified], 2.5–4 months of age, were given 2-acetylaminofluorene intragastrically at a dose of 2.5 mg/rat three times a week for 6 weeks and methylthiouracil [purity not specified] in the drinking-water at a concentration of 0.01% for a total experimental period of 71 weeks. Combined exposure to 2-acetylaminofluorene, methylthiouracil and a low-iodine diet produced thyroid adenomas in 100% of the rats that lived for 5 months or longer [number not stated], compared with 0/30 rats treated with 2-acetylaminofluorene alone and 1/25 rats treated with methylthiouracil alone (Lapis & Vekerdi, 1962).

In a study published since the previous evaluation, 75 female Wistar rats weighing 150 g [age not specified] were given a single oral dose of 40 mg/kg bw N-methyl-N-nitrosourea (MNU) on 3 consecutive days followed 4 weeks later by methylthiouracil [purity not specified] in the drinking-water at a concentration of 0.1% up to week 60 of the experiment. Thyroid tumours were observed from week 16 and carcinomas from week 24. After 30 weeks, 13 rats had tumours with metastases to the lungs (Schäffer & Müller, 1980). [The Working Group noted that the numbers of rats sampled at various times were not given, nor was the incidence, but the latter was inferred to be 100%.]

In a multigeneration study published since the previous evaluation, groups of white random-bred female rats [initial numbers and age not specified] received an intra-peritoneal injection of MNU at 20 mg/kg bw in 0.9% saline on day 21 of gestation. Groups of rats of the F_1 generation received either no further treatment or methyl-thiouracil in their drinking-water at a concentration of 0.1% (about 100 mg/kg bw per day) for life. Two additional groups of rats with no transplacental exposure to MNU received either methylthiouracil alone as above or no treatment (control group). Methylthiouracil caused a statistically significant increase ($p < 0.01$) in the incidence of MNU-induced thyroid tumours, from 4/100 with MNU alone to 33/43 with MNU plus methylthiouracil, but decreased ($p < 0.01$) the incidence of MNU-induced kidney and nervous system tumours. The incidences of thyroid tumours in rats given methyl-thiouracil are reported in section 3.1.2 (Alexandrov et al., 1989).

4. Other Data Relevant to an Evaluation of Carcinogenicity and its Mechanisms

4.1 Absorption, distribution, metabolism and excretion

4.1.1 Humans

No data were available to the Working Group.

4.1.2 Experimental systems

After intravenous injection of a single dose of 5 mg methylthiouracil, 84–90% of the dose could be recovered from the carcasses of animals killed after 1 min and 55–60% from the carcasses of animals killed after 3 h. At 3 h, the concentration of methylthiouracil in the thyroid was approximately 1 mg/g of tissue (Williams & Kay, 1947).

Methylthiouracil crossed the placental barrier and was excreted in the milk of lactating rats (Napalkov & Alexandrov, 1968).

After male Sprague-Dawley rats were given an intraperitoneal injection of [^{35}S]methylthiouracil in alkaline saline (pH 8.0), accumulation of radiolabel was observed in the thyroid, with a thyroid:plasma ratio of 43 (Marchant *et al.*, 1972).

4.2   Toxic effects

4.2.1   *Humans*

Use of methylthiouracil is associated with a high frequency of agranulocytosis (Westwick *et al.*, 1972). Use of this drug by a 21-year-old woman led to a bullous haemorrhagic rash (Cox *et al.*, 1985).

4.2.2   *Experimental systems*

Methylthiouracil (0.03%) given in the drinking-water to male Wistar rats had increased the plasma concentrations of thyroid-stimulating hormone by 1 week after the start of the treatment; however, the plasma concentrations of triiodothyronine and thyroxine were markedly decreased by 2 weeks (Tohei *et al.*, 1997).

Male Wistar/Holtzman rats given an intraperitoneal injection of 40 mg of methyl-thiouracil showed acute increases in the secretion of thyroid-stimulating hormone and interference with the recycling of iodide (Onaya *et al.*, 1973).

Male and female C57BL mice were given diets containing methylthiouracil at a concentration of 0.3 or 0.5% *ad libitum* for 2 weeks. Mice with hypothalamic lesions had decreased goitre development (Moll *et al.*, 1969).

Methylthiouracil given at a concentration of 0.1% in the drinking-water to male Wistar rats for 3 weeks led to disappearance of thyroid peroxidase activity from the follicular cells, measured by histochemistry; however, the activity reappeared after prolonged treatment for 6 months (Christov & Stoichkova, 1977).

Wistar rats treated with 0.1% methylthiouracil in their drinking-water had a fourfold increase in thyroid weights within 3 months and a 10-fold increase within 15 months. The mitotic index had increased by 10–15-fold in hyperplastic and malignant cells at 9 months (Christov, 1985).

4.3   Reproductive and developmental effects

No data were available to the Working Group.

4.4   Effects on enzyme induction or inhibition and gene expression

No data were available to the Working Group.

4.5   Genetic and related effects

4.5.1   *Humans*

No data were available to the Working Group

4.5.2   *Experimental systems* (see Table 1 for references)

Methylthiouracil was not mutagenic to *Salmonella typhimurium* in an assay with preincubation when tested with or without metabolic activation. It induced somatic recombination in eye cells in all three strains of *Drosophila melanogaster* tested when administered continuously in feed to larvae.

Methylthiouracil did not induce micronucleus formation in male mice after intra-peritoneal injection or oral gavage [details not provided]. When the drug was administered orally in two doses to pregnant mice, it appeared to increase the frequency of micronucleated polychromatic erythrocytes in the fetuses, but no micronucleus formation was seen in maternal bone-marrow cells. However, it is not clear that the same or similar cell populations were observed in the control and treated groups (the percentages of nucleated cells were quite different), and there was no significant increase in the number of micronucleated cells at doses of 5–100 mg/kg bw.

4.6   Mechanistic considerations

Inadequate data were available on the genotoxicity of methylthiouracil.

Methylthiouracil belongs to a class of drugs used in the treatment of hyper-thyroidism. The mode of action is inhibition of thyroid peroxidase, which decreases thyroid hormone production and increases follicular-cell proliferation by increasing the secretion of thyroid-stimulating hormone. This is assumed to be the basis of the tumorigenic activity of methylthiouracil in the thyroid in experimental animals; however, the lack of adequate data limits the confidence with which conclusions can be drawn.

The lack of adequate data on genotoxicity for methylthiouracil precludes a con-clusion regarding the mechanism of carcinogenesis.

5.   Summary of Data Reported and Evaluation

5.1   Exposure data

Methylthiouracil is a thionamide anti-thyroid drug, introduced in the 1940s, which has been used in the treatment of hyperthyroidism. Little is known about its current use.

Table 1. Genetic and related effects of methylthiouracil

Test system	Result[a]		Dose[b] (LED/HID)	Reference
	Without exogenous metabolic system	With exogenous metabolic system		
Salmonella typhimurium TA100, TA1535, TA98, TA97, reverse mutation	–	–	10 000 µg/plate	Zeiger et al. (1992)
Drosophila melanogaster, somatic recombination, *w/w* locus	+		71 µg/mL in feed	Rodriguez-Arnaiz (1998)
Micronucleus formation, peripheral blood cells of male CD-1 mice *in vivo*	–		2000 ip × 2 or po × 1	Morita et al. (1997)
Micronucleus formation, blood cells of fetal AG$_2$ mice, transplacental exposure *in vivo*	(+)		5 po × 2	Ioan (1980)
Micronucleus formation, bone-marrow cells of pregnant AG$_2$ mice *in vivo*	–		100 po × 2	Ioan (1980)

[a] +, positive; –, negative; (+), weak positive
[b] LED, lowest effective dose; HID, highest ineffective dose; in-vitro tests, µg/mL; in-vivo tests, mg/kg bw/day; ip, intraperitoneal injection; po, oral gavage

5.2   Human carcinogenicity studies

No epidemiological data on use of methylthiouracil and cancer were found. However, two analyses were published of one cohort study conducted in the United Kingdom and the USA of the cancer risk of patients, mainly women, with hyper-thyroidism who had been treated with anti-thyroid drugs. The earlier analysis showed more malignant thyroid neoplasms in patients receiving these drugs than in those treated with surgery or ^{131}I, but the excess may have been due to closer surveillance of the patients given drugs owing to more frequent use of thyroidectomy. In the later analysis, patients with hyperthyroidism treated only with anti-thyroid drugs had a modest increase in the risk for death from cancer, due chiefly to oral cancer and cancer of the brain. Neither report provided information on the type, quantity or dates of anti-thyroid drug use.

Two case–control studies of cancer of the thyroid showed no significant association with treatment with anti-thyroid medications.

5.3   Animal carcinogenicity data

Although no conventional bioassay of carcinogenicity in rodents has been reported, methylthiouracil has produced tumours in three species of laboratory rodents after oral administration. In two studies in mice, multiple studies in rats and one study in hamsters, methylthiouracil produced thyroid follicular-cell adenomas and/or carcinomas after oral administration. In initiation–promotion studies with the known carcinogens 2-acetylaminofluorene and N-methyl-N-nitrosourea, methylthiouracil increased the incidence of thyroid follicular-cell tumours.

5.4   Other relevant data

Little is known about the disposition of methylthiouracil in humans. In rats, methylthiouracil was found to accumulate in the thyroid. The compound crosses the placental barrier and is transferred rapidly across the placenta throughout gestation.

Human exposure to methylthiouracil is associated with a high frequency of agranulocytosis.

The available data on the mechanism of action of methylthiouracil in experimental animals is limited, but inhibition of thyroid peroxidase and increased secretion of thyroid-stimulating hormone may be the basis of its tumorigenic activity in the thyroid.

No data were available on reproductive or developmental effects of methyl-thiouracil.

Methylthiouracil was not mutagenic in single studies of reverse mutation in bacteria and bone-marrow micronucleus formation in rodents. It induced chromo-somal recombination in somatic cells of insects. It gave an inconclusive response in a test for micronucleus formation in fetal mouse blood cells.

5.5   Evaluation

There is *inadequate evidence* in humans for the carcinogenicity of methyl-thiouracil.

There is *sufficient evidence* in experimental animals for the carcinogenicity of methylthiouracil.

Overall evaluation

Methylthiouracil is *possibly carcinogenic to humans (Group 2B)*.

6.   References

Alexandrov, V.A., Popovich, I.G., Anisimov, V.N. & Napalkov, N.P. (1989) Influence of hormonal disturbances on transplacental and multigeneration carcinogenesis in rats. In: Napalkov, N.P., Rice, J.M., Tomatis. L. & Yamasaki, H., eds, *Perinatal and Multigeneration Carcinogenesis* (IARC Scientific Publications No. 96), Lyon, IARC*Press*, pp. 35–49

Batjoens, P., De Brabander, H.F. & De Wasch, K. (1996) Rapid and high-performance analysis of thyreostatic drug residues in urine using gas chromatography–mass spectrometry. *J. Chromatogr.*, **A750**, 127–132

Blanchflower, W.J., Hughes, P.J., Cannavan, A., McCoy, M.A. & Kennedy, D.G. (1997) Determination of thyreostats in thyroid and urine using high-performance liquid chromato-graphy–atmospheric pressure chemical ionization mass spectrometry. *Analyst*, **122**, 967–972

Budavari, S., ed. (2000) *The Merck Index*, 12th Ed., Version 12:3, Whitehouse Station, NJ, Merck & Co. & Boca Raton, FL, Chapman & Hall/CRC [CD-ROM]

Buick, R.K., Barry, C., Traynor, I.M., McCaughey, W.J. & Elliott, C.T. (1998) Determination of thyreostat residues from bovine matrices using high-performance liquid chromato-graphy. *J. Chromatogr. B. Biomed. Sci. Appl.*, **720**, 71–79

Centrich Escarpenter, F. & Rubio Hernández, D. (1990) [Analysis of thyrostatics in the thyroid glands by thin layer chromatography and HPLC-UV.] *An. Bromatol.*, **42**, 337–344 (in Spanish)

Christov, K. (1985) Cell population kinetics and DNA content during thyroid carcinogenesis. *Cell Tissue Kinet.*, **18**, 119–131

Christov, K. & Raichev, R. (1972a) Experimental thyroid carcinogenesis. *Curr. Top. Pathol.*, **56**, 79–114

Christov, K. & Raichev, J.R. (1972b) Thyroid carcinogenesis in hamsters after treatment with 131-iodine and methylthiouracil. *Z. Krebsforsch.*, **77**, 171–179

Christov, K. & Stoichkova, N. (1977) Cytochemical localization of peroxidase activity in normal, proliferating and neoplastic thyroid tissues of rats. An ultrastructural study. *Acta histochem.*, **58**, 275–289

CIS Information Services (2000a) *Directory of World Chemical Producers (Version 2000.1)*, Dallas, TX [CD-ROM]

CIS Information Services (2000b) *Worldwide Bulk Drug Users Directory (Version 2000)*, Dallas, TX [CD-ROM]

Cox, N.H., Dunn, L.K. & Williams, J. (1985) Cutaneous vasculitis associated with long-term thiouracil therapy. *Clin. exp. Dermatol.*, **10**, 292–295

De Brabander, H.F., Batjoens, P. & Van Hoof, J. (1992) Determination of thyreostatic drugs by HPTLC with confirmation by GC-MS. *J. planar Chromatogr. Mod. TLC*, **5**, 124–130

Dobyns, B.M., Sheline, G.E., Workman, J.B., Tompkins, E.A., McConahey, W.M. & Becker, D.V. (1974) Malignant and benign neoplasms of the thyroid in patients treated for hyperthyroidism: A report of the Cooperative Thyrotoxicosis Therapy Follow-up Study. *J. clin. Endocrinol. Metab.*, **38**, 976–998

Doniach, I. (1970) Experimental thyroid tumours. In: Smithers, D., ed., *Neoplastic Disease at Various Sites*, Vol. 6, *Tumours of the Thyroid Gland*, Edinburgh, E. & S. Livingstone, pp. 73–99

Esteve-Romero, J., Escrig-Tena, I., Simó-Alfonso, E.F. & Ramis-Ramos, G. (1999) Determination of thyreostatics in animal feed by micellar electrokinetic chromatography. *Analyst*, **124**, 125–128

Field, J.B., McCammon, C.J., Valentine, R.J., Bernick, S., Orr, C. & Starr, P. (1959) Failure of radioiodine to induce thyroid cancer in the rat. *Cancer Res.*, **19**, 870–873

Hallquist, A., Hardell, L., Degerman, A. & Boquist, L. (1994) Thyroid cancer: Reproductive factors, previous diseases, drug intake, family history and diet. A case–control study. *Eur. J. Cancer Prev.*, **3**, 481–488

Herbrand, K.G. (2000) *Pharmaceutical Specialties for the Treatment of Thyroid Diseases (Hyperthyroidism)*, Gengenbach, Germany [www.herbrand-pharma.de]

Hooijerink, H. & De Ruig, W.G. (1987) Determination of thyreostatics in meat by reversed-phase liquid chromatography with ultraviolet and electrochemical detection. *J. Chromatogr.*, **394**, 403–407

IARC (1974) *IARC Monographs on the Evaluation of Carcinogenic Risk of Chemicals to Man*, Vol. 7, *Some Anti-thyroid and Related Substances, Nitrofurans and Industrial Chemicals*, Lyon, IARCPress, pp. 53–65

IARC (1987) *IARC Monographs on the Evaluation of Carcinogenic Risks to Humans*, Suppl. 7, *Overall Evaluations of Carcinogenicity: An Updating of* IARC Monographs *Volumes 1 to 42*, Lyon, IARCPress, p. 66

Ioan, D. (1980) The mutagenic effect of carbimazol and methylthiouracil detected by the transplacental micronucleus test. *Rev. Roum. Med. Endocrinol.*, **18**, 247–250

Jemec, B. (1977) Studies of the tumorigenic effect of two goitrogens. *Cancer*, **40**, 2188–2202

Jemec, B. (1980) Studies of the goitrogenic and tumorigenic effect of two goitrogens in combination with hypophysectomy or thyroid hormone treatment. *Cancer*, **45**, 2138–2148

Junik, R., Lacka, K., Sowinski, J., Horst-Sikorska, W. & Gembicki, M. (1987) [Antithyroid antibodies and thyroglobulin in the serum of patients with hyperthyroidism treated with methylthiouracil.] *Polski Togodnik Lek.*, **42**, 1120–1123 (in Polish)

Krivánková, L., Krásenský, S. & Bocek, P. (1996) Application of capillary zone electrophoresis for analysis of thyreostatics. *Electrophoresis*, **17**, 1959–1963

Lapis, K. & Vekerdi, L. (1962) Simultaneous histological, autoradiographic and biochemical examination of experimentally induced thyroid tumour. *Acta morphol. sci. hung.*, **11**, 267–283

Le Bizec, B., Monteau, F., Maume, D., Montrade, M.-P., Gade, C. & Andre, F. (1997) Detection and identification of thyreostats in the thyroid gland by gas chromatography–mass spectrometry. *Anal. chim. Acta*, **340**, 201–208

Lide, D.R. & Milne, G.W.A. (1996) *Properties of Organic Compounds*, Version 5.0, Boca Raton, FL, CRC Press [CD-ROM]

Marchant, B., Alexander, W.D., Lazarus, J.H., Lees, J. & Clark, D.H. (1972) The accumulation of ^{35}S-antithyroid drugs by the thyroid gland. *J. clin. Endocrinol. Metab.*, **34**, 847–851

Medical Products Agency (2000) Uppsala

Medicines Control Agency (2000) London

Medicines Evaluation Board Agency (2000) The Hague

Moll, J., Martens, E. & Jansen, H.G. (1969) Development of goitre after methylthiouracil treatment of mice with hypothalamic lesions. *J. Endocrinol.*, **45**, 483–488

Moretti, G., Amici, M. & Cammarata, P. (1986) [Determination of methylthiouracil and analogous thyrostatics in animal tissues by HPTLC after solid-phase purification.] *Riv. Soc. ital. Sci. aliment.*, **15**, 35–39 (in Italian)

Moretti, G., Amici, M., Cammarata, P. & Fracassi, F. (1988) Identification of thyrostatic drug residues in animal thyroids by high-performance thin-layer chromatography and fluorescence reaction detection. *J. Chromatogr.*, **442**, 459–463

Moretti, G., Betto, R., Cammarata, P., Fracassi, F., Giambenedetti, M. & Borghese, A. (1993) Determination of thyreostatic residues in cattle plasma by high-performance liquid chromatography with ultraviolet detection. *J. Chromatogr.*, **616**, 291–296

Morita, T., Asano, N., Awogi, T., Sasaki, Y.F., Sato, S., Shimada, H., Sutou, S., Suzuki, T., Wakata, A., Sofuni, T. & Hayashi, M. (1997) Evaluation of the rodent micronucleus assay in the screening of IARC carcinogens (Groups 1, 2A and 2B). The summary report of the 6th collaborative study by CSGMT/JEMS.MMS. *Mutat. Res.*, **389**, 3–122

Napalkov, N.P. & Alexandrov, V.A. (1968) On the effects of blastomogenic substances on the organism during embryogenesis. *Z. Krebsforsch.*, **71**, 32–50

Onaya, T., Yamada, T. & Halmi, N.S. (1973) Intrathyroidal recycling of iodide in the rat: Effects of goitrogens. *Proc. Soc. exp. Biol. Med.*, **143**, 181–184

Rodriguez-Arnaiz, R. (1998) Biotransformation of several structurally related 2B compounds to reactive metabolites in the somatic w/w^+ assay of *Drosophila melanogaster*. *Environ. mol. Mutag.*, **31**, 390–401

Ron, E., Kleinerman, R.A., Boice, J.D., Jr, LiVolsi, V.A., Flannery, J.T. & Fraumeni, J.F., Jr (1987) A population-based case–control study of thyroid cancer. *J. natl Cancer Inst.*, **79**, 1–12

Ron, E., Doody, M.M., Becker, D.V., Brill, A.B., Curtis, R.E., Goldman, M.B., Harris, B.S.H., Hoffman, D.A., McConahey, W.M., Maxon, H.R., Preston-Martin, S., Warshauer, E., Wong, F.L. & Boice, J.D., Jr for the Cooperative Thyrotoxicosis Therapy Follow-up Study Group (1998) Cancer mortality following treatment for adult hyperthyroidism. *J. Am. med. Assoc.*, **280**, 347–355

Royal Pharmaceutical Society of Great Britain (2000) *Martindale, The Extra Pharmacopoeia*, 13th Ed., London, The Pharmaceutical Press [MicroMedex Online]

Sadtler Research Laboratories (1980) *Sadtler Standard Spectra, 1980 Cumulative Molecular Formula Index*, Philadelphia, PA, p. 61

Saldaña Monllor, L., Carbonell Martín, G. & Alonso Fuente, C. (1980) [*Thin-layer Chromato-graphic Separation and Identification of 2-Thiouracil, 4(6)-Methyl-2-thiouracil and 6(4)-Propyl-2-thiouracil in Feed Additives and Biological Materials by Thin-layer Chromatography.*], Madrid, Instituto National de Investigationes Agrarias (in Spanish)

Schäffer, R. & Müller, H.-A. (1980) On the development of metastasizing tumors of the rat thyroid gland after combined administration of nitrosomethylurea and methylthiouracil. *J. Cancer Res. clin. Oncol.*, **96**, 281–285

Swiss Pharmaceutical Society, ed. (2000) *Index Nominum, International Drug Directory*, 16th Ed., Stuttgart, Medpharm Scientific Publishers [MicroMedex Online]

Tohei, A., Akai, M., Tomabechi, T., Mamada, M. & Taya, K. (1997) Adrenal and gonadal function in hypothyroid adult male rats. *J. Endocrinol.*, **152**, 147–154

Van der Laan, W.P. & Storrie, V.M. (1955) A survey of factors controlling thyroid function, with especial reference to newer views on antithyroid substances. *Pharm. Rev.*, **7**, 301–334

Vargas, G., Havel, J. & Frgalová, K. (1998) Capillary zone electrophoresis determination of thyreostatic drugs in urine. *J. capillary Electrophor.*, **5**, 9–12

Westwick, W.J., Allsop, J. & Watts, R.W. (1972) A study of the effect of some drugs which cause agranulocytosis on the biosynthesis of pyrimidines in human granulocytes. *Biochem. Pharmacol.*, **15**, 1955–1966

Williams, R.H. & Kay, G.A. (1947) Thiouracils and thioureas: Comparisons of the absorption, distribution, destruction and excretion. *Arch. intern. Med.*, **80**, 37–52

Yu, G.Y.F., Murby, E.J. & Wells, R.J. (1997) Gas chromatographic determination of residues of thyreostatic drugs in bovine muscle tissue using combined resin mediated methylation and extraction. *J. Chromatogr. B. Biomed. Sci. Appl.*, **703**, 159–166

Zeiger, E., Anderson, B., Haworth, S., Lawlor, T. & Mortelmans, K. (1992) *Salmonella* muta-genicity tests: V. Results from the testing of 311 chemicals. *Environ. mol. Mutag.*, **19** (Suppl. 21), 2–141

PROPYLTHIOURACIL

This substance was considered by previous working groups, in 1974 (IARC, 1974) and 1987 (IARC, 1987). Since that time, new data have become available, and these have been incorporated into the monograph and taken into consideration in the present evaluation.

1. Exposure Data

1.1 Chemical and physical data

1.1.1 *Nomenclature*

Chem. Abstr. Serv. Reg. No.: 51-52-5
Deleted CAS Reg. No.: 500-50-5
Chem. Abstr. Name: 2,3-Dihydro-6-propyl-2-thioxo-4(1*H*)-pyrimidinone
IUPAC Systematic Name: 6-Propyl-2-thiouracil
Synonyms: 6-*n*-Propyl-2-thiouracil; 6-*n*-propylthiouracil; 6-propyl-2-thio-2,4-(1*H*,3*H*)pyrimidinedione; 6-propylthiouracil; PTU; 2-thio-4-oxy-6-propyl-1,3-pyrimidine; 2-thio-6-propyl-1,3-pyrimidin-4-one

1.1.2 *Structural and molecular formulae and relative molecular mass*

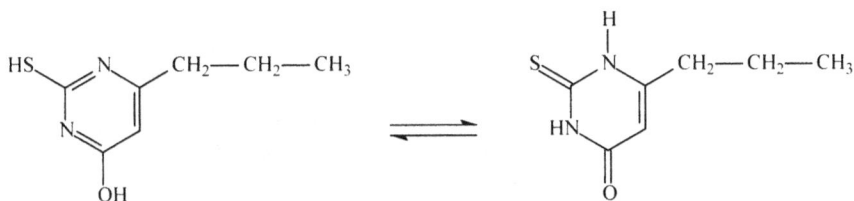

$C_7H_{10}N_2OS$

Relative molecular mass: 170.24

1.1.3   *Chemical and physical properties of the pure substance*

    (*a*) *Description*: White to pale-cream crystals or microcrystalline powder (Aboul-Enein, 1977; Lide & Milne, 1996; Budavari, 2000)

    (*b*) *Melting-point*: 219 °C (Lide & Milne, 1996)

    (*c*) *Spectroscopy data*: Infrared [prism (25719), grating (1591)], ultraviolet (9305), nuclear magnetic resonance [proton (8367)] and mass spectral data have been reported (Sadtler Research Laboratories, 1980; Lide & Milne, 1996).

    (*d*) *Solubility*: Slightly soluble in water, chloroform and ethanol; insoluble in benzene and diethyl ether (Lide & Milne, 1996)

1.1.4   *Technical products and impurities*

Propylthiouracil is available as 25- or 50-mg tablets (Gennaro, 1995; American Hospital Formulary Service, 2000; Herbrand, 2000).

Trade names for propylthiouracil include Procasil, Propacil, Propycil, Propyl-Thiocil, Propyl-Thyracil, Propylthiorit, Prothiucil, Prothiurone, Prothycil, Prothyran, Protiural, Thiuragyl, Thyreostat II and Thiotil.

1.1.5   *Analysis*

Several international pharmacopoeias specify infrared absorption spectrophotometry with comparison to standards, thin-layer chromatography and colorimetry as methods for identifying propylthiouracil; potentiometric titration and titration with sodium hydroxide are used to assay its purity. In pharmaceutical preparations, propylthiouracil is identified by infrared and ultraviolet absorption spectrophotometry and high-performance liquid chromatography (HPLC) with ultraviolet detection; HPLC with ultraviolet detection and titration with sodium hydroxide or mercury nitrate are used to assay for propylthiouracil content (British Pharmacopoeial Commission, 1993; Society of Japanese Pharmacopoeia, 1996; Council of Europe, 1997; AOAC International, 1998; US Pharmacopeial Convention, 1999).

Methods have been reported for the analysis of propylthiouracil in biological fluids (blood, milk, serum, urine), tissues, dried animal feed, feed additives and drugs. The methods include potentiometric titration, capillary zone electrophoresis with ultraviolet detection, micellar electrokinetic chromatography, thin-layer chromatography, high-performance thin-layer chromatography, HPLC with atmospheric pressure chemical ionization mass spectrometry, reversed-phase HPLC with ultraviolet detection and gas chromatography with mass spectrometry (Saldaña Monllor *et al.*, 1980; Moretti *et al.*, 1986, 1988; Centrich Escarpenter & Rubio Hernández, 1990; De Brabander *et al.*, 1992; Moretti *et al.*, 1993; Krivánková *et al.*, 1996; Blanchflower *et al.*, 1997; Ciesielski & Zakrzewski, 1997; Le Bizec *et al.*, 1997; Yu *et al.*, 1997; Buick *et al.*, 1998; Vargas *et al.*, 1998; Esteve-Romero *et al.*, 1999).

1.2 Production

Propylthiouracil can be prepared by the condensation of ethyl β-oxocaproate with thiourea (Anderson *et al.*, 1945).

Information available in 2000 indicated that propylthiouracil was manufactured by three companies in Germany, two companies in Japan and one company in Brazil (CIS Information Services, 2000a).

Information available in 2000 indicated that propylthiouracil was used in the formulation of pharmaceutical drugs by four companies in the USA, three companies in Germany, two companies each in Austria, Canada, Thailand and the United Kingdom and one company each in Australia, Belgium, Brazil, Israel, Japan, Portugal, the Republic of Korea, Singapore, Sweden, Switzerland and Turkey (CIS Information Services, 2000b).

1.3 Use

Propylthiouracil has been used since the 1940s in the treatment of hyperthyroidism. The starting doses are usually 100–150 mg three times a day orally; higher doses, up to 2400 mg/day, have been used in severe thyrotoxicosis. There are no intravenous preparations, but rectal use has been reported (Cooper, 1998). The dose of propylthiouracil is not different for infants, children or the elderly, and it is considered unnecessary to alter the dose for patients with hepatic or renal disease (Cooper, 2000). In the USA, propylthiouracil is used as the primary therapy for hyperthyroidism in pregnancy (Masiukiewicz & Burrow, 1999). The doses used are similar to those for non-pregnant women, with an effort to minimize them when possible to avoid fetal hypothyroidism. Propylthiouracil has also been deemed safe for use by lactating women (Cooper, 1987; Momotani *et al.*, 2000).

Anti-thyroid drugs, including propylthiouracil, may be given for several weeks up to 1–2 years for the treatment of hyperthyroidism. After initiation of therapy, thyroid function improves slowly, returning to normal only by 6–12 weeks of treatment (Okamura *et al.*, 1987). The time that it takes a patient to achieve a euthyroid state depends on a variety of clinical factors, including the severity of the hyperthyroidism at baseline, the size of the thyroid (correlated with intrathyroidal hormonal stores) and the dose of the anti-thyroid drug. Often, as thyroid function improves, the doses of anti-thyroid drug can be reduced. For example, maintenance doses of 50–150 mg of propylthiouracil per day may be adequate to control thyroid function for an extended period. Low doses of anti-thyroid drugs are most successfully used in areas of the world with marginal iodine sufficiency, as high intrathyroidal iodine concentrations would be expected to offset the effects of the drugs (Azizi, 1985).

Propylthiouracil has been investigated as a possible therapy for alcoholic hepatitis (Orrego *et al.*, 1987), the rationale being that the induction of a hypothyroid state might decrease hepatic oxygen requirements, or that propylthiouracil might function as a free-radical scavenger. However, this use has not gained much support (Orrego *et al.*, 1994).

By inducing hypothyroidism, propylthiouracil can increase the body weight of cattle (Thrift *et al.*, 1999), but the use of thyrostatic drugs for this purpose is forbidden in the European Union (European Commission, 1981) and by the Department of Agriculture (2000) in the USA.

1.4   Occurrence

1.4.1   *Occupational exposure*

According to the 1981–83 National Occupational Exposure Survey (National Institute for Occupational Safety and Health, 2000), about 3300 workers, comprising mainly pharmacists and laboratory workers in health services, were potentially exposed to propylthiouracil in the USA.

1.4.2   *Environmental occurrence*

No data were available to the Working Group.

1.5   Regulations and guidelines

Propylthiouracil is listed in the pharmacopoeias of China, France, Germany, Japan, the United Kingdom and the USA and also in the European and International Pharmacopoeias (Society of Japanese Pharmacopoeia, 1996; Council of Europe, 1997; Royal Pharmaceutical Society of Great Britain, 2000; Swiss Pharmaceutical Society, 2000), and it is registered for human use in Norway, Sweden, Portugal and the United Kingdom (Instituto Nacional de Farmacia e do Medicamento, 2000; Medical Products Agency, 2000; Medicines Control Agency, 2000; Medicines Evaluation Board Agency, 2000; Norwegian Medicinal Depot, 2000).

2.   Studies of Cancer in Humans

No information was available specifically on propylthiouracil.

2.1   Cohort studies

Dobyns *et al.* (1974) followed up 34 684 patients treated in England and the USA for hyperthyroidism between 1946 and 1964, 1238 of whom had been treated for at least 1 year with unspecified anti-thyroid drugs. No malignant thyroid neoplasm was found within 1 year of treatment. By 1968, more cases of thyroid neoplasm were found at follow-up among patients initially treated with anti-thyroid drugs (4 malignant tumours and 18 adenomas in 1238 patients) than among those initially treated with [131]I (19 malignant tumours and 41 adenomas in 21 714 patients) or (partial) thyroidectomy (4 malignant tumours and 14 adenomas in 11 732 patients). The authors suggested that more neoplasms were found in the drug-treated patients because subsequent thyroidectomy was more frequent in this group (30% of drug-treated patients, as compared with 0.5% of those initially treated with ^{131}I and 1.2% of those treated with primary thyroidectomy), which provided more opportunity for identification of neoplasms. [The Working Group noted that rates could not be calculated because person–years were not provided, and the ages of the groups were not given.]

Ron et al. (1998) updated the report of Dobyns et al. (1974) and followed-up 35 593 patients treated for hyperthyroidism between 1946 and 1964 in 25 clinics in the USA and one in the United Kingdom. By December 1990, about 19% had been lost to follow-up, and 50.5% of the study cohort had died. A total of 1374 patients (1094 women) had been treated with anti-thyroid drugs only, 10 439 (7999 women) with ^{131}I and drugs, 10 381 (8465 women) with thyroidectomy and drugs, 2661 (2235 women) with a combination of the three types of treatment and the remainder by other means. The drugs used during the study period were chiefly thiourea derivatives and iodine compounds. One year or more after the start of the study, the standardized mortality ratio (SMR) in comparison with the general population for the patients treated with anti-thyroid drugs only was 1.3 (95% confidence interval [CI], 1.1–1.6) for deaths from all cancers, which was chiefly due to significantly more deaths from oral cancer (4.2; 95% CI, 1.3–9.7; five cases) and brain tumours (3.7; 95% CI, 1.2–8.6; five cases). The excess risk for death from brain cancer persisted after exclusion of cases prevalent at the time of entry into the study. No deaths from thyroid carcinoma were recorded. The SMR for all cancers was approximately 1.0 in patients treated with ^{131}I or surgery (with or without anti-thyroid drugs), but the SMR for thyroid cancer was fourfold higher (3.9; 95% CI, 2.5–5.9; 24 cases observed) among patients who had been treated with ^{131}I with or without drugs. The authors noted that the group treated with drugs only was small; the type, quantity and dates of drug use were generally not available; and many patients had cancer before entry into the study, suggesting that some, but not all, of the excess could be attributed to the selection of patients with health problems for drug therapy. [The Working Group noted that the expected number of deaths from thyroid carcinomas was not reported, although it would almost certainly have been less than 1.0. Results were given separately for patients treated only with drugs and not for those given drugs with other treatment.]

2.2   Case–control studies

Ron et al. (1987) conducted a study of 159 cases of thyroid cancer and 285 population controls in Connecticut, USA, between 1978 and 1980. The use of anti-thyroid medications was not associated with an increased risk [relative risks not shown].

In a study carried out in northern Sweden between 1980 and 1989, 180 cases of thyroid cancer and 360 population controls were evaluated (Hallquist *et al.*, 1994). Use of anti-thyroid drugs (two cases and two controls) was associated with a relative risk of 2.0 (95% CI, 0.2–21).

3.   Studies of Cancer in Experimental Animals

Propylthiouracil was evaluated in a previous monograph (IARC, 1974). Because there have been only four new studies on the carcinogenicity of propylthiouracil in animals and none that are conventional bioassays in rodents, the most relevant studies from the previous monograph were analysed in greater depth. Studies on the carcinogenicity of anti-thyroid chemicals, including propylthiouracil, in experimental animals have been reviewed (Doniach, 1970; Christov & Raichev, 1972; Paynter *et al.*, 1988).

3.1   Oral administration

Mouse: Groups of male strain A mice [initial numbers not specified, but presumed to be four], 4–6 weeks of age, received a commercial diet containing 0.8% propyl-thiouracil [purity not specified] for up to 534 days. Thyroid follicular-cell carcinomas (two of which metastasized to the lungs) were present in all four propylthiouracil-treated mice and chromophobe adenomas of the anterior lobe of the pituitary gland in three of these mice. The anterior pituitary glands of a similar group of surgically thyroidectomized mice were normal (Moore *et al.*, 1953). [The Working Group noted the small numbers of animals in the groups.]

Groups of 60 C57BL mice [sex not specified], 4–5 weeks of age, were fed a diet containing propylthiouracil [purity not specified] at a concentration of 0 (control), 10 or 12 g/kg of diet for 17 months. The survival rate in all groups was approximately 50%. Pituitary adenomas occurred in 15/24 and 21/29 mice at the two concentrations, respectively, and in 0/28 control mice. Thyroid follicular-cell hyperplasia was grossly apparent in the treated mice. Administration of 2,4-dinitrophenol (an inhibitor of thyrotropin release) at 0.5 g/kg of diet in conjunction with the two doses of propyl-thiouracil reduced the incidence of pituitary tumours by at least 75% in each case, and no thyroid hyperplasia was apparent in these mice (King *et al.*, 1963).

Rat: Two groups of young adult white rats [number per group, sex, age and strain not specified] were given drinking-water containing propylthiouracil [purity not specified] at a concentration of 0.1%. One of the groups received propylthiouracil and potassium iodide alternately, the latter at a concentration of 0.01% in the drinking-water [exact protocol not stated]. The study was terminated within 1 year, when the total survival rate in the two groups was 44 of the original 100 rats. Thyroid follicular-cell tumours occurred in 4/15 survivors given propylthiouracil alone and in 20/29 survivors treated with propylthiouracil and potassium iodide alternately. All but one of the tumours were thyroid adenomas, the exception being a thyroid carcinoma in a rat given propylthiouracil plus potassium iodide (Zimmerman *et al.*, 1954).

Groups of male and female Wistar rats [group size presumed to be 55 of each sex], 6–8 weeks of age, received propylthiouracil [purity not specified] at a concentration of 0.2% in their drinking-water alone or after a single intraperitoneal injection of 30 μCi of ^{131}I. Because of a high mortality rate, the concentration of propylthiouracil given to both groups was reduced to 0.1% at 3 months, 0.05% at 6 months and 0.025 % at 1 year. In a second part of the experiment, 25 rats [number of each sex not specified] received a low concentration of propylthiouracil in their drinking-water, adjusted to provide a dose of 7 mg/kg bw per day initially (approximately equivalent to the human clinical dose) and then reduced to 1 mg/kg bw per day over 3 months. The control groups comprised 20 untreated male and 20 untreated female rats on normal diet. The treatments were continued until termination at 18 months, but control rats were continued until approximately 20 months of age. In the groups receiving 0.2% propyl-thiouracil alone, thyroid follicular-cell adenomas occurred in 11/18 males and 20/30 females and thyroid carcinomas in 3/18 males and 4/30 females. In the groups receiving 0.2% propylthiouracil plus ^{131}I, thyroid adenomas occurred in 9/15 males and 16/24 females and thyroid carcinomas in 4/15 males and 6/24 females. In the groups that initially received propylthiouracil at 7 mg/kg bw per day, thyroid adenomas occurred in 2/5 males and 7/13 females and thyroid carcinomas in 1/5 males and 2/13 females. In the untreated control groups, thyroid adenomas occurred in 2/20 males and 1/20 females, but there were no carcinomas in either sex (Willis, 1961).

Groups of 99–112 male Long Evans rats, 6 weeks of age, were fed a diet containing propylthiouracil [purity not specified] at a concentration of 0.1% (100 rats), the same diet after a single intraperitoneal injection of 25 μCi of ^{131}I in 0.5 mL of distilled water (112 rats), propylthiouracil in combination with ^{131}I plus dessicated thyroid powder at a concentration of 250 mg/kg of diet (99 rats) or propylthiouracil plus dessicated thyroid powder (99 rats). Additional groups consisted of untreated controls (101 rats), rats receiving ^{131}I only (106 rats), rats receiving dessicated thyroid powder only (103 rats) and rats receiving ^{131}I plus dessicated thyroid powder (106 rats). Each group was maintained on its specific diet for 1 year, at which time the study was terminated. In the group receiving 0.1% propylthiouracil alone, thyroid follicular-cell adenomas occurred in 16/33 survivors. With propylthiouracil in combination with ^{131}I, 23/35 rats had thyroid adenomas, while in the group given propylthiouracil plus ^{131}I plus dessicated thyroid powder, 64/65 rats developed thyroid tumours, of which 51 were adenomas and 13 carcinomas. In the group given propylthiouracil plus dessicated thyroid powder, 43/60 rats developed thyroid tumours, of which 39 were adenomas and 4 carcinomas. None of 68 untreated control rats had adenomas or papillary or follicular carcinomas (Lindsay *et al.*, 1966).

In a study published since the previous evaluation, groups of four to six male albino rats, 4 months of age, were given propylthiouracil [purity not specified] in the drinking-water at a concentration of 60 μg/mL for 3, 5, 7 or 9 months 1 week after a single intra-peritoneal injection of 25 μCi of ^{131}I in 0.5 mL of saline with or without L-thyroxine in the drinking-water at a concentration of 0.5 μg/mL. Control groups of four rats received no irradiation, propylthiouracil or thyroxine. In the groups given ^{131}I plus propylthio-uracil, thyroid tumours occurred in 1/4, 5/5 and 6/6 rats at 5, 7 and 9 months, respec-tively. In the groups given ^{131}I plus propylthiouracil plus thyroxine, thyroid follicular-cell tumours occurred in 1/4 and 5/5 rats at 7 and 9 months, respectively. There were no thyroid tumours in the control rats (Al-Hindawi *et al.*, 1977). [The Working Group noted the small numbers of animals in each group.]

Hamster: Groups of 214 male and 197 female Syrian golden hamsters, 3 months of age, were given drinking-water containing propylthiouracil [purity not specified] at a concentration of 0.2% for up to 133 weeks for males and 113 weeks for females. A control group of 205 males and 146 females were fed a diet with no propylthiouracil. The survival rate was reported not to be markedly influenced by treatment, the mean lifespans being 636, 500, 568 and 500 days for control males and females and treated males and females, respectively. Twelve animals per group were selected for eight interim killings for biochemical analyses. Thyroid follicular-cell cancer was diagnosed in 13/58 males and 9/44 females exposed to propylthiouracil, and an additional four males and six females had thyroid cancer that had metastasized to the lungs or lymph nodes. The thyroid tumour incidence in the control hamsters was not given, but a historical control incidence of 1.5% was cited (Fortner *et al.*, 1960). The combined tumour incidence for males and females treated with propylthiouracil was statistically significantly greater than 1.5% ($p < 0.01$) (Sichuk *et al.*, 1968). [The Working Group noted the lack of data on concurrent controls.]

Guinea-pig: Groups of 20 male guinea-pigs weighing 600–900 g [age and strain not specified] were given propylthiouracil [purity not specified] in their drinking-water at a concentration of 0.03% for up to 24 months, with or without a series of seven subcutaneous injections of 1 mL of thyroid-lipid extract emulsified in physio-logical saline given over the course of the study. Two groups of five control animals received the same regimen but without propylthiouracil. The survival rate at the end of the study at 24 months was 30–35% in the propylthiouracil-treated groups and 60% in the control groups. The incidence of animals with thyroid follicular-cell adenomas was 3/20 with propylthiouracil only and 12/20 with propylthiouracil plus thyroid-lipid extract, in contrast to none in either control group (Hellwig & Welch, 1963).

3.2   Administration with known carcinogens

Four studies in which rats were treated with propylthiouracil in combination with known carcinogens have been published since the previous evaluation.

Groups of female Fischer 344 rats, 50 days of age, received a single intravenous injection of N-methyl-N-nitrosourea (MNU) at a dose of 50 mg/kg bw. Five days later, groups of 30 rats were given propylthiouracil [purity not specified] in their drinking-water at concentrations of 0.3, 1.0 or 3.0%. A control group of 12 rats received no treatment, and 43 rats received the initiating dose of MNU alone. The incidence of thyroid follicular-cell tumours was increased from 0/12 controls and 0/43 receiving MNU only to 12/30, 30/30 and 30/30 with the increasing doses of propylthiouracil, respectively (Milmore *et al.*, 1982).

Two groups of 21 male inbred Wistar rats, 6 weeks of age, were fed basal diet containing propylthiouracil [purity not specified] at a concentration of 0.15% either alone or in combination with a single intraperitoneal injection of N-nitrosobis(2-hydroxypropyl)amine (NBHPA) at the start of the study at a dose of 2.8 g/kg bw. Two additional groups received the initiating dose of NBHPA alone or basal diet alone (control group). The animals were maintained for 20 weeks, at which time the survival rate was 100%. Thyroid follicular-cell tumours occurred in 21/21 rats given NBHPA plus propylthiouracil, 4/21 given NBHPA only ($p < 0.05$) and 0/21 given propylthiouracil only or no treatment. Of the rats given NBHPA plus propylthiouracil, seven of those bearing thyroid tumours had thyroid carcinomas (Kitahori *et al.*, 1984).

Two groups of 20 male inbred Wistar rats, 8 weeks of age, were given basal diet containing propylthiouracil [purity not specified] at a concentration of 0.1% for 19 weeks either alone or in combination with a single intraperitoneal injection of NBHPA (purity, 99.8%) at 7 weeks of age at a dose of 2.8 g/kg bw. Two additional groups received the initiating dose of NBHPA alone or basal diet alone. The survival rate at the end of the experiment was 100% for all groups. Thyroid follicular-cell adenomas occurred in 19/20 rats receiving NBHPA plus propylthiouracil, 1/20 treated with NBHPA alone ($p < 0.05$) and 0/20 receiving propylthiouracil or basal diet alone (Hiasa *et al.*, 1987).

Female Sprague-Dawley rats, 50–60 days of age, were given 7,12-dimethyl-benz[*a*]anthracene (DMBA) in sesame oil by oral gavage at a dose of 6.5, 10, 13.5 or 15 mg per animal. Propylthiouracil was given in the drinking-water at concentrations between 0.5 and 4.0 mg/100 mL for various times before and after the DMBA treatment, ranging from 17 days before DMBA up to the end of the study at 4 months. Severe hypothyroidism produced by administration of propylthiouracil at the higher dose from 7 days before DMBA up to study termination reduced the mammary tumour incidence from 68/108 in rats given DMBA only to 3/45 in those given DMBA plus propylthiouracil (Goodman *et al.*, 1980).

4.   Other Data Relevant to an Evaluation of Carcinogenicity and its Mechanisms

4.1   Absorption, distribution, metabolism and excretion

4.1.1   *Humans*

In seven healthy persons (six men and one woman) given an intravenous injection of 400 mg of propylthiouracil, the average half-time of the drug was 77 min. In a two-compartmental equation, the total clearance was calculated to be 112 mL/min per m². When the same dose was given orally, the average maximum serum concentration of propylthiouracil was 9.1 µg/mL and was reached at 57 min (average for the seven subjects). The total volume of distribution was calculated to be 30% of the body weight, and the bioavailability of propylthiouracil was determined to be 77% (range, 53–88%) (Kampmann & Skovsted, 1974). After intravenous infusion of propylthiouracil into three men and one woman, the half-time and total body clearance were similar to those after injection, but the total volume of distribution (40%) was slightly larger (Kampmann, 1977). In another study, oral administration of a smaller dose of propyl-thiouracil (200 mg) to six subjects showed a similar half-time, *viz* 1.1 h (Sitar & Hunninghake, 1975). Ringhand *et al.* (1980) calculated a half-time of 1.24–1.4 h after oral administration of propylthiouracil.

In a study in which propylthiouracil was given as a single oral dose of 300 mg to eight healthy volunteers (five women and three men) in either the fasting state or after a standardized breakfast, absorption of the drug was found to be influenced by inter-individual variation but to only a minor extent by food intake (Melander *et al.*, 1977). The severity of hyperthroidism and prior exposure to propylthiouracil were reported to affect the rate of elimination after oral administration of 3 mg/kg bw to 10 women and seven men. In patients with mild to moderate hyperthyroidism, elimination of the first dose of propylthiouracil was faster than the elimination in the same individual after 1 month of therapy, whereas in patients with severe hyperthyroidism, elimination of the first dose was inhibited. No changes in absorption rate were reported (Sitar *et al.*, 1979).

When patients undergoing thyroidectomy were given [³⁵S]propylthiouracil orally at 100 µCi 3–48 h before surgery, the compound accumulated in the thyroid but not in thyroid neoplasms (Marchant *et al.*, 1972).

In one person given 51 mg of [³⁵S]propylthiouracil orally, propylthiouracil glucu-ronide was the major excretion product (86%) in urine between 0 and 6 h, whereas at 8.8–23 h, a sulfate conjugate was the major urinary metabolite (Taurog & Dorris, 1988).

Placental transfer of [³⁵S]propylthiouracil was examined in four women who were 8–16 weeks pregnant and undergoing therapeutic abortions. The women were given 15 mg (100 µCi) of propylthiouracil orally. The average fetal:maternal serum ratio of radiolabel, obtained for two women, was 0.31. Accumulation of radiolabel in the fetal thyroid was noted (Marchant *et al.*, 1977). Six pregnant hyperthyroid women were given an oral dose of 100 mg of propylthiouracil. The serum profiles of the drug during the third trimester of pregnancy were qualitatively similar to those in non-pregnant women, but the concentrations were consistently lower in the late third trimester than those seen *post partum*. The cord serum concentrations were higher than those in maternal serum collected simultaneously (Gardner *et al.*, 1986).

In isolated, perfused, term human placentae, propylthiouracil at doses of 4 and 40 μg/mL in either a protein-free perfusate or a perfusate containing 40 g/L bovine serum albumin readily crossed the placenta and reached equilibrium within 2 h. The binding of propylthiouracil to bovine serum albumin, measured by ultrafiltration, was 94.5% and that to human serum albumin was 60.6%. The transfer of propylthiouracil was similar to that of methimazole (Mortimer *et al.*, 1997).

4.1.2   *Experimental systems*

In male Sprague-Dawley rats given [^{14}C]propylthiouracil intravenously, intraperito-neally or orally at a dose of 20 mg/kg bw, equilibrium dialysis indicated that 57% of the drug in plasma was bound to protein. No particular affinity for any tissue was noted. Between 75% and 90% of the administered radiolabel was excreted in the urine and approximately 15% in the bile. The half-time was 4–6 h by all routes of administration. Between 9 and 15% of the initial dose was excreted unchanged within 24 h. The major urinary metabolite was propylthiouracil glucuronide (40–48% in 24-h urine samples), but a different glucuronide conjugate of propylthiouracil appeared to be excreted in bile (Sitar & Thornhill, 1972). Another group of rats given [^{35}S]propylthiouracil intraperi-toneally at 1.2 μmol [204 μg] per animal showed accumulation of the propylthiouracil in the thyroid (Marchant *et al.*, 1972). Other authors have reported a similar bile meta-bolite (Papapetrou *et al.*, 1972; Lindsay *et al.*, 1974; Taurog & Dorris, 1988). Taurog and Dorris (1988) reported that propylthiouracil was the main excretion product, accounting for 34% of the administered radiolabel, and propylthiouracil glucuronide accounted for 32%. In a study with both [^{14}C]- and [^{35}S]propylthiouracil in the same strain of rats, unaltered propylthiouracil comprised 42% of the total urinary output, an unidentified metabolite 22% and propylthiouracil glucuronide 16%. Additional minor metabolites have been reported in both urine and bile (Lindsay *et al.*, 1974).

In CD rats given drinking-water containing propylthiouracil at concentrations of 0.0001–0.01% for 1 week or 1 month, the compound was cleared from the serum by bi-exponential disappearance, and an initial increase in the thyroid content of propyl-thiouracil was seen. Thereafter, the concentration in the thyroid declined linearly (Cooper *et al.*, 1983).

In the same strain of rats and with a radioimmunoassay specific for propylthiouracil, the serum concentration was reported to be a linear function of the dose (0.0001–0.05% in drinking-water), while the thyroid concentration was a linear function of the logarithm of the dose. The serum propylthiouracil concentrations were higher after

1 month of treatment than after 1 week. These results were consistent with a multi-compartmental model for the distribution of propylthiouracil (Halpern *et al.*, 1983).

Placental transfer of ^{14}C-labelled propylthiouracil was demonstrated in pregnant rats on day 14 of gestation after injection of 1 μCi of the compound. The label was cleared from the fetus within 24 h (Hayashi *et al.*, 1970).

When Sprague-Dawley rats were given intravenous injections of [^{14}C]propyl-thiouracil (4.1 μmol [698 μg]) on days 19 and 20 of gestation, the fetal:maternal serum concentration ratio was < 1 during 2 h after injection (Marchant *et al.*, 1977).

Nakashima *et al.* (1978) reported that the intrathyroidal metabolism of propyl-thiouracil in male Sprague-Dawley rats was strongly influenced by the dose (0.18–59 μmol [31 μg–10 mg] intraperitoneally). Propylthiouracil inhibited its own intra-thyroidal metabolism.

Metabolism of propylthiouracil in activated neutrophils resulted in three oxidized metabolites: propylthiouracil-disulfide, propyluracil-2-sulfinate and propyluracil-2-sulfonate. The metabolism was inhibited by sodium azide and catalase and by propyl-thiouracil itself (Waldhauser & Uetrecht, 1991).

The metabolism of the drug was either reversible or irreversible, depending on iodination conditions, in an in-vitro system containing thyroid peroxidase. Propyl-thiouracil disulfide was the earliest detectable metabolite (Taurog *et al.*, 1989).

4.1.3   *Comparison of animals and humans*

In both humans and laboratory animals, propylthiouracil is quickly absorbed and uniformly distributed, apart from concentration in the thyroid of adults and fetuses. It is rapidly excreted, the main metabolite being a glucuronide in both humans and rats.

4.2   Toxic effects

4.2.1   *Humans*

(*a*)   *Effects on thyroid function at therapeutic doses*

Propylthiouracil is commonly used to treat hyperthyroidism. It inhibits intra-thyroidal synthesis of thyroid hormones by interfering with thyroid peroxidase-mediated iodine utilization. As a result, the concentrations of thyroxine (T4) and triiodothyronine (T3) in serum are decreased. In addition, and unlike methimazole, propylthiouracil inhibits type-1 deiodinase which converts T4 to T3 in the liver and other tissues (Cooper, 2000). Therefore, serum T3 concentrations fall rapidly after administration of propyl-thiouracil, sooner than would be expected on the basis of inhibition of thyroidal hormone synthesis.

In some studies, hyperthyroid patients became hypothyroid if the dose of propyl-thiouracil was not monitored carefully. In one study, 56% of patients became hypo-thyroid within 12 weeks while taking 400 mg/day (Kallner *et al.*, 1996). With respect to its effects on T4 deiodination, both normal and hyperthyroid patients showed marked decreases in serum T3 concentrations within a few hours of ingesting 50–300 mg of propylthiouracil. The concentration of T3 decreased by up to 50% in hyperthyroid patients, and that of reverse T3 (rT3), an inactive metabolite of T4 that is cleared by type-1 deiodinase (see Figure 1, General Remarks), increased by up to 50% (Cooper *et al.*, 1982). Ten patients with primary hypothyroidism (eight women and two men), who had been receiving 0.1 or 0.2 mg of T4 daily for ≥ 2 months, were given 1000 mg of propylthiouracil daily in combination with 0.1 mg of T4 for 7 days. The average serum T3 concentration decreased from approximately 80 to 60 ng/100 mL, the average concentration of thyroid-stimulating hormone (TSH) increased gradually from approximately 30 to 40 μU/mL (not statistically significant for the whole group), and no changes occurred in T4 concentrations (Saberi *et al.*, 1975). Similar changes were seen when six healthy volunteers (three men and three women) who had been treated with T4 at 200–250 μg/day for 9 days were given 150 mg of propylthiouracil orally four times a day for 5 days. Thus, the T3 serum concentration was reduced and that of rT3 was enhanced. The concentrations rapidly returned to normal after cessation of treatment with propylthiouracil (Westgren *et al.*, 1977). Similar effects were noted when a dose of 200 mg of propylthiouracil was given orally four times a day for 5 days to 19 hypothyroid patients (six men and 13 women) who had been taking 50–200 μg of T4 per day for ≥ 2 months before the study; however, no changes in TSH concentration were seen (Siersbaek-Nielsen *et al.*, 1978).

(b)   Other studies in humans

Most of the toxic effects of propylthiouracil are considered to be allergenic, including fever, skin rashes and arthralgia, which occur in 1–10% of patients. Agranulocytosis is the most significant major side-effect, occurring in 0.1–0.5% of patients. (Van der Klauw *et al.*, 1998; Cooper, 1999). Other rare but serious reactions include toxic hepatitis (Williams *et al.*, 1997), vasculitis (often antineutrophil cyto-plasmic antibody-positive) (Gunton *et al.*, 1999) and a drug-induced lupus syndrome.

4.2.2   Experimental systems

In female NMRI mice fed a low-iodine diet, administration of drinking-water containing 0.1% propylthiouracil impaired thyroidal uptake of ^{125}I (Ahrén & Rerup, 1987).

The inhibition of thyroid iodide peroxidase (TPO) by propylthiouracil was studied *in vivo* and *in vitro* by measuring oxidized iodide. Propylthiouracil was given at a dose of 10 mg by intraperitoneal injection to Wistar rats weighing about 150 g. The activity of TPO in the thyroid gland isolated after 3 h was significantly decreased before dialysis and restored after dialysis. *In vitro*, the activity of TPO was decreased by incu-bation with propylthiouracil and restored by dialysis and by dilution. Propylthiouracil interacted directly with the product of TPO (the oxidized iodide) without significantly affecting the activity of TPO itself. At a concentration of 2×10^{-6} mol/L, 50% inhibition occurred (Nagasaka & Hidaka, 1976). In male CD rats given propyl-thiouracil by intraperitoneal injection at 10–50 mg/kg bw in the absence of oxidizable substrates, irreversible inhibition of TPO was observed. When iodide or thiocyanate was present, inhibition was prevented, suggesting that the initial action of propyl-thiouracil is to block iodination by trapping oxidized iodide (Davidson *et al.*, 1978). In an iodination system, inactivation of TPO by propylthiouracil involved a reaction between propylthiouracil and the oxidized haem group produced by interaction between TPO and H_2O_2 (Engler *et al.*, 1982a). A specific inhibitory effect of propyl-thiouracil on coupling was demonstrated in an incubation system in which TPO catalysed conversion of diiodotyrosine to T4 (Engler *et al.*, 1982b).

When male Sprague-Dawley rats maintained on T4 at 20 or 50 µg/kg bw per day were given propylthiouracil, the conversion of T4 to T3 was inhibited (Oppenheimer *et al.*, 1972). Frumess and Larsen (1975) further studied the role of the conversion of T4 to T3 in thyroidectomized, hypothyroid male Sprague-Dawley rats that were given a subcutaneous injection of T4 at 8 or 16 µg/kg bw per day, with or without an intra-peritoneal injection of propylthiouracil at 10 mg/kg bw per day. The rats were killed after 5, 10, 12 or 15 days. At 5 days, propylthiouracil treatment had increased the serum T4 concentration (from 4.9 to 5.7 µg/100 mL) and decreased that of T3 (from 37 to 19 ng/100 mL), resulting in a marked increase in the serum T4:T3 ratio (from 134 to 329). The serum TSH concentration was increased from 165 to 339 µU/mL in propylthiouracil-treated groups, and their weight gain was slower. When daily doses of 30 mg/kg bw were administered orally for 5 weeks to male Sprague-Dawley rats, both the T3 and T4 concentrations in serum were decreased, and a decrease in iodine incorporation was also noted. Increases in TSH concentration, thyroid weight and hyperplasia of the follicular cells were also reported (Takayama *et al.*, 1986). When propylthiouracil was administered to rats in the diet at 30 mg/kg from 3 up to 90 days, it reduced the T3 concentration by 60% and that of T4 by 90%, and increased the thyroid weight (fivefold) and the TSH concentration by more than eightfold. Thyroid-cell proliferation increased by up to 8.5-fold during the first week but had returned to control levels by 45 days (Hood *et al.*, 1999a). Hood *et al.* (1999b) also correlated TSH concentrations with thyroid weight and with the rate of thyroid follicular-cell proliferation in male Sprague-Dawley rats treated with propylthiouracil (1–300 mg/kg of diet) for 21 days. They suggested that small increases in TSH concentration are sufficient to stimulate thyroid follicular-cell proliferation.

Male Wistar rats were given drinking-water containing 0.01% propylthiouracil for 6 months. The drug first acted on the peripheral metabolism of T4 and subsequently on that of TSH. This induced a rapid increase in plasma TSH concentration during the first week, similar to increases seen in other strains of rats. The TSH plasma concen-tration had returned to normal by day 17, but then increased continuously until the end of treatment. The pituitary TSH concentration decreased after 24 h of treatment and remained low for 3 weeks, then recovered to normal after 1 month. The thyroid weight increased regularly throughout treatment, and the intrathyroid iodine concentration had decreased by 30-fold after 1 month. Secretion of TSH from the pituitary was found to decrease during the first week of treatment, to recover between 17 days and 1 month, and then to increase again by fourfold with continued treatment. The half-time of TSH was shown to be prolonged by propylthiouracil treatment (Griessen & Lemarchand-Béraud, 1973).

In other studies in male Wistar rats on the secretion of thyroid hormones, infusion of propylthiouracil for 4 h at a rate of 2 mg/h increased the excretion of rT3 in the bile of rats that had also received an infusion of T4, starting 2 h before the propylthiouracil treatment. Infusion of propylthiouracil at 0.05–0.4 mg over 2 h after a pulse of 1 μg of rT3 by intravenous injection increased excretion of rT3 in bile in a dose-dependent manner (Langer & Gschwendtová, 1992). Propylthiouracil at 0.05% in the diet also stimulated excretion of T4 in the bile and faeces of Wistar rats. The compound also stimulated uptake of T4 in liver tissue *in vitro* (Yamada *et al.*, 1976).

In male Wistar rats given propylthiouracil at a concentration of 0.1% in drinking-water for 20 days (calculated intake, 16 mg/day) and an intraperitoneal injection of 100 μCi of ^{125}I 24 h before sacrifice, the amount of soluble thyroglobulin was decreased by > 50% and the proportion of particulate thyroglobulin was slightly increased. The thyroglobulin from treated animals was poorly iodinated. Incubation of thyroid tissue with propylthiouracil *in vitro* inhibited thyroglobulin biosynthesis (Monaco *et al.*, 1980).

In liver homogenates from male Wistar rats, the conversion of T4 to T3 was lower in those from rats given 0.05% propylthiouracil in a low-iodine diet. A graded dose of T4 failed to restore conversion activity in these rats (Aizawa & Yamada, 1981). In monolayers of freshly isolated rat hepatocytes, outer-ring deiodination of an intermediate in thyroid hormone metabolism (3,3′-diiodothyronine sulfate) was completely inhibited by 10^{-4} mol/L propylthiouracil, essentially with no effect on overall 3,3′-diiodothyronine clearance (Otten *et al.*, 1984).

Using a sensitive, specific radioimmunoassay for propylthiouracil, Cooper *et al.* (1983) examined the effects of propylthiouracil at 0.0001–0.01% in drinking-water for 1 week or 1 month in CD rats. A strong inverse relationship was found between the dose of propylthiouracil and both thyroid hormone biosynthesis and peripheral T4 deiodination. The time for recovery from long-term (1 month) treatment was greater than that from short-term (1 week) treatment (2.8 *vs* 1.1 days), although the two treatments had quantitatively similar effects on thyroid function.

Whereas 30 mg/kg bw propylthiouracil given to rats daily for 5 weeks increased thyroid weight sevenfold and decreased both T3 and T4 concentrations by 70%, the same treatment produced no changes in the thyroid in squirrel monkeys (*Saimiri sciureus*). The concentration of propylthiouracil required to inhibit thyroid peroxidase *in vitro* in microsomes isolated from thyroids was markedly higher for the monkeys (4.1×10^{-6} mol/L) than for rats (8.1×10^{-8} mol/L) (Takayama *et al.*, 1986). These findings suggest that rats are more sensitive to the anti-thyroid effects of propylthiouracil than primates and that inhibition of thyroid peroxidase plays an important role in the anti-thyroid effect of propylthiouracil.

Male Sprague-Dawley rats given 0.05% propylthiouracil in the drinking-water for 17 days showed a decreased (40%) proportion of suppressor T cells in the spleen (Pacini *et al.*, 1983).

Intraperitoneal administration of propylthiouracil at 0.5–1.5 mmol/kg bw (85–255 mg/kg bw) to male Sprague-Dawley rats resulted in dose-related decreases in body and spleen weight and an increase in liver weight. Leukocyte counts were markedly reduced. Histologically, congestion of red pulp in the spleen and vacuolization of the liver were noted (Kariya *et al.*, 1983).

Female Fischer 344 rats were given 0.1% propylthiouracil in the drinking-water for 3, 7, 14 or 28 days and observed 3, 7 and 14 days after cessation of treatment. During propylthiouracil ingestion, growth hormone-producing cells in the pituitary gland lost their secretory granules, became enlarged and displayed progressive dilatation of rough endoplasmic reticulum, becoming thyroidectomy cells. This effect was reversible: 14 days after treatment ceased, the normal pituitary structure was seen (Horvath *et al.*, 1990).

Young (3 months) and aged (26 months) male Lewis rats were given drinking-water containing 0.05% propylthiouracil for 4 weeks. In the younger animals, propyl-thiouracil increased the percentage of sphingomyelin in synaptosomes from the cerebral cortex. In contrast, a decrease in glycerophosphocholine concentration and an increase in that of cholesterol were noted in aged rats (Salvati *et al.*, 1994).

4.3   Reproductive and developmental effects

4.3.1   *Humans*

A review of the clinical literature resulted in limited information on the risk of propylthiouracil-induced malformations in newborns, but the authors noted that an estimated 1–5% of women treated with propylthiouracil during pregnancy have infants who develop significant transient hypothyroidism (Friedman & Polifka, 1994).

Neonatal goitre was observed in one of a dizygotic set of twins whose mother had received propylthiouracil during pregnancy at an initial dose of 400 mg/day, which was subsequently reduced to 100 mg/day. The reason for the apparently selective effect of propylthiouracil on one of the twins was not clear. The goitre receded within 2 weeks, without therapy (Refetoff *et al.*, 1974).

In 20 women who had received propylthiouracil during the third trimester of pregnancy at doses of 50–400 mg/day, four cases of neonatal goitre, one of thyro-toxicosis, three pregnancy losses and two malformations occurred (Mujtaba & Burrow, 1975). [The Working Group noted that many of these outcomes may have been related to the underlying condition.] In a follow-up study, the intellectual capacity of 18 children whose mothers received propylthiouracil during pregnancy was compared with that of 17 siblings who had not been exposed. The two groups did not differ in a standard intelligence test, the Peabody test, the Goodenough test or on a number of physical characteristics (Burrow *et al.*, 1968). Similarly, no differences were noted in the distribution of IQs in a group of 28 children who had been exposed to propyl-thiouracil *in utero* (23 exposed at least in the third trimester) due to treatment of maternal Graves disease and in 32 unexposed siblings (Burrow *et al.*, 1978).

In six pregnant hyperthyroid women who received a daily oral dose of 50, 100 or 150 mg of propylthiouracil, a significant inverse correlation ($r = -0.92$; $p = 0.026$) was found between the area under the curve for concentration–time for maternal serum propylthiouracil in the third trimester and the index of free T4 in cord serum (Gardner *et al.*, 1986).

In a study of 34 women with Graves hyperthyroidism who received propyl-thiouracil during pregnancy, 6% (2/34) of cord blood samples contained free T4 at concentrations below the normal range, while 21% (7/34) had concentrations of TSH above the normal range. All the infants with low free T4 or high TSH concentrations were clinically euthyroid and none had goitre at birth (Momotani *et al.*, 1997).

Transient neonatal hypothyroidism was seen in the offspring of 11 women who had received propylthiouracil at a dose of 100–200 mg/day at term [route unspecified] for Graves disease during pregnancy. The controls were 40 infants born around the same time. The free and total serum T4 concentrations, but not that of T3, were significantly lower in the exposed infants 1 and 3 days after birth (Cheron *et al.*, 1981).

4.3.2 *Experimental systems*

Testicular growth and serum testosterone concentrations were studied in groups of 8–24 male offspring at 90, 135, 160 and 180 days of age after administration of propyl-thiouracil in the drinking-water at 0.1% w/v to their lactating Sprague-Dawley dams from the day of parturition until day 25. The growth of treated offspring was reduced up to 25 days of age and then generally paralleled that of control animals, but their body weight remained lower than that of the controls. At all ages studied, the testis weights were increased in the propylthiouracil-exposed groups, despite reductions in body weights. For example, at 90 days of age, the testis weight was increased by 41%, while the body weight was reduced by 22%. Histologically, there was evidence of enhancement of normal spermatogenesis. Epidydymal, seminal vesicle and ventral prostate weights were also increased, but this effect was not apparent until 135 days of age. The weights of non-reproductive organs (e.g. brain, liver, pituitary and salivary glands) were reduced in the exposed groups. There was no effect on serum T4, T3 or testosterone concentration at any adult age, and there were no obvious histological changes in any tissue. Administration of T4 at 15 μg/kg bw per day and T3 at 10 μg/kg bw per day to pups during exposure to propylthiouracil abolished the effects on testi-cular growth (Cooke & Meisami, 1991). A subsequent study showed an increase in daily sperm production of 83–136%, depending on age (Cooke *et al.*, 1991). The increases in testis weight and daily sperm production could not be induced by prenatal exposure to propylthiouracil (gestation day 16 to birth) or by exposure beginning after postnatal day 8 (Cooke *et al.*, 1992). While the serum testosterone concentration was not permanently affected by this treatment, the circulating gonadotropin concentration remained 30–50% lower than that in controls throughout adulthood, an effect related to impairment of gonadal feedback and gonadotrope synthetic ability (Kirby *et al.*, 1997). These results suggest a direct impairment of gonadotropin-releasing hormone regulation of gonadotrope development.

Of six interstitial cell types, only Leydig cells showed an increased mitotic labelling index in male pups of rat dams given propylthiouracil at 0.1% in the drinking-water from the day of parturition to the time of weaning 24 days *post partum* (Hardy *et al.*, 1996). The total number of Leydig cells in the testes of 180-day-old male offspring of dams given propylthiouracil at 0.1% in the drinking-water for the first 25 days of their life was increased by about 70%, while luteinizing hormone-stimulated testosterone production and the steroidogenic potential from 22(R)-hydroxycholesterol — measured as testosterone production — were reduced by 55% and 73%, respectively (Hardy *et al.*, 1993). A similar doubling of the number of Leydig cells was reported in 135-day-old male Sprague-Dawley rats made hypothyroid by the addition of 0.1% propylthiouracil to the drinking-water of their dams from parturition through postnatal day 25, in contrast to a lower average volume and steroid production per Leydig cell (Mendis-Handagama & Sharma, 1994). Examination of 1-, 7-, 14- and 21-day-old male rats exposed to 0.1% propylthiouracil in their dams' drinking-water showed that, while the number of fetal Leydig cells did not differ from that in controls at any age, there was a delay in the appearance of adult-type Leydig cells (11β-hydroxysteroid dehydrogenase-positive cells) at day 21. In parallel with the morphological delay, luteinizing hormone-stimulated androstenedione production from testis *in vitro* increased from day 14 to day 21 in samples from controls but not in those from propylthiouracil-treated rats (Mendis-Handagama *et al.*, 1998). A decrease in the relative proportion of Leydig cells (identified by morphology and 3β-hydroxysteroid dehydrogenase staining) in interstitial cells were also observed between day 12 and day 16 in propylthiouracil-exposed Wistar rats (Teerds *et al.*, 1998).

Ultrastructural analysis of Sertoli cells provided evidence of an approximate 10-day delay in development in 25-day-old propylthiouracil-treated male rats, including the presence of mitotic Sertoli cells not present in 25-day-old control males (De Franca *et al.*, 1995). The observed effects on Sertoli cell development confirmed earlier work in Wistar rats exposed to 0.1% propylthiouracil in the drinking-water from birth through day 26. The authors found a cessation of proliferation of control Sertoli cells by day 20, as measured by a bromodeoxyuridine-labelling index, whereas propylthiouracil-treated animals had significantly enhanced labelling indices beginning on day 12 and continuing through at least day 26. As a result, there was an 84% increase in the number of Sertoli cells by day 36 (Van Haaster *et al.*, 1992).

In parallel with the delays in Leydig and Sertoli cell development, the development of germ cells was also impaired by neonatal exposure to propylthiouracil. When Sprague-Dawley rats were given 0.1% propylthiouracil in the drinking-water on days 1–25 of postnatal life, decreases in the numbers of spermatocytes and round spermatids were observed at days 20 and 30 in the testes of propylthiouracil-treated rats when compared with controls (Simorangkir *et al.*, 1997).

Further examination of this experimental model of increased testis weight and function after exposure of rats to propylthiouracil during days 1–24 of life indicated that the testis weights were reduced between 10 and 60 days of age, after which time the increase became apparent (Kirby *et al.*, 1992). Serum luteinizing and follicle-stimulating hormone concentrations were reduced to 50–70% of control levels throughout life, the changes being noticeable early after onset of exposure to propylthiouracil. The serum concentrations of growth hormone, prolactin and T4, which were depressed during exposure, returned to control levels at 40–50 days of age — i.e. within a few weeks after cessation of treatment — as did the increase in TSH concentration. The dose–response characteristics of the effect on testes were evaluated in 90-day-old male rats given 0, 0.0004, 0.0015, 0.006, 0.012 or 0.1% propylthiouracil in their drinking-water from birth to postnatal day 25. Both testis weight and daily sperm production were significantly increased at all concentrations. The testis weight reached a plateau and the daily sperm production a peak value at the 0.006% concentration. Maternal water consumption was significantly reduced at 0.1% propylthiouracil during days 1–13 *post partum* and only slightly reduced at 0.006% (Cooke *et al.*, 1993).

Overall, these data support the conclusion that neonatal hypothyroidism in rats allows a prolonged period of proliferation of Sertoli cells, which ultimately leads to increased numbers of Leydig cells, increased testis weights and increased daily sperm production in adults. While most of the studies were conducted by giving drinking-water containing 0.1% propylthiouracil on days 1–25 of postnatal life, one study suggested that the effects would probably occur at concentrations down to at least 0.0004% propylthiouracil in water.

In order to study the effects of propylthiouracil on prostate weight, the offspring of Sprague-Dawley rats maintained on 0.1% propylthiouracil in the drinking-water from parturition until they were 25 days of age were examined between days 14 and 180. The ventral prostate weights were lower than those of controls up to 95 days of age but increased from day 95, and the glands were about 40% heavier at 180 days of age. The increase in weight was at least partially due to the presence of new ductal structures. The histological appearance of the prostate was normal at all ages, but a transient increase in amiloride-inhibitable plasminogen activator activity was seen in the ventral and dorso-lateral prostate at 42 days of age. These activities had returned to control levels by 90 days. Treatment with propylthiouracil also increased the activity of metalloprotease in the ventral prostate at 21–42 days of age. and in the dorso-lateral prostate at 21 and 28 days of age (Wilson *et al.*, 1997).

Examination of female Wistar rats that received 0.1% propylthiouracil in the drinking-water from birth through day 40 indicated that their body weights were significantly reduced by 12 days of age and their ovarian weights by 21 days of age; by day 40, there were signs of altered follicular development. In contrast to effects seen in males, the follicle-stimulating hormone concentration was not reduced in propylthiouracil-treated females (Dijkstra *et al.*, 1996).

Groups of 70–114-day-old female Sprague-Dawley rats were exposed to propyl-thiouracil in the diet (0.3%) and drinking-water (0.001%) from parturition until their pups were 30 days of age. There were four litters per group. The serum T4 concentrations of the dams were depressed through 120 days of age, and their body weight was diminished by about 20%. Neuroanatomical effects in 90-day-old offspring of treated dams included thinning of the cerebellar cortex and fewer synapses in Purkinje cells. In behavioural assessments which included differential reinforcement of low-rate learning, escape and avoidance tasks and motor activity and exploration, control rats learned the escape and avoidance tasks faster and were hyperactive (Schalock *et al.*, 1977).

The effects of propylthiouracil on heart and kidney development were studied in Sprague-Dawley rats by treating their dams by subcutaneous injection of 20 mg/kg bw from gestation day 17 to lactation day 5, and by direct injection of the pups on post-natal days 1–5. Body and organ weights and organ DNA and protein content were determined in groups of 7–12 animals on multiple days between birth and day 50. Propylthiouracil significantly impaired body growth and heart and kidney weights (by 10–25%), although the weights had returned to control levels by 50 days of age. The changes in the DNA content of these two organs were similar to the body weight effects, recovery taking longer in the kidney than in the heart; cell size was reduced to a greater extent and for longer periods than cell number (Slotkin *et al.*, 1992).

Coronary arterioles were examined in 12-, 28- and 80-day-old Sprague-Dawley rats of dams that had received 0.05% propylthiouracil in their drinking-water on postnatal days 2–28. The body weights of the offspring were significantly depressed after day 20, while their heart rates were significantly depressed at 12 and 28 days of age. Long-term depression of the cardiac mass was also noted, in the presence of capillary proliferation and marked attenuation of arteriolar growth (Heron & Rakusan, 1996).

Female Wistar rats received 0.1% propylthiouracil in the drinking-water from the beginning of gestation through lactation [precise treatment period not indicated], and brain development was evaluated in 6–10 offspring per group on postnatal days 5, 20 and 48. Propylthiouracil significantly reduced the live litter size and pup weight at all ages and also significantly reduced the volume of the neocortex. Further analysis indicated reduced numbers of glial cells in the neocortex only at day 48, while the numbers of neurons were not significantly reduced at any age (Behnam-Rassoli *et al.*, 1991).

The auditory response (brainstem-response audiometry) to frequencies of 4 and 16 kHz was evaluated in Sprague-Dawley rats 12, 16, 25 and 125 days of age that had been exposed to propylthiouracil during various 10-day periods of development. For exposure during gestation, 0.05% propylthiouracil was given in the drinking-water; for exposure after birth, 7 mg/kg bw were given by subcutaneous injection. Hypothyrodism was confirmed by a hormone assay. After neonatal exposure, the concentrations of thyroid hormones were reduced to about 20% of the control levels and that of TSH was about 10-fold higher. The hormone concentrations were not significantly reduced when exposure began at 28 or 120 days of age. Treatment with propylthiouracil significantly increased the latency of wave 1 (representing the cochlear nerve compound action potential) of the brainstem response when given from 3 days before parturition through 6 days of age, but had no permanent effect when given for 10 days starting 10 days after birth (Hébert et al., 1985).

The effects of propylthiouracil on growth, motor development and auditory function were evaluated in Long Evans rats (six to eight litters per group) exposed via the drinking-water to propylthiouracil at 0, 1, 5 or 25 mg/L from gestation day 18 to postnatal day 21. No effects were observed at 1 mg/L. At 5 and 25 mg/L, the serum T4 concentration was sharply reduced on days 1, 7, 14 and 21 after birth, while that of T3 was reduced on days 7, 14 and 21 at 25 mg/L and on day 21 at 5 mg/L. Pups exposed to 25 mg/L had reduced body weights, delayed eye opening, delayed preweaning motor activity and persistent postweaning hyperactivity. Slight effects on eye opening and motor activity were noted at 5 mg/L. Adult offspring that had been exposed to 5 or 25 mg/L showed auditory startle deficits at all frequencies tested (range, 1–40 kHz) (Goldey et al., 1995).

Reproductive development was studied after subcutaneous injection of 0 or 50 mg/kg bw per day propylthiouracil to groups of 10–15 ICR mice from postnatal day 1 until day 28. No effects on growth were seen in the offspring. The plasma T3 concentration was reduced by 40–50% [period not stated]. Histologically, the ovaries of propylthiouracil-treated females showed decreased numbers of primordial, multilaminar and Graafian follicles as folliculogenesis occurred during days 14–28. In males, there was evidence of reduced numbers of seminiferous tubules, but the histological appearance was normal. The fertility of both male and female treated mice was normal (Chan & Ng, 1995).

Daily exposure by oral gavage to propylthiouracil at 0 or 50 mg/kg bw of groups of six male and female CD rats on days 26–96 affected the growth rates of animals of each sex, altered the estrous cycles of females (with a predominance of diestrous stages), increased the weights of the thyroid, pituitary and testis and decreased the weight of the adrenals (Baksi, 1973).

4.4   Effects on enzyme induction or inhibition and gene expression

4.4.1   *Humans*

No data were available to the Working Group.

4.4.2   *Experimental systems*

Hepatic and renal 5′-deiodinase activities were strongly inhibited in microsomal preparations from male Sprague-Dawley rats that had been given propylthiouracil orally at 10 mg/kg bw per day for 7 or 14 days (de Sandro *et al.*, 1991). The inhibition could be reversed by increasing amounts of glutathione (Yamada *et al.*, 1981).

Propylthiouracil significantly decreased cytochrome *c* reductase and aniline hydroxylase activity in male Wistar rat microsomes (Raheja *et al.*, 1985).

Propylthiouracil inhibited glutathione transferases in a concentration-dependent manner, a 10-mmol/L concentration causing 25% inhibition. The *S*-oxides of propyl-thiouracil were even more potent inhibitors: the 2-sulfonate inhibited the enzyme activity by 80% (Kariya *et al.*, 1986).

Propylthiouracil given at 0.05% in drinking-water for 4 weeks to young and aged male Lewis rats (3 and 26 months, respectively) resulted in increased synaptosomal acetylcholinesterase activity in both groups, an increased density of muscarinic receptor sites in the young rats and an increase in synaptosomal cholesterol concen-tration in the aged animals (Salvati *et al.*, 1994).

Propylthiouracil increased thyroglobulin mRNA levels in the Fischer rat thyroid cell line FRTL-5 and resulted in accumulation of thyroglobulin in the medium. The total RNA levels were not affected. The effects were suppressed by iodide and did not occur when protein synthesis was inhibited by cycloheximide (Leer *et al.*, 1991).

4.5   Genetic and related effects

4.5.1   *Humans*

No data were available to the Working Group.

4.5.2   *Experimental systems* (see Table 1 for references)

Propylthiouracil did not induce gene mutations in bacteria, or DNA strand breaks in primary cultures of rat or human hepatocytes. It was marginally mutagenic to yeast. Chromosomal aberrations were not induced in a mouse mammary carcinoma-derived cell line or in cultured thyroid cells [not otherwise defined] derived from male Wistar rats given drinking-water containing propylthiouracil at 0.06 mg/L for 10 or 15 weeks. It did not induce somatic recombination in eye cells of *Drosophila melanogaster* when administered continuously in feed to larvae.

4.6   Mechanistic considerations

There are insufficient data to evaluate the genotoxicity of propylthiouracil.

The main effect of propylthiouracil in humans and rodents is inhibition of thyroid peroxidase, which results in decreased plasma concentrations of T3 and T4 and an

Table 1. Genetic and related effects of propylthiouracil

Test system	Result[a] Without exogenous metabolic system	Result[a] With exogenous metabolic system	Dose[b] (LED/HID)	Reference
Escherichia coli Sd-4-73, reverse mutation	–	NT	NR	Szybalski (1958)
Saccharomyces cerevisiae D6, petite mutation	(+)	NT	1000	Wilkie & Gooneskera (1980)
Drosophila melanogaster, somatic recombination, *w/w+* locus	–		170 µg/mL in feed	Rodriguez-Arnaiz (1998)
DNA damage, rat hepatocytes *in vitro*	–	NT	953	Martelli *et al.* (1992)
Chromosomal aberrations, FM3A mouse mammary carcinoma cell line *in vitro*	–	NT	1073	Kodama *et al.* (1980)
Chromosomal aberrations, Wistar rat thyroid cells *ex vivo*	–	NT	0.06 mg/L in drinking-water, 15 weeks	Speight *et al.* (1968)
DNA damage, human hepatocytes *in vitro*	–	NT	953	Martelli *et al.* (1992)

[a] –, negative; NT, not tested; (+), weak positive
[b] LED, lowest effective dose; HID, highest ineffective dose; in-vitro tests, µg/mL; NR, not reported

increased concentration of TSH, with consequent thyroid follicular-cell proliferation and growth. Squirrel monkeys are much less sensitive to the effect of propylthiouracil on thyroid peroxidase than rats. Another effect of propylthiouracil is inhibition of conversion of T4 to T3 by inhibiting type-1 deiodinase. Alteration of thyroid hormone production is the presumptive mechanism for thyroid tumour formation in rodents.

The lack of adequate data on genotoxicity for propylthiouracil precludes a conclusion regarding the mechanism of carcinogenicity.

5. Summary of Data Reported and Evaluation

5.1   Exposure data

Propylthiouracil is a thionamide anti-thyroid drug that has been widely used since the 1940s in the treatment of hyperthyroidism. It has been used as a fattening agent in cattle, but this use has been banned.

5.2   Human carcinogenicity studies

No epidemiological data on use of propylthiouracil and cancer were found. However, two analyses were published of one cohort study conducted in the United Kingdom and the USA of the cancer risk of patients, mainly women, with hyperthyroidism who had been treated with anti-thyroid drugs. The earlier analysis showed more malignant thyroid neoplasms in patients receiving these drugs than in those treated with surgery or ^{131}I, but the excess may have been due to closer surveillance of the patients given drugs owing to more frequent use of thyroidectomy. In the later analysis, patients with hyperthyroidism treated only with anti-thyroid drugs had a modest increase in the risk for death from cancer, due chiefly to oral cancer and cancer of the brain. Neither report provided information on the type, quantity or dates of anti-thyroid drug use.

Two case–control studies of cancer of the thyroid showed no significant association with treatment with anti-thyroid medications.

5.3   Animal carcinogenicity data

Although no conventional bioassay of carcinogenicity in rodents has been reported, propylthiouracil has produced tumours in multiple species. In two small studies in mice, oral administration of propylthiouracil produced thyroid follicular-cell carcinomas and tumours of the anterior pituitary. In multiple studies with various strains of rats, propyl-thiouracil produced thyroid follicular-cell adenomas and carcinomas. In single studies, propylthiouracil produced thyroid follicular-cell adenomas and carcinomas in hamsters and adenomas in guinea-pigs. In initiation–promotion models of thyroid carcinogenesis in rats, propylthiouracil increased the incidence of thyroid follicular-cell tumours initiated by *N*-methyl-*N*-nitrosourea or *N*-nitrosobis(2-hydroxypropyl)amine.

5.4   Other relevant data

The elimination of propylthiouracil in both humans and experimental animals is relatively rapid, and the major metabolic pathway is glucuronidation and excretion in the urine.

The main effect of propylthiouracil in humans and rodents is interference with thyroid peroxidase-mediated iodination of thyroglobulin, which results in decreased plasma concentrations of triiodothyronine and thyroxine and increases in those of thyroid-stimulating hormone, with consequent thyroid follicular-cell proliferation and thyroid growth. This is a plausible mechanism of propylthiouracil-induced tumorigenesis in the thyroid.

Propylthiouracil is not considered to be a human teratogen, although a small percentage of infants whose mothers received the drug during pregnancy developed transient hypothyroidism. Follow-up of small numbers of offspring exposed prenatally did not suggest impairment of intellectual development. Experimental studies on the effects of propylthiouracil focused on the consequences of the induction of hypothyroidism during the early postnatal period on the development and functioning of the brain and reproductive tract. Hyperactivity, auditory deficits and increased sperm production have been observed in rats. The latter outcome is the result of a prolonged period of proliferation of Sertoli cells, and subsequently Leydig cells, in the testes that allows additional spermatogonia in adulthood.

Propylthiouracil has not been adequately tested for gene mutation induction. It did not induce mutations in bacteria, and it was only marginally mutagenic in yeast. Propylthiouracil did not induce chromosomal recombination in insects, DNA strand breaks in rat or human hepatocytes or chromosomal aberrations in a mouse mammary carcinoma-derived cell line. It did not induce chromosomal aberrations in thyroid cells of rats exposed *in vivo* via the drinking-water.

5.5   Evaluation

There is *inadequate evidence* in humans for the carcinogenicity of propylthiouracil.

There is *sufficient evidence* in experimental animals for the carcinogenicity of propylthiouracil.

Overall evaluation

Propylthiouracil is *possibly carcinogenic to humans (Group 2B).*

6. References

Aboul-Enein, H.Y. (1977) Propylthiouracil. *Anal. Profiles Drug Subst.*, **6**, 457–486

Ahrén, B. & Rerup, C. (1987) Kinetics of radioiodine released from prelabelled thyroid gland *in vivo*: Influence of propylthiouracil. *Pharmacol. Toxicol.*, **61**, 69–71

Aizawa, T. & Yamada, T. (1981) Effects of thyroid hormones, antithyroid drugs and iodide on *in vitro* conversion of thyroxine to triiodothyronine. *Clin. exp. Pharmacol. Physiol.*, **8**, 215–225

Al-Hindawi, A.Y., Black, E.G., Brewer, D.B., Griffiths, S.G. & Hoffenberg, R. (1977) Measurement of thyroid hormone in experimental thyroid tumours in rats. *J. Endocrinol.*, **75**, 245–250

American Hospital Formulary Service (2000) *AHFS Drug Information® 2000*, Bethesda, MD, American Society of Health-System Pharmacists [AHFSfirst CD-ROM]

Anderson, G.W., Halverstadt, I.F., Miller, W.H. & Roblin, R.O., Jr (1945) Antithyroid compounds. Synthesis of 5- and 6-substituted 2-thiouracils from β-oxo esters and thiourea. *J. Am. chem. Soc.*, **67**, 2197–2200

AOAC International (1998) AOAC Official Method 952.27. Propylthiouracil in drugs. In: *Official Methods of Analysis of AOAC International*, 15th Ed., Gaithersburg, MD [CD-ROM]

Azizi, F. (1985) Environmental iodine intake affects the response to methimazole in patients with diffuse toxic goiter. *J. clin. Endocrinol. Metab.*, **61**, 374–377

Baksi, S.N. (1973) Effect of propylthiouracil-induced hypothyroidism on serum levels of luteinizing hormone and follicle-stimulating hormone in the rat. *J. Endocrinol.*, **59**, 655–656

Behnam-Rassoli, M., Herbert, L.C., Howard, V., Pharoah, P.O.D. & Stanisstreet, M. (1991) Effect of propylthiouracil treatment during prenatal and early postnatal development on the neocortex of rat pups. *Neuroendocrinology*, **53**, 321–327

Blanchflower, W.J., Hughes, P.J., Cannavan, A., McCoy, M. & Kennedy, D.G. (1997) Determination of thyreostats in thyroid and urine using high-performance liquid chromatography–atmospheric pressure chemical ionization mass spectrometry. *Analyst*, **122**, 967–972

British Pharmacopoeia Commission (1993) *British Pharmacopoeia 1993*, Vols I & II, London, Her Majesty's Stationery Office, pp. 557–558, 1083

Budavari, S., ed. (2000) *The Merck Index*, 12th Ed., Version 12:3, Whitehouse Station, NJ, Merck & Co. & Boca Raton, FL, Chapman & Hall/CRC [CD-ROM]

Buick, R.K., Barry, C., Traynor, I.M., McCaughey, W.J. & Elliott, C.T. (1998) Determination of thyreostat residues from bovine matrices using high-performance liquid chromatography. *J. Chromatogr. B. Biomed. Sci. appl.*, **720**, 71–79

Burrow, G.N., Bartsocas, C., Klatskin, E.H. & Grunt, J.A. (1968) Children exposed *in utero* to propylthiouracil. Subsequent intellectual and physical development. *Am. J. Dis. Child.*, **116**, 161–165

Burrow, G.N., Klatskin, E.H. & Genel, M. (1978) Intellectual development in children whose mothers received propylthiouracil during pregnancy. *Yale J. Biol. Med.*, **51**, 151–156

Centrich Escarpenter, F. & Rubio Hernández, D. (1990) Analysis of thyrostatics in the thyroid glands by thin layer chromatography and HPLC–UV. *An. Bromatol.*, **42**, 337–344

Chan,W.Y. & Ng, T.B. (1995) Effect of hypothyroidism induced by propylthiouracil and thiourea on male and female reproductive systems of neonatal mice. *J. exp. Zool.*, **273**, 160–169

Cheron, R.G., Kaplan, M.M., Larsen, P.R., Selenkow, H.A. & Crigler, J.F. (1981) Neonatal thyroid function after propylthiouracil therapy for maternal Graves' disease. *New Engl. J. Med.*, **304**, 525–528

Christov, K. & Raichev, R. (1972) Experimental thyroid carcinogenesis. *Curr. Top. Pathol.*, **56**, 79–114

Ciesielski, W. & Zakrzewski, R. (1997) Potentiometric and coulometric titration of 6-propyl-2-thiouracil. *Analyst*, **122**, 491–494

CIS Information Services (2000a) *Directory of World Chemical Producers (Version 2000.1)*, Dallas, TX [CD-ROM]

CIS Information Services (2000b) *Worldwide Bulk Drug Users Directory (Version 2000)*, Dallas, TX [CD-ROM]

Cooke, P.S. & Meisami, E. (1991) Early hypothyroidism in rats causes increased adult testis and reproductive organ size but does not change testosterone levels. *Endocrinology*, **129**, 237–243

Cooke, P.S., Hess, R.A., Porcelli, J. & Meisami, E. (1991) Increased sperm production in adult rats after transient neonatal hypothyroidism. *Endocrinology*, **129**, 244–248

Cooke, P.S., Porcelli, J. & Hess, R.A. (1992) Induction of increased testis growth and sperm production in adult rats by neonatal administration of the goitrogen propylthiouracil (PTU): The critical period. *Biol. Reprod.*, **46**, 146–154

Cooke, P.S., Kirby, J.D. & Porcelli, J. (1993) Increased testis growth and sperm production in adult rats following transient neonatal goitrogen treatment: Optimization of the propylthiouracil dose and effects of methimazole. *J. Reprod. Fertil.*, **97**, 493–499

Cooper, D.S. (1987) Antithyroid drugs: To breast feed or not to breast feed? *Am. J. Obstet. Gynecol.*, **157**, 234–235

Cooper, D.S. (1998) Antithyroid drugs for the treatment of hyperthyroidism caused by Graves' disease. *Endocrinol. Metab. Clin. N. Am.*, **27**, 225–247

Cooper, D.S. (1999) The side effects of antithyroid drugs (Abstract). *Endocrinologist*, **9**, 457

Cooper, D.S. (2000) The treatment of hyperthyroidism. In: Braverman, L.E. & Utiger, R.D., eds, *Werner & Ingbar's. The Thyroid. A Fundamental and Clinical Text*, 8th Ed., Philadelphia, PA, J.B. Lippincott, pp. 691–715

Cooper, D.S., Saxe, V.C., Meskell, M., Maloof, F. & Ridgway, E.C. (1982) Acute effects of propylthiouracil (PTU) on thyroidal iodide organification and peripheral iodothyronine deiodination: Correlation with serum PTU levels measured by radioimmunoassay. *J. clin. Endocrinol. Metab.*, **54**, 101–107

Cooper, D.S., Kieffer, J.D., Halpern, R., Saxe, V., Mover, H., Maloof, F. & Ridgway, E.C. (1983) Propylthiouracil (PTU) pharmacology in the rat. II. Effects of PTU on thyroid function. *Endocrinology*, **113**, 921–928

Council of Europe (1997) *European Pharmacopoeia*, 3rd Ed., Strasbourg, pp. 1400–1401

Davidson, B., Soodak, M., Neary, J.T., Strout, H.V., Kieffer, J.D., Mover, H. & Maloof, F. (1978) The irreversible inactivation of thyroid peroxidase by methylmercaptoimidazole, thiouracil, and propylthiouracil *in vitro* and its relationship to *in vivo* findings. *Endocrinology*, **103**, 871–882

De Brabander, H.F., Batjoens, P. & Van Hoof, J. (1992) Determination of thyreostatic drugs by HPTLC with confirmation by GC–MS. *J. planar Chromatogr.*, **5**, 124–30

De Franca, L.R., Hess, R.A., Cooke, P.S. & Russell, L.D. (1995) Neonatal hypothyroidism causes delayed Sertoli cell maturation in rats treated with propylthiouracil: Evidence that the Sertoli cell controls testis growth. *Anat. Rec.*, **242**, 57–69

Department of Agriculture (2000) *Thyrostatic Drugs*, Washington DC, Food Safety and Inspection Service [http://www.fsis.usda.gov]

Dijkstra, G., de Rooij, D.G., de Jong, F.H. & van den Hurk, R. (1996) Effect of hypothyroidism on ovarian follicular development, granulosa cell proliferation and peripheral hormone levels in the prepubertal rat. *Eur. J. Endocrinol.*, **134**, 649–654

Dobyns, B.M., Sheline, G.E., Workman, J.B., Tompkins, E.A., McConahey, W.M. & Becker, D.V. (1974) Malignant and benign neoplasms of the thyroid in patients treated for hyperthyroidism: A report of the Cooperative Thyrotoxicosis Therapy Follow-up Study. *J. clin. Endocrinol. Metab.*, **38**, 976–998

Doniach, I. (1970) Experimental thyroid tumours. In: Smithers, D., ed., *Neoplastic Disease at Various Sites*, Vol. 6, *Tumours of the Thyroid Gland*, Edinburgh, E. & S. Livingstone, pp. 73–99

Engler, H., Taurog, A. & Nakashima, T. (1982a) Mechanism of inactivation of thyroid peroxidase by thioureylene drugs. *Biochem. Pharmacol.*, **31**, 3801–3806

Engler, H., Taurog, A. & Dorris, M. (1982b) Preferential inhibition of thyroxine and 3,5,3'-triiodothyronine formation by propylthiouracil and methylmercaptoimidazole in thyroid peroxidase-catalyzed iodination of thyroglobulin. *Endocrinology*, **10**, 190–197

Esteve-Romero, J., Escrig-Tena, I., Simo-Alfonso, E.F. & Ramis-Ramos, G. (1999) Determination of thyreostatics in animal feed by micellar electrokinetic chromatography. *Analyst*, **124**, 125–128

European Commission (1981) Council Directive of 31 July 1981 concerning the prohibition of certain substances having a hormonal action and of any substances having a thyrostatic action. *Off. J. Eur. Comm.*, **L222**, 32–33

Fortner, J.G., George, P.A. & Sternberg, S.S. (1960) Induced and spontaneous thyroid cancer in the Syrian (golden) hamster. *Endocrinology*, **66**, 364–376

Friedman, J. & Polifka, J. (1994) *Teratogenic Effects of Drugs: A Resource for Clinicians*, Baltimore, The Johns Hopkins University Press, pp. 530–532

Frumess, R.D. & Larsen, P.R. (1975) Correlation of serum triiodothyronine (T3) and thyroxine (T4) with biologic effects of thyroid hormone replacement in propylthiouracil-treated rats. *Metabolism*, **24**, 547–554

Gardner, D.F., Cruikshank, D.D., Hays, P.M. & Cooper, D.S. (1986) Pharmacology of propylthiouracil (PTU) in pregnant hyperthyroid women: Correlation of maternal PTU concentrations with cord serum thyroid function tests. *J. clin. Endocrinol. Metab.*, **62**, 217–220

Gennaro, A.R. (1995) *Remington: The Science and Practice of Pharmacy*, 19th Ed., Vol. II, Easton, PA, Mack Publishing Co., p. 1087

Goldey, E.S., Kehn, L.S., Rehnberg, G.L. & Crofton, K.M. (1995) Effects of developmental hypothyroidism on auditory and motor function in the rat. *Toxicol. appl. Pharmacol.*, **135**, 67–76

Goodman, D.A., Hoekstra, S.J. & Marsh, P.S. (1980) Effects of hypothyroidism on the induction and growth of mammary cancer induced by 7,12-dimethylbenz(*a*)anthracene in the rat. *Cancer Res.*, **40**, 2336–2342

Griessen, M. & Lemarchand-Béraud, T. (1973) Thyrotropin secretion and metabolism in rats during propylthiouracil treatment. *Endocrinology*, **92**, 166–173

Gunton, J.E., Stiel, J., Caterson, R.J. & McElduff, A. (1999) Anti-thyroid drugs and anti-neutrophil cytoplasmic antibody positive vasculitis. A case report and review of the literature. *J. clin. Endocrinol. Metab.*, **84**, 13–16

Hallquist, A., Hardell, L., Degerman, A. & Boquist, L. (1994) Thyroid cancer: Reproductive factors, previous diseases, drug intake, family history and diet. A case–control study. *Eur. J. Cancer Prev.*, **3**, 481–488

Halpern, R., Cooper, D.S., Kieffer, J.D., Saxe, V., Mover, H., Maloof, F. & Ridgway, E.C. (1983) Propylthiouracil (PTU) pharmacology in the rat. I. Serum and thyroid PTU measurements by radioimmunoassay. *Endocrinology*, **113**, 915–920

Hardy, M.P., Kirby, J.D., Hess, R.A. & Cooke, P.S. (1993) Leydig cells increase their numbers but decline in steroidogenic function in the adult rat after neonatal hypothyroidism. *Endocrinology*, **132**, 2417–2420

Hardy, M.P., Sharma, R.S., Arambepola, N.K., Sottas, C.M., Russell, L.D., Bunick, D., Hess, R.A. & Cooke, P.S. (1996) Increased proliferation of Leydig cells induced by neonatal hypothyroidism in the rat. *J. Androl.*, **17**, 231–238

Hayashi, T.T., Teubner, J. & Gilling, B. (1970) Study of placental transfer of thiouracil derivatives. *Am. J. Obstet. Gynecol.*, **108**, 723–728

Hébert, R., Langlois, J.-M. & Dussault, J.H. (1985) Permanent defects in rat peripheral auditory function following perinatal hypothyroidism: Determination of a critical period. *Dev. Brain Res.*, **23**, 161–170

Hellwig, C.A. & Welch, J.W. (1963) Drug-induced tumors of the thyroid in guinea pigs with experimental thyroiditis. *Growth*, **27**, 305–315

Herbrand, K.G. (2000) *Pharmaceutical Specialties for the Treatment of Thyroid Diseases (Hyperthyroidism)*, Gengenbach, Germany [www.herbrand-pharma.de]

Heron, M. & Rakusan, K. (1996) Short- and long-term effects of neonatal hypo- and hyperthyroidism on coronary arterioles in rat. *Am. J. Physiol.*, **271**, H1746–H1754

Hiasa, Y., Kitahori, Y., Kato, Y., Ohshima, M., Konishi, N., Shimoyama, T., Sakaguchi, Y., Hashimoto, H., Minami, S. & Murata, Y. (1987) Potassium perchlorate, potassium iodide, and propylthiouracil: Promoting effect on the development of thyroid tumors in rats treated with *N*-bis(2-hydroxypropyl)nitrosamine. *Jpn. J. Cancer Res.*, **78**, 1335–1340

Hood, A., Liu, J. & Klaassen, C.D. (1999a) Effects of phenobarbital, pregnenolone-16α-carbonitrile, and propylthiouracil on thyroid follicular cell proliferation. *Toxicol. Sci.*, **50**, 45–53

Hood, A., Liu, Y.P., Gattone, V.H., II & Klaassen, C.D. (1999b) Sensitivity of thyroid gland growth to thyroid stimulating hormone (TSH) in rats treated with antithyroid drugs. *Toxicol. Sci.*, **49**, 263–271

Horvath, E., Lloyd, R.V. & Kovacs, K. (1990) Propylthiouracyl-induced hypothyroidism results in reversible transdifferentiation of somatotrophs into thyroidectomy cells. *Lab. Invest.*, **63**, 511–520

IARC (1974) *IARC Monographs on the Evaluation of Carcinogenic Risk of Chemicals to Man*, Vol. 7, *Some Anti-thyroid and Related Substances, Nitrofurans and Industrial Chemicals*, Lyon, IARC*Press*, pp. 67–76

IARC (1987) *IARC Monographs on the Evaluation of Carcinogenic Risks to Humans*, Suppl. 7, *Overall Evaluations of Carcinogenicity: An Updating of* IARC Monographs *Volumes 1 to 42*, Lyon, IARC*Press*, pp. 329–330

Instituto Nacional de Farmacia e do Medicamento (2000) Lisbon

Kallner, G., Vitols, S. & Ljunggren, J.G. (1996) Comparison of standardized initial doses of two antithyroid drugs in the treatment of Graves' disease. *J. intern. Med.*, **239**, 525–529

Kampmann, J.P. (1977) Pharmacokinetics of propylthiouracil in man after intravenous infusion. *J. Pharmacokinet. Biopharm.*, **5**, 435–443

Kampmann, J.P. & Skovsted, L. (1974) The pharmacokenetics of propylthiouracil. *Acta pharmacol. toxicol.*, **35**, 361–369

Kariya, K., Dawson, E. & Neal, R.A. (1983) Toxic effects of propylthiouracil in the rat. *Res. Commun. chem. Pathol. Pharmacol.*, **40**, 333–336

Kariya, K., Sawahate, T., Okuno, S. & Lee, E. (1986) Inhibition of hepatic glutathione transferases by propylthiouracil and its metabolites. *Biochem. Pharmacol.*, **35**, 1475–1479

King, D.W., Bock, F.G. & Moore, G.E. (1963) Dinitrophenol inhibition of pituitary adenoma formation in mice fed propylthiouracil. *Proc. Soc. exp. Biol. Med.*, **112**, 365–366

Kirby, J.D., Jetton, A.E., Cooke, P.S., Hess, R.A., Bunick, D., Ackland, J.F., Turek, F.W. & Schwartz, N.B. (1992) Developmental hormonal profiles accompanying the neonatal hypothyroidism-induced increase in adult testicular size and sperm production in the rat. *Endocrinology*, **131**, 559–565

Kirby, J.D., Arambepola, N., Porkka-Heiskanen, T., Kirby, Y.K., Rhoads, M.L., Nitta, H., Jetton, A.E., Iwamoto, G., Jackson, G.L., Turek, F.W. & Cooke, P.S. (1997) Neonatal hypothyroidism permanently alters follicle-stimulating hormone and luteinizing hormone production in the male rat. *Endocrinology*, **138**, 2713–2721

Kitahori, Y., Hiasa, Y., Konishi, N., Enoki, N., Shimoyama, T. & Miyashiro, A. (1984) Effect of propylthiouracil on the thyroid tumorigenesis induced by N-bis(2-hydroxypropyl)-nitrosamine in rats. *Carcinogenesis*, **5**, 657–660

Kodama, F., Fukushima, K. & Umeda, M. (1980) Chromosome aberrations induced by clinical medicines. *J. toxicol. Sci.*, **5**, 141–149

Krivánková, L., Krásensky, S. & Bocek, P. (1996) Application of capillary zone electrophoresis for analysis of thyreostatics. *Electrophoresis*, **17**, 1959–1963

Langer, P. & Gschwendtová, K. (1992) Immediate and dose–response related increase of biliary excretion of reverse triiodothyronine after propylthiouracil administration. *Exp. clin. Endocrinol.*, **99**, 18–20

Le Bizec, B., Monteau, F., Maume, D., Montrade, M.-P., Gade, C. & Andre, F. (1997) Detection and identification of thyreostats in the thyroid gland by gas chromatography–mass spectrometry. *Anal. chim. Acta*, **340**, 201–208

Leer, L.M., Cammenga, M. & De Vijlder, J.M. (1991) Methimazole and propylthiouracil increase thyroglobulin gene expression in FRTL-5 cells. *Mol. cell. Endocrinol.*, **82**, R25–R30

Lide, D.R. & Milne, G.W.A. (1996) *Properties of Organic Compounds*, Version 5.0, Boca Raton, FL, CRC Press [CD-ROM]

Lindsay, S., Nichols, C.W. & Chaikoff, I.L. (1966) Induction of benign and malignant thyroid neoplasms in the rat. *Arch. Pathol.*, **81**, 308–316

Lindsay, R.H., Hill, J.B., Kelly, K. & Vaughn, A. (1974) Excretion of propylthiouracil and its metabolites in rat bile and urine. *Endocrinology*, **94**, 1689–1698

Marchant, B., Alexander, W.D., Lazarus, J.H., Lees, J. & Clark, D.H. (1972) The accumulation of ^{35}S-antithyroid drugs by the thyroid gland. *J. clin. Endocrinol. Metab.*, **34**, 847–851

Marchant, B., Brownlie, B.E.W., McKay Hart, D., Horton, P.W. & Alexander, W.D. (1977) The placental transfer of propylthiouracil, methimazole and carbimazole. *J. clin. Endocrinol. Metab.*, **45**, 1187–1193

Martelli, A., Allavena, A. & Brambilla, G. (1992) Comparison of the DNA-damaging activity of 15 carcinogens in primary cultures of human and rat hepatocytes (Abstract). *Proc. Am. Assoc. Cancer Res.*, **33**, 178

Masiukiewicz, U.S. & Burrow, G.N. (1999) Hyperthyroidism in pregnancy: Diagnosis and treatment. *Thyroid*, **7**, 647–652

Medical Products Agency (2000) Uppsala

Medicines Control Agency (2000) London

Medicines Evaluation Board Agency (2000) The Hague

Melander, A., Wåhlin, E., Danielson, K. & Hanson, A. (1977) Bioavailability of propylthiouracil: Interindividual variation and influence of food intake. *Acta med. scand.*, **201**, 41–44

Mendis-Handagama, S.M.L.C. & Sharma, O.P. (1994) Effects of neonatal administration of the reversible goitrogen propylthiouracil on the testis interstitium in adult rats. *J. Reprod. Fertil.*, **100**, 85–92

Mendis-Handagama, S.M.L.C., Ariyaratne, H.B.S., Teunissen van Manen, K.R. & Haupt, R.L. (1998) Differential of adult Leydig cells in the neonatal rat testis is arrested by hypothyroidism. *Biol. Reprod.*, **59**, 351–357

Milmore, J.E., Chandrasekaran,V. & Weisburger, J.H. (1982) Effects of hypothyroidism on development of nitrosomethylurea-induced tumors of the mammary gland, thyroid gland, and other tissues. *Proc. Soc. exp. Biol. Med.*, **169**, 487–493

Momotani, N., Noh, J.Y., Ishikawa, N. & Ito, K. (1997) Effects of propylthiouracil and methimazole on fetal thyroid status in mothers with Graves' hyperthyroidism. *J. clin. Endocrinol. Metabol.*, **82**, 3633–3636

Momotani, N., Yamashita, R., Makino, F., Noh, J.Y., Ishikawa, N. & Ito, K. (2000) Thyroid function in wholly breast-feeding infants whose mothers take high doses of propylthiouracil. *Clin. Endocrinol.*, **53**, 177–181

Monaco, F., Santolamazza, C., De Ros, I. & Andreoli, A. (1980) Effects of propylthiouracil and methylmercaptoimidazole on thyroglobulin synthesis. *Acta endocrinol.*, **93**, 32–36

Moore, G.E., Brackney, E.L. & Bock, F.G. (1953) Production of pituitary tumors in mice by chronic administration of a thiouracil derivative. *Proc. Soc. exp. Biol. Med.*, **82**, 643–645

Moretti, G., Amici, M. & Cammarata, P. (1986) [Determination of methylthiouracil and analogous thyrostatics in animal tissues by HPLC after solid-phase purification.] *Riv. Soc. ital. Sci. aliment.*, **15**, 35–39 (in Italian)

Moretti, G., Amici, M., Cammarata, P. & Fracassi, F. (1988) Identification of thyrostatic drug residues in animal thyroids by high-performance thin-layer chromatography and fluorescence reaction detection. *J. Chromatogr.*, **442**, 459–463

Moretti, G., Betto, R., Cammarata, P., Fracassi, F., Giambenedetti, M. & Borghese, A. (1993) Determination of thyreostatic residues in cattle plasma by high-performance liquid chromatography with ultraviolet detection. *J. Chromatogr.*, **616**, 291–296

Mortimer, R.H., Cannell, G.R., Addison, R.S., Johnson, L.P., Roberts, M.S. & Bernus, I. (1997) Methimazole and propylthiouracil equally cross the perfused human term placental lobule. *J. clin. Endocrinol. Metab.*, **82**, 3099–3102

Mujtaba, Q. & Burrow, G.N. (1975) Treatment of hyperthyroidism in pregnancy with propyl-thiouracil and methimazole. *Obstet. Gynecol.*, **46**, 282–286

Nagasaka, A. & Hidaka, H. (1976) Effect of antithyroid agents 6-propyl-2-thiouracil and 1-methyl-2-mercaptoimidazole on human thyroid iodide peroxidase. *J. clin. Endocrinol. Metab.*, **43**, 152–158

Nakashima, T., Taurog, A. & Riesco, G. (1978) Mechanism of action of thioureylene anti-thyroid drugs: Factors affecting intrathyroidal metabolism of propylthiouracil and methi-mazole in rats. *Endocrinology*, **103**, 2187–2197

National Institute for Occupational Safety and Health (2000) *National Occupational Exposure Survey 1981–83*, Cincinnati, OH, Department of Health and Human Services, Public Health Service

Norwegian Medicinal Depot (2000) Oslo

Okamura, K., Ikenoue, H., Shiroozu, A., Sato, K., Yoshinari, M. & Fujishima, M. (1987) Reevaluation of the effects of methylmercaptoimidazole and propylthiouracil in patients with Graves' hyperthyroidism. *J. clin. Endocrinol. Metab.*, **65**, 719–723

Oppenheimer, J.H., Schwartz, H.L. & Surks, M.I. (1972) Propylthiouracil inhibits the conversion of L-thyroxine to L-triiodothyronine. *J. clin. Invest.*, **51**, 2493–2497

Orrego, H., Blake, J.E., Blendis, L.M., Compton, K.V. & Israel, Y. (1987) Long-term treatment of alcoholic liver disease with propylthiouracil. *New Engl. J. Med.*, **317**, 1421–1427

Orrego, H., Blake, J.E., Blendis, L.M., Compton, K.V., Volpe, R. & Israel, Y. (1994) Long-term treatment of alcoholic liver disease with propylthiouracil. Part 2: Influence of drop-out rates and of continued alcohol consumption in a clinical trial. *J. Hepatol.*, **20**, 343–349

Otten, M.H., Hennemann, G., Docter, R. & Visser, T.J. (1984) Metabolism of 3,3'-diiodothyronine in rat hepatocytes: Interaction of sulfation with deiodination. *Endocrinology*, **115**, 887–894

Pacini, F., Nakamura, H. & DeGroot, L.J. (1983) Effect of hypo- and hyperthyroidism on the balance between helper and suppressor T cells in rats. *Acta endocrinol.*, **103**, 528–534

Papapetrou, P.D., Marchant, B., Gavras, H. & Alexander, W.D. (1972) Biliary excretion of ^{35}S-labelled propylthiouracil, methimazole and carbimazole in untreated and pentobarbitone pretreated rats. *Biochem. Pharmacol.*, **21**, 363–377

Paynter, O.E., Burin, G.J., Jaeger, R.B. & Gregorio, C.A. (1988) Goitrogens and thyroid folli-cular cell neoplasia: Evidence for a threshold process. *Regul. Toxicol. Pharmacol.*, **8**, 102–119

Raheja, K.L., Linscherr, W.G., Chijiiwa, K. & Iba, M. (1985) Inhibitory effect of propyl-thiouracil-induced hypothyroidism in rat on oxidative drug metabolism. *Comp. Biochem. Physiol.*, **82C**, 17–19

Refetoff, S., Ochi, Y., Selenkow, H.A. & Rosenfield, R.L. (1974) Neonatal hypothyroidism and goiter in one infant of each of two sets of twins due to maternal therapy with antithyroid drugs. *Pediatr. Pharmacol. Ther.*, **85**, 240–244

Ringhand, H.P., Ritschel, W.A., Meyer, M.C., Straughn, A.B. & Hardt, T. (1980) Pharmaco-kinetics of propylthiouracil upon p.o. administration in man. *Int. J. clin. Pharmacol. Ther. Toxicol.*, **18**, 488–493

Rink, T., Wieg, C., Schroth, H., Helisch, A. & Bertram, U. (1999) [Hyperthyroidism in a pre-mature infant due to transplacental passage of maternal thyrotropin-receptor antibodies.] *Nuklearmedizin*, **38**, 156–159 (in German)

Rodriguez-Arnaiz, R. (1998) Biotransformation of several structurally related 2B compounds to reactive metabolites in the somatic *w/w+* assay of *Drosophila melanogaster*. *Environ. mol. Mutag.*, **31**, 390–401

Ron, E., Kleinerman, R.A., Boice, J.D., Jr, LiVolsi, V.A., Flannery, J.T. & Fraumeni, J.F., Jr (1987) A population-based case–control study of thyroid cancer. *J. natl Cancer Inst.*, **79**, 1–12

Ron, E., Doody, M.M., Becker, D.V., Brill, A.B., Curtis, R.E., Goldman, M.B., Harris, B.S.H., Hoffman, D.A., McConahey, W.M., Maxon, H.R., Preston-Martin, S., Warshauer, E., Wong, L. & Boice, J.D., Jr for the Cooperative Thyrotoxicosis Therapy Follow-up Study Group (1998) Cancer mortality following treatment for adult hyperthyroidism. *J. Am. med. Assoc.*, **280**, 347–355

Royal Pharmaceutical Society of Great Britain (2000) *Martindale, The Extra Pharmacopoeia*, 13th Ed., London, The Pharmaceutical Press [MicroMedex Online]

Saberi, M., Sterling, F.H. & Utiger, R.D. (1975) Reduction in extrathyroidal triiodothyronine production by propylthiouracil in man. *J. clin. Invest.*, **55**, 218–223

Sadtler Research Laboratories (1980) *Sadtler Standard Spectra, 1980 Cumulative Molecular Formula Index*, Philadelphia, PA, p. 171

Saldaña Monllor, L., Carbonell Martin, G. & Alonso Fuente, C. (1980) [*Thin-layer Chromatographic Separation and Identification of 2-Thiouracil, 4(6)-Methyl-2-thiouracil and 6(4)-Propyl-2-thiouracil in Feed Additives and Biological Materials by Thin-layer Chromatography.*], Madrid, Instituto Nacional de Investigationes Agrarias (in Spanish)

Salvati, S., Attorri, L., Campeggi, L.M., Olivieri, A., Sorcini, M., Fortuna, S. & Pintor, A. (1994) Effect of propylthiouracil-induced hypothyroidism on cerebral cortex of young and aged rats: Lipid composition of synaptosomes, muscarinic receptor sites, and acetyl-cholinesterase activity. *Neurochem. Res.*, **19**, 1181–1186

de Sandro, V., Chevrier, M., Boddaert, A., Melcion, C., Cordier, A. & Richert, L. (1991) Comparison of the effects of propylthiouracil, amiodarone, diphenylhydantoin, pheno-barbital, and 3-methylcholanthrene on hepatic and renal T4 metabolism and thyroid gland function in rats. *Toxicol. appl. Pharmacol.*, **111**, 263–278

Schalock, R.L., Brown, W.J. & Smith, R.L. (1977) Long term effects of propylthiouracil-induced neonatal hypothyroidism. *Dev. Psychobiol.*, **12**, 187–199

Sichuk, G., Money, W.L., Der, B.K. & Fortner, J.G. (1968) Cancer of the thyroid, goitrogenesis and thyroid function in Syrian (golden) hamsters. *Cancer*, **21**, 952–963

Siersbaek-Nielsen, K., Kirkegaard, C., Rogowski, R., Faber, J., Lumholtz, B. & Friis, T. (1978) Extrathyroidal effects of propylthiouracil and carbimazole on serum T_4, T_3, reverse T_3 and TRH-induced TSH-release in man. *Acta endocrinol.*, **87**, 80–87

Simorangkir, D.R., Wreford, N.G. & De Kretser, D.M. (1997) Impaired germ cell development in the testes of immature rats with neonatal hypothyroidism. *J. Androl.*, **18**, 186–193

Sitar, D.S. & Hunninghake, D.B. (1975) Pharmacokinetics of propylthiouracil in man after a single oral dose. *J. clin. Endocrinol. Metab.*, **26**, 26–29

Sitar, D.S. & Thornhill, D.P. (1972) Propylthiouracil: Absorption, metabolism and excretion in the albino rat. *J. Pharmacol. exp. Ther.*, **183**, 440–448

Sitar, D.S., Abu-Bakare, A., Gardiner, R.J. & Ogilvie, R.I. (1979) Effect of chronic therapy with propylthiouracil on its disposition in hyperthyroid patients. *Clin. invest. Med.*, **2**, 93–97

Slotkin, T.A., Seidler, F.J., Kavlock, R.J. & Bartolome, J.V. (1992) Thyroid hormone differentially regulates cellular development in neonatal rat heart and kidney. *Teratology*, **45**, 303–312

Society of Japanese Pharmacopoeia (1996) *The Japanese Pharmacopoeia JP XIII*, 13th Ed., Tokyo, pp. 597–598

Speight, J.W., Baba, W.I. & Wilson, G.M. (1968) Effect of propylthiouracil and ^{131}I on rat thyroid chromosomes. *J. Endocrinol.*, **42**, 267–275

Swiss Pharmaceutical Society, ed. (2000) *Index Nominum, International Drug Directory*, 16th Ed., Stuttgart, Medpharm Scientific Publishers [MicroMedex Online]

Szybalski, W. (1958) Special microbiological systems. II. Observations on chemical mutagenesis in microorganisms. *Ann. N.Y. Acad. Sci.*, **76**, 475–489

Takayama, S., Aihara, K., Onodera, T. & Akimoto, T. (1986) Antithyroid effects of propylthiouracil and sulfamonomethoxine in rats and monkeys. *Toxicol. appl. Pharmacol.*, **82**, 191–199

Taurog, A. & Dorris, M.L. (1988) Propylthiouracil and methimazole display contrasting pathways of peripheral metabolism in both rat and human. *Endocrinology*, **122**, 592–601

Taurog, A., Dorris, M.L., Guziec, F.S., Jr & Uetrecht, J.P. (1989) Metabolism of [35]S- and ^{14}C-labeled propylthiouracil in a model in vitro system containing thryoid peroxidase. *Endocrinology*, **124**, 3030–3037

Teerds, K.J., de Rooij, D.G., de Jong, F.H. & van Haaster, L.H. (1998) Development of the adult-type Leydig cell population in the rat is affected by neonatal thyroid hormone levels. *Biol. Reprod.*, **59**, 344–350

Thrift, T.A., Bernal, A., Lewis, A.W., Neuendorff, D.A., Willard, C.C. & Randel, R.D. (1999) Effects of induced hypothyroidism on weight gains, lactation, and reproductive performance of primiparous Brahman cows. *J. Anim. Sci.*, **77**, 1844–1850

US Pharmacopeial Convention (1999) *The 2000 US Pharmacopeia*, 24th rev./*The National Formulary*, 19th rev., Rockville, MD, pp. 1436, 2288

Van der Klauw, M.M., Wilson, J.H. & Stricker, B.H. (1998) Drug-associated agranulocytosis: 20 years of reporting in The Netherlands (1974–1994). *Am. J. Hematol.*, **57**, 206–211

Van Haaster, L.H., De Jong, F.H., Docter, R. & De Rooij, D.G. (1992) The effect of hypothyroidism on Sertoli cell proliferation and differentiation and hormone levels during testicular development in the rat. *Endocrinology*, **131**, 1574–1576

Vargas, G., Havel, J. & Frgalová, K. (1998) Capillary zone electrophoresis determination of thyreostatic drugs in urine. *J. Capillary Electrophor.*, **5**, 9–12

Waldhauser, L. & Uetrecht, J. (1991) Oxidation of propylthiouracil to reactive metabolites by activated neurophils. *Drug Metab. Disposition*, **19**, 354–359

Westgren, U., Melander, A., Wåhlin, E. & Lindgren, J. (1977) Divergent effects of 6-propylthiouracil on 3,5,3'-triiodothyronine (T_3) and 3,3',5'-triiodothyronine (RT_3) serum levels in man. *Acta endocrinol.*, **85**, 345–350

Wilkie, D. & Gooneskera, S. (1980) The yeast mitochondrial system in carcinogen testing. *Chem. Ind.*, **21**, 847–850

Williams, K.V., Nayak, S., Becker, D., Reyes, J. & Burmeister, L.A. (1997) Fifty years of experience with propylthiouracil-associated hepatotoxicity: What have we learned? *J. clin. Endocrinol. Metab.*, **82**, 1727–1733

Willis, J. (1961) The induction of malignant neoplasms in the thyroid gland of the rat. *J. Pathol. Bacteriol.*, **82**, 23–27

Wilson, M.J., Kirby, J.D., Zhato, Y., Sinha, A.A. & Cooke, P.S. (1997) Neonatal hypothyroidism alters the pattern of prostatic growth and differentiation, as well as plasminogen activator and metalloprotease expression, in the rat. *Biol. Reprod.*, **56**, 475–482

Yamada, T., Koizumi, Y. & Kojima, A. (1976) An increase of liver uptake of thyroxine, an initial step of an increased fecal loss of thyroxine in response to propylthiouracil in rats. *Arch. int. Pharmacodyn.*, **224**, 21–29

Yamada, T., Chopra, I.J. & Kaplowitz, N. (1981) Inhibition of rat hepatic thyroxine 5'-monodeiodinase by propylthiouracil: Relation to site of interaction of thyroxine and glutathione. *J. Endocrinol. Invest.*, **4**, 379–387

Yu, G.Y.F., Murby, E.J. & Wells, R.J. (1997) Gas chromatographic determination of residues of thyreostatic drugs in bovine muscle tissue using combined resin mediated methylation and extraction. *J. Chromatogr.*, **B703**, 159–166

Zimmerman, L.M., Shubik, P., Baserga, R., Ritchie, A.C. & Jacques, L. (1954) Experimental production of thyroid tumors by alternating hyperplasia and involution. *J. clin. Endocrinol.*, **14**, 1367–1373

THIOURACIL

This substance was considered by previous working groups, in 1974 (IARC, 1974) and 1987 (IARC, 1987). Since that time, new data have become available, and these have been incorporated into the monograph and taken into consideration in the present evaluation.

1. Exposure Data

1.1 Chemical and physical data

1.1.1 *Nomenclature*

Chem. Abstr. Serv. Reg. No.: 141-90-2
Deleted CAS Reg. Nos: 156-82-1; 4401-53-0; 4401-54-1; 107646-88-8; 107646-89-9
Chem. Abstr. Name: 2,3-Dihydro-2-thioxo-4(1*H*)-pyrimidinone
IUPAC Systematic Name: 2-Thiouracil
Synonyms: 4-Hydroxy-2-mercaptopyrimidine; 6-hydroxy-2-mercaptopyrimidine; 4-hydroxy-2-pyrimidinethiol; 2-mercapto-4-hydroxypyrimidine; 2-mercapto-4-pyrimidinol; 2-mercapto-4-pyrimidinone

1.1.2 *Structural and molecular formulae and relative molecular mass*

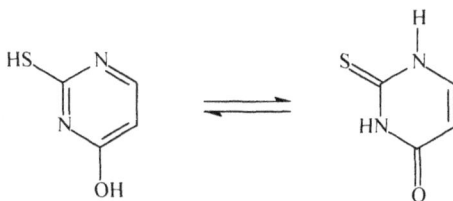

$C_4H_4N_2OS$ Relative molecular mass: 128.15

1.1.3   Chemical and physical properties of the pure substance

(a) *Description*: Prisms from water or ethanol (Lide & Milne, 1996)

(b) *Melting-point*: > 340 °C (decomposes) (Lide & Milne, 1996)

(c) *Spectroscopy data*: Infrared [prism (9400), grating (29954)], ultraviolet (2508), nuclear magnetic resonance [proton (9191)] and mass spectral data have been reported (Sadtler Research Laboratories, 1980; Lide & Milne, 1996).

(d) *Solubility*: Slightly soluble in water and ethanol; soluble in anhydrous hydrofluoric acid and alkaline solutions (Lide & Milne, 1996; Budavari, 2000)

1.1.4   Technical products and impurities

Trade names for thiouracil include Antagothyroil, Deracil and Nobilen.

1.1.5   Analysis

Methods have been reported for the analysis of thiouracil in biological fluids (blood, milk, serum, urine), tissues, incubation material, dried animal feed, feed additives and drugs. The methods include potentiometric titration, capillary zone electrophoresis with ultraviolet detection, flow injection analysis with chemiluminescent detection, micellar electrokinetic chromatography, thin-layer chromatography, high-performance thin-layer chromatography, high-performance liquid chromatography (HPLC) with atmospheric pressure chemical ionization mass spectrometry, reversed-phase HPLC with ultraviolet and electrochemical detection and gas chromatography with negative-ion chemical-ionization mass spectrometry (Saldaña Monllor *et al.*, 1980; Moretti *et al.*, 1986; Hooijerink & De Ruig, 1987; Moretti *et al.*, 1988; Centrich Escarpenter & Rubio Hernández, 1990; Watson *et al.*, 1991; De Brabander *et al.*, 1992; López García *et al.*, 1993; Moretti *et al.*, 1993; Vinas *et al.*, 1993; Batjoens *et al.*, 1996; Krivánková *et al.*, 1996; Blanchflower *et al.*, 1997; Le Bizec *et al.*, 1997; Yu *et al.*, 1997; Buick *et al.*, 1998; Vargas *et al.*, 1998; Esteve-Romero *et al.*, 1999; Ciesielski & Zakrzewski, 2000).

1.2   Production

Thiouracil can be prepared by condensing ethyl formylacetate with thiourea (Budavari, 2000).

Information available in 2000 indicated that thiouracil was manufactured by six companies in China and one company in Switzerland (CIS Information Services, 2000).

1.3   Use

Thiouracil was introduced in 1943 as the first thionamide anti-thyroid drug. The usual dose was 1–2 g/day in divided doses. Owing to a high frequency of adverse reactions, especially agranulocytosis, its use was abandoned in favour of other, less toxic drugs, such as propylthiouracil and methimazole (see monographs in this volume). Thiouracil is not currently used as a thyrostatic drug in humans (Astwood & VanderLaan, 1945; Stanley & Astwood, 1949).

Thiouracil also has been reported to be used as a chemical intermediate (IARC, 1974) and in metal plating.

1.4   Occurrence

1.4.1   *Occupational exposure*

According to the 1981–83 National Occupational Exposure Survey (National Institute for Occupational Safety and Health, 2000), about 1800 technicians and metal-plating machine operators working in the manufacture of instruments and related products were potentially exposed to thiouracil in the USA.

1.4.2   *Environmental occurrence*

Thiouracil occurs in seeds of Brassica and Cruciferae (Budavari, 2000).

1.5   Regulations and guidelines

No data were available to the Working Group.

2.   Studies of Cancer in Humans

No information was available specifically on thiouracil.

2.1   Cohort studies

Dobyns *et al.* (1974) followed up 34 684 patients treated in England and the USA for hyperthyroidism between 1946 and 1964, 1238 of whom had been treated for at least 1 year with unspecified anti-thyroid drugs. No malignant thyroid neoplasm was found within 1 year of treatment. By 1968, more cases of thyroid neoplasm were found at follow-up among patients initially treated with anti-thyroid drugs (4 malignant tumours and 18 adenomas in 1238 patients) than among those initially treated with ^{131}I (19 malignant tumours and 41 adenomas in 21 714 patients) or (partial) thyroidectomy (4 malignant tumours and 14 adenomas in 11 732 patients). The authors suggested that more neoplasms were found in the drug-treated patients because subsequent thyroidectomy was more frequent in this group (30% of drug-treated patients, as compared with 0.5% of those initially treated with ^{131}I and 1.2% of those treated with primary thyroidectomy), which provided more opportunity for identification of neoplasms. [The Working Group noted that rates could not be calculated because person–years were not provided, and the ages of the groups were not given.]

Ron *et al.* (1998) updated the report of Dobyns *et al.* (1974) and followed-up 35 593 patients treated for hyperthyroidism between 1946 and 1964 in 25 clinics in the USA and one in the United Kingdom. By December 1990, about 19% had been lost to follow-up, and 50.5% of the study cohort had died. A total of 1374 patients (1094 women) had been treated with anti-thyroid drugs only, 10 439 (7999 women) with ^{131}I and drugs, 10 381 (8465 women) with thyroidectomy and drugs, 2661 (2235 women) with a combination of the three types of treatment and the remainder by other means. The drugs used during the study period were chiefly thiourea derivatives and iodine compounds. One year or more after the start of the study, the standardized mortality ratio (SMR) in comparison with the general population for the patients treated with anti-thyroid drugs only was 1.3 (95% confidence interval [CI], 1.1–1.6) for deaths from all cancers, which was chiefly due to significantly more deaths from oral cancer (4.2; 95% CI, 1.3–9.7; five cases) and brain tumours (3.7; 95% CI, 1.2–8.6; five cases). The excess risk for death from brain cancer persisted after exclusion of cases prevalent at the time of entry into the study. No deaths from thyroid carcinoma were recorded. The SMR for all cancers was approximately 1.0 in patients treated with ^{131}I or surgery (with or without anti-thyroid drugs), but the SMR for thyroid cancer was fourfold higher (3.9; 95% CI, 2.5–5.9; 24 cases observed) among patients who had been treated with ^{131}I with or without drugs. The authors noted that the group treated with drugs only was small; the type, quantity and dates of drug use were generally not available; and many patients had cancer before entry into the study, suggesting that some, but not all, of the excess could be attributed to the selection of patients with health problems for drug therapy. [The Working Group noted that the expected number of deaths from thyroid carcinomas was not reported, although it would almost certainly have been less than 1.0. Results were given separately for patients treated only with drugs and not for those given drugs with other treatment.]

2.2   Case–control studies

Ron *et al.* (1987) conducted a study of 159 cases of thyroid cancer and 285 population controls in Connecticut, USA, between 1978 and 1980. The use of anti-thyroid medications was not associated with an increased risk [relative risks not shown].

In a study carried out in northern Sweden between 1980 and 1989, 180 cases of thyroid cancer and 360 population controls were evaluated (Hallquist *et al.*, 1994). Use of anti-thyroid drugs (two cases and two controls) was associated with a relative risk of 2.0 (95% CI, 0.2–21).

3.   Studies of Cancer in Experimental Animals

Thiouracil was evaluated in a previous monograph (IARC, 1974). Because there have been no new studies on its carcinogenicity in animals, the most relevant studies from the previous monograph were analysed in greater depth. One study in which thiouracil was administered with a known carcinogen which had been published since the previous evaluation is summarized. Studies on the carcinogenicity of anti-thyroid chemicals, including thiouracil, in experimental animals have been reviewed (Doniach, 1970; Christov & Raichev, 1972; Paynter *et al.*, 1988).

3.1   Oral administration

Mouse: Groups of 28 A, 29 C57 and 24 I mice [sex unspecified], 1–3 months of age, were fed diets containing thiouracil [purity not specified] at a concentration of 0.1% for various periods up to 81 weeks. Groups of 36 untreated A, 51 untreated C57 and 35 untreated I mice served as controls. In 69 treated mice of all three strains examined at various intervals, the author described thyroid follicular-cell hyperplasia from 40 days of treatment, which developed into follicular cystic or nodular lesions after 180 days. The author interpreted these lesions as non-malignant. In seven treated A strain mice, pulmonary foci very similar to the hyperplastic thyroid tissue were present (Gorbman, 1947). [The Working Group considered that, under current histopathological criteria, the thyroid and pulmonary lesions described in the study might be diagnosed as thyroid neoplasia and metastases of thyroid neoplasia.]

A total of 143 female C3H mice, approximately 10 weeks of age, were divided into two approximately equal groups; one was fed basal diet and served as controls, and the other received thiouracil in the diet at an initial concentration of 0.375%, increased later to 0.5%. The animals were killed at selected intervals or when moribund. The authors described the development of thyroid follicular-cell hyperplasia in treated mice during the first 12 months of the study but diagnosed no neoplasia. However, 10/23 mice treated for 362–464 days developed pulmonary metastases of thyroid tissue, which were interpreted by the authors as 'benign metastasizing thyroid tissue' (Dalton *et al.*, 1948). [The Working Group noted that, under current histopathological criteria, the pulmonary lesions might be regarded as metastases of thyroid neoplasia.]

Groups of male and female C3H mice and an inbred strain designated TM [initial numbers not specified], 1 month of age, were fed a diet containing 0.3% thiouracil [purity not specified] for 17 months. Thiouracil produced 'hepatomas' in 12/13 male and 14/16 female C3H mice but not in 22 male or 22 female TM mice. In the control groups, hepatomas occurred in 2/32 male and 0/24 female C3H mice and in 0/20 male and 0/20 female TM mice (Casas, 1963).

Rat: Groups of 6–20 male and 7–15 female Stanford albino rats, of an average age of 55 and 45 days, respectively, were fed diets containing thiouracil [purity not specified] at a concentration of 0.1% for various periods from 120 up to 312 days. Nodular hyperplasia (solitary or multiple nodules) of the thyroid was observed in 20/56 male rats examined at 169 days and in 17/55 female rats examined at 120 days. The nodular lesions were considered by the author to be benign (Laqueur, 1949). [The Working Group noted the lack of a control group.]

In a study of the combined effects of thiouracil and 2-acetylaminofluorene on the thyroid gland, 20 male and female Sherman strain rats, weighing 75–100 g [age not specified], were given thiouracil [purity not specified] in the drinking-water at a concentration of 0.05 or 0.1% for 245–884 days. Thyroid tumours occurred in 12/20 rats [not separated on the basis of dose], 11 of which had adenomas and one a carcinoma. In the group receiving thiouracil and 0.03% 2-acetylaminofluorene in the diet simultaneously and killed after only 22–45 weeks, the incidences of thyroid follicular-cell adenomas and carcinomas were 28/28 and 5/28, respectively (Paschkis et al., 1948). [The Working Group noted that there was no untreated control group.]

A group of 35 male Sprague-Dawley rats, weighing on average 61 g [age not specified], was given thiouracil [purity not specified] in the drinking-water at a concentration of 0.2% for 24 months. A control group of 25 males was available. Two rats from each group were killed at 6, 14 and 18 months, and the remaining 26 treated and 17 control rats were killed at 2 years. Thyroid adenomas were diagnosed in approximately 65% of the treated rats, but the tumour incidence in the control group was not reported (Clausen, 1954). [The Working Group noted the limited information provided in the report.]

In a complex study of carcinogen interactions in various target organs, groups of 23–24 male and female Fischer 344 rats [age not specified] were fed diets containing thiouracil ['checked for purity'] at a concentration of 83, 250 or 750 mg/kg for 104 weeks. A control group comprised 214 male and 214 female rats. At 725 days, the numbers of survivors were 191/214, 19/24, 21/24 and 4/24 males at 0, 83, 250 and 750 mg/kg, respectively, and 184/214, 21/23, 18/24 and 17/24 females, respectively. The incidences of malignant thyroid follicular-cell tumours over the study period were 5/214, 6/24, 14/24 and 5/24 males and 5/214, 2/23, 6/24 and 18/24 females in the four groups, respectively. No malignant liver or kidney tumours were found (Fears et al., 1989).

3.2 Administration with known carcinogens

Gerbil: Groups of 20 male and 11 female gerbils [age not specified but stated as equal across groups] were given diets containing thiouracil [purity not specified] at a concentration of 0.2% in combination with a subcutaneous injection of 23 mg/kg bw N-nitrosodiethylamine (NDEA) once a week for life. Additional groups of 20 males and 19 females received NDEA only, and 12 males and 12 females received the thiouracil diet only; a vehicle control group of 11 males and 10 females received 0.9% saline only. The average survival times were 37 weeks for males and 24 weeks for females given NDEA only, 54 weeks for males and 45 weeks for females given NDEA plus thiouracil,

79 weeks for males and 81 weeks for females given thiouracil only and 80 weeks for males and 69 weeks for females given saline. Thiouracil given in conjunction with NDEA inhibited the development of cholangiocarcinomas induced by NDEA alone, the incidences being 17/20 males and 16/19 females given NDEA only and 0/20 males and 0/11 females given NDEA plus thiouracil. Some cholangiomas were also observed, the incidences being 0/20 males and 0/19 females given NDEA only and 13/20 males and 4/11 females given NDEA plus thiouracil. The incidence of nasal cavity adenocarcinomas induced by NDEA was not influenced by thiouracil, and no tumours of any type were observed in the group given thiouracil alone (Green & Ketkar, 1978).

4. Other Data Relevant to an Evaluation of Carcinogenicity and its Mechanisms

4.1 Absorption, distribution, metabolism and excretion

4.1.1 *Humans*

No data were available to the Working Group.

4.1.2 *Experimental systems*

In male Sprague-Dawley rats given a single intraperitoneal injection of 5 mg of [^{35}S]thiouracil, thyroid accumulation of the label began at 4 h and reached a peak at 10 h. The concentration gradient between thyroid tissue and plasma was 7.5 at 10 h and 156 after 48 h. Five ^{35}S-labelled compounds were detected in the thyroid by thin-layer chromatography: [^{35}S]sulfate, protein-bound ^{35}S, unmetabolized thiouracil and two unidentified metabolites (Lees *et al.*, 1973). Accumulation of [^{35}S]thiouracil in the thyroid of rats was also reported by Marchant *et al.* (1972).

Rapid placental transfer of [^{14}C]thiouracil was demonstrated in rabbits given a single intravenous injection of 0.01–0.03 mmol [1.3–3.8 mg] on days 31–33 of gestation and in dogs injected with a dose of 0.05 mmol [6.4 mg] on days 61–63 of gestation. An equilibrium was reached between maternal and fetal blood within 30 min, but the concentrations in maternal and fetal thyroid increased for 3 and 6 h after treatment in rabbits and dogs, respectively. The radiolabel in the fetal thyroid appeared to be associated with the parent compound (Quinones *et al.*, 1972).

After intraperitoneal injection of [^{14}C]thiouracil to pregnant Sprague-Dawley rats on day 10, 12, 14, 17 or 20 of gestation, placental transfer was found at all stages but was most pronounced at late stages of gestation (Sabbagha & Hayashi, 1969).

Autoradiographic analysis of the fate of about 0.07 mg of [^{14}C]thiouracil injected intravenously into pregnant NMRI mice in a late stage of gestation [gestational age not indicated] revealed accumulation in the fetal thyroid (Slanina *et al.*, 1973).

4.2   Toxic effects

4.2.1   *Humans*

When thiouracil was used as an anti-thyroid drug, a high frequency of adverse reactions was seen (VanderLaan & Storrie, 1955), including agranulocytosis.

4.2.2   *Experimental systems*

Thiouracil increased the iodide content of the salivary glands and decreased that of the thyroid of white male rats [strain not specified] fed a diet containing 0.035% thiouracil for 3 months (Hassanein & Almallah, 1978).

Male Fischer rats fed a low-iodine diet containing 0.25% thiouracil developed hyperplasia of the thyroid gland within 3 days, and the capsule of the gland increased to a substantial multilayered structure (Wollmann & Herveg, 1978).

Enlargement of the adipose tissue pads on the thyroid of male Fischer rats during ingestion of a diet containing 0.25% thiouracil for 10 days was probably due to an elevated concentration of circulating thyroid-stimulating hormone and not to a direct effect of thiouracil (Smeds & Wollman, 1983).

4.3   Reproductive and developmental effects

4.3.1   *Humans*

No data were available to the Working Group.

4.3.2   *Experimental systems*

Perinatal thyroid deficiency induced by thiouracil (2 mg/kg of diet) given to pregnant rats [strain not specified] during the last 15 days of gestation and the first 15 days after parturition caused a chronic hypermetabolic state in both male and female offspring. In female rats, a mild hyperthyroid condition occasionally persisted (Davenport & Hennies, 1976).

The adrenal weights of 15-day-old Sprague-Dawley rats made hypothyroid by administration of 0.25% thiouracil in the diet of dams from the day of conception through lactation were reduced by 23%, but they showed no change in adrenal corticosterone secretion or corticosterone secretion per milligram of adrenal tissue. The corticotropin-releasing factor-like activity of the median eminence was reduced (Meserve & Pearlmutter, 1983). A similar response was observed in genetically hypothyroid (*hyt/hyt*) mice born to heterozygous dams, but the effect was not apparent until 30 days of age, i.e. after weaning, suggesting a role of maternal thyroid hormones in the maintenance of hypothalamic corticotropin-releasing factor (Meserve, 1987). A time-course study of corticosterone release after corticosterone stimulation in 15-day-old Sprague-Dawley rats made hypothyroid by dietary exposure of the dams to 0.25%

thiouracil from conception indicated that the hypothalamic response was attenuated and not ablated (Meserve & Juárez de Ku, 1993).

4.4   Effects on enzyme induction or inhibition and gene expression

4.4.1   *Humans*

No data were available to the Working Group.

4.4.2   *Experimental systems*

In male CD rats given an intraperitoneal injection of 10–50 mg/kg bw thiouracil, in the absence of oxidizable substrates, irreversible inhibition of thyroid iodide peroxidase occurred. When iodine or thiocyanate was present, the inhibition was prevented, suggesting that the initial action of thiouracil is to block iodination by trapping oxidized iodide (Davidson *et al.*, 1978).

Female Sprague-Dawley rats fed a diet containing 0.2% thiouracil for 14 days had increased (approximately threefold) NADH duroquinone (2,3,5,6-tetramethyl-1,4-benzoquinone) reductase activity and decreased (by ~ 20%) α-glycerophosphate de-hydrogenase activity compared with controls (Ruzicka & Rose, 1981).

Chopra *et al.* (1982) studied the structure–activity relationships of the inhibition of hepatic monodeiodination of thyroxine to triiodothyronine by thiouracil and other related compounds in liver homogenates from male Sprague-Dawley rats. The results suggested that the thiourea moiety is insufficient to inhibit the conversion.

In rat liver microsomal systems, thiouracil at 0.5 or 1 μmol/L [64 or 128 μg/L] was a non-competitive inhibitor with respect to substrate and a competitive inhibitor with respect to cofactors of iodothyronine-5′-deiodinase (Visser, 1979). Inactivation of iodo-thyronine-5′-deiodinase by thiouracil required a substrate (Visser & van Overmeeren-Kaptein, 1981).

Thiouracil inhibited peroxidase in a microsomal preparation from the gastric mucosa of male Swiss mice (Banerjee & Datta, 1981).

4.5   Genetic and related effects

4.5.1   *Humans*

No data were available to the Working Group.

4.5.2   *Experimental systems* (see Table 1 for reference)

Thiouracil did not induce DNA strand breaks in cultured mammalian cells in the only study in which thiouracil was tested alone for genotoxicity.

Table 1. Genetic and related effects of thiouracil

Test system	Result[a]		Dose[b] (LED/HID)	Reference
	Without exogenous metabolic system	With exogenous metabolic system		
DNA strand breaks, L5178Y mouse lymphoma cells *in vitro*	–	NT	1282	Garberg *et al.* (1988)

[a] –, negative; NT, not tested
[b] LED, lowest effective dose; HID, highest ineffective dose; in-vitro tests, µg/mL

Irradiation of *Escherichia coli recA⁻* cells in the presence of thiouracil resulted in greater cytotoxicity than in wild-type or *uvrA⁻* cells. Furthermore, thiouracil enhanced the incidence of mutations induced by ultraviolet A irradiation in *E. coli uvrA⁻*, but not *recA⁻* cells, while irradiation of *Salmonella* cells with ultraviolet A in the presence of thiouracil led to increased expression of *umuDC* (Komeda *et al.*, 1997). Thiouracil enhanced the DNA-strand breaking effect of 334-nm ultraviolet radiation in purified bacterial DNA (Peak *et al.*, 1984).

4.6 Mechanistic considerations

Thiouracil belongs to a class of drugs used in the treatment of hyperthyroidism which act by interfering with thyroid peroxidase functioning, thus decreasing thyroid hormone production and increasing proliferation by increasing the concentration of thyroid-stimulating hormone. This is the probable basis of the tumorigenic activity of thiouracil in the thyroid of experimental animals.

The lack of adequate data on genotoxicity for thiouracil precludes a conclusion regarding the mechanism of carcinogenicity.

5. Summary of Data Reported and Evaluation

5.1 Exposure data

Thiouracil was used briefly in the 1940s as the first thionamide anti-thyroid drug.

5.2 Human carcinogenicity studies

No epidemiological data on use of thiouracil and cancer were found. However, two analyses were published of one cohort study conducted in the United Kingdom and the USA of the cancer risk of patients, mainly women, with hyperthyroidism who had been treated with anti-thyroid drugs. The earlier analysis showed more malignant thyroid neoplasms in patients receiving these drugs than in those treated with surgery or ^{131}I, but the excess may have been due to closer surveillance of the patients given drugs owing to more frequent use of thyroidectomy. In the later analysis, patients with hyperthyroidism treated only with anti-thyroid drugs had a modest increase in the risk for death from cancer, due chiefly to oral cancer and cancer of the brain. Neither report provided information on the type, quantity or dates of anti-thyroid drug use.

Two case–control studies of cancer of the thyroid showed no significant association with treatment with anti-thyroid medications.

5.3   Animal carcinogenicity data

Several early studies in mice showed that oral administration of thiouracil induced nodular thyroid follicular-cell hyperplasia, including some pulmonary metastases suggestive of thyroid neoplasia by current histopathological criteria. In one study in one strain of mice, thiouracil produced hepatocellular tumours. In one adequate study in rats, thiouracil produced thyroid follicular-cell adenomas and carcinomas. In one study in gerbils, thiouracil inhibited the progression of *N*-nitrosodiethylamine-induced cholangiomas into cholangiocarcinomas.

5.4   Other relevant data

Little is known about the disposition of thiouracil in humans. In rats and fetal rats, thiouracil accumulated in the thyroid. Thiouracil acts by inhibiting thyroid peroxidase, thus decreasing thyroid hormone production, and it increases proliferation by increasing the secretion of thyroid-stimulating hormone. This is the probable basis of its tumo-rigenic activity in the thyroid of experimental animals.

No data were available on the developmental or reproductive effects of thiouracil in humans. The only studies in experimental animals indicated altered adrenal function in young rats made hypothyroidal from birth.

In the only study in which thiouracil was tested for genotoxicity, it did not induce DNA strand breaks in cultured mammalian cells. It has not been tested for mutageni-city or clastogenicity.

5.5   Evaluation

There is *inadequate evidence* in humans for the carcinogenicity of thiouracil.

There is *sufficient evidence* in experimental animals for the carcinogenicity of thiouracil.

Overall evaluation

Thiouracil is *possibly carcinogenic to humans (Group 2B)*.

6.   References

Astwood, E.B. & VanderLaan, W.P. (1945) Thiouracil derivatives of greater activity for the treatment of hyperthyroidism. *J. clin. Endocrinol.*, **5**, 424–430

Banerjee, R.K. & Datta, A.J. (1981) Gastric peroxidase — Localization, catalytic properties and possible role in extrathyroidal thyroid hormone formation. *Acta endocrinol.*, **96**, 208–214

Batjoens, P., De Brabander, H.F. & De Wasch, K. (1996) Rapid and high-performance analysis of thyreostatic drug residues in urine using gas chromatography–mass spectrometry. *J. Chromatogr.*, **A750**, 127–132

Blanchflower, W.J., Hughes, P.J., Cannavan, A., McCoy, M. & Kennedy, D.G. (1997) Determination of thyreostats in thyroid and urine using high-performance liquid chromatography–atmospheric pressure chemical ionization mass spectrometry. *Analyst*, **122**, 967–972

Budavari, S., ed. (2000) *The Merck Index*, 12th Ed., Version 12:3, Whitehouse Station, NJ, Merck & Co. & Boca Raton, FL, Chapman & Hall/CRC [CD-ROM]

Buick, R.K., Barry, C., Traynor, I.M., McCaughey, W.J. & Elliott, C.T. (1998) Determination of thyreostat residues from bovine matrices using high-performance liquid chromatography. *J. Chromatogr.*, **B720**, 71–79

Casas, C.B. (1963) Induction of hepatomas by thiouracil in inbred strains of mice. *Proc. Soc. exp. Biol. Med.*, **113**, 493–494

Centrich Escarpenter, F. & Rubio Hernández, D. (1990) Analysis of thyrostatics in the thyroid glands by thin layer chromatography and HPLC–UV. *An. Bromatol.*, **42**, 337–344

Chopra, I.J., Teco, G.N.C., Eisenberg, J.B., Wiersinga, W.M. & Solomon, D.H. (1982) Structure–activity relationships of inhibition of hepatic monodeiodination of thyroxine to 3,5,3'-triiodothyronine by thiouracil and related compounds. *Endrocrinology*, **110**, 163–168

Christov, K. & Raichev, R. (1972) Experimental thyroid carcinogenesis. *Curr. Top. Pathol.*, **56**, 79–114

Ciesielski, W. & Zakrzewski, R. (2000) Iodimetric determination of 2-thiouracils. *Chem. Anal.*, **45**, 135–144

CIS Information Services (2000) *Directory of World Chemical Producers (Version 2000.1)*, Dallas, TX [CD-ROM]

Clausen, H.J. (1954) Experimental production of struma fibrosa. *Arch. Pathol.*, **58**, 222–226

Dalton, A.J., Morris, H.P. & Dubnick, C.S. (1948) Morphologic changes in the organs of female C3H mice after long-term ingestion of thiourea and thiouracil. *J. natl Cancer Inst.*, **9**, 201–223

Davenport, J.W. & Hennies, R.S. (1976) Perinatal hypothyroidism in rats: Persistent motivational and metabolic effects. *Dev. Psychobiol.*, **9**, 67–82

Davidson, B., Soodak, M., Neary, J.T., Strout, H.V., Kieffer, J.D., Mover, H. & Maloof, F. (1978) The irreversible inactivation of thyroid peroxidase by methylmercaptoimidazole, thiouracil, and propylthiouracil *in vitro* and its relationship to in vivo findings. *Endocrinology*, **103**, 871–882

De Brabander, H.F., Batjoens, P. & Van Hoof, J. (1992) Determination of thyreostatic drugs by HPTLC with confirmation by GC–MS. *J. planar Chromatogr.*, **5**, 124–30

Dobyns, B.M., Sheline, G.E., Workman, J.B., Tompkins, E.A., McConahey, W.M. & Becker, D.V. (1974) Malignant and benign neoplasms of the thyroid in patients treated for hyperthyroidism: A report of the Cooperative Thyrotoxicosis Therapy Follow-up Study. *J. clin. Endocrinol. Metab.*, **38**, 976–998

Doniach, I. (1970) Experimental thyroid tumours. In: Smithers, D., ed., *Neoplastic Disease at Various Sites*, Vol. 6, *Tumours of the Thyroid Gland*, Edinburgh, E. & S. Livingstone, pp. 73–99

Esteve-Romero, J., Escrig-Tena, I., Simo-Alfonso, E.F. & Ramis-Ramos, G. (1999) Determination of thyreostatics in animal feed by micellar electrokinetic chromatography. *Analyst*, **124**, 125–128

Fears, T.R., Elashoff, R.M. & Schneiderman, M.A. (1989) The statistical analysis of a carcinogen mixture experiment. III. Carcinogens with different target systems, aflatoxin B$_1$, *N*-butyl-*N*-(4-hydroxybutyl)nitrosamine, lead acetate, and thiouracil. *Toxicol. ind. Health*, **5**, 1–22

Garberg, P., Akerblom, E.-L. & Bolcsfoldi, G. (1988) Evaluation of a genotoxicity test measuring DNA-strand breaks in mouse lymphoma cells by alkaline unwinding and hydroxyapatite elution. *Mutat. Res.*, **203**, 155–176

Gorbman, A. (1947) Thyroidal and vascular changes in mice following chronic treatment with goitrogens and carcinogens. *Cancer Res.*, **7**, 746–758

Green, U. & Ketkar, M. (1978) The influence of diazepam and thiouracil upon the carcinogenic effect of diethylnitrosamine in gerbils. *Z. Krebsforsch.*, **92**, 55–62

Hallquist, A., Hardell, L., Degerman, A. & Boquist, L. (1994) Thyroid cancer: Reproductive factors, previous diseases, drug intake, family history and diet. A case–control study. *Eur. J. Cancer Prev.*, **3**, 481–488

Hassanein, R.R. & Almallah, A.K. (1978) The effect of antithyroid and iodide compounds on the iodide content of both thyroid and salivary glands of rats. *Zbl. vet. Med. A.*, **25**, 241–246

Hooijerink, H. & De Ruig, W.G. (1987) Determination of thyreostatics in meat by reversed-phase liquid chromatography with ultraviolet and electrochemical detection. *J. Chromatogr.*, **394**, 403–407

IARC (1974) *IARC Monographs on the Evaluation of Carcinogenic Risk of Chemicals to Man*, Vol. 7, *Some Anti-Thyroid and Related Substances, Nitrofurans and Industrial Chemicals*, Lyon, IARCPress, pp. 85–94

IARC (1987) *IARC Monographs on the Evaluation of Carcinogenic Risks to Humans*, Suppl. 7, *Overall Evaluations of Carcinogenicity: An Updating of* IARC Monographs *Volumes 1 to 42*, Lyon, IARCPress, p. 72

Komeda, K., Iwamoto, S., Kominami, S. & Ohnishi, T. (1997) Induction of cell killing, mutation, and *umu* gene expression by 6-mercaptopurine or 2-thiouracil with UVA irradiation. *Photochem. Photobiol.*, **65**, 115–118

Krivánková, L., Krásenský, S. & Bocek, P. (1996) Application of capillary zone electrophoresis for analysis of thyreostatics. *Electrophoresis*, **17**, 1959–1963

Laqueur, G.L. (1949) Nodular hyperplasia of thyroid glands induced by thiouracil. *Cancer Res.*, **9**, 247–255

Le Bizec, B., Monteau, F., Maume, D., Montrade, M.P., Gade, C. & Andre, F. (1997) Detection and identification of thyreostats in the thyroid gland by gas chromatography–mass spectrometry. *Anal. chim. Acta*, **340**, 201–208

Lees, J., Alexander, W.D. & Marchant, B. (1973) Accumulation of ^{35}S-thiouracil by the rat thyroid gland. *Endocrinology*, **93**, 162–171

Lide, D.R. & Milne, G.W.A. (1996) *Properties of Organic Compounds*, Version 5.0, Boca Raton, FL, CRC Press [CD-ROM]

López García, I., Viñas, P. & Martínez Gil, J.A. (1993) FIA titrations of sulfide, cysteine and thiol-containing drugs with chemiluminescent detection. *Fresenius J. anal. Chem.*, **345**, 723–726

Marchant, B., Alexander, W.D., Lazarus, J.H., Lees, J. & Clark, D.H. (1972) The accumulation of ^{35}S-antithyroid drugs by the thyroid gland. *J. clin. Endocrinol. Metab.*, **34**, 847–851

Meserve, L.A. (1987) Hypothalamic CRF immunoreactivity in genetically hypothyroid (*hyt/hyt*) mice. *Proc. Soc. exp. Biol. Med.*, **185**, 335–338

Meserve, L.A. & Juárez de Ku, L.M. (1993) Effect of thiouracil-induced hypothyroidism on time course of adrenal response in 15 day old rats. *Growth Dev. Aging*, **57**, 25–30

Meserve, L.A. & Pearlmutter, A.F. (1983) Perinatal thiouracil exposure depresses cortico-tropin-releasing factor activity in 15 day old rats. *Horm. Metab. Res.*, **15**, 488–490

Moretti, G., Amici, M. & Cammarata, P. (1986) [Determination of methylthiouracil and analogous thyrostatics in animal tissues by HTLC after solid-phase purification.] *Riv. Soc. ital. Sci. aliment.*, **15**, 35–39 (in Italian)

Moretti, G., Amici, M., Cammarata, P. & Fracassi, F. (1988) Identification of thyrostatic drug residues in animal thyroids by high-performance thin-layer chromatography and fluorescence reaction detection. *J. Chromatogr.*, **442**, 459–463

Moretti, G., Betto, R., Cammarata, P., Fracassi, F., Giambenedetti, M. & Borghese, A. (1993) Determination of thyreostatic residues in cattle plasma by high-performance liquid chromatography with ultraviolet detection. *J. Chromatogr. Biomed. Appl.*, **616**, 291–296

National Institute for Occupational Safety and Health (2000) *National Occupational Exposure Survey 1981–83*, Cincinnati, OH, Department of Health and Human Services, Public Health Service

Paschkis, K.E., Cantarow, A. & Stasney, J. (1948) Influence of thiouracil on carcinoma induced by 2-acetaminofluorene. *Cancer Res.*, **8**, 257–263

Paynter, O.E., Burin, G.J., Jaeger, R.B. & Gregorio C.A. (1988) Goitrogens and thyroid follicular cell neoplasia: Evidence for a threshold process. *Regul. Toxicol. Pharmacol.*, **8**, 102–119

Peak, J.G., Peak, M.J. & MacCoss, M. (1984) DNA breakage caused by 334-nm ultraviolet light is enhanced by naturally occurring nucleic acid components and nucleotide coenzymes. *Photochem. Photobiol.*, **39**, 713–716

Quinones, J.D., Boyd, C.M., Beierwaltes, W.H. & Poissant, G.R. (1972) Transplacental transfer and tissue distribution of ^{14}C-2-thiouracil in the fetus. *J. nucl. Med.*, **13**, 148–154

Ron, E., Kleinerman, R.A., Boice, J.D., Jr, LiVolsi, V.A., Flannery, J.T. & Fraumeni, J.F., Jr (1987) A population-based case–control study of thyroid cancer. *J. Natl Cancer Inst.*, **79**, 1–12

Ron, E., Doody, M.M., Becker, D.V., Brill, A.B., Curtis, R.E., Goldman, M.B., Harris, B.S.H., Hoffman, D.A., McConahey, W.M., Maxon, H.R., Preston-Martin, S., Warshauer, E., Wong, L. & Boice, J.D., Jr for the Cooperative Thyrotoxicosis Therapy Follow-up Study Group (1998) Cancer mortality following treatment for adult hyperthyroidism. *J. Am. med. Assoc.*, **280**, 347–355

Ruzicka, F.J. & Rose, D.P. (1981) The influence of thyroidal status on rat hepatic mitochondrial NADH duroquinone reductase. *Endocrinology*, **109**, 664–666

Sabbagha, R.E. & Hayashi, T.T. (1969) Transfer of ^{14}C-thiouracil during pregnancy. *Am. J. Obst. Gynecol.*, **103**, 121–127

Sadtler Research Laboratories (1980) *Sadtler Standard Spectra, 1980 Cumulative Molecular Formula Index*, Philadelphia, PA, p. 31

Saldaña Monllor, L., Carbonell Martín, G. & Alonso Fuente, C. (1980) [*Thin-layer Chromatographic Separation and Identification of 2-Thiouracil, 4(6)-Methyl-2-thiouracil and 6(4)-Propyl-2-thiouracil in Feed Additives and Biological Materials by Thin-layer Chromatography.*], Madrid, Instituto Nacional de Investigaciones Agriarias, p. 8 (in Spanish)

Slanina, P., Ullberg, S. & Hammarström, L. (1973) Distribution and placental transfer of ^{14}C-thiourea and ^{14}C-thiouracil in mice studied by whole-body autoradiography. *Acta pharmacol. toxicol.*, **32**, 358–368

Smeds, S. & Wollman, S.H. (1983) Capillary endothelial cell multiplication in adipose tissue pads on the thyroid during the feeding of thiouracil. *Endocrinology*, **112**, 1718–1722

Stanley, M.M. & Astwood, E.B. (1949) Notes and comments. 1-Methyl-2-mercaptoimidazole: An antithyroid compound highly active in man. *Endocrinology*, **44**, 588–589

VanderLaan, W.P. & Storrie, V.M. (1955) A survey of factors controlling thyroid function, with especial reference to newer views on antithyroid substances. *Pharm. Rev.*, **7**, 301–334

Vargas, G., Havel, J. & Frgalová, K. (1998) Capillary zone electrophoresis determination of thyreostatic drugs in urine. *J. Capillary Electrophor.*, **5**, 9–12

Vinas, P., Lopez Garcia, I. & Martinez, G.J.A. (1993) Determination of thiol-containing drugs by chemiluminescence–flow injection analysis. *J. Pharm. biomed. Anal.*, **11**, 15–20

Visser, T. (1979) Mechanism of action of iodothyronine-5′-deiodinase. *Biochim. biophys. Acta*, **569**, 302–308

Visser, T. & van Overmeeren-Kaptein, E. (1981) Substrate requirement for inactivation of iodothyronine-5′-deiodinase activity by thiouracil. *Biochim. biophys. Acta*, **658**, 202–208

Watson, D.G., Bates, C.D., Skellern, G.G., Mairs, R. & Martin, S. (1991) Analysis of thiocarbamides by gas chromatography–negative-ion chemical-ionization mass spectrometry. *Rapid Commun. mass Spectrom.*, **5**, 141–142

Wollman, S.H. & Herveg, J.P. (1978) Thyroid capsule changes during the development of thyroid hyperplasia in the rat. *Am. J. Pathol.*, **93**, 639–654

Yu, G.Y.F., Murby, E.J. & Wells, R.J. (1997) Gas chromatographic determination of residues of thyreostatic drugs in bovine muscle tissue using combined resin mediated methylation and extraction. *J. Chromatogr.*, **B703**, 159–166

SEDATIVES

DOXYLAMINE SUCCINATE

1. Exposure Data

1.1 Chemical and physical data

1.1.1 *Nomenclature*

Chem. Abstr. Serv. Reg. No.: 562-10-7
Deleted CAS Reg. No.: 121367-03-1
Chem. Abstr. Name: Butanedioic acid, compd. with *N,N*-dimethyl-2-[1-phenyl-1-(2-pyridinyl)ethoxy]ethanamine (1:1); *N,N*-dimethyl-2-[1-phenyl-1-(2-pyridinyl)-ethoxy] ethanamine, butanedioate (1:1)
IUPAC Systematic Name: Pyridine, 2-[α-[2-(dimethylamino)ethoxy]-α-methyl-benzyl]-, succinate (1:1); succinic acid, compd. with 2-[α-[2-(dimethylamino)-ethoxy]-α-methylbenzyl]pyridine (1:1)
Synonyms: Doxylamine succinate (1:1); histadoxylamine succinate

1.1.2 *Structural and molecular formulae and relative molecular mass*

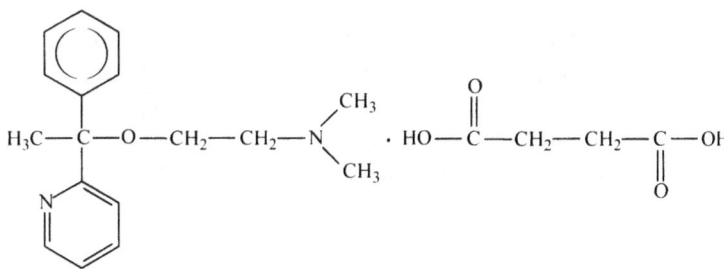

$C_{17}H_{22}N_2O.C_4H_6O_4$ Relative molecular mass: 388.46

1.1.3 *Chemical and physical properties of the pure substance*

(*a*) *Description*: White or creamy-white powder (Gennaro, 1995)
(*b*) *Melting-point*: 100–104 °C (Budavari, 2000)

(c) *Solubility*: Very soluble in water (1000 g/L at 25 °C) and chloroform; soluble in ethanol; slightly soluble in benzene and diethyl ether (Gennaro, 1995; American Hospital Formulary Service, 2000; Budavari, 2000)

(d) *Spectroscopy data*: Infrared [proton (9383), grating [45206P] spectral data have been reported (Sadtler Research Laboratories, 1980).

(e) *Ionization constants*: pKa, 5.8 and 9.3 (American Hospital Formulary Service, 2000)

1.1.4   *Technical products and impurities*

Doxylamine is currently formulated exclusively as the succinate salt. Doxylamine succinate is commercially available as an over-the-counter 25-mg tablet and a 50-mg liquid-filled capsule; it is also available in combination with antitussives and decongestants. Inactive ingredients in commercial formulations may include dibasic calcium phosphate, FD&C Blue No. 1, aluminium lake, magnesium stearate, microcrystalline cellulose and sodium starch glycolate (Gennaro, 1995; American Hospital Formulary Service, 2000; Medical Economics Co., 2000).

Trade names for doxylamine succinate include Alsadorm, Decapryn, Donormyl, Dormacil, Dormidina, Doxised, Doxy-Sleep-Aid, Dozile, Duebien, Evigoa D, Gittalun, Hewedormir, Hoggar N, Lidène, Mereprine, Munleit, Nighttime Sleep Aid, Noctyl, Nytol, Restaid, Sanalepsi, SchlafTabs-ratiopharm, Sedaplus, Sleep Aid, Sleep Easy and Unisom (Royal Pharmaceutical Society of Great Britain, 2000; Swiss Pharmaceutical Society, 2000; Vidal, 2000).

Doxylamine succinate is also used in over 50 pharmaceutical preparations in combination with other drugs.

1.1.5   *Analysis*

The *US Pharmacopeia* specifies ultraviolet absorption spectrophotometry with comparison to standards as the method for identifying doxylamine succinate; titration with perchloric acid is used to assay its purity. In pharmaceutical preparations, doxylamine succinate is identified by infrared absorption spectrophotometry; ultraviolet absorption spectrophotometry and high-performance liquid chromatography are used to assay for content (US Pharmacopeial Convention, 1999).

1.2   Production

Doxylamine can be prepared by converting methylphenyl-2-pyridylcarbinol into its sodium alcoholate and refluxing in toluene or in the presence of sodamide in xylene with 2-(*N,N*-dimethylamino)ethyl chloride. The doxylamine thus formed is converted to its succinate salt by reaction with an equimolar quantity of succinic acid in warm acetone (Gennaro, 1995; Budavari, 1998).

Information available in 2000 indicated that doxylamine succinate was manufactured by three companies in Germany and one company each in Ireland, Italy,
Mexico and Spain (CIS Information Services, 2000a).

Information available in 2000 indicated that doxylamine succinate was used in the
formulation of pharmaceuticals by 12 companies in South Africa, nine companies in
Germany, seven companies in Spain, six companies in India, five companies in
Australia, four companies each in Brazil, Canada, Taiwan and the United Kingdom,
three companies in Chile, two companies each in Egypt, France, the Republic of
Korea, Switzerland, Turkey and the USA and one company each in Indonesia,
Thailand, Philippines and Venezuela (CIS Information Services, 2000b).

1.3   Use

Doxylamine succinate, an ethanolamine-based antihistamine, shares the actions and
uses of other antihistamines. Because of its sedative effect, it is used in the short-term
management of insomnia. It is used for the symptomatic relief of hypersensitivity
reactions and in the treatment of pruritic skin disorders. It is also used in combination
with antitussives and decongestants (e.g., dextromethorphan, pseudoephedrine, phenyl-
propanolamine) for the temporary relief of cough and cold symptoms (Gennaro, 1995;
American Hospital Formulary Service, 2000; Medical Economics Co., 2000; Royal
Pharmaceutical Society of Great Britain, 2000).

Since 1956, doxylamine succinate has been used in the management of nausea and
vomiting during pregnancy, in combination with pyridoxine hydrochloride and
dicyclomine hydrochloride until the mid-1970s (Reynolds, 1996) and then in combination with pyridoxine alone until the early 1980s in most countries. The combination
drug was known as Bendectin® or Debendox®. A formulation known as Diclectin® is
apparently still available in Canada (Mitchell *et al.*, 1983; Tyl *et al.*, 1988; Royal
Pharmaceutical Society of Great Britain, 2000).

The usual oral dose of doxylamine succinate as an antihistamine for adults and
children 12 years and older is 7.5–12.5 mg every 4–6 h, not to exceed 75 mg within 24 h.
Under the direction of a physician, these patients may receive up to 25 mg every 4–6 h
[or 2 mg/kg bw or 60 mg/m^2 daily in divided doses], not to exceed 150 mg within 24 h.
The usual oral dose for children 6–12 years old is 3.75–6.25 mg every 4–6 h, not to
exceed 37.5 mg within 24 h. Under the direction of a physician, these paediatric patients
may receive up to 12.5 mg every 4–6 h [or 2 mg/kg bw or 60 mg/m^2 daily in divided
doses], not to exceed 75 mg within 24 h. Under the direction of a physician, children
aged 2 to < 6 years may receive an antihistaminic dose of 1.9–3.125 mg every 4–6 h,
not to exceed 18.75 mg in 24 h. The drug is contraindicated for neonates (Gennaro,
1995; American Hospital Formulary Service, 2000).

1.4   Occurrence

No data were available to the Working Group.

1.5   Regulations and guidelines

Doxylamine succinate is listed in the pharmacopoeias of France, Germany and the USA (US Pharmacopeial Convention, 1999; Royal Pharmaceutical Society of Great Britain, 2000; Swiss Pharmaceutical Society, 2000; Vidal, 2000). It is also registered for human use in Ireland, Italy, Portugal, Spain and the United Kingdom (Instituto Nacional de Farmacia e do Medicamento, 2000; Irish Medicines Board, 2000; Medicines Control Agency, 2000; Ministry of Health, Department of Drugs Assessment and Monitoring, 2000; Spanish Medicines Agency, 2000).

2.   Studies of Cancer in Humans

2.1   Case report

In a series of 200 children included in a case–control study of primary intracranial neoplasm, the authors mention 'the surprising coincidence' of two girls with a posterior fossa pilocytic astrocytoma whose mothers had taken Bendectin® [which contains doxylamine, dicyclomine and pyridoxine] (Giuffrè et al., 1990).

2.2   Case–control studies

In a study of childhood cancer in England, 615 cases and 1230 controls were considered to be eligible for the study (Birch et al., 1985). The parents of 555 children (response rate, 90%) in whom an incident cancer (171 leukaemias, 74 lymphomas, 78 central nervous system tumours and 232 other cancers) had been diagnosed in the regional paediatric oncology clinics of three Health Service regions of England were interviewed (McKinney et al., 1985). For each case, two controls matched on age and sex were selected, one on the list of the same general practitioner as the case child and the other from paediatric hospital admissions, with response rates of 72% and 64%, respectively. Controls who refused to participate were replaced, to obtain a total of 1110 controls. Information on the drug use of the mother during pregnancy was obtained by interview and also, whenever possible, from the combined information from obstetric records (88%) and general practitioners' notes (91%). The odds ratio for all cancers associated with use of Debendox® during pregnancy as reported by the mother was 0.69 and that obtained from medical records was 0.99. Although the odds ratio was significantly increased in relation to medically recorded use for 1–2 months (odds ratio, 10; 95% confidence interval [CI], 1.8–57), there was no dose–response relationship, the odds ratios being 0.75 for 2–6 months' use and 0.50 for > 6 months. The odds ratios for use of Debendox® reported by the mother were below 1 for any duration of use. For the group of leukaemias and lymphomas combined, the odds ratio was 1.0 with both exposure ascertainment methods, and those for other cancers were 0.47 with the mothers' recall and 0.95 with medical records.

A case–control study was conducted on patients under 18 years in the member and affiliate institutions of the Children Cancers Study Group in Canada and the USA in whom acute non-lymphoblastic leukaemia had been diagnosed between 1980 and 1984 (Robison *et al.*, 1989). For each case, one control was selected by random-digit dialling and matched on age, race and telephone area code. Of the 262 eligible patients, 204 (78%) were interviewed, as were 78% of the 260 eligible controls. The two parents were interviewed separately by telephone on a wide range of topics. The matched-pair odds ratio for maternal use of Bendectin® or other tablets for morning sickness during pregnancy was 1.8 (95% CI, 0.98–3.2), although the mothers of patients did not report morning sickness more frequently than mothers of controls (odds ratio, 0.80). The risk increased with increasing duration of use ($p = 0.05$; test for trend), and the odds ratio for use for more than 10 weeks compared with less than 1 week was 2.8 ($p < 0.05$).

3. Studies of Cancer in Experimental Animals

3.1 Oral administration

Mouse: Groups of 48 male and 48 female B6C3F$_1$ mice, 31–40 days of age, were fed diets containing doxylamine succinate (purity, 100%) at a concentration of 0, 190, 375 or 750 mg/kg (dose based on the free amine) for 104 weeks. Additionally, groups of 12 males and 12 females were fed the same concentrations for 65 weeks, at which time all surviving animals were killed. The survival rates in each group at the end of 104 weeks varied from 88 to 96% for males and from 85 to 98% for females. Increased incidences of hepatocellular adenoma were seen in both males (6/60 control, 12/60 low dose, 17/59 mid dose ($p < 0.01$; Fisher's exact test) and 31/60 high dose ($p < 0.001$)) and females (0/58, 3/60, 0/60 and 9/60 ($p < 0.01$), respectively). Thyroid follicular-cell adenomas were observed in both males (1/58, 0/57, 11/57 ($p < 0.01$) and 5/58) and females (0/56, 0/60, 2/57 and 8/59 ($p < 0.01$)). Dose-related increases in the incidence of follicular-cell hyperplasia were also observed in both male and female mice (Jackson & Sheldon, 1993).

Rat: Groups of 48 male and 48 female Fischer 344 rats, 31–40 days of age, were fed diets containing doxylamine succinate (purity, 100%) at a concentration of 0, 500, 1000 or 2000 mg/kg (dose based on the free amine) for 104 weeks. Additional groups of nine males and nine females received the same concentrations for 65 weeks, at which time animals were killed. The survival rates in each group at 104 weeks varied from 40 to 58% in males and from 56 to 69% in females. When compared with controls, the final body weight of high-dose males was reduced by 8.4% and that of females by 22.8%, suggesting that the maximal tolerated dose had been exceeded for the females. The incidence of hepatocellular adenoma and carcinoma combined in males was: control, 0/57; low dose, 0/57, mid dose, 0/57 and high dose, 5/57 ($p \leq 0.05$; Fisher's exact test). The five liver tumours in males at the high dose comprised two adenomas and three carcinomas. There was no increase in the incidence of neoplasms in female rats (Jackson & Blackwell, 1993).

4. Other Data Relevant to an Evaluation of Carcinogenicity and Its Mechanisms

4.1   Absorption, distribution, metabolism and excretion

4.1.1   *Humans*

The pharmacokinetics of doxylamine succinate was determined in 16 healthy male volunteers after administration of a single oral dose of 25 mg. The mean peak plasma concentration was 99 ng/mL, the peak time was 2.4 h after the dose, the elimination half-time was 10.1 h, and the apparent oral clearance was 217 mL/min (Friedman & Greenblatt, 1985). Clearance of a single oral dose of 25 mg of doxylamine succinate was slower (174 versus 240 mL/min) in older men (60–87 years) than in younger men (20–43 years), but no difference was seen in women (Friedman *et al.*, 1989).

N-Desmethyldoxylamine, N,N-didesmethyldoxylamine and their respective N-acetyl conjugates were identified as urinary metabolites after oral administration of 50 mg of doxylamine succinate to a single volunteer (Ganes & Midha, 1987). Approximately 1% of an oral dose of 75–100 mg of doxylamine succinate was recovered in the urine of male volunteers as quaternary ammonium-linked glucuronides (Luo *et al.*, 1991).

4.1.2   *Experimental systems*

Total urine and faecal recovery of radiolabel after oral administration of [^{14}C]-doxylamine succinate at 13.3 or 133 mg/kg bw to male and female Fischer 344 rats was > 90%, regardless of sex and dose. The identified unconjugated urinary metabolites (representing 36–44% of the radiolabel) included doxylamine N-oxide, N-desmethyl-doxylamine, N,N-didesmethyldoxylamine and ring-hydroxylated products of doxyl-amine and desmethyldoxylamine (Holder *et al.*, 1987). The identified conjugated meta-bolites (representing 44–55% of the radiolabel) included doxylamine O-glucuronide, N-desmethyldoxylamine O-glucuronide and N,N-didesmethyldoxylamine O-glucu-ronide (Holder *et al.*, 1990). N-Acetyl conjugates of N-desmethyl- and N,N-dides-methyldoxylamine were tentatively identified in rat urine (Ganes *et al.*, 1986).

[14]C-Doxylamine succinate given as a single oral dose of 13 mg/kg bw to four female rhesus monkeys (*Macaca mullata*) was metabolized by at least four pathways: a major pathway to mono- and didesmethyldoxylamine via successive *N*-demethylation; a major pathway to side-chain cleavage products via direct side-chain oxidation and/or deamination; a minor pathway to the *N*-oxide; and a minor pathway to unknown polar metabolites (Slikker *et al.*, 1986). In two male squirrel monkeys (*Saimiri sciureus*) given 20 mg of doxylamine succinate orally twice daily for 1 week, only the *N*-acetyl conjugate of *N,N*-didesmethyldoxylamine was detected in the urine (Ganes *et al.*, 1986). Repeated oral administration of 7 mg/kg bw per day of Bendectin® during days 22–50 of gestation to three cynomolgus monkeys (*Macaca fascicularis*), four rhesus monkeys (*Macaca mulatta*) and five baboons (*Papio cynocephalus*) did not alter the pharmacokinetics of doxylamine (Rowland *et al.*, 1989).

Analysis of fetal plasma samples by high-performance liquid chromatography demonstrated the presence of doxylamine and metabolites after a single intravenous injection of 13.3 mg/kg bw doxylamine succinate to three rhesus monkeys in late-term pregnancy (Slikker *et al.*, 1987, 1989).

4.1.3 *Comparison of animals and humans*

Similar demethylated metabolites and their *N*-acetylated derivatives have been determined in the urine of humans, monkeys and rats after oral doses of doxylamine succinate. In addition, rats metabolized the compound by *N*-oxidation, aromatic hydroxylation and ether cleavage.

4.2 Toxic effects

4.2.1 *Humans*

In 109 cases of intoxication with doxylamine preparations, the most frequent symptoms included impaired consciousness, seizures, tachycardia, mydriasis and a psychosis-like state similar to catatonic stupor. A serious complication may be rhabdomyolysis with subsequent impairment of renal function and acute renal failure (Köppel *et al.*, 1987).

4.2.2 *Experimental systems*

Administration of feed containing doxylamine succinate at a concentration of 0, 40, 375, 750 or 1500 mg/kg (expressed as free amine) to male and female B6C3F$_1$ mice for 7 or 15 days resulted in decreased serum thyroxine concentrations (approximately 80% of control) with compensatory increases (fourfold) in those of serum thyroid stimulating hormone, as also seen with phenobarbital at a concentration of 375 mg/kg of diet (expressed as free acid). No clear changes in serum triiodothyronine concentration were apparent (Bookstaff *et al.*, 1996).

Groups of 12 male and female Fischer 344 rats were given diets containing doxyl-amine succinate at a concentration of 0, 162, 405, 1012, 2530 or 6325 ppm (expressed as free amine) for 90 days. The only histopathological changes seen were cytoplasmic vacuo-lization or fatty change in the liver and cytomegaly in the parotid salivary glands (Jackson & Blackwell, 1988a). In groups of 12 male and female B6C3F$_1$ mice given diets containing doxylamine succinate at a concentration of 0, 80, 162, 325, 750 or 1500 ppm (expressed as free amine) for 90 days, the liver was the only organ affected. The histological lesions consisted of mild to severe cytomegaly and/or karyomegaly and a high incidence of hepatocellular necrosis in animals of each sex at the highest concentration in feed, although necrosis was also observed at lower concentrations (Jackson & Blackwell, 1988b)

4.3   Reproductive and developmental effects

4.3.1   *Humans*

Doxylamine succinate has rarely been used on its own, but it has been used exten-sively in pregnancy in combination with pyridoxine as Bendectin® for the treatment of nausea and vomiting. Reviews of the extensive literature on Bendectin® use, covering many thousands of women exposed during pregnancy, have concluded that the drug is not a human teratogen (Shiono & Klebanoff, 1989; McKeigue *et al.*, 1994; Brent, 1995).

4.3.2   *Experimental systems*

No satisfactory studies on doxylamine alone were available to the Working Group. Studies of Bendectin® in rats and non-human primates were available.

Groups of 37–41 pregnant CD Sprague–Dawley rats were given 0, 200, 500 or 800 mg/kg bw Bendectin® by gavage daily on days 6–15 of gestation (day 0 being considered that on which a positive vaginal smear was found) and were killed on day 20 for examination of their fetuses by standard teratological techniques. The highest dose was very toxic to the dams, killing 17%, and a marked reduction in body-weight gain was observed at the two higher doses. The lowest dose was minimally toxic. A small increase in the frequency of resorptions was seen at the highest dose and reduced fetal weight and reduced skeletal ossification at 500 and 800 mg/kg bw per day. There was no increase in the number of fetuses with malformations, but the number of litters with malformed fetuses was increased at the highest dose, due mainly to an increase in the number of fetuses with short 13th ribs. No increase in the incidence of external or visceral malformations was observed in any group (Tyl *et al.*, 1988).

Groups of 21–24 pregnant cynomolgus monkeys (*Macaca fascicularis*) were given Bendectin® at an approximate dose of 0, 1.3, 3.3 or 13.3 mg/kg bw (as 2/5, 1 and 4 tablets/day per animal, corresponding to two, five and 20 times the human dose) by nasogastric intubation daily on days 22–50 of gestation. The fetuses were removed surgically just prior to term for examination. No maternal toxicity and no embryofetal toxicity or teratogenicity was observed (Hendrickx *et al.*, 1985).

4.4   Effects on enzyme induction or inhibition and gene expression

4.4.1   *Humans*

A randomized, placebo-controlled study was conducted in 48 healthy male volunteers to compare the effects of doxylamine succinate on the pharmacokinetics of antipyrine metabolites and the urinary excretion of 6β-hydroxycortisol. Normal renal function, an age between 18 and 40 years and a normal diet were the criteria for inclusion. Groups of 16 men received 12.5 mg of doxylamine succinate, placebo or 30 mg of phenobarbital orally every 6 h for 17 days. No statistically significant differences indicative of enzyme induction were observed (Thompson *et al.*, 1996).

4.4.2   *Experimental systems*

Doxylamine succinate caused a dose-dependent increase (up to 2.6-fold) in liver microsomal cytochrome P450 (CYP) enzyme activity in male and female $B6C3F_1$ mice (aged 45–52 days) after 7 or 15 days on a diet containing the compound at a concentration of 0, 40, 375, 750 or 1500 mg/kg (expressed as free amine). Doxyl-amine succinate caused marked induction of CYP2B enzymes, as demonstrated by a large increase in the *O*-dealkylation of 7-pentoxyresorufin (up to 38-fold) and in the 16β-hydroxylation of testosterone (up to 6.9-fold). In addition, treatment resulted in a modest induction of CYP3A and CYP2A and a 50% increase in thyroxine glucuro-nosyltransferase activity. No induction of CYP1A, CYP2E or CYP4A was found. These results suggest that doxylamine is a phenobarbital-type inducer of liver micro-somal CYP enzymes in $B6C3F_1$ mice (Bookstaff *et al.*, 1996).

Doxylamine inhibited aminopyrine *N*-demethylation by rat liver microsomes, with a median inhibitory concentration of 73 μmol/L (Brandes *et al.*, 1994).

4.5   Genetic and related effects

4.5.1   *Humans*

No data were available to the Working Group.

4.5.2   *Experimental systems* (see Table 1 for references)

Doxylamine succinate did not induce mutations in *Salmonella typhimurium*. It weakly induced unscheduled DNA synthesis in primary rat hepatocytes *in vitro* in the absence of an exogenous metabolic system. It inhibited gap-junctional intercellular communication, measured as metabolic cooperation, in Chinese hamster V79 cells. It

Table 1. Genetic and related effects of doxylamine succinate

Test system	Result[a] Without exogenous metabolic system	Result[a] With exogenous metabolic system	Dose[b] (LED/HID)	Reference
Salmonella typhimurium TA100, T1535, TA98, reverse mutation	–	–	10 000 µg/plate	Zeiger *et al* (1987)
Unscheduled DNA synthesis, Fischer 344 primary rat hepatocytes *in vitro*	(+)	NT	194	Budroe *et al.* (1984)
Inhibition of gap-junctional intercellular communication, Chinese hamster V79 cells *in vitro*	+	NT	80	Toraason *et al.* (1992)
Sister chromatid exchange, human lymphocytes *in vitro*	–	–	15 930	Müller *et al.* (1989)
Micronucleus formation, Chinese hamster bone marrow *in vivo*	–		400 po × 1	Müller *et al.* (1989)
Chromosomal aberrations, transplacental exposure, NMRI mouse embryo *in vivo* (whole-body suspension)	+		150 po × 1	Müller *et al.* (1989)
Sister chromatid exchange, transplacental exposure, NMRI mouse embryo *in vivo* (whole-body suspension)	–		300 po × 1	Müller *et al.* (1989)
Micronucleus formation, transplacental exposure, fetal blood, NMRI mice *in vivo*	–		300 po × 1	Müller *et al.* (1989)

[a] +, positive; (+), weak positive; –, negative; NT, not tested; po, orally

[b] LED, lowest effective dose; HID, highest ineffective dose; in-vitro tests, µg/mL; in-vivo tests, mg/kg bw per day

did not induce sister chromatid exchange in human lymphocytes *in vitro* or micro-nucleus formation in hamster bone-marrow cells. In a transplacental system, a small dose-dependent induction of chromosomal aberrations, but no sister chromatid exchange or micronucleus formation, was found in the embryos of mice treated on day 11 of gestation[1].

4.6   Mechanistic considerations

Doxylamine succinate is considered not to be genotoxic.

It is a potent phenobarbital-type inducer of hepatic CYP2B enzymes in B6C3F$_1$ mice. In contrast, male volunteers given doxylamine succinate repeatedly showed no evidence of CYP enzyme induction. Doxylamine succinate, like phenobarbital, also induced thyroxine glucuronosyltransferase activity in mice, accompanied by decreased serum concentrations of thyroxine and increased serum concentrations of thyroid-stimulating hormone.

The lack of increased activity of liver enzymes associated with thyroxine meta-bolism and the increased thyroid-stimulating hormone concentrations in humans exposed to doxylamine succinate for longer than therapeutically recommended indicate that the compound would not be expected to produce thyroid tumours in humans at therapeutic doses. Doxylamine succinate damaged the liver in mice, and this effect may be related to its hepatocarcinogenicity.

5.   Summary of Data Reported and Evaluation

5.1   Exposure data

Doxylamine succinate is an ethanolamine-based antihistamine used in the management of insomnia and, in combination with antitussives and decongestants, in the relief of cough and cold symptoms. It was widely used until the early 1980s in combination with other drugs to control nausea associated with pregnancy and is still registered for this use in at least one country.

5.2   Human carcinogenicity data

Two studies addressed the association between use of an anti-emetic drug containing doxylamine succinate during pregnancy and cancer during childhood in the offspring. The study in England showed no association with childhood cancer in

---

[1] The Working Group was aware of unpublished studies of sister chromatid exchange and chromosomal aberrations in Chinese hamster ovary cells *in vitro*, which showed no effect of doxylamine succinate.

general or with lymphohaematopoietic neoplasms, and no evidence of a dose–response relationship. The study from Canada and the USA on children with acute non-lympho-blastic leukaemia found an increased risk of borderline significance for self-reported use of a drug containing doxylamine succinate or other tablets for morning sickness during pregnancy and a trend of borderline significance with duration of use.

5.3   Animal carcinogenicity data

Doxylamine succinate was tested by oral administration in one study each in mice and rats. In mice, it increased the incidences of hepatocellular and thyroid follicular-cell adenomas in males and females, although the thyroid response was not dose-related in males. In rats, doxylamine succinate marginally increased the incidence of hepatocellular adenomas and carcinomas combined only in males.

5.4   Other relevant data

Doxylamine is converted to demethylated metabolites and their N-acetylated derivatives in humans, monkeys and rats. In rats, doxylamine is also metabolized via N-oxidation, aromatic hydroxylation and ether cleavage pathways. Doxylamine is a potent, phenobarbital-type inducer of cytochrome P450 enzymes in mice. No evidence of enzyme induction has been found in humans. Doxylamine succinate causes liver damage in mice; this effect may be related to its hepatocarcinogenicity. Doxylamine induces thyroxine glucuronidation in mice, with concomitant decreases in serum thyroxine and increases in serum thyroid stimulating hormone concentrations. This is the probable mechanism of action for the induction of thyroid tumours in animals. It has not been shown to be teratogenic in humans or experimental animals.

No data were available on the genetic and related effects of doxylamine succinate in humans. It did not induce micronucleus formation in mice when given trans-placentally or in hamsters. It did, however, induce chromosomal aberrations in mice treated transplacentally. Doxylamine succinate induced DNA damage in primary rat hepatocytes and inhibited intercellular communication, but it did not induce sister chromatid exchange in mammalian cells in culture or induce mutations in bacteria. Doxylamine succinate is considered not to be genotoxic.

5.5   Evaluation

There is *inadequate evidence* in humans for the carcinogenicity of doxylamine succinate.

There is *limited evidence* in experimental animals for the carcinogenicity of doxylamine succinate.

Overall evaluation

Doxylamine succinate is *not classifiable as to its carcinogenicity to humans (Group 3)*.

6. References

American Hospital Formulary Service (2000) *AHFS Drug Information® 2000*, Bethesda, MD, American Society of Health-System Pharmacists [AHFSfirst CD-ROM]

Birch, J.M., Mann, J.R., Cartwright, R.A., Draper, G.J., Waterhouse, J.A., Hartley, A.L., Johnston, H.E., McKinney, P.A., Stiller, C.A. & Hopton, P.A. for the IRESCC Group (1985) The Inter-Regional Epidemiological Study of Childhood Cancer (IRESCC). Study design, control selection and data collection. *Br. J. Cancer*, **52**, 915–922

Bookstaff, R.C., Murphy, V.A., Skare, J.A., Minnema, D., Sanzgiri, U. & Parkinson, A. (1996) Effects of doxylamine succinate on thyroid hormone balance and enzyme induction in mice. *Toxicol. appl. Pharmacol.*, **141**, 584–594

Brandes, L.J., Warrington, R.C., Arron, R.J., Bogdanovic, R.P., Fang, W., Queen, G.M., Stein, D.A., Tong, J., Zaborniak, C.L.F. & LaBella, F.S. (1994) Enhanced cancer growth in mice administered daily human-equivalent doses of some H₁-antihistamines: Predictive in vitro correlates. *J. natl Cancer Inst.*, **86**, 770–775

Brent, R.L. (1995) Bendectin: Review of the medical literature of a comprehensively studied human nonteratogen and the most prevalent tortogen-litigen. *Reprod. Toxicol.*, **9**, 337–349

Budavari, S., ed. (1998) *The Merck Index*, 12th Ed., Version 12:2, Whitehouse Station, NJ, Merck & Co. [CD-ROM] [Monograph: 3497]

Budavari, S., ed. (2000) *The Merck Index*, 12th Ed., Version 12:3, Whitehouse Station, NJ, Merck & Co. & Boca Raton, FL, Chapman & Hall/CRC [CD-ROM]

Budroe, J.D., Shaddock, J.G. & Casciano, D.A. (1984) A study of the potential genotoxicity of methapyrilene and related antihistamines using the hepatocyte/DNA repair assay. *Mutat. Res.*, **135**, 131–137

CIS Information Services (2000a) *Directory of World Chemical Producers (Version 2000-1)*, Dallas, TX [CD-ROM]

CIS Information Services (2000b) *Worldwide Bulk Drug Users Directory (Version 2000)*, Dallas, TX [CD-ROM]

Friedman, H. & Greenblatt, D.J. (1985) The pharmacokinetics of doxylamine: Use of automated gas chromatography with nitrogen-phosphorus detection. *J. clin. Pharmacol.*, **25**, 448–451

Friedman, H., Greenblatt, D.J., Scavone, J.M., Burstein, E.S., Ochs, H.R., Harmatz, J.S. & Shader, R.I. (1989) Clearance of the antihistamine doxylamine: Reduced in elderly men but not in elderly women. *Clin. Pharmacokin.*, **16**, 312–316

Ganes, D.A. & Midha, K.K. (1987) Identification in in vivo acetylation pathway for N-dealkylated metabolites of doxylamine in humans. *Xenobitotica*, **17**, 993–999

Ganes, D.A., Hindmarsh, K.W. & Midha, K.K. (1986) Doxylamine metabolism in rat and monkey. *Xenobiotica*, **16**, 781–794

Gennaro, A.R. (1995) *Remington: The Science and Practice of Pharmacy*, 19th Ed., Vol. II, Easton, PA, Mack Publishing Co., p. 1226

Giuffrè, R., Liccardo, G., Pastore, F.S., Spallone, A. & Vagnozzi, R. (1990) Potential risk factors for brain tumors in children. An analysis of 200 cases. *Child's Nerv. Syst.*, **6**, 8–12

Hendrickx, A.G., Cukierski, M., Prahalada, S., Janos, G., Booher, S. & Nyland, T. (1985) Evaluation of Bendectin embryotoxicity in nonhuman primates: II. Double-blind study in term cynomolgus monkeys. *Teratology*, **32**, 191–194

Holder, C.L, Thompson, H.C., Jr, Gosnell, A.B., Siitonen, P.H., Korfmacher, W.A., Cerniglia, C.E., Miller, D.W., Casciano, D.A. & Slikker, W., Jr (1987) Metabolism of doxylamine succinate in Fischer 344 rats. Part II: Nonconjugated urinary and fecal metabolites. *J. anal. Toxicol.*, **11**, 113–121

Holder, C.L., Siitonen, P.H., Slikker, W., Jr, Branscomb, C.J., Korfmacher, W.A., Thompson, H.C., Jr, Cerniglia, C.E., Gosnell, A.B. & Lay, J.O., Jr (1990) Metabolism of doxylamine succinate in Fischer 344 rats. Part III: Conjugated urinary and fecal metabolites. *J. anal. Toxicol.*, **14**, 247–251

Instituto Nacional de Farmacia e do Medicamento (2000) Lisbon

Irish Medicines Board (2000) Dublin

Jackson, C.D. & Blackwell, B.-N. (1988a) Subchronic studies of doxylamine in Fischer 344 rats. *Fundam. appl. Toxicol.*, **10**, 243–253

Jackson, C.D. & Blackwell, B.-N. (1988b) Subchronic studies of doxylamine in B6C3F$_1$ mice. *Fundam. appl. Toxicol.*, **10**, 254–261

Jackson, C.D. & Blackwell, B.-N. (1993) 2-Year toxicity study of doxylamine succinate in the Fischer 344 rat. *J. Am. Coll. Toxicol.*, **12**, 1–11

Jackson, C.D. & Sheldon, W.S. (1993) Two-year toxicity study of doxylamine succinate in B6C3F1 mice. *J. Am. Coll. Toxicol.*, **12**, 311–321

Köppel, C., Tenczer, J. & Ibe, K. (1987) Poisoning with over-the-counter doxylamine preparations: An evaluation of 109 cases. *Hum. Toxicol.*, **6**, 355–359

Luo, H., Hawes, E.M., McKay, G., Korchinski, E.D. & Midha, K.K. (1991) N$^+$-Glucuronidation of aliphatic tertiary amines, a general phenomenon in the metabolism of H$_1$-antihistamines in humans. *Xenobiotica*, **21**, 1281–1288

McKeigue, P.M., Lamm, S.H., Linn, S. & Kutcher, J.S. (1994) Bendectin and birth defects: I. A meta-analysis of the epidemiologic studies. *Teratology*, **50**, 27–37

McKinney, P.A., Cartwright, R.A., Stiller, C.A., Hopton, P.A., Mann, J.R., Birch, JM., Harley, A.L., Waterhouse, J.A. & Johnston, H.E. (1985) Inter-Regional Epidemiological Study of Childhood Cancer (IRESCC): Childhood cancer and the consumption of Debendox and related drugs in pregnancy. *Br. J. Cancer*, **52**, 923–929

Medical Economics Co. (2000) *PDR®: Physicians' Desk Reference*, 53rd Ed., Montvale, NJ, Medical Economics Data Production Co. [http://druginfo.cc.nih.gov/mdxcgi/]

Medicines Control Agency (2000) London

Ministry of Health, Department of Drugs Assessment and Monitoring (2000) Rome

Mitchell, A.A., Schwingl, P.J., Rosenberg, L., Louik, C. & Shapiro, S. (1983) Birth defects in relation to Bendectin use in pregnancy. II. Pyloric stenosis. *Am. J. Obstet. Gynecol.*, **147**, 737–742

Müller, L., Korte, A. & Madle, S. (1989) Mutagenicity testing of doxylamine succinate, an antinauseant drug. *Toxicol. Lett.*, **49**, 79–86

Reynolds, J.E.F., ed. (1996) *Martindale, The Extra Pharmacopoieia*, 31st Ed., London, Royal Pharmaceutical Society, p. 428

Robison, L.L., Buckley, J.D., Daigle, A.E., Wells, R., Benjamin, D., Arthur, D.C. & Hammond, G.D. (1989) Maternal drug use and risk of childhood nonlymphoblastic leukemia among offspring. *Cancer*, **63**, 1904–1911

Rowland, J.M., Slikker, W., Jr, Holder, C.L., Denton, R., Prahalada, S., Young, J.F. & Hendrickx, A.G. (1989) Pharmacokinetics of doxylamine given as Bendectin® in the pregnant monkey and baboon. *Reprod. Toxicol.*, **3**, 197–202

Royal Pharmaceutical Society of Great Britain (2000) *Martindale, The Extra Pharmacopoeia*, 31st Ed., London, The Pharmaceutical Press [MicroMedex Online]

Sadtler Research Laboratories (1980) *Sadtler Standard Spectra, 1980 Cumulative Alphabetical Index*, Philadelphia, PA, p. 597

Shiono, P.H. & Klebanoff, M.A. (1989) Bendectin and human congenital malformations. *Teratology*, **40**, 151–155

Slikker, W., Jr, Holder, C.L., Lipe, G.W., Korfmacher, W.A., Thompson, H.C., Jr & Bailey, J.R. (1986) Metabolism of ^{14}C-labeled doxylamine succinate (Bendectin®) in the rhesus monkey (*Macaca mulatta*). *J. anal. Toxicol.*, **10**, 87–92

Slikker, W., Jr, Bailey, J.R., Holder, C.L. & Lipe, G.W. (1987) Transplacental disposition of doxylamine succinate in the late-term rhesus monkey. *Pharmacokinetics in Teratogenesis*, **1**, 193–202

Slikker, W., Jr, Holder, C.L., Lipe, G.W., Bailey, J.R. & Young, J.F. (1989) Pharmacokinetics of doxylamine, a component of Bendectin®, in the rhesus monkey. *Reprod. Toxicol.*, **3**, 187–196

Spanish Medicines Agency (2000) Madrid

Swiss Pharmaceutical Society, ed. (2000) *Index Nominum, International Drug Directory*, 16th Ed., Stuttgart, Medpharm Scientific Publishers [MicroMedex Online]

Thompson, G.A., St Peter, J.V., Heise, M.A., Horowitz, Z.D., Salyers, G.C., Charles, T.T., Brezovic, C., Russell, D.A., Skare, J.A. & Powell, J.H. (1996). Assessment of doxylamine influence on mixed function oxidase activity upon multiple dose oral administration to normal volunteers. *J. pharm. Sci.*, **85**, 1242–1247

Toraason, M., Bohrman, J.S., Krieg, E., Combes, R.D., Willington, S.E., Zajac, W. & Langenbach, R. (1992) Evaluation of the V79 cell metabolic co-operation assay as a screen *in vitro* for developmental toxicants. *Toxicol. In Vitro*, **6**, 165–174

Tyl, R.W., Price, C.J., Marr, M.C. & Kimmel, C.A. (1988) Developmental toxicity evaluation of Bendectin in CD rats. *Teratology*, **37**, 539–552

US Pharmacopeial Convention (1999) *The 2000 US Pharmacopeia*, 24th rev./*The National Formulary*, 19th rev., Rockville, MD, pp. 612–613, 1853, 2268

Vidal (2000) *Le Dictionnaire*, 76th ed., Paris, Editions du Vidal

Zeiger E., Anderson, B., Haworth, S., Lawlor, T., Mortelmans, K. & Speck, W. (1987) *Salmonella* mutagenicity tests: III. Results from the testing of 255 chemicals. *Environ. Mutag.*, **9** (Suppl. 9), 1–110

PHENOBARBITAL AND ITS SODIUM SALT

This substance was considered by previous working groups, in 1976 (IARC, 1977) and 1987 (IARC, 1987). Since that time, new data have become available, and these have been incorporated into the monograph and taken into consideration in the present evaluation.

1. Exposure Data

1.1 Chemical and physical data

1.1.1 *Nomenclature*

Phenobarbital

> *Chem. Abstr. Serv. Reg. No.*: 50-06-6
> *Deleted CAS Reg. Nos*: 11097-06-6; 46755-67-3
> *Chem. Abstr. Name*: 5-Ethyl-5-phenyl-2,4,6($1H,3H,5H$)-pyrimidinetrione
> *IUPAC Systematic Name*: 5-Ethyl-5-phenylbarbituric acid
> *Synonyms*: Phenobarbitone; phenobarbituric acid; phenylethylbarbituric acid; 5-phenyl-5-ethylbarbituric acid; phenylethylmalonylurea

Sodium phenobarbital

> *Chem. Abstr. Serv. Reg. No.*: 57-30-7
> *Deleted CAS Reg. Nos*: 125-36-0; 8050-96-2
> *Chem. Abstr. Name*: 5-Ethyl-5-phenyl-2,4,6($1H,3H,5H$)-pyrimidinetrione, mono-sodium salt
> *IUPAC Systematic Name*: 5-Ethyl-5-phenylbarbituric acid, sodium salt
> *Synonyms*: 5-Ethyl-5-phenylbarbituric acid sodium; phenobarbital sodium; phenobarbitone sodium; sodium ethylphenylbarbiturate; sodium 5-ethyl-5-phenylbarbiturate; sodium phenobarbitone; sodium phenylethylbarbiturate; sodium phenylethylmalonylurea; sol phenobarbital; sol phenobarbitone; soluble phenobarbital; soluble phenobarbitone

1.1.2   *Structural and molecular formulae and relative molecular masses*

Phenobarbital

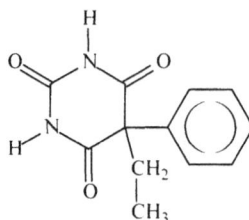

$C_{12}H_{12}N_2O_3$ Relative molecular mass: 232.24

Sodium phenobarbital

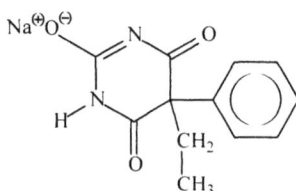

$C_{12}H_{11}N_2NaO_3$ Relative molecular mass: 254.22

1.1.3   *Chemical and physical properties of the pure substances*

Phenobarbital

(a) *Description*: White, crystalline plates with three different phases (Gennaro, 1995; Lide & Milne, 1996; Budavari, 2000)

(b) *Melting-point*: 174 °C (Lide & Milne, 1996)

(c) *Spectroscopy data*: Infrared [prism (483), grating (21015)], ultraviolet (171), nuclear magnetic resonance [proton (6644), C-13 (4431)] and mass spectral data have been reported (Sadtler Research Laboratories, 1980; Lide & Milne, 1996).

(d) *Solubility*: Slightly soluble in water (1 g/L); insoluble in benzene; soluble in alkali hydroxides, carbonates, diethyl ether and ethanol (Gennaro, 1995; Lide & Milne, 1996; Budavari, 2000)

(e) *Dissociation constants*: pK_1, 7.3; pK_2, 11.8 (Chao *et al.*, 1978)

Sodium phenobarbital

(a) *Description*: Slightly hygroscopic crystals or white powder (Gennaro, 1995; Budavari, 2000)

(b) *Spectroscopy data*: Infrared [prism (8775), grating (28039), ultraviolet (19554) and nuclear magnetic resonance [proton 14710] and spectral data have been reported (Sadtler Research Laboratories, 1980).

(c) *Solubility*: Very soluble in water (1 kg/L) and ethanol; insoluble in chloroform and diethyl ether (Budavari, 2000)

1.1.4 *Technical products and impurities*

Phenobarbital is available as 8-, 16-, 32-, 65- and 100-mg tablets, as a 16-mg capsule and as a 15- or 20-mg/5 mL elixir. Sodium phenobarbital is available as 30-, 60-, 65- and 130-mg/mL injections and as a sterile powder in 120-mg ampules (Gennaro, 1995).

Trade names for phenobarbital include Adonal, Agrypnal, Amylofene, Barbenyl, Barbiphenyl, Barbipil, Barbita, Barbivis, Blu-phen, Cratecil, Dormiral, Doscalun, Duneryl, Eskabarb, Etilfen, Euneryl, Fenemal, Gardenal, Gardepanyl, Hysteps, Lepinal, Lepinaletten, Liquital, Lixophen, Lubergal, Lubrokal, Luminal, Neurobarb, Noptil, Nunol, Phenaemal, Phenemal, Phenobal, Phenoluric, Phenonyl, Phenyral, Phob, Sedonal, Sedophen, Sevenal, Somonal, Stental Extentabs, Teolaxin, Triphenatol and Versomnal. Trade names for sodium phenobarbital include Gardenal sodium, Linasen, Luminal sodium, PBS, Phenemalum, Phenobal sodium and Sodium luminal.

1.1.5 *Analysis*

Several international pharmacopoeias specify infrared absorption spectrophotometry with comparison to standards, thin-layer chromatography, high-performance liquid chromatography (HPLC) with ultraviolet detection and colorimetry as the methods for identifying phenobarbital; HPLC and titration with ethanolic potassium hydroxide are used to assay its purity. In pharmaceutical preparations, phenobarbital is identified by infrared absorption spectrophotometry, HPLC and colorimetry; HPLC and titration with ethanolic potassium hydroxide or silver nitrate are used to assay for phenobarbital content (British Pharmacopoeia Commission, 1993; Society of Japanese Pharmacopoeia, 1996; Council of Europe, 1997; US Pharmacopeial Convention, 1999).

Several international pharmacopoeias specify infrared absorption spectrophotometry with comparison to standards, thin-layer chromatography and HPLC as the methods for identifying sodium phenobarbital; HPLC with ultraviolet detection and potentiometric titration are used to assay its purity. In pharmaceutical preparations, sodium phenobarbital is identified by infrared absorption spectrophotometry and HPLC; HPLC with ultraviolet detection is used to assay for sodium phenobarbital content (British Pharmacopoeia Commission, 1993; Council of Europe, 1997; US Pharmacopeial Convention, 1999).

1.2   Production

The introduction of barbital in 1903 and phenobarbital in 1912 initiated the predominance of barbiturates, and for over half a century they reigned as the pre-eminent sedative-hypnotic agents. Although several so-called 'non-barbiturates' were introduced to displace barbiturates from time to time, it was not until chlordiazepoxide was marketed in 1961 that their position was challenged seriously. During the ensuing quarter of a century, the benzodiazepines displaced the barbiturates as the sedative-hypnotics of choice (Hardman *et al.*, 1996).

Two general methods of synthesis have been used for phenobarbital. The first is based on condensation of α-ethylbenzenepropanedioic acid ester (methyl or ethyl ester) with urea in the presence of sodium ethoxide. The second comprises condensation of benzeneacetonitrile with diethyl carbonate in ether solution to form α-cyanobenzene-acetic ester, followed by ethylation of this ester to α-cyano-α-ethylbenzeneacetic acid ester, which is further condensed with urea to yield iminobarbituric acid, and hydrolysis of iminobarbituric acid to phenobarbital (Chao *et al.*, 1978).

Sodium phenobarbital is obtained by dissolving phenobarbital in an ethanolic solution of an equivalent quantity of sodium hydroxide and evaporating at low temperature (Gennaro, 1995).

Information available in 2000 indicated that phenobarbital was manufactured by three companies each in China and India, by two companies in the Russian Federation and by one company each in Armenia, Germany, Hungary, Latvia, Switzerland and the USA (CIS Information Services, 2000a).

Information available in 2000 indicated that phenobarbital and its salts (unspecified) were formulated as a pharmaceutical by 31 companies in India, 18 companies in France, 12 companies in the USA, 11 companies each in Chile and South Africa, 10 companies each in Taiwan, Turkey and the United Kingdom, nine companies in Argentina, eight companies each in Brazil, Italy and Spain, six companies each in China and Poland, five companies each in Hungary and Japan, four companies each in Canada, Germany, the Islamic Republic of Iran, Portugal, the Republic of Korea and Switzerland, three companies each in Australia, Belgium, Bulgaria, Ecuador, Greece, Peru and Venezuela, two companies each in the Czech Republic, Egypt, Lithuania, Mexico, Romania, the Russian Federation, Thailand and Viet Nam and one company each in Hong Kong, Indonesia, Ireland, Malta, Norway, the Philippines, Singapore, the Slovak Republic, Surinam, Sweden, the Ukraine and Yugoslavia (CIS Information Services, 2000b).

Information available in 2000 indicated that sodium phenobarbital was manu-factured by one company each in China, Germany, Hungary, Latvia and the United Kingdom (CIS Information Services, 2000a) and that it was formulated as a pharma-ceutical by seven companies in India, four companies in Italy, two companies each in Argentina, Australia, Chile, Ecuador, France, the United Kingdom and the USA and one company each in Belgium, Bulgaria, Germany, Hungary, Indonesia, the Islamic

Republic of Iran, Japan, the Philippines, Poland, South Africa, Taiwan, Thailand and Venezuela (CIS Information Services, 2000b).

1.3 Use

Phenobarbital is a sedative, hypnotic and anti-epileptic drug. In appropriate doses, it is used in the treatment of neuroses and related tension states when mild, prolonged sedation is indicated, as in hypertension, coronary artery disease, functional gastro-intestinal disorders and pre-operative apprehension. In addition, it has specific use in the symptomatic therapy of epilepsy, particularly for patients with generalized tonic–clonic seizures (grand mal) and complex partial (psychomotor) seizures. Pheno-barbital is also included in the treatment and prevention of hyperbilirubinaemia in neonates. Because of its slow onset of action, phenobarbital is not generally used orally to treat insomnia but is used to help withdraw people who are physically dependent on other central nervous system depressants. With the exception of metharbital and mephobarbital, it is the only barbiturate effective in epilepsy (Gennaro, 1995).

Sodium phenobarbital, because it is soluble in water, may be administered paren-terally. It is given by slow intravenous injection for control of acute convulsive syndromes (Gennaro, 1995).

The usual adult oral dose of phenobarbital as a sedative is 30–120 mg in two to three divided doses, that as a hypnotic is 100–320 mg and that as an anticonvulsant is 50–100 mg two or three times a day. The usual dose is 30–600 mg/day. The usual paediatric oral dose of phenobarbital as a sedative is 2 mg/kg bw or 60 mg/m^2 three times a day, that as a hypnotic is individualized by the physician and that as an anti-convulsant or antidyskinetic is 3–5 mg/kg bw or 125 mg/m^2 a day until a blood concentration of 10–15 µg/mL is attained (Gennaro, 1995).

The usual adult oral dose of sodium phenobarbital as a sedative is the same as that for phenobarbital, that as an intramuscular or intravenous sedative is 100–130 mg, that as an anticonvulsant is 200–300 mg repeated within 6 h if necessary, that as a pre-operative medication is 130–200 mg every 6 h and that as a post-operative sedative is 32–100 mg. The usual paediatric dose of sodium phenobarbital as an intramuscular sedative is 60 mg/m^2 three times a day, that as an anticonvulsant is 125 mg/m^2 per dose, that as a pre-operative medication is 16–100 mg and that as a post-operative sedative is 8–30 mg (Gennaro, 1995).

Phenobarbital ranked 63rd among the 200 generic drugs most frequently sold by prescription in the USA in 1999 (Anon., 2000).

1.4   Occurrence

1.4.1   *Occupational exposure*

According to the 1981–83 National Occupational Exposure Survey (National Institute for Occupational Safety and Health, 2000), about 23 000 workers, including 20 000 nurses, nursing aides, health aides, pharmacists and laboratory workers in health services and 2900 chemical industry workers, were potentially exposed occupationally to phenobarbital in the USA.

1.4.2   *Environmental occurrence*

No data were available to the Working Group.

1.5   Regulations and guidelines

Phenobarbital is listed in the pharmacopoeias of Austria, China, the Czech Republic, France, Germany, Italy, Japan, Poland, the United Kingdom and the USA, and in the European and International pharmacopoeias (US Pharmacopeial Convention, 1999; Royal Pharmaceutical Society of Great Britain, 2000; Swiss Pharmaceutical Society, 2000; Vidal, 2000). It is registered for human use in Ireland, the Netherlands, Norway, Spain and Sweden (Irish Medicines Board, 2000; Medical Products Agency, 2000; Medicines Evaluation Board Agency, 2000; Norwegian Medicinal Depot, 2000; Spanish Medicines Agency, 2000).

Sodium phenobarbital is listed in the pharmacopoeias of Austria, China, the Czech Republic, Germany, Italy, Japan, Poland, the United Kingdom and the USA, and in the European and International pharmacopoeias (Royal Pharmaceutical Society of Great Britain, 2000; Swiss Pharmaceutical Society, 2000).

2.   Studies of Cancer in Humans

2.1   Cohort studies

2.1.1   *Studies of patients with seizures* (see Table 1)

A cohort of (initially) 9136 patients hospitalized for epilepsy in the Filadelfia treatment community in Denmark between 1933 and 1962 was followed for cancer incidence from 1943 to 1967 (Clemmesen *et al.*, 1974). Throughout the study period, phenobarbital was the basic therapeutic drug, given in daily doses of 100–300 mg. In the 1940s, phenytoin was introduced at the treatment centre, either alone or in combination with phenobarbital, and in the mid-1950s primidone was also used. Primidone is partly metabolized to phenobarbital. The files of the Danish Cancer Registry, established in

Table 1. Cohort studies of cancer incidence or mortality in epilepsy patients, generally treated with phenobarbital

Studies of patients with seizures

Country (reference)	Population; outcome measure (size); recruitment period/ follow-up period	Treatment modality	Cancer site	Relative risk (95% CI)	Comments
Denmark (Clemmesen & Hjalgrim-Jensen, 1981) (Update of Clemmesen et al., 1974)	Epilepsy patients; SIR (8077); 1933–62/1943–76	Anticonvulsants including phenobarbital	All cancers	[1.1] [1.0–1.2]	Benign brain tumours included; initial 4 weeks of follow-up excluded
			Brain	[5.3] [4.1–6.6]	
			Latency period (years):		
			0–9	[12] [8.5–16]	
			10–14	[5.4] [2.9–9.2]	
			15–19	[1.8] [0.5–4.5]	
			20–24	[2.7] [0.9–6.2]	
			25–29	[1.4] [0.2–5.1]	
			30–34	[2.1] [0.2–7.6]	
			≥ 35	[0.0] [0.0–5.8]	
			Liver	[3.8] [2.0–6.5]	Thorotrast exposure in 10/13 liver cancer cases
			Lung	[1.3] [1.0–1.7]	
Denmark (Olsen et al., 1989) (update of Clemmesen et al., 1974)	Epilepsy patients; SIR (7864); 1933–62/1943–84	Anticonvulsants including phenobarbital	All cancers	1.2 (1.1–1.3)	Followed-up from date of first hospitalization for epilepsy; 140 patients known to have received Thorotrast were excluded.
			Brain	5.7 (4.7–6.8)	
			Latency period (years):		
			0–9	20 (16–26)	
			10–19	4.1 (2.5–6.2)	
			20–29	1.5 (0.7–2.8)	
			≥ 30	1.3 (0.5–2.8)	
			All except brain	1.0 (0.97–1.1)	
			Lung	1.4 (1.2–1.7)	
			Liver	1.9 (0.9–3.6)	
			Thyroid	1.2 (0.3–3.2)	
			Non-Hodgkin lymphoma	1.4 (0.8–2.3)	
			Leukaemia	0.8 (0.4–1.4)	
			Bladder	0.6 (0.3–0.9)	
			Melanoma	0.5 (0.2–1.0)	

Table 1 (contd)

Country (reference)	Population; outcome measure (size); recruitment period/ follow-up period	Treatment modality	Cancer site	Relative risk (95% CI)	Comments
England (White et al., 1979)	Epilepsy patients; SMR (1980); 1931–71/1951–77	Anticonvulsants (long term) including phenobarbital	All cancers	1.5 (1.2–1.9)	
			Brain	4.1 (1.5–8.9)	
			All except brain	1.4 (1.1–1.8)	
			Lung	1.4 (0.9–2.1)	
			Liver	0.0 (0.0–12)	~ 0.3 cases expected
			Lymphoma and leukaemia	1.3 (0.5–2.1)	
USA, Minnesota (Shirts et al., 1986)	Patients with seizure disorders; SIR (959); 1935–79/1935–82	Not specified	All cancers	1.4 (1.1–1.8)	
			Brain	24 (14–39)	
			Length of follow-up (years)		
			0–4	47 (26–82)	
			5–9	12 (1.4–43)	
			≥ 10	5.9 (0.7–21)	
			All except brain	1.1 (0.8–1.4)	
			Lung	2.7 (1.2–5.2)	Seven of nine lung cancers diagnosed during first 5 years of follow-up
			Liver	No cases observed	
			Lymphoma and leukaemia	2.9 (1.0–5.0)	
		Medication:	All except brain		Primarily phenobarbital and phenytoin
		Yes		0.9 (0.6–1.4)	
		No		1.3 (0.8–2.0)	

Table 1 (contd)

Country (reference)	Population; outcome measure (size); recruitment period/ follow-up period	Treatment modality	Cancer site	Relative risk (95% CI)		Comments
Transplacental exposure						
Denmark (Olsen et al., 1990)	Offspring of epilepsy patients; SIR (3727) 1933–62/1943–86	Born after mother's first admission for epilepsy (2579)	All cancers Brain	1.0 1.4	(0.6–1.7) (0.3–4.0)	
		Born before mother's first admission (1148)	All cancers	0.9	(0.6–1.2)	

1942, were used to identify incident cases of cancer, including benign brain tumours and bladder papillomas (Olsen *et al.*, 1989), in the patients. The expected numbers of cases were calculated from national cancer incidence rates, similarly based on the files of the Cancer Registry. In two updated reports with extended follow-up (Clemmesen & Hjalgrim-Jensen, 1977, 1981), the original roster was revised to include 8078 and 8077 subjects, respectively. The reduction of the cohort by 12% was due to exclusion of non-Danish citizens, patients who died before 1943 when the follow-up began, duplicate registrations and persons whose diagnosis of epilepsy was not sustained. In the most recent update (Clemmesen & Hjalgrim-Jensen, 1981), the period of follow-up was from 4 weeks after first admission to the treatment community or 1 January 1943, whichever came last, to the day of death or the end of 1976, whichever came first. A total of 467 cases of cancer were observed when 419.5 were expected [yielding an overall standardized incidence ratio (SIR) of 1.1; 95% confidence interval (CI), 1.0–1.2; or 1.25 (95% CI, 1.1–1.4) among men and 0.99 (95% CI, 0.87–1.13) among women]. The overall increase was due mainly to the observation of 71 tumours of the brain and nervous system when 13.4 were expected [yielding a significantly increased SIR of 5.3; 5.8 among men and 4.8 among women]. Excess rates of brain tumour were seen in particular during the first 15 years of follow-up [with SIRs of 12, 5.4, 1.8, 2.7, 1.4, 2.1 and 0.0 for latency periods of 0–9, 10–14, 15–19, 20–24, 25–29, 30–34 and ≥ 35 years, respectively]. The authors suggested that the seizures of some patients were early symptoms of their brain tumours. Thirteen cases of primary liver cancer were observed, when 3.44 cases were expected [SIR, 3.8; 95% CI, 2.0–6.5]. This excess of liver cancer, which was particularly evident in patients followed for 15 years or more, was ascribed to use of radioactive thorium dioxide (Thorotrast) for cerebral angiography in a subgroup of patients during diagnostic work-up. Only three of the 13 patients with primary liver cancer had had no documented exposure to Thorotrast, which was in agreement with the 3.4 cases expected among all cohort members. Finally, the increased SIR for lung cancer among male patients [SIR, 1.3; 95% CI, 0.94–1.7] was considered most likely to be due to a higher prevalence of smokers.

The Danish cohort was further evaluated by Olsen *et al.* (1989), who extended follow-up for cancer incidence from 1976 through 1984. Exclusion of additional duplicate admissions, non-Danish citizens and patients for whom the data were incomplete and the inclusion of patients hospitalized for fewer than 4 weeks reduced the cohort to 8004 patients. Of these, 140 had had documented exposure to Thorotrast. Linkage of the records of the remaining 7864 patients not known to have received this contrast medium with the files of the national Cancer Registry resulted in identification of 789 cancers, with 663.7 expected (SIR, 1.2; 95% CI, 1.1–1.3). A sixfold increased risk was seen for brain cancer on the basis of 118 observed cases; 43 were seen within 1 year of admission (SIR, 88). The risk for brain tumours in childhood was especially high. A significant excess also occurred for cancer of the lung, but with no clear trend over time. Non-significantly increased risks were seen for cancers of the liver (SIR, 1.9) and biliary tract (SIR, 1.7) on the basis of 9 and 11 observed cases, respectively. It was suggested by the authors that these non-significant increases in risk among patients not known to have received Thorotrast might be related to undocumented exposure to this hepatocarcinogen. Four cases of thyroid cancer were observed, with 3.2 cases expected (SIR, 1.2; 95% CI, 0.3–3.2). Significant deficits of bladder cancer (SIR, 0.6; 18 cases) and melanoma (SIR, 0.5; 7 cases) were observed. In the subgroup of 140 patients with documented exposure to Thorotrast, 17 cases of liver cancer (SIR, 202) and three cases of biliary-tract cancer (SIR, 28) were reported.

White *et al.* (1979) evaluated mortality among patients admitted to one treatment centre for epilepsy in England between 1931 and 1971. Patients were included in the study if their notes stated a diagnosis of epilepsy not due to trauma or progressive disease and if they had been prescribed long-term anti-convulsant drug therapy. Most of the patients severely affected by epilepsy had been treated with phenobarbital and phenytoin. After exclusion of patients who were known to have discontinued anti-convulsant drug therapy within 6 months of starting, 2099 subjects were linked to the files of the National Health Service Central Register of the United Kingdom for information on vital status and migration; for those who had died, a copy of the death certificate was provided by the Office of Population Censuses and Surveys. Personal data on 38 subjects (2%) could not be verified, and 81 were known to have died before the period of follow-up (1951–77), leaving 1980 patients for the analysis of mortality. A total of 78 deaths from cancer was recorded when 51.5 were expected on the basis of the age-, sex- and calendar year-specific rates for England and Wales (standardized mortality ratio [SMR],1.5; 95% CI, 1.2–1.9). Neoplasms of the brain and central nervous system accounted for six of the deaths, with 1.5 expected (SMR, 4.1; 95% CI, 1.5–8.9). When these neoplasms were excluded as possibly being associated with epilepsy, the SMR was 1.4, which was still significantly high (95% CI, 1.1–1.8), but there was no trend over time and no significant excess of deaths was associated with cancer at a particular site. A non-significantly increased risk of 1.4 was seen for lung cancer.

Through a medical records system in Rochester, Minnesota (USA), providing access to all medical contacts of citizens of the area covered by the system, Shirts *et al.* (1986) identified 959 patients in whom an unprovoked seizure disorder had been diagnosed between 1935 and 1979. On the basis of the same records system, patients were followed for new diagnoses of cancer from the date of the initial diagnosis of seizure to death, last contact or the end of 1982: on average, 13 years. A total of 65 primary cancers were diagnosed when 45.9 were expected from the age- and sex-specific incidence rates of the background population, yielding an overall SIR of 1.4 (95% CI, 1.1–1.8). The increased risk was largely attributable to 17 primary brain cancers, for which the expected number was < 1; an SIR of 47 (13 cases) during the first 5 years of follow-up decreased gradually to 12 (two cases) and 5.9 (two cases) in the subsequent 5–9 years and 10 or more years of follow-up, respectively. The risk for lung cancer was also significantly elevated, with an SIR of 2.7 (95% CI, 1.2–5.2); however, seven of the nine cases were observed during the first 5 years of follow-up, limiting the excess to this early period. Marginally significant increased risks were seen for breast cancer (SIR, 2.0; 95% CI, 0.98–3.8; 10 cases) and cancers of the lymphatic and haematopoietic system (SIR, 2.9; 1.0–5.0; seven cases), with no clear trends in risk over time. [The Working Group noted that no information was given on the completeness of follow-up.] The SIR for all cancers except primary brain cancers was 0.9 (95% CI, 0.6–1.4) for users of anticonvulsants and 1.3 (0.8–2.0) for non-users.

2.1.2   *Studies of transplacental exposure*

Annegers *et al.* (1979) reported on the occurrence of brain tumours in 177 individuals born in Rochester, Minnesota (USA), between 1939 and 1976 who had been exposed *in utero* to anti-convulsants during the first trimester of gestation. Barbiturates had been prescribed for the mothers of 135 of these patients. No case of brain tumour was observed during follow-up. [The Working Group noted that the expected number of brain tumours was not estimated, and that the number of person–years of follow-up was not provided]

Olsen *et al.* (1990) conducted a separate study of the incidence of cancer among 3727 offspring of 3758 women admitted for epilepsy to the Filadelfia treatment community in Denmark between 1933 and 1962. A survey of drug use by 130 of the patients indicated that 76% had been treated with phenobarbital and 30% with primidone. The records of the offspring, who were identified from hospital charts, population listings and parish registers, were linked with the files of the Danish Cancer Registry in order to follow-up for cancer through 1986. The expected age-, sex- and calendar time-specific cancer incidence rates for the general population were also derived from the Registry. Overall, 49 cancers were identified, with 53.8 expected, yielding an SIR of 0.9 (95% CI, 0.7–1.2). Among the 2579 children born after their mother's first admission for epilepsy, and thus presumably exposed *in utero* to anticonvulsant drugs, 14 cases of cancer were identified (average follow-up period, 22.4 years; maximum, 50 years), with 13.8 expected (SIR, 1.0; 95% CI, 0.6–1.7). This sub-cohort of offspring showed no excess risk for any specific tumour type, including brain tumours (3 observed cases, 2.2 expected). Among the group of 1148 offspring born before the first admission of the mother to the treatment community, 35 developed cancer (average follow-up period, 37.5 years; maximum, 65 years), with 40.0 expected (SIR, 0.9; 95% CI, 0.6–1.2). No significant increase in the risk for any cancer was found.

2.1.3   *Studies in the general population*

Phenobarbital was included in a hypothesis-generating cohort study designed to screen a large number (215) of drugs for possible carcinogenicity, which covered more than 140 000 subscribers enrolled between July 1969 and August 1973 in a prepaid medical care programme in northern California (USA). Computer records of persons to whom at least one drug prescription has been dispensed were linked to the cancer records of hospitals covered by the medical care programme and the regional cancer registry. The observed numbers of cancers were compared with those expected, standardized for age and sex, for the entire cohort. Three publications summarized the findings for follow-up periods of up to 7 years (Friedman & Ury, 1980), up to 9 years (Friedman & Ury, 1983) and up to 15 years (Selby *et al.*, 1989). Among 5834 persons who received phenobarbital, mostly as a sedative, associations were noted in the 7-year report for cancers of the lung (44 cases observed, 28.9 expected; $p < 0.05$), ovary (seven cases observed, 2.7 expected; $p < 0.05$) and gall-bladder (four cases observed, 1.0 expected; $p < 0.05$) and in the 9-year report for cancer of the lung [figures not given] and gall-bladder and biliary tract (six cases observed, 1.8 expected; $p < 0.05$). In the 15-year report, associations were noted with cancers of the gall-bladder (eight cases observed, 3.2 expected; $p < 0.05$) and bone (three cases observed, 0.6 observed; $p < 0.05$), but not for cancer of the lung. [The Working Group noted, as did the authors, that, since some 12 000 comparisons were made in this hypothesis-generating study, the associations should be verified independently. Data on duration of use were generally not provided.]

In a post-hoc evaluation of the finding of lung cancer in the 7-year follow-up, Friedman (1981) merged this group with 2156 users of pentobarbital and 2884 users of secobarbital, two other commonly used barbiturates. In the combined group of 9816 users of one of these three barbiturates, the author observed 87 cases of lung cancer when 50.2 were expected (SIR, 1.7; $p < 0.002$). Data on smoking habits, collected at regular health check-ups, were available for 49% of the members of the combined cohort, and information on histological subtype of lung cancer was obtained from the medical charts of cancer patients. The resulting SIRs for lung cancer among barbiturate users were 1.5 [95% confidence interval (CI), 0.4–3.8] for non-smokers, 1.4 [0.5–3.0] for ex-smokers and 1.6 [1.1–2.3] for smokers. There was no change in the risk for lung cancer after the incorporation of a lag time of 1 or 2 years in the analysis. There was no particular association with any of the major sub-types of lung cancer.

The risk pattern for lung cancer was evaluated by Friedman and Habel (1999), who extended follow-up through to 1992 and further added users of mixtures of barbiturates, resulting in a group of 10 213 exposed individuals. An initially elevated SIR of 1.6 (95% CI, 1.3–1.9) for lung cancer for the combined group of barbiturate users with 3–7 years of follow-up, unadjusted for smoking habits, gradually decreased and stabilized at about 1.3 [1.2–1.4] after 11–15 years of follow-up. An initial, non-significant increase in the risk for lung cancer of 80% among people who had never smoked decreased to near unity in later periods of follow-up. A dose–response trend was observed, on the basis of the number of prescriptions dispensed, with an SIR of 3.4 (95% CI, 2.0–5.4) for individuals receiving the highest dose (20 or more prescriptions of barbiturates). Adjustment for smoking habits in a Cox model in the subgroup for which this information was available reduced, but did not eliminate, the dose–response trend. [The Working Group noted that the last two analytical studies were post-hoc evaluations of a finding of lung cancer in a large surveillance study with multiple testing. These studies did not include the results for phenobarbital users specifically but rather for the combined group of barbiturate users.]

In a companion study, based on the 10 368 users of barbiturates, Habel *et al.* (1998) observed 34 cases of bladder cancer in the 1992 follow-up, yielding an overall SIR of 0.71 (95% CI, 0.51–1.0). The SIRs for current smokers and former smokers were 0.56 (0.23–1.2) and 0.68 (0.27–1.4), respectively, whereas the SIR for people who had never smoked was 1.04 (0.48–2.0), indicating an inverse association between barbiturate treatment and bladder cancer risk only among current and former smokers.

2.2   Case–control studies (see Table 2)

In order to evaluate the relationships between cancer in children and drugs given to their mothers during pregnancy, Sanders and Draper (1979) studied 11 169 matched case–control pairs of children aged up to 15 years included in the Oxford Survey of Childhood Cancers. A history of epilepsy was reported by 39 case mothers [0.35%] and 22 control mothers [0.20%]; a review of available medical records (for 30 case mothers and 18 control mothers) showed no difference in the proportions of mothers in the two groups who had received phenobarbital (67% and 67%). Six of the 39 tumours in children of mothers with epilepsy were lymphomas, when four cases would have been expected on the basis of the proportion of lymphomas among childhood cancers in the population. [The Working Group noted that the number of children with brain tumours of the 39 mothers with epilepsy was not given.]

In a case–control study by Gold *et al.* (1978), all children under 20 years of age in whom brain tumours had been diagnosed in the Baltimore area, Maryland (USA), between 1965 and 1975 were ascertained from multiple data sources, including hospital tumour registries and death certificates. Of a total of 127 children who were eligible for the study, 84 were included (response rate, 66%) after completion of an interview with the parents. The parents of 76 population controls [response rate not provided] selected from birth certificates and matched to case children by race, sex and date of birth and 112 cancer controls [response rate not provided] selected from the same data sources as the cases and matched by race, sex and date and age at diagnosis were also interviewed [the items included in the interview were not fully characterized]. These subjects formed 73 matched pairs of brain tumour patients and population controls and 78 matched pairs of brain tumour patients and cancer controls, which were analysed separately. In the substudy in which population controls were used, maternal intake of barbiturates during the index pregnancy was associated with an odds ratio of 2.0 (95% CI, 0.3–22). Use of barbiturates by the children themselves was associated with an odds ratio of 2.5 (0.4–26). In the sub-study of matched pairs with cancer controls, the association with prenatal exposure became significant (lower 95% confidence bound, 1.5). Any use of barbiturates pre- or postnatally was significantly associated with brain tumours in the analysis with cancer controls (odds ratio, 5.5; 95% CI, 1.2–51), but not in that with population controls (3.0; 0.8–17). [The Working Group noted that neither

Table 2. Case–control studies of barbiturates, primarily phenobarbital, by cancer site

Country (reference)	Subjects	Exposure estimates	Odds ratio (95% CI)	Comments
Childhood cancers				
England (Sanders & Draper, 1979)	11 169 patients 11 169 cancer controls	Epilepsy in mother	[0.35%] [0.20%]	Formal risk estimates were not provided. Similar proportions of case and control mothers with epilepsy took phenobarbital.
Childhood brain tumours				
USA, Maryland (Gold et al., 1978)	73 patients	Prenatal (maternal) intake of barbiturates	2.0	(0.3–22)	No information available on specific use of phenobarbital
	73 population controls	Postnatal Both	2.5 3.0	(0.4–26) (0.8–17)	
	78 patients	Prenatal	∞	(1.5–∞)	
	78 cancer controls	Postnatal Both	2.5 5.5	(0.4–26) (1.2–51)	
USA, California (Goldhaber et al., 1990)	237 patients 474 controls	Prenatal	1.0	(0.5–1.9)	Based on records for 86 mothers; phenobarbital was the predominant barbiturate used.
		Postnatal Unadjusted Adjusted	1.8 1.4	(1.2–2.7) (0.9–2.2)	Epilepsy of the child included in the adjusted estimate

Table 2 (contd)

Country (reference)	Subjects	Exposure estimates	Odds ratio (95% CI)		Comments
Childhood neuroblastoma					
USA (Kramer et al., 1987)	104 patients 104 controls	Mothers' phenobarbital use	[2.9%] [0.0%] 2.8	(1.3–6.0)	Formal risk estimates were not provided. 90% CI
		Neurally active drugs			
Lung cancer					
Denmark (Olsen et al., 1993)	104 patients 200 controls	Phenobarbital treatment Ever versus never 1–749 g ≥ 750 g	1.2 1.6 1.0	(0.7–2.2) (0.8–3.0) (0.5–1.8)	
Bladder cancer					
Denmark (Olsen et al., 1993)	18 patients 33 controls	Phenobarbital treatment Ever versus never 1–749 g ≥ 750 g	0.3 0.6 0.2	(0.1–0.9) (0.1–2.7) (0.0–0.9)	
Primary liver cancer					
Denmark (Olsen et al., 1995)	26 patients 49 controls	Phenobarbital treatment Ever versus never 5–749 g ≥ 750 g	2.0 0.4 3.2	(0.5–7.2) (0.1–3.4) (0.7–14)	

Table 2 (contd)

Country (reference)	Subjects	Exposure estimates	Odds ratio (95% CI)		Comments
Biliary-tract cancer					
Denmark	13 patients	Phenobarbital treatment			
(Olsen *et al.*, 1995)	24 controls	Ever versus never	1.5	(0.4–6.7)	
		5–749 g	1.3	(0.3–7.0)	
		≥ 750 g	1.6	(0.3–8.9)	
Malignant lymphoma					
Denmark	21 patients	Phenobarbital treatment			
(Olsen *et al.*, 1995)	98 controls	Ever versus never	1.5	(0.5–5.0)	

the type nor duration of the exposure of mothers or children to barbiturates was described.]

In a population-based study in the USA (Kramer *et al.*, 1987), 181 children with newly diagnosed, histologically confirmed neuroblastomas were identified from either the files of the Greater Delaware Valley Pediatric Tumour Registry or the Children's Hospital of Philadelphia for the period 1970–79. Of the 139 children eligible for study, 18 could not be traced and 17 refused, leaving 104 for inclusion (response rate, 75%). One population control per case was selected by random-digit dialling and matched to the case by area of residence, race and date of birth (plus or minus 3 years). The response rate of those eligible and invited was 57%. Interviews, conducted over the telephone with mothers of study subjects, included questions on health history and exposure to alcohol, drugs and other treatments. Three case mothers and no control mothers reported use of phenobarbital at some time during pregnancy. When use of phenobarbital was combined with use during pregnancy of other 'neurally active drugs', defined by the authors to include other barbiturates, amphetamines, narcotics, tranquillizers, diet pills and muscle relaxants, there was a statistically significant, positive association with neuroblastoma in the children, with an odds ratio for the matched pairs of 2.8 (90% CI, 1.3–6.0).

Goldhaber *et al.* (1990) identified 304 children aged 0–19 years, notified with malignant intracranial or spinal cord tumours between 1960 and 1983, from a computerized information system on patients discharged from hospitals run by a prepaid medical care programme in northern California (USA) and the files of the Cancer Registry of the San Francisco Bay Area. The 237 that were included were those for which the diagnosis had been confirmed in a medical record review and whose family had belonged to the programme for at least 6 months. For each study child, two control children were selected from the membership list and matched to the case on year of birth, sex and initial date of membership of the health care programme. The medical charts of the mothers, from the respective birth departments (inside or outside the medical care programme), were reviewed for information on barbiturate use during pregnancy, and the available medical charts on the children after birth were reviewed. Fifty-five cases (23%) and 72 (15%) controls had a history of childhood exposure to barbiturates, yielding an odds ratio of 1.8 (1.2–2.7). In a subgroup of 86 women for whom prenatal records were available, there was no difference between cases and controls with regard to exposure to barbiturates, 19 (22%) case mothers and 39 (23%) control mothers having taken barbiturates during pregnancy, yielding a matched-pair odds ratio of 1.0 (95% CI, 0.5–1.9). Phenobarbital, alone or in combination, was the predominant barbiturate used. Gastrointestinal disorder was the most common indication for barbiturate use for the mothers of both cases (38%) and controls (29%). Epilepsy in the child was associated with an odds ratio for brain cancer of 5.1 (1.8–14). Adjustment for epilepsy in a conditional logistic regression model reduced the odds ratio for brain cancer associated with barbiturate use from 1.8 to 1.4 (0.9–2.2).

Olsen *et al.* (1993) conducted a case–control study of lung and bladder cancer nested in the Danish cohort of epileptic patients described above (Olsen *et al.*, 1989), in order to address the effects of phenobarbital specifically. A total of 111 cases of lung cancer (SIR, 1.5; 95% CI, 1.2–1.8) and 19 cases of bladder cancer (0.6; 0.4–0.9) observed during follow-up of cohort members through 1984 were each matched to two cancer-free cohort members on the basis of sex, year of birth and time from year of first admittance to the treatment centre for epilepsy. Eight cases (6.2%) and 13 controls (5.0%) were excluded because medical records could not be obtained. An additional 14 controls for which the case had been excluded were also dropped, leaving 104 lung cancer cases with 200 lung cancer controls and 18 bladder cancer cases with 33 bladder cancer controls for study. Information on use of phenobarbital, primidone and other anti-convulsants was abstracted from the medical records at the epilepsy centre, and indications of exposure to Thorotrast were obtained from the files of the Danish Thorotrast study. In a conditional logistic regression analysis for matched sets, with adjustment for concurrent use of other anti-convulsants, any use of phenobarbital was associated with odds ratios of 1.2 (95% CI, 0.7–2.2) for lung cancer and 0.3 (0.1–0.9) for bladder cancer. Dose–response analyses revealed no consistent relationship between lung cancer and cumulative exposure to phenobarbital. The risk for bladder cancer declined significantly with increasing cumulative exposure to phenobarbital. Exclusion from the analysis of five cases of lung cancer and two controls for cases of bladder cancer with exposure to Thorotrast did not change the results appreciably.

On the basis of the same cohort of 8004 epileptic patients, Olsen *et al.* (1995) conducted a nested case–control study of hepatobiliary cancer and malignant lymphoma. A total of 26 cases of primary liver cancer (SIR, 4.7; 95% CI, 3.2–6.8), 14 of biliary-tract cancer (2.2; 1.2–3.5), 17 of non-Hodgkin lymphoma (1.5; 0.9–2.3) and six of Hodgkin disease (0.9; 0.4–2.0) observed during follow-up of cohort members through 1984 were each matched to two (hepatobiliary cancers) or five (lymphomas) cancer-free controls on the basis of sex, year of birth and time from year of first admittance to the treatment centre for epilepsy. Three cases (4.8%) and 12 controls (6.2%) were excluded because medical records were missing; an additional 12 controls that were no longer matched to a case were excluded, leaving 60 cases and 171 controls for study. Overall, administration of phenobarbital, adjusted for the effect of other anti-convulsant therapy, was associated with non-significantly increased rates for cancers of the liver (odds ratio, 2.0) and biliary tract (odds ratio, 1.5). A separate, but unadjusted, matched analysis after exclusion of individuals exposed to Thorotrast revealed no increase in risk for liver cancer (odds ratio, 1.0) or for biliary-tract cancers (odds ratio, 0.8) in association with exposure to phenobarbital. The relative risk for malignant lymphomas was 1.5 (95% CI, 0.5–5.0).

3.   Studies on Cancer in Experimental Animals

Phenobarbital has been evaluated previously (IARC, 1977). The Working Group was aware of numerous studies involving long-term oral administration of pheno-barbital to mice and chose a number of well-conducted studies of carcinogenicity in various strains, in which adequate numbers of animals, several doses and an adequate duration were used.

3.1   Oral administration

Mouse: Groups of 17–37 male and 16–39 female C3Hf/Anl (C3H) mice, 1–3 months of age, were fed a control diet or a diet containing 0.05% phenobarbital [purity not specified] for 12 months. Male mice on the control diet had a higher incidence of hepatic tumours (neoplastic hepatic nodules) than females, and an increased tumour inci-dence in animals of each sex was found when the number of mice per cage was decreased from five to one (control males: for five mice/cage, 7/17 (41%); and for one mouse/cage, 25/37 (68%); control females: for five mice/cage, 1/16 (6%); and for one mouse/cage, 5/39 (13%)). Dietary administration of phenobarbital increased the inci-dence of hepatic tumours in animals of each sex (males: 35/36 (97%) for one mouse/ cage and 16/17 (94%) for five mice/cage; females: 29/29 (100%) for one mouse/cage and 10/16 (63%) for five mice/cage). An increase in the multiplicity of tumours was also observed in phenobarbital-treated mice of each sex (males: 6.33 versus 1.62 for one mouse/cage and 4.47 versus 0.41 for five mice/cage; female: 6.66 versus 0.13 for one mouse/cage and 1.44 versus 0.06 for five mice/cage). Treatment with phenobarbital did not affect the histological characteristics or degree of differentiation of hepatic tumours (Peraino *et al.*, 1973a). [The Working Group noted that no statistical methods were used to compare the tumour incidence or multiplicity in treated and untreated groups.]

Groups of 30 male and 30 female CF-1 mice, 4 weeks of age, were fed a diet containing sodium phenobarbital (purity > 97%) at 500 mg/kg for up to 109 weeks. The control groups comprised 45 animals of each sex. Liver tumours were found in 11/45 male and 10/44 female controls and in 24/30 males and 21/28 females treated with phenobarbital. Histologically, the tumours were classified as type A (tumours in which the parenchymal structure was basically retained) and type B (tumours in which the parenchymal structure was distorted). In the treated group, 16 type A tumours and eight type B tumours were found in males and 12 type A and nine type B tumours in females, whereas only two type B tumours were found in control males, and all the other tumours in the control group were type A (Thorpe & Walker, 1973). [The Working Group interpreted type A tumours as adenomas and type B tumours as carcinomas.]

Groups of male and female CF-1 mice were given drinking-water containing 0.05% sodium phenobarbital [purity not specified] (112 males, 74 females) or normal water (49 males and 47 females) from the time of weaning until 120 weeks of age. The average age at death of mice with hepatomas was much lower in treated males (84.9 weeks) than in the controls (106 weeks). The incidences of hepatomas in treated mice were much higher than those in the control groups (treated males, 77/98; treated females, 45/73; control males, 12/44; control females, 0/47). The first hepatoma was found in a treated male at 48 weeks of age, and the first hepatoma was seen in a control male at 79 weeks (Ponomarkov *et al.*, 1976). [The Working Group noted that no statistical methods were used to compare the results in treated and control groups.]

Groups of 30 male and 30 female BALB/c mice, 8 weeks of age, were given drinking-water containing 0.05% sodium phenobarbital (purity, 99%) for life. Fifty male and 50 female mice were used as untreated controls. No liver tumours were observed in either treated or control mice during their lifetime (110–120 weeks). The incidence of lung tumours in treated males (8/30) and females (6/30) was not statistically different from that of control males (19/50) and females (7/50) (Cavaliere *et al.*, 1986).

Groups of male A^{vy}/A (yellow) and agouti A/a (C3H/HeN-MTV/Nctr × VY/WffC3Hf/Nctr-A^{vy})F$_1$ mice, 7–8 weeks of age, were fed a diet containing sodium phenobarbital [purity not specified] at a concentration of 500 mg/kg for 510–593 days. Index groups of 12 treated yellow mice were killed after 12, 15 and 18 months of treatment. No significant difference was seen in the incidence of hepatocellular adenomas between untreated yellow and agouti males at terminal sacrifice. Sodium phenobarbital increased the incidence of hepatocellular adenomas in yellow male mice from 23/193 (12%) in controls to 105/192 (55%) in treated animals. The incidence of hepatocellular adenomas in treated yellow males was significantly greater than that in treated agouti males (105/192 versus 46/192) [*p* value not given in table or text]. Treatment with sodium phenobarbital decreased the incidence of carcinoma significantly (*p* = 0.0001) from that observed in the untreated groups of both yellow (6/192 treated versus 26/193 untreated; *p* = 0.0002) and agouti (15/192 treated versus 28/189 untreated; *p* = 0.03) mice (Wolff *et al.*, 1986).

Groups [initial numbers not specified] of male germ-free (Gf) and conventional (Cv) C3H/He mice, 6 weeks of age, were given an irradiated basal diet containing phenobarbital [purity not specified] at 200 mg/kg until 12 months of age. The incidence and number of liver nodules per mouse in treated Gf mice was significantly higher than that in untreated Gf animals (67% (14/21) versus 30% (42/139); *p* < 0.01; tumour nodules/mouse, 2.0 versus 0.4; *p* < 0.001). The incidence of liver tumour nodules and their average number in phenobarbital-treated Cv mice were also significantly higher than those in untreated mice (100% (31/31) versus 75% (42/56); *p* < 0.01; average number, 4.5 versus 1.3; *p* < 0.001) (Mizutani & Mitsuoka, 1988).

Groups of male C3H/He and C57BL/6 mice, 8 weeks old, were given diets containing sodium phenobarbital [purity not specified] to provide a daily intake of 85 mg/kg bw. Groups of five control and five treated mice of each strain were killed at 5, 30, 40 and 80 weeks, and two additional groups of 20 control and 20 treated animals of each strain were killed at 60 weeks. Further groups of 190 C3H/He and C57BL/6 control and 90 C3H/He and 125 C57BL/6 treated mice were killed *in extremis* or at the end of the respective experiments, i.e. at 91 weeks for C3H/He and 100 weeks for the C57BL/6 mice. In addition, 25 animals of each strain were treated for 60 weeks and then returned to the control diet, and the survivors were killed at the end of the respective experiments. Nodules were seen in both treated and control C3H/He mice as early as 30 weeks, and were numerous in both these groups at the final kill at 91 weeks. In control animals, all the nodules were of the basophilic type, while in the treated group both basophilic and eosinophilic nodules were found. The majority of treated animals bore eosinophilic nodules. By 91 weeks, 80% (16/20) of the control animals and 40% (8/20) of the treated animals bore basophilic nodules, while all the treated animals and none of the controls (0/20) also developed multiple eosinophilic nodules (20/20). C3H/He mice given sodium phenobarbital for 60 weeks and then returned to the control diet bore fewer nodules at 91 weeks than treated mice killed at 60 or 91 weeks. Nodules did not develop in C57BL/6 mice until week 60 in the treated group and not until week 100 among control animals. In C57BL/6 mice treated with sodium phenobarbital, 2/20 mice developed eosinophilic nodules by week 60, and 50% of them bore this type of nodule at 100 weeks; however, fewer eosino-philic nodules were found than in C3H/He mice at 91 weeks (26 in 10 C57 BL/6 mice versus 68 in 20 C3H/He mice). The cumulative incidence of carcinomas in control C3H/He and C57BL/6 mice was 28 and 4%, respectively. The incidence of carcinomas was not increased by treatment with sodium phenobarbital in either strain (30% in C3H/He and 5% in C57BL/6 treated mice). The authors concluded that the two strains of mouse reacted in a qualitatively similar manner to administration of sodium pheno-barbital, although they showed considerable quantitative differences in terms of the time and number of nodules (Evans *et al.*, 1992).

Genetically modified mouse: Groups of single transgenic c-*myc* mice (over-expressing the c-*myc* oncogene), double transgenic c-*myc*/HGF mice (overexpressing c-*myc* and co-expressing the hepatocyte growth factor) and wild-type mice [initial numbers and sex not specified] were given a diet containing 0.05% phenobarbital from 3 weeks to 10 months of age. At 6 months, the incidence of hepatocellular adenomas was 5/10 in c-*myc* mice fed phenobarbital, 0/5 in wild-type mice and 0/10 in c-*myc* mice on basal diet. At 8 months, the incidence of hepatocellular adenomas was 8/10 in c-*myc* mice fed phenobarbital, 0/5 in wild-type mice and 2/10 in c-*myc* mice on basal diet. At 10 months, the incidence of hepatocellular adenomas was 10/10 in c-*myc* mice fed phenobarbital, 0/5 in wild-type mice and 4/12 in *c-myc* mice on basal diet. At 8 months, hepatocellular carcinoma occurred only in c-*myc* mice fed phenobarbital (2/10). At 10 months, the incidence of hepatocellular carcinomas was 4/10 in c-*myc* mice fed phenobarbital, 0/5 in wild-type mice and 1/12 in c-*myc* mice fed basal diet. In contrast to the single transgenic c-*myc* mice, no liver tumours were found in 10 c-*myc*/ HGF mice killed at 6, 8 or 10 months after treatment with phenobarbital, nor were there any liver tumours in the control c-*myc*/HGF animals (10 mice killed at 6 and 8 months and 12 mice at 10 months) (Thorgeirsson & Santoni-Rugiu, 1996; Thorgeirsson *et al.*, 1997).

Groups of 15 male and 15 female $p53$ heterozygous (C57BL/6TacfBR-[KO]$p53^{+/-}$) and wild-type (C57BL/6TacfBR) mice [age unspecified] were fed diets containing phenobarbital at 0, 500 or 1000 mg/kg for 26 weeks. All groups, including those fed normal diet, had a 97% survival rate. All mice fed phenobarbital showed a significant increase in absolute and relative liver weights; no difference in the liver weights was seen between heterozygous and wild type mice. There were no tumours in mice of either sex or genotype treated with phenobarbital, although the livers of all animals showed moderate to marked centrilobular hepatocellular hypertrophy (Sagartz *et al.*, 1998).

Groups of 15 transgenic male MT42 mice harbouring a mouse metallothionein promoter and a human transforming growth factor α (TGFα) cDNA transgene, and 15 non-transgenic male CD-1 mice were given drinking-water containing 0.05% (w/v) sodium phenobarbital from 6 weeks of age for 26 weeks. Five mice from each group were killed at 12, 24 and 32 weeks. The TGFα-transgenic MT42 mice had no tumours at 12 weeks, and the incidence of hepatocellular tumours (adenomas plus carcinomas) after 24 weeks was 4/5 (2/5 mice with carcinomas) and that after 32 weeks was 3/4 (all with carcinomas). No liver tumours appeared in the non-transgenic CD-1 mice at any time during the experiment (Takagi *et al.*, 1993).

Rat: Groups of 34–36 male and female Wistar rats, 7 weeks of age, were given drinking-water containing 0 (control) or 500 mg/L sodium phenobarbital up to 152 weeks of age, when the survivors were killed. No significant differences were found in body-weight gain or survival between groups. Sodium phenobarbital induced hepato-cellular adenomas late in life, the first tumour being diagnosed at 77 weeks. The average age at death of rats with liver tumours was 132 weeks for males and 125 weeks for females. In males and females, respectively, the liver tumour incidences were 1/22 and 2/28 before 99 weeks of age, 5/18 and 2/19 between 100 and 129 weeks and 7/8 and 5/12 from 130 weeks. The cumulative incidences of liver adenomas throughout the study were 0/35 for control and 13/36 for treated males and 0/32 for control and 9/29 for treated females. Among older rats, the numbers of nodules per rat in the treated groups were 11.0 ± 5.5 for males and 14.2 ± 6.0 for females. The hepatocellular nodules were larger in treated females than in males (10.1 ± 3.1 mm versus 5.3 ± 1.1 mm) [no statistical analysis provided] (Rossi *et al.*, 1977).

Fifty male Fischer 344 rats [age unspecified] were placed on a diet containing sodium phenobarbital at 500 mg/kg for 1 week, after which the concentration was increased to 1000 mg/kg of diet and was maintained at this level for 103 weeks. Twenty-five male rats maintained on a normal diet for 2 years served as controls. Of the 33 treated rats that lived 80 weeks or more, 11 (33%) developed small foci of nodular hyperplasia; none developed in the controls. Only one treated animal killed at 102 weeks had a lesion, which compressed the surrounding liver without local invasion or metastasis [an adenoma by recent criteria] (Butler, 1978).

Two groups of 30 male Fischer 344/NCr rats (874 days of age on average) were given drinking-water containing 500 mg/L sodium phenobarbital for up to 233 days. Although there was no significant difference in the number of rats with hepatocellular adenomas between the control (10/30) and the treated group (14/30), the total numbers of hepatocellular adenomas were greater in the treated than the control group (sodium phenobarbital: five basophilic, 64 eosinophilic; control: 14 basophilic, two eosinophilic). Of the 47 hepatocellular adenomas in treated rats that were examined, 36 were positive for γ-glutamyl transpeptidase (γ-GT), while none of the 11 adenomas in control rats were positive for this enzyme. The hepatocellular carcinomas in sodium phenobarbital-treated (2/30) and control rats (2/30) were all negative for the enzyme (Ward, 1983).

Groups of 20 male Fischer 344/DuCrj rats [age unspecified] were fed diets containing sodium phenobarbital at a concentration of 0 (control), 8, 30, 125 or 500 mg/kg for 104 weeks. No treatment-related changes in clinical signs, survival rates, body weight, food consumption or haematological or blood biochemical end-points were observed at any concentration; however, significantly elevated liver weights (relative to body weight) were noted in groups fed 125 and 500 mg/kg of diet ($2.50\% \pm 1.24$ and $3.03\% \pm 0.19$ versus $2.30\% \pm 0.30$, $p < 0.05$ and 0.01, respectively). Hypertrophy of hepatocytes was also seen at these concentrations. Regenerative hyperplasia was observed in 11/20 rats at the highest concentration. Although foci positive for gluta-thione S-transferase (placental form) were found in all groups at termination, the numbers per cm^2 and areas (mm^2/cm^2) in rats fed the two higher concentrations of sodium phenobarbital were significantly higher than control values (average number, > 25 and > 30 versus > 11, $p < 0.01$ for both groups; average area, > 4 and > 8 versus > 1, $p < 0.01$ for both groups). No hepatocellular adenomas were found, and hepato-cellular carcinomas occurred in only one rat each at 8 and 125 mg/kg of diet. At the concentrations given, no changes were observed in any other organ (including thyroid) (Hagiwara et al., 1999).

3.2   Exposure in utero

Mouse: In a study to determine the possible carcinogenic effects of sodium phenobarbital on the offspring of mice exposed both before and during gestation, 12 BALB/c/Cb/Se mice, 10 weeks of age, were given 1 mg of sodium phenobarbital per day by stomach tube for 10 days before and throughout gestation. Twelve mice of the same sex and age given water alone under identical conditions served as controls. During the observation period of 80 weeks, no increase in the incidence of tumours of the liver (control, 0/56; sodium phenobarbital, 0/60 [males and females combined]), lung (control, 13/56; sodium phenobarbital, 18/60) or any other organ was found in exposed offspring compared with those of controls (Cavaliere et al., 1985). [The Working Group noted the small numbers of animals.]

3.3   Administration with known carcinogens and modifying agents

Numerous studies have shown the tumour promoting activity of phenobarbital in mouse and rat liver and rat thyroid, although there is less evidence of such activity in rat lung (Pollard & Luckert, 1997), bladder (Wang *et al.*, 1983; Imaida & Wang, 1986; Diwan *et al.*, 1989a) and male accessory glands (Pollard *et al.*, 1995). The results of the numerous studies of initiation–promotion show that the primary promoting effect of phenobarbital in mice and rats is on the liver and thyroid.

In mice, inhibition or enhancement of hepatocarcinogenesis by phenobarbital depends on the strain, sex, age at the start of exposure and type of initiator used (Uchida & Hirono, 1979; Diwan *et al.*, 1984; Pereira *et al.*, 1985, 1986; Klaunig *et al.*, 1988a,b; Weghorst *et al.*, 1989, 1994).

Selected studies of liver and thyroid tumour promotion are summarized below, while studies of initiation–promotion by phenobarbital in the liver of various species are summarized in Table 3. Table 4 lists similar studies on the thyroid, and Table 5 shows those on other organs.

3.3.1   *Promotion in mouse liver*

(*a*)   *Studies in adult mice*

Groups of 10–12 male mice of strains C57 BL/6NCr (C57BL/6), C3H/HeNCr^{MTV-} (C3H), and DBA/2NCr (DBA/2), 8 weeks of age, were given a single intraperitoneal injection of 90 mg/kg bw *N*-nitrosodiethylamine (NDEA). Beginning 2 weeks later, groups of mice were given drinking-water containing 0.05% phenobarbital, and 10 mice per group were killed at 12, 24, 36 and 52 weeks of age. Phenobarbital significantly increased the incidence of hepatocellular tumours after 24 weeks of treatment in NDEA-initiated C3H mice (from 20% to 70%) and DBA/2 mice (from 0% to 90%). When the mice were 36 weeks of age, the incidence of liver tumours in mice given NDEA alone was 10% for DBA/2, 10% for C57 BL/6 and 50% for C3H mice and those in mice given NDEA plus phenobarbital was 90% in DBA/2 and 100% in C3H mice, but no such increase was observed in C57BL/6 mice. At 52 weeks, the low incidence of hepatocellular tumours in C57BL/6 mice given NDEA was not significantly increased by subsequent exposure to phenobarbital (from 20% to 30%), but DBA/2 mice were especially susceptible (incidence increased from 40% to 100%) (Diwan *et al.*, 1986a).

In order to analyse the genetics of susceptibility to promotion of hepatocarcinogenesis in DBA/2NCr (susceptible) and C57BL/6NCr (resistant) mice by phenobarbital, groups of 40 reciprocal F_1 hybrid male B6D2F$_1$ and D2B6F$_1$, 5 weeks of age, were given an intraperitoneal injection of 90 mg/kg bw NDEA or an equal volume of tricaprylin. Two weeks later, the groups received 0.05% phenobarbital continuously in the drinking-water or drinking-water alone. Ten mice from each group were killed at 33 weeks of age, and the remaining mice were killed when found moribund or at

Table 3. Promotion of preneoplastic and neoplastic liver lesions by phenobarbital (PB) or sodium phenobarbital (NaPB) in mice, rats, hamsters and monkeys initiated by various carcinogens

Strain (sex)	Initiator, dose, route and duration	Interval between initiator and promoter	Dose and duration of PB or NaPB and route	Promoting or anti-promoting effects on preneoplastic or neoplastic hepatocellular lesions	Reference
Mouse					
C57BL/6, C3H and DBA2 (M)	NDEA, 90 mg/kg bw, ip × 1	2 weeks	PB, 0.05% in water, 52 weeks	Percentage of mice with tumours C57BL/6: NDEA, 20%; NDEA + PB, 30% C3H: NDEA, 90%; NDEA + PB, 100% DBA/2: NDEA, 40%; NDEA + PB, 100%	Diwan et al. (1986a)
D2B6F$_1$ (M)	NDEA, 90 mg/kg bw, ip × 1	2 weeks	PB, 0.05% diet up to 53 weeks (NDEA alone, 110 weeks)	Percentage of mice with tumours NDEA: adenomas, 97%; carcinomas, 40%; hepatoblastomas, 10% NDEA + PB: adenomas, 96%; carcinomas, 90%; hepatoblastomas, 77%	Diwan et al. (1995)
C3H, C57BL/6 and BALB/c (M)	NDEA 20 h after PH, 20 mg/kg bw, ip × 1	6 h	PB, 0.05% diet, 20 weeks	Total volume of EAIs: C3H: NDEA, 710/cm³, NDEA + PB, 83824/cm³ C57BL/6: NDEA, 83/cm³; NDEA + PB, 131/cm³ BALB/c: NDEA, 140/cm³; NDEA + PB, 5452/cm³	Lee et al. (1989)
B6C3F$_1$ (M)	NDEA, 35 mg/kg bw, ip × 2/week/8 weeks	12 weeks	PB, 0.05% diet, 60 days	Altered foci per liver (NDEA, 407; NDEA + PB, 696); PB removed for 30 days (NDEA + PB, 95)	Kolaja et al. (1996a)

Table 3 (contd)

Strain (sex)	Initiator, dose, route and duration	Interval between initiator and promoter	Dose and duration of PB or NaPB and route	Promoting or anti-promoting effects on preneoplastic or neoplastic hepatocellular lesions	Reference
Transgenic mice					
TGF-α transgenic (MT42) and non-transgenic CD1 (M)	NDEA, 5 mg/kg bw, ip × 1 at 15 days of age	2 weeks	PB, 0.05% diet, 35 weeks	MT42: NDEA or NDEA + PB, 80–100% carcinomas; PB alone, 33%; CD1: NDEA + PB, 40% carcinomas; NDEA or PB alone, no tumours	Tamano et al. (1994)
$Cx32^{y/+}$, $Cx32^{y/-}$	NDEA, 90 mg/kg, ip × 1	NR	PB, 0.05% diet, 39 weeks	Promotion of liver tumours in $Cx32^{y/+}$ mice but not in $Cx32^{y/-}$ mice	Moennikes et al. (2000)
Rat					
SD/Anl [Anl66] (NR)	AAF, 0.02% diet, 11, 16, 21 or 26 days	None	PB, 0.05% diet, 260 days	Highest incidence of hepatomas in group initiated for 26 days (AAF, 27/103; AAF + PB, 86/108)	Peraino et al. (1971)
Sprague-Dawley (M)	AAF, 0.02% diet, 18 days	Various intervals (up to 120 days)	PB, 0.05% diet, up to 407 days	Final tumour incidences influenced by duration of post-AAF treatment and not length of treatment-free intervals	Peraino et al. (1977)
Fischer 344 (NR)	AAF, 0.02% for 13 weeks + iron-loading diet	0 days	PB, 0.05% diet, 24 weeks	Iron accumulation-resistant foci; when AAF discontinued, foci disappear; AAF followed by PB, foci reappear	Watanabe & Williams (1978)

Table 3 (contd)

Strain (sex)	Initiator, dose, route and duration	Interval between initiator and promoter	Dose and duration of PB or NaPB and route	Promoting or anti-promoting effects on preneoplastic or neoplastic hepatocellular lesions	Reference
Sprague-Dawley (M)	B[a]P, 4 mg/rat ig × 6 (24 h after PH)	2 weeks	PB, 0.05% diet, 50 weeks	B[a]P given ig followed by PB produced tumours in 6/15 rats; PB alone, 0/10	Kitagawa et al. (1980)
Donryu (M)	3'-Me-DAB, 0.06% diet, 3 weeks	2 weeks	PB, 0.05% diet with initiator and/or given as a promoter for 35 weeks	Inhibition of EAIs when given with initiator; promotion when given after initiation	Narita et al. (1980)
CD1 (M)	AAF, 0.02% diet, 2 weeks	1 week	PB, 0.002–0.25% diet (various concentrations), 78–84 weeks	Dose-dependent tumour-promoting effects	Peraino et al. (1980)
ACI (M and F)	Cycasin, 100 mg/kg bw, ig × 1	1 week	PB, 0.05% diet, up to 480 days	γ-GT-positive foci; incidence significantly greater in females than in males	Uchida & Hirono (1981)
CD (F)	N-OH-AABP or N-OH-FABP, 0.4 mmol/kg bw, ip × 1 (24 h after PH)	2 days	PB, 0.05% diet, 64 weeks	γ-GT-positive foci; no growth with PB alone; growth initiated by PH + PB	Shirai et al. (1981)
Sprague-Dawley (M)	NDEA, 40 or 50 mg/kg bw, ip (18 h after PH)	1 week	PB 0.06% with choline-sufficient diet for 6 or 7 weeks or choline-deficient diet for 8 weeks	γ-GT-positive foci; choline-sufficient + PB, increased; choline-deficient + PB, synergistic promoting action	Shinozuka et al. (1982)
Wistar (M)	NDEA, ~ 10 mg/kg bw in water, 2, 4 or 6 weeks	1 week	PB, ~ 15 mg/kg bw per day in water, 4, 6 or 8 weeks	PB treatment reduced latency for development of neoplastic nodules by 3–6 months	Barbason et al. (1983)

Table 3 (contd)

Strain (sex)	Initiator, dose, route and duration	Interval between initiator and promoter	Dose and duration of PB or NaPB and route	Promoting or anti-promoting effects on preneoplastic or neoplastic hepatocellular lesions	Reference
Sprague-Dawley (M)	NMOR, 120 mg/L, in water, 7 weeks	0 days	PB, 0.75, 0.075 or 0.0075 g/L, drinking-water, 16 weeks	γ-GT, G6PDH, ATPase-deficient foci; dose-dependent promotion by PB	Moore et al. (1983)
Fischer 344 (M)	FANFT, 0.2% diet, 6 weeks	1 week	PB, 0.05% diet, 86 weeks	No phenotype given; promotion by PB	Wang et al. (1983)
Sprague-Dawley (M)	NMOR, 80 mg/L, in water, 7 weeks	5 weeks	PB, 0.05% diet for 10 weeks, before or after NMOR	γ-GT-positive foci; slight inhibition before NMOR; promotion after NMOR	Schwarz et al. (1983)
Sprague-Dawley (M)	NMOR, 200 mg/L, in water, 3 weeks	1 week	PB, 0.05% diet, 12, 24, 36 or 48 weeks	γ-GT-, G6PDH-, ATPase-positive foci; time-dependent in number and size of foci; PB increased homogeneity and number of foci; increased G6PDH activity	Ito et al. (1984)
Donryu (M)	3'-Me-DAB, diet, 3 weeks	None	PB, 5–500 mg/kg of diet, 21 weeks	Dose-dependent increase in number and size of EAIs	Kitagawa et al. (1984)
Fischer 344 (M)	AAF, 0.02% diet, 8 weeks	4 weeks	PB, 0.05% diet, for 24 weeks, after or before AAF (4-week interval between PB and AAF)	PB had promoting but not syncarcinogenic effect.	Williams & Furuya (1984)
Fischer 344 (M and F)	MNU, 0.05 mmol/kg bw, iv × 1/week, 4 weeks	2 weeks	PB, 0.05% in water, 71 weeks	MNU alone, no liver tumours; MNU + PB, 50% males and 40% females developed liver tumours	Diwan et al. (1985)
Sprague-Dawley (F)	NDEA, 10 mg/kg bw, ig × 1, 24 h after PH	2–6 weeks	PB, 0.00005–0.2% diet, 7–8 months	Dose-dependent increase in number and size of foci; NOAEL at 0.001%	Goldsworthy et al. (1984)

Table 3 (contd)

Strain (sex)	Initiator, dose, route and duration	Interval between initiator and promoter	Dose and duration of PB or NaPB and route	Promoting or anti-promoting effects on preneoplastic or neoplastic hepatocellular lesions	Reference
Fischer 344 (M)	NDEA, 200 mg/kg bw or N-OH-AAF, 30 mg/kg bw or AFB₁, 0.5 or 1.0 mg/kg bw, ip	2 weeks	PB, 0.05% diet, 6 weeks; PH end of third week of the experiment	γ-GT-positive foci; growth only in NDEA-initiated rats	Shirai et al. (1985)
Wistar (M)	NDEA 10 mg/kg bw per day + PB 15 mg/ rat, for 2, 4 or 6 weeks	None (simultaneous administration)	PB, 15 mg/rat, for 2, 4 or 6 weeks	PAS-positive; at 6 weeks significant decrease in number of foci with NDEA + PB	Barbason et al. (1986)
Wistar (M)	NDEA, 1.1, 3.3, 10 or 30 mg/kg bw, ip × 1	1 week	NaPB, 40, 100 or 1000 μg/mL in water, 12–18 months	Liver carcinomas (38%) seen only after 1000 μg/mL PB promotion and 30 mg/kg bw NDEA	Driver & McLean (1986a)
CD (F)	NDEA, 10 mg/kg bw, ig, 20 h after PH	1 week	PB, 0.05% diet, 6 months; PB withdrawn for 10 days	γ-GT-positive foci; growth with PB; decrease in number and size of foci after withdrawal of PB	Glauert et al. (1986)
	NDEA, 10 mg/kg bw, ig, 20 h after PH	1 week	PB, 0.05% diet, 3 months, then high- or low-fat diet for 8 months	At 3 months, promotion of mostly γ-GT-positive foci; high- or low-fat diet decreased number and size of foci	
Fischer 344 (F)	NDEA, 10 mg/kg bw ig × 1, 24 h after PH	1 week	PB, 0.05% diet, 4 months; groups of rats withdrawn from PB for 5–180 days; re-administration of PB for 10–90 days	Altered hepatocellular foci; withdrawal of PB decreased total number; re-administration of PB increased number	Hendrich et al. (1986)

Table 3 (contd)

Strain (sex)	Initiator, dose, route and duration	Interval between initiator and promoter	Dose and duration of PB or NaPB and route	Promoting or anti-promoting effects on preneoplastic or neoplastic hepatocellular lesions	Reference
Fischer 344 (M)	NBHPA, 1000 mg/kg bw ip × 1 + (250 mg/kg bw ip × 3, fortnightly, 3 weeks later)	1 week	PB, 0.05% in water, 22 weeks	γ-GT-positive foci; promotion by PB	Moore et al. (1986)
Sprague-Dawley (M/F)	NDEA, 4, 8 or 16 mg/kg bw, ip at day 1	20 days	PB, 0.05% diet, 8 weeks	γ-GT-positive foci, increase in number and size of foci (similar in both sexes); γ-GT-positive/Fe-resistant foci, greater in F	Peraino et al. (1987)
Fischer 344 (F)	NDEA, 10 mg/kg bw, ig × 1, 24 h after PH	2 weeks	PB, 0.001–0.5% diet (various concentrations), 6 months	Dose-dependent increase in number and volume of foci; threshold at 0.005%	Pitot et al. (1987)
Fischer 344 (M)	NBHPA, 0.2% in water, 1 week	1 week	PB, 0.05% diet, 50 weeks	No phenotype given; promotion by PB	Shirai et al. (1988)
Fischer 344 (M)	IQ, 0.025, 0.05 or 0.1% diet, 2 weeks (PH at end of first week)	1 week	PB, 0.05% diet, 83 weeks	IQ, no carcinomas; IQ + PB, 35–50% carcinomas; increase in γ-GT-positive foci	Tsuda et al. (1988)

Table 3 (contd)

Strain (sex)	Initiator, dose, route and duration	Interval between initiator and promoter	Dose and duration of PB or NaPB and route	Promoting or anti-promoting effects on preneoplastic or neoplastic hepatocellular lesions	Reference
Fischer 344 (M)	NDEA, 1 × 100 mg/kg bw (day 1) + MNU, 4 × 20 mg/kg bw (days 2, 5, 8, 11), ip + NBHPA, 0.1% in water, 2 weeks (weeks 3–4)	0 day	NaPB, 0.05% diet, 14 or 20 weeks	GST-P-positive foci; increase in number and size of foci	Shibata et al. (1990)
Fischer 344 (M and F)	NDEA, 10 mg/kg bw × 1 (24 h after PH) at 4 weeks, 6 or 12 months of age, ig	2 weeks	PB, 0.05%, 6 months	γ-GT-positive foci; growth more effective at 6 months than when initiated at 4 weeks or 12 months; males more susceptible	Xu et al. (1990)
Wistar (F)	NDEA, 10 mg/kg bw, ig	10 days	PB, 20, 50, 100, 200 and 200 mg/L in water for 70, 23, 11, 9, 5 weeks, respectively	ATPase-deficient foci; not increased at 20 mg/L; no effect at 50, 100 mg/L; inhibitory effect at 200 mg/L	Appel et al. (1991)
Fischer 344 (M)	NBHPA, 1000 mg/kg bw × 2 (week 1), ip; NEHEA, 1500 mg/kg bw × 2 (week 2), ip; DMAB, 75 mg/kg bw (week 3), sc × 2	1 week	PB, 0.05% diet, 12 weeks	GST-P-positive foci; promotion by PB	Uwagawa et al. (1992)
Fischer 344/DuCrj (M)	NDEA, 100 mg/kg bw, ip	1 week	PB, 1, 4, 16, 75, 300 or 1200 mg/L in water, 39 weeks	γ-GT-positive, GST-P-positive foci; dose-dependent promotion by PB from 75 to 1200 mg/L	Maekawa et al. (1992)

Table 3 (contd)

Strain (sex)	Initiator, dose, route and duration	Interval between initiator and promoter	Dose and duration of PB or NaPB and route	Promoting or anti-promoting effects on preneoplastic or neoplastic hepatocellular lesions	Reference
SPF Wistar (M/F)	AFB$_1$, 2 mg/kg bw (M), 5 mg/kg bw (F), ig	3 weeks	PB, 50 mg/kg diet for 70 weeks (F) and 55–59 weeks (M)	GST subunits; mostly eosinophilic clear-cell foci with elevated levels of mu (Yb1, Yb2) and pi (Yp) family subunits	Grasl-Kraupp et al. (1993)
Fischer 344 (M)	PB, 0.1% in water, AFB$_1$, 1 mg/kg bw, ip	–	PB, 1 week before AFB$_1$	GST-P-positive foci; inhibition of AFB$_1$-induced foci by PB	Gopalan et al. (1993)
Fischer 344 (M)	NBHPA, 2000 mg/kg bw, sc	1 week	PB, 1000 mg/kg bw or (PB, 500 mg/kg bw diet + thiourea, 0.05% in water), 19 weeks	Eosinophilic, basophilic, clear-cell foci; increase with PB; synergistic with thiourea	Shimo et al. (1994)
Sprague-Dawley (F)	NDEA, 10 mg/kg bw	1 week	PB, 500 mg/kg diet for 170 or 240 days; + TCDD (150 μg/kg diet) from 170 to 240 days or 240 to 450 days	Eosinophilic foci; PB alone, no effect; PB + TCDD, increase in number and size	Sills et al. (1994)
Wistar (M)	Tamoxifen, 420 mg/kg diet, 3 months	0 days	PB, 0.1% in water for 3, 6, 9, 12 months or lifetime	GST-P-positive foci; increased at 6 and 9 months	Carthew et al. (1995)
Fischer 344 (M)	^{192}Ir seeds	None	PB, 0.05% diet, 20, 40 or 60 weeks	PB promoted development of EAIs initiated by ^{192}Ir	Ida et al. (1995)
Sprague-Dawley (F)	NDEA, 10 mg/kg bw, ip at 5 days of age	16 days	PB, 10, 100 or 500 mg/kg diet and/or mestranol, 0.02 or 0.2 mg/kg diet, 8 months	GST-P-positive foci; growth at low mestranol + 10 or 100 mg/kg diet PB; no growth at low mestranol + 500 mg/kg diet PB; high mestranol effective only with 100 mg/kg diet PB	Dragan et al. (1996)

Table 3 (contd)

Strain (sex)	Initiator, dose, route and duration	Interval between initiator and promoter	Dose and duration of PB or NaPB and route	Promoting or anti-promoting effects on preneoplastic or neoplastic hepatocellular lesions	Reference
Fischer 344 (M)	NDEA, 150 mg/kg bw, ip × 2	4 months	PB, 10, 100 or 500 mg/kg diet for 7, 30 or 60 days	Eosinophilic foci; growth at 100 (7 and 60 days), 500 (30 and 60 days) mg/kg diet; at 10 mg/kg diet, PB was ineffective	Kolaja et al. (1996b)
Fischer 344 (M)	NDEA, 100 mg/kg bw, ip × 1/week, 3 weeks	1 week	PB, 500 mg/kg diet, 20 weeks or PB + 100 mg/kg diet MMTS, 20 weeks	GST-P-positive foci; promotion with PB; inhibition with PB + MMTS	Sugie et al. (1997)
Fischer 344 (M)	NDEA, 200 mg/kg bw, ip; 2 weeks later, D-galactosamine, 300 mg/kg bw, ip at the end of weeks 2 and 5	2 weeks	PB, 500 mg/kg diet, weeks 3–8	GST-P-positive foci; promotion by PB; multiple injection of D-galactos-amine as effective as PH	Kim et al. (1997)
Fischer 344 (M)	NDEA, 200 mg/kg ip, PH at week 3	2 weeks	PB, 1, 2, 4, 7.5, 15 or 500 mg/kg diet, 6 weeks	GST-P- and TGF-α-positive foci; promotion at 500 mg/kg diet; inhibition at 1, 2, 4, 7.5 mg/kg diet	Kitano et al. (1998)
			PB, 0.01, 0.1 or 0.5 mg/kg diet, 6 weeks	No promotion	
			PB, 1, 2, 4, 7.5, 15, 30, 60, 125, 250 or 500 mg/kg diet, 6 weeks	GST-positive foci; promotion at doses higher than 15 mg/kg diet; inhibition at 2 and 4 mg/kg diet	

Table 3 (contd)

Strain (sex)	Initiator, dose, route and duration	Interval between initiator and promoter	Dose and duration of PB or NaPB and route	Promoting or anti-promoting effects on preneoplastic or neoplastic hepatocellular lesions	Reference
Hamster					
Syrian golden (M)	NDEA, 100 mg/kg bw, ip × 1 or MAMA, 20 mg/kg bw × 1	2 weeks	PB, 0.05% in water, up to 62 weeks	Percentage of mice with tumours: NDEA alone, 37% adenomas; MAMA alone, 63% adenomas, 11% carcinomas; NDEA + PB, 27% adenomas; MAMA + PB, 67% adenomas, 11% carcinomas	Diwan et al. (1986b)
Syrian golden (NR)	NDMA, 6 mg/kg bw, ip × 1	1 week	PB, 0.05% diet, 31 weeks	NDMA alone, 1/15 adenomas; NDMA + PB, 3/15 adenomas	Tanaka et al. (1987)
Monkey					
Erythrocebus patas (M and F)	NDEA (to pregnant monkeys), 0.6–3.2 mmol/kg bw (cumulative), iv	4 years	PB (to mother and offspring), 15 mg/kg bw per day in water, up to 43 months	NDEA alone, no tumours; NDEA + PB, 11.6 adenomas per mother, 5.6 adenomas per offspring	Rice et al. (1989)
	NDEA, 0.1–0.4 mmol/kg bw, ip (at 14-day intervals) × 20	2 weeks	PB, 15 mg/kg bw in water, 9 months	NDEA alone, 1.6 adenomas per monkey and 0.3 carcinomas per monkey; NDEA + PB, 17.25 adenomas per monkey and 2.0 carcinomas per monkey	

Table 3 (contd)

AAF, 2-acetylaminofluorene
AFB$_1$, aflatoxin B$_1$
B[a]P, benzo[a]pyrene
DMAB, 3,3'-dimethyl-4-aminobiphenyl
EAI, enzyme-altered island
F, female
FANFT, N-[4-(5-nitro-2-furyl)-2-thiazolyl]formamide
G6PDH, glucose 6-phosphate dehydrogenase
γ-GT, γ-glutamyl transferase
GST, glutathione S-transferase
GST-P, glutathione S-transferase placental form
ig, intragastrically
ip, intraperitoneally
IQ, 2-amino-3-methylimidazo[4,5-f]quinoline
iv, intravenously
M, male
MAMA, methylazoxymethanol acetate
3'-Me-DAB, 3'-methyl-4-(dimethylamino)azobenzene

MMTS, S-methyl methanethiosulfonate
MNU, N-methyl-N-nitrosourea
NBHPA, N-nitrosobis(2-hydroxypropyl)amine
NDEA, N-nitrosodiethylamine
NEHEA, N-nitrosoethyl-N-hydroxyethylamine
NMOR, N-nitrosomorpholine
NOAEL, no-observed-adverse-effect level
N-OH-AABP, N-hydroxy-4-acylaminobiphenyl
N-OH-AAF, N-hydroxy-2-acetylaminofluorene
N-OH-FABP, N-hydroxy-4-formylaminobiphenyl
NR, not reported
PAS, periodic acid-Schiff
PH, partial hepatectomy
sc, subcutaneously
SPF, specific pathogen-free
TCDD, 2,3,7,8-tetrachloro-$para$-dibenzodioxin
TGF-α, transforming growth factor α

Table 4. Promotion of thyroid tumours in rats initiated by various carcinogens and promoted by phenobarbital (PB) or sodium phenobarbital (NaPB)

Strain (sex)	Initiator, dose, route and duration	Interval between initiator and promoter	Dose, route and duration of PB or NaPB	Promoting effects on preneoplastic and/or neoplastic thyroid lesions	Reference
Wistar (M)	NBHPA, 70 mg/kg bw per week, sc × 1 per week, 6 weeks	1 week	PB, 500 mg/kg diet, 12 weeks	Follicular-cell neoplasms; NBHPA, 23%; NBHPA + PB, 100%	Hiasa et al. (1982)
Wistar (M)	NBHPA, 2800 mg/kg bw, sc	1 week	PB, 500 mg/kg diet, 6, 12 or 19 weeks	Follicular-cell adenomas at 19 weeks: NBHPA, 37%; NBHPA + PB, 87%	Hiasa et al. (1983)
Wistar (M and F)	NBHPA, 2100 mg/kg bw (M), 4200 mg/kg bw (F), ip	1 week	PB, 20, 100, 500 or 2500 mg/kg diet, 19 weeks	Thyroid tumours; 500 mg/kg diet, 3-fold yield in M only; 2500 mg/kg diet, 8-fold in M and 3-fold in F	Hiasa et al. (1985)
Wistar (M), castrated at week 2 or at beginning	NBHPA, 2100 mg/kg bw, ip, week 1	1 week	PB, 500 mg/kg diet, 38 weeks	Follicular-cell adenomas; NBHPA, 20%; NBHPA + PB, 75%; castrated at week 2, 30%; castrated at beginning, 20%	Hiasa et al. (1987)
Fischer 344 (M)	NDEA, 75 mg/kg bw × 1, ip	2 weeks	PB, 500 mg/kg diet, 45–71 weeks	Follicular-cell tumours at 71 weeks NDEA, 0/15; NDEA + PB, 5/15	Diwan et al. (1988)
Fischer 344 (M and F)	MNU, 0.05 mmol/kg bw, iv × 1 per week, 4 weeks, or 0.2 mmol/kg bw, iv × 1	None, 2 or 5 weeks	PB, 0.05% in water with or following MNU	Follicular-cell tumours; PB promotion by both simultaneous and subsequent administration	Diwan et al. (1985)
Fischer 344 (M)	NBHPA, 1000 mg/kg bw, ip × 1 + (250 mg/kg bw, ip × 3, fortnightly, 3 weeks later)	1 week	PB, 0.05% in water, 22 weeks	Follicular-cell adenomas; NBHPA, 3/15; NBHPA + PB, 9/15	Moore et al. (1986)

Table 4 (contd)

Strain (sex)	Initiator, dose, route and duration	Interval between initiator and promoter	Dose, route and duration of PB or NaPB	Promoting effects on preneoplastic and/or neoplastic thyroid lesions	Reference
CD (SD) BR (M and F)	NBHPA, 700 mg/kg bw × 1 per week, sc, 5 weeks	2 weeks	PB, 500 mg/kg diet and/or thyroxine, 15 weeks	Follicular-cell adenomas; M: NBHPA, 6/16; NBHPA + PB, 15/18; NBHPA + PB + thyroxine, 5/20; F: NBHPA + PB, 1/20	McClain et al. (1988)
Fischer 344 (M)	NBHPA, 0.2% in water	1 week	PB, 500 mg/kg diet, 50 weeks	Follicular-cell adenomas	Shirai et al. (1988)
Fischer 344 (M)	IQ, 0.025, 0.05 or 0.1% diet, 2 weeks	1 week	PB, 0.05% diet	Papillar adenomas and carcinomas; IQ (0.1%), 5.3%; IQ + PB, 44–64%	Tsuda et al. (1988)
Fischer 344 (M)	NDMA.OAc, 0.05 nmol/kg bw, ip	2 weeks	PB, 500 mg/L in drinking-water, 50 or 78 weeks	Follicular-cell tumours at 78 weeks; NDMA.OAc, 1/15; NDMA.OAc + PB, 7/15	Diwan et al. (1989c)
Fischer 344/DuCrj (M)	NBHPA, 2800 mg/kg bw, sc	1 week	PB, 0.05% in water, 25 weeks	Multiple thyroid neoplasms; NBHPA, 3/30; NBHPA + PB, 14/30	Kanno et al. (1990)
Fischer 344 (M)	NDEA, 100 mg/kg bw, ip × 1 (day 1) + MNU, 20 mg/kg bw, ip × 4 (day 2, 5, 8 and 11) + NBHPA, 0.1% in water, 2 weeks (weeks 3–4)	0 day	NaPB, 500 mg/kg diet, 20 weeks	Follicular-cell hyperplasia and adenoma: initiated rats, 5/15 and 4/15; initiated rats given NaPB, 14/15 and 12/15	Shibata et al. (1990)

Table 4 (contd)

Strain (sex)	Initiator, dose, route and duration	Interval between initiator and promoter	Dose, route and duration of PB or NaPB	Promoting effects on preneoplastic and/or neoplastic thyroid lesions	Reference
Fischer 344 (M)	NBHPA, 1000 mg/kg bw, ip × 2 (week 1) + NEHEA, 1500 mg/kg bw, ig × 2 (week 2) + NEHEA, 75 mg/kg bw, sc × 2 (week 3)	1 week	PB, 0.05% in diet, 12 weeks	Follicular-cell hyperplasia (no adenoma): NBHPA + NEHEA + DMAB, 0/15; NBHPA + NEHEA + DMAB + PB, 5/15	Uwagawa et al. (1992)

DMAB, 3,3'-dimethyl-4-aminobiphenyl
F, female
ip, intraperitoneally
IQ, 2-amino-3-methylimidazo[4,5-f]quinoline
iv, intravenously
M, male
MNU, N-methyl-N-nitrosourea
NBHPA, N-nitrosobis(2-hydroxypropyl)amine
NDEA, N-nitrosodiethylamine
NDMA.OAc, N-nitrosomethyl(acetoxymethyl)amine
NEHEA, N-nitrosoethyl-N-hydroxyethylamine
sc, subcutaneously

Table 5. Tumours in other organs initiated by various carcinogens and promoted by phenobarbital (PB) or sodium phenobarbital (NaPB)

Strain (sex)	Initiator, dose, route and duration	Interval between initiator and promoter	Dose, route and duration of PB or NaPB	Promoting effects on pre-neoplastic and/or neoplastic lesions	Reference
Lung					
Mouse					
Swiss (M and F)	Urethane, 4%, 1 mL, sc × 1	0 day	PB, 2%, 0.1 mL, sc × 1/day, 6 days, before urethane; PB, 2%, 0.1 mL, sc × 1/day, 8 days	PB before urethane: inhibition of tumour formation; PB after urethane: no effect	Adenis *et al.* (1970)
ddy (pregnant)	ENU, 50 mg/kg bw, ip × 1, on gestation day 16	4 weeks	PB, 0.05% diet to offspring, 4 weeks to 6 months of age	No promotion by PB	Tsuchiya *et al.* (1984)
Rat					
Wistar (NR)	MNU, 30 mg/kg bw, iv × 1	7 months	PB, 0.5% diet or NaPB, 0.05% in water, 15–16 months	Promotion by PB and NaPB	Pollard & Luckert (1997)
Bladder					
Mouse					
C57BL/6 (M/F)	NBHPA, 0.022% or NDBA, 0.024% in water for life	None	NaPB, 1 mg/mL in water, starting 1 week before initiation and continued concurrently	No effect on NBHPA-induced tumours; prolonged tumour induction by NDBA	Bertram & Craig (1972)
Rat					
Fischer 344 (M)	FANFT, 0.2% diet, 6 weeks	1 week	PB, 0.05% diet, 86 weeks	PB promoted bladder carcinogenesis	Wang *et al.* (1983)

Table 5 (contd)

Strain (sex)	Initiator, dose, route and duration	Interval between initiator and promoter	Dose, route and duration of PB or NaPB	Promoting effects on pre-neoplastic and/or neoplastic lesions	Reference
Fischer 344 (M)	FANFT, 0.2% diet or NDBA, 0.005% in water, 4 weeks	1 week	NaPB, 0.05% or 0.15% diet, 95 weeks	NaPB promoted bladder carcinogenesis initiated with FANFT but not with NDBA	Imaida & Wang (1986)
Fischer 344 (M)	FANFT, 0.2% diet, 2 or 6 weeks	2 weeks	NaPB, 0.1% diet, 60 weeks	NaPB promoted preneoplastic bladder lesions in rats fed FANFT for 6 weeks	Diwan *et al.* (1989a)
Skin					
Mouse					
HRS/J/Anl (F)	DMBA, 250 µg, topical × 1/week, 6 weeks	1 week	PB, 0.05% diet, 49 weeks	PB had no effect on skin tumour development	Grube *et al.* (1975)
	DMBA, 250 µg, topical × 1/week, 12 weeks	None	PB, 0.05% diet, 49 weeks (starting week 7)	PB decreased skin tumour development after 10 weeks of DMBA	
Brain					
Rat					
Fischer 344 (pregnant)	ENU, 3.5 mg/kg bw, iv × 1, day 20 of gestation	4 weeks	PB, 0.05% in water, 74 weeks	PB had no effect on ENU-induced neurogenic tumours	Walker & Swenberg (1989)

Table 5 (contd)

Strain (sex)	Initiator, dose, route and duration	Interval between initiator and promoter	Dose, route and duration of PB or NaPB	Promoting effects on pre-neoplastic and/or neoplastic lesions	Reference
Male accessory glands					
Rat					
Wistar (M)	MNU, 30 mg/kg bw, iv × 1	7 months	PB, 500 mg/kg diet, 7 months	PB promoted MNU-induced male accessory gland carcinogenesis (prostate and seminal vesicle)	Pollard *et al.* (1995)
Gastrointestinal tract					
Rat					
Wistar (M)	MNNG, 100 mg/L in water, 8 weeks	0 day	PB, 0.05% diet, 32 weeks	PB had not effect on MNNG-induced gastro-duodenal tumours	Takahashi *et al.* (1984)
Fischer 344 (M)	NDMA.OAc, 0.05 nmol/kg bw, ip × 1	2 weeks	PB, 0.05% in water, 78 weeks	PB had no effect on NDMA.OAc-induced intestinal tumours	Diwan *et al.* (1989c)

Table 5 (contd)

DMBA, 7,12-dimethylbenz[*a*]anthracene
ENU, *N*-ethyl-*N*-nitrosourea
F, female
FANFT, *N*-[4-(5-nitro-2-furyl)-2-thiazolyl]formamide
ip, intraperitoneally
iv, intravenous;y
M, male

MNNG, *N*-methyl-*N'*-nitro-*N*-nitrosoguanidine
MNU, *N*-methyl-*N*-nitrosourea
NBHPA, *N*-nitrosobis(2-hydroxypropyl)amine
NDBA, *N*-nitrosodibutylamine
NDMA.OAc, *N*-nitrosodimethyl(acetoxymethyl)amine
NR, not reported
sc, subcutaneously

47 weeks of age. At 33 weeks, 9/10 D2B6F$_1$ mice given NDEA followed by phenobarbital had hepatocellular adenomas (3.8 ± 1.0/mouse) versus 2/10 (1.0 ± 0) with NDEA alone. Administration of phenobarbital significantly increased the incidence (from 30% to 100%, $p < 0.05$) and the number of tumours (average number, 5.2 versus 2.0/mouse, $p < 0.05$) initiated by NDEA in the reciprocal F$_1$ cross B6D2F$_1$ mice. By 47 weeks, all mice of reciprocal F$_1$ hybrids D2B6F$_1$ and B6D2F$_1$ that had received phenobarbital after administration of NDEA had multiple hepatocellular tumours, including both adenomas (12.5 and 15/mouse, respectively) and carcinomas (2.6 and 2.7/mouse, respectively). Thus, the susceptibility to promotion of hepatocarcinogenesis by phenobarbital was a dominant trait in crosses between DBA/2 and C57BL/6, and the two reciprocal F$_1$ hybrids responded similarly to promotion by phenobarbital. Interestingly, however, 8/10 D2B6F$_1$ mice but only 1/10 B6D2F$_1$ mice given phenobarbital after NDEA developed single or multiple (1.75 ± 0.4) hepatoblastomas between 33 and 47 weeks. No hepatoblastomas were found in mice given only NDEA or phenobarbital (Diwan et al., 1989b).

Eight groups of 30 male weanling C3H/HeN mice were given either a normal diet or a diet containing 1.0% choline chloride, 1.5% DL-methionine or both DL-methionine and choline chloride with or without 0.05% phenobarbital for 52 weeks. A further eight groups of 30 mice each were given a single intraperitoneal injection of 150 mg/kg bw NDEA and received the same dietary supplements with or without 0.05% phenobarbital. Treatment with NDEA resulted in a 63% suppression in the body weight gained at 15 weeks (maximum growth period) when all groups of mice receiving NDEA were combined and compared with all groups not receiving NDEA (6.0 versus 16.2 g weight gain, respectively [no p value given]). NDEA decreased the survival time of mice in all treated groups ($p < 0.005$ compared with untreated controls) except for one NDEA-treated group without phenobarbital and supplemented with methionine only. The first death from liver cancer occurred at 20 weeks after initiation for the group given NDEA plus phenobarbital, at 25 weeks for the group given NDEA only, at 42 weeks for that given phenobarbital only and at 49 weeks for the untreated control group. Animals given phenobarbital only with both methionine and choline had longer survival than mice receiving no supplementation when analysed on the basis of deaths with tumours ($p < 0.0005$). Groups receiving the initiating dose of NDEA and no phenobarbital showed similar trends. Combined treatment with methionine lowered the relative liver weights of the mice given NDEA plus phenobarbital from 19.5% ± 1.6 to 13.8% ± 1.5 of body weight ($p < 0.05$). Treatment with phenobarbital only resulted in incidences of hepatocellular carcinoma of 79% in animals on the normal diet, 74% in those on choline-supplemented diet, 60% with methionine supplementation and 31% with methionine plus choline supplementation. In mice initiated with NDEA and promoted with phenobarbital, dietary supplementation with methionine and choline also protected against the formation of liver carcinomas; however, the total incidence of liver tumours (adenomas and carcinomas) was not altered. Metastases of hepatocellular carcinomas to the lungs were found only in mice receiving NDEA plus phenobarbital; the incidence was reduced from 16% in the group receiving no supplement to 6% in the group receiving choline supplementation and to 0% in groups of mice receiving diets supplemented with methionine alone or with choline and methionine (Fullerton *et al.*, 1990).

To confirm the promoter-dependent development of hepatoblastomas in mice, groups of 30 male D2B6F$_1$ mice, 5 weeks of age, were given a single intraperitoneal injection of 90 mg/kg bw NDEA and then 2 weeks later were given either a normal diet or a diet containing 500 mg/kg phenobarbital for 53 weeks. Mice exposed to NDEA alone and to phenobarbital alone were maintained for 110 weeks. Hepato-cellular tumours (adenomas and carcinomas) occurred in 97% of D2B6F$_1$ mice given NDEA alone. The incidence of hepatocellular carcinomas in NDEA-treated mice (37%) was significantly enhanced by subsequent administration of phenobarbital (96%). Multiple hepatocellular adenomas and carcinomas developed in 77% of mice exposed to phenobarbital alone. Only 10% of the mice treated with NDEA alone developed hepatoblastomas, while subsequent administration of phenobarbital resulted in an increased incidence (77%) and multiplicity (2.8 ± 1.5) of such tumours. Multiple hepatoblastomas also occurred in 11/30 (37%) mice that received pheno-barbital only. Thus, in D2B6F$_1$ mice, the development of hepatoblastoma from its precursor cells (adenoma and carcinoma cells) is strongly increased in the presence of a promoting agent (Diwan *et al.*, 1995).

(b)   Studies in juvenile mice

Groups of male and female pups of DDD strain mice [total initial number not given] were given either an intraperitoneal injection of 0.025 mL of 0.12% *N*-nitroso-dimethylamine (NDMA) 24 h after birth followed by 0.05% phenobarbital in the drinking-water from 4 weeks of age (36 newborn mice), NDMA alone (24 newborn mice), a single intraperitoneal injection of saline (0.9% NaCl) followed by pheno-barbital (38 newborn mice) or a single intraperitoneal injection of saline alone (24 newborn mice). The experiment was terminated 16 weeks after birth. Survival was not affected in any group. Liver tumours occurred in 27/35 (77%) mice exposed to NDMA plus phenobarbital, with a multiplicity of 4.3 per mouse. Twenty-four had type A tumours (simple nodular growth of liver parenchymal cells) and three male mice had type B tumours (areas of papilliform or adenoid growth of tumour cells with a distorted parenchymal structure). None of the tumours metastasized. In mice that received NDMA alone, liver tumours (all type A) occurred in 8/24 (33%) mice, with an average number of 0.4 tumours per mouse. No sex difference was found in the incidence, type or multiplicity of tumours in mice given NDMA alone or NDMA plus phenobarbital. None of the mice exposed to saline and phenobarbital or saline alone developed tumours (Uchida & Hirono, 1979). [The Working Group noted the short duration of exposure.]

Groups of 40 male B6C3F$_1$ mice, 15 days of age, were given a single intraperitoneal dose of 5 mg/kg bw NDEA. Starting 2 weeks later, groups of mice received 500 mg/L phenobarbital continuously in the drinking-water until 36 weeks of age. Three animals from each group were killed at 4, 20 and 28 weeks, and six animals from each group were killed at 12, 36 and 44 weeks of age. Half of the remaining animals were killed at 52 weeks and the remainder at 60 weeks of age. NDEA alone induced multiple focal hepatic lesions, including hepatocellular foci, adenomas (average, 34/mouse at 44 weeks, 16/mouse at 52 weeks and 13/mouse at 60 weeks) and carcinomas (3/mouse at 44 weeks, 8/mouse at 52 weeks and 12/mouse at 60 weeks). Subsequent exposure to phenobarbital suppressed the development of focal hepatic lesions, decreased the number of adenomas (5/mouse at 44 weeks, 6/mouse at 52 weeks and 8/mouse at 60 weeks) and carcinomas (0 at 44 weeks, 0 at 52 weeks and 1/mouse at 60 weeks) and prolonged the latency or significantly slowed the rate at which hepatocellular tumours developed in these mice (Diwan *et al.*, 1984).

Groups of CD-1 mice [initial numbers unspecified; sex ratio presumably equal], 15 days of age, received an intraperitoneal injection of 0, 5 or 20 mg/kg bw N-ethyl-N-nitrosourea (ENU). At 5 weeks of age, they received 500 mg/L sodium phenobarbital in the drinking-water until 51 weeks of age, and the experiment was terminated 1 week later. ENU induced lung and liver tumours in a dose-dependent fashion. Sodium phenobarbital promoted the hepatocarcinogenesis initiated by ENU in females (at the high dose of ENU: 6/33 adenomas ($p \leq 0.01$), 7/33 carcinomas ($p \leq 0.01$; adenomas plus carcinomas); at the low dose of ENU: 4/32 adenomas ($p \leq 0.05$), 2/32 carcinomas; ($p \leq 0.05$; adenomas plus carcinomas); ENU alone: no liver tumours). Males were more susceptible than females to the carcinogenicity of ENU, and subsequent treatment with sodium phenobarbital increased the hepatocellular carcinoma incidence (high dose of ENU: 22/30 adenomas and 10/30 carcinomas; low dose of ENU: 8/39 adenomas and 2/39 carcinomas; high dose of ENU plus sodium phenobarbital: 22/25 adenomas, 17/25 carcinomas ($p \leq 0.05$); low dose of ENU plus sodium phenobarbital, 14/36 adenomas, 10/36 carcinomas; $p \leq 0.01$). Subsequent treatment with sodium phenobarbital also promoted the development of spontaneous liver tumours. Sodium phenobarbital treatment did not, however, alter the incidence of lung tumours induced by ENU (Pereira *et al.*, 1985).

In a study to compare the effect of sodium phenobarbital on the development of liver tumours in juvenile and adult mice, 6-week-old male B6C3F$_1$ mice (20–24 per group) received 15 or 45 mg/L NDEA in the drinking-water for 4 weeks. One week later, they were given 500 mg/L sodium phenobarbital in the drinking-water until termination of the study at 50 weeks of age. In a second experiment, 15-day-old male BALB/c and B6C3F$_1$ mice received a single intraperitoneal injection of 25 mg/kg bw NDEA or the vehicle alone. At 4 weeks of age, they were given 500 mg/L sodium phenobarbital in the drinking-water until 20 or 28 weeks of age. In the first experiment, both concentrations of NDEA induced hepatocellular adenomas (25 and 65%, respectively) and carcinomas (13 and 30%, respectively). Subsequent treatment with sodium phenobarbital increased the incidence of both hepatocellular adenomas (100% with both initiating concentrations of NDEA; $p \leq 0.01$ at 15 mg/L) and carcinomas (81 and 70% at 45 and 15 mg/L of

NDEA, respectively; $p \leq 0.01$). In the second experiment, BALB/c mice given NDEA alone had a high incidence (66%) of hepatocellular adenomas (2.4 ± 0.72 adenomas/ mouse) at 28 weeks. Subsequent administration of sodium phenobarbital increased both the incidence (88% at 20 weeks, $p \leq 0.01$, and 100% at 28 weeks) and the number of adenomas per mouse (1.70 ± 0.82 at 20 weeks, $p \leq 0.05$, and 18.9 ± 1.23 at 28 weeks, $p \leq 0.01$). Sodium phenobarbital alone did not produce any liver tumours. In B6C3F$_1$ mice, NDEA alone induced both hepatocellular adenomas (100%) and carcinomas (30%) by 28 weeks. Subsequent administration of sodium phenobarbital decreased the incidence of hepatocellular carcinomas (0%) and the number of adenomas per mouse (51.8 ± 3.0 versus 7.0 ± 0.56, $p \leq 0.01$). The authors concluded that inhibition or enhancement of hepatocarcinogenesis by phenobarbital is dependent on both the mouse strain and the age at the start of exposure (Pereira et al., 1986).

Groups of infant male BALB/c mice, 15 days of age, received a single intra-peritoneal injection of 2.5, 10, 25 or 50 mg/kg bw NDEA, and at weaning (28 days) were given either tap-water or water containing 500 mg/L sodium phenobarbital for 40 weeks. Ten mice per group were killed at 12 weeks, 15 at 24 weeks and 20 at 40 weeks after weaning. No significant differences were seen in the body weights of the groups. Both NDEA and sodium phenobarbital alone increased the liver: body weight ratios at all times examined. At 12 weeks, hepatic adenomas were seen only with the highest dose of NDEA alone, but when NDEA treatment was followed by sodium phenobarbital, mice in all treated groups developed hepatocellular adenomas (4/10 at 2.5 mg/kg bw and 80–100% at higher doses). Sodium phenobarbital thus decreased the latency to hepatic adenoma formation in NDEA-initiated mice. Hepatocellular trabecular carcinomas occurred at 40 weeks in 1/20 (5%) and 2/20 (10%) mice exposed to 25 and 50 mg/kg bw of NDEA, respectively; phenobarbital treatment decreased the time to appearance of carcinomas and increased the incidence (20 and 30%, respectively) of such lesions over that in mice exposed to NDEA alone, but this effect was not significant. Subsequent administration of phenobarbital did not alter the incidence or multiplicity of lung adenomas induced by NDEA (Klaunig et al., 1988a).

Groups of 10 male B6C3F$_1$ mice, 15 days of age, were given a single intraperi-toneal injection of either NDEA or NDMA (5 mg/kg bw) and, after weaning at 4 weeks of age, were exposed to 500 mg/L phenobarbital in the drinking-water or given tap-water for 24 weeks. Control groups received a single intraperitoneal injection of saline at 15 days of age and at weaning were exposed to either tap-water or 500 mg/L phenobarbital. No significant difference in body weights was seen between different groups. Exposure to NDEA only induced a 100% incidence of hepatocellular adenomas, with a mean of 14.8 adenomas/mouse; subsequent adminis-tration of phenobarbital significantly decreased this number to 6.4/mouse ($p < 0.05$). In contrast, phenobarbital treatment after exposure to NDMA significantly increased the incidence (from 60% to 100%; $p < 0.05$) and number of adenomas per liver (0.80 to 5.70; $p < 0.05$). Phenobarbital treatment increased the percentage of eosinophilic adenomas in both NDEA- (from 8% to 20%) and NDMA- (from 0% to 72%) treated mice. No hepatocellular foci or adenomas were seen in groups given phenobarbital only or no treatment. The type of initiator therefore appears to be important in determining whether 15-day-old initiated male B6C3F$_1$ mice respond to the promoting effects of phenobarbital (Klaunig *et al.*, 1988b). [The Working Group noted the short duration of exposure and the small number of animals per group.]

Groups of male C57BL, C3H and B6C3F$_1$ mice [total initial number not given], 15 days of age, were given either a single intraperitoneal injection of 5 mg/kg bw NDEA or an equal volume of saline. At 28 days of age (at weaning), they received either normal drinking-water (controls) or drinking-water containing 500 mg/L phenobarbital for 28 weeks. In a second study, NDMA was used as the initiator instead of NDEA under identical experimental conditions. All three strains of mice exposed to phenobarbital after NDEA developed hepatocellular foci, but their incidence, number and size did not differ from those in mice given NDEA only. All C3H mice exposed to NDEA only or NDEA plus phenobarbital developed hepatocellular adenomas, but the number of adenomas in the latter group (52.5 ± 18.2) was significantly higher ($p < 0.05$) than that in mice given NDEA only (29.8 ± 13.6). B6C3F$_1$ mice exposed to NDEA plus phenobarbital, however, showed a significant decrease ($p < 0.05$) in the number of hepatic adenomas (6.4 ± 4.1) as compared with the group given NDEA only (15.0 ± 5.4), although no difference was found in the incidence or size of the tumours. In C57BL/6 mice, phenobarbital treatment decreased the incidence of adenomas in those given NDEA from 90% to 50% ($p < 0.05$). The number (18.5 ± 5.4) and size of the adenomas (20.8 ± 6.5 mm) in C3H mice given NDMA plus phenobarbital were significantly greater than in the NDMA-treated group (number, 1.7 ± 1.0, $p < 0.05$; size, 12.3 ± 3.4 mm, $p < 0.05$). In B6C3F$_1$ mice, the number but not the size of adenomas in animals given NDMA plus phenobarbital was significantly greater than in mice given NDMA only (6.2 ± 4.3 versus 0.8 ± 0.8; $p < 0.05$). In C57/BL mice treated with NDMA plus phenobarbital, the size of the adenomas was significantly decreased as compared with the group given NDMA only (6.5 ± 1.1 versus 11.0 ± 2.8 mm; $p < 0.05$). Thus, the strain of the mouse and the initiating carcinogen determine the ability of phenobarbital to either inhibit or promote hepatocellular carcinogenesis in 15-day-old mice (Weghorst *et al.*, 1989). [The Working Group noted the small number of mice per group.]

Groups of male and female B6C3F$_1$ mice, 15 days of age, were given either a single intraperitoneal injection of 5 mg/kg bw NDEA or an equal volume of saline. At weaning (28 days of age), some groups received drinking-water containing 500 mg/L phenobarbital, while others received deionized water, for 24 weeks. All mice were killed at 28 weeks of age. Hepatocellular foci and adenomas were found only in groups that received NDEA or NDEA plus phenobarbital. In males, NDEA plus phenobarbital caused a significant decrease ($p < 0.05$) in the total number and size of hepatocellular adenomas when compared with the group given NDEA only (number, 15.5 ± 4.8 with NDEA only, 6.4 ± 4.1 with NDEA plus phenobarbital; size, 13.9 ± 1.7 with NDEA only and 10.7 ± 3.0 with NDEA plus phenobarbital). None of the female mice exposed to NDEA only developed adenomas, but 100% of those exposed to NDEA plus phenobarbital had multiple hepatocellular adenomas which were exclusively eosinophilic. In male mice exposed to NDEA plus phenobarbital, the percentage of basophilic adenomas was smaller than in mice given NDEA only (65% versus 97% of all adenomas). The authors concluded that the sex of mice was important in determining their susceptibility to promotion by phenobarbital (Weghorst & Klaunig, 1989). [The Working Group noted the small number of mice per group.]

Groups of male and female C3H/HeNCr mice [total initial number not given], 15 days of age, were given either a single intraperitoneal injection of 5 mg/kg bw NDEA or saline, and at 4 weeks of age, received either 500 mg/L phenobarbital in the drinking-water or normal drinking-water for 24 weeks. At 28 weeks of age, 8/10 male and 0/10 female mice exposed to NDEA only developed adenomas. The adenomas in phenobarbital-promoted male (10/10) and female mice (7/10) were predominantly eosinophilic, while these lesions in mice given NDEA only were typically basophilic. Treatment with phenobarbital significantly increased the number and size of hepato-cellular adenomas in NDEA-initiated male mice, the number of adenomas with NDEA only being 7.1 ± 5.7 and that with NDEA plus phenobarbital being 19.8 ± 14.8 ($p < 0.05$); the volume (mm^3) of adenomas with NDEA only was 1.33 ± 0.47 and that with NDEA plus phenobarbital was 1.83 ± 0.18 ($p < 0.05$). Thus, both male and female young C3H/HeNCr mice are susceptible to the promoting effect of phenobarbital (Weghorst et al., 1994).

(c)   Studies in transgenic mice

Groups of 110 TGF-α transgenic MT42 mice and 112 CD-1 mice [sex unspecified], 15 days of age, were given a single intraperitoneal injection of 5 mg/kg bw NDEA and either a normal diet or, 2 weeks later, a diet containing 0.05% phenobarbital, from 4 weeks of age for 35 weeks. Control groups received a single intraperitoneal injection of saline alone and normal diet or the diet containing phenobarbital. At 10, 23 and 37 weeks after the start of the experiment, 5–10 mice from each group were killed. The mean body weights of MT42 mice given NDEA plus phenobarbital decreased from week 16, while that of mice given NDEA only decreased from 26 weeks. No remarkable changes in body weight were seen in CD-1 mice. The first death from a liver tumour was that of an MT42 mouse given NDEA plus phenobarbital at week 21, and the effective numbers of animals were determined on the basis of those alive after that time. Almost all (9/10) MT42 mice given NDEA plus phenobarbital died of liver tumours in weeks 21–34, and 8/8 given NDEA only died of liver tumours in weeks 29–34. All CD-1 mice and all control MT42 mice lived to 37 weeks. A time-related increase in the liver weights of MT42 mice given NDEA plus phenobarbital or NDEA only was observed which was due mainly to a large number of coalescing liver tumours. The livers of MT42 control mice were also heavier than those of control CD-1 mice. Hepatocellular carcinomas developed in 10/10 MT42 mice given NDEA plus phenobarbital by week 23, and in only 2/5 CD-1 mice by week 37. Hepatocellular carcinomas were also observed at week 23 in 8/10 MT42 mice given NDEA only, but the number per liver and the volume per cent of hepatocellular carcinomas were significantly greater in those receiving NDEA plus phenobarbital (number, 11.7 ± 1.0 versus 4.0 ± 1.1, $p < 0.001$; volume %, 54.2 ± 3.6 versus 20.8 ± 5.5, $p < 0.001$). Adenomas and preneoplastic foci were induced by phenobarbital alone at week 23, while only one control MT42 mouse developed foci at that time. By week 37, 5/5 MT42 mice given NDEA only and 2/6 given phenobarbital only had developed hepatocellular carcinomas and adenomas. In CD-1 mice, NDEA initiation and phenobarbital promotion significantly increased the numbers per liver and volume per cent of adenomas and foci at 23 weeks when compared with those given NDEA alone (number of foci, 30.7 ± 9.8 versus 5.4 ± 3.8, $p < 0.05$; foci volume, $0.16\% \pm 0.06$ versus $0.03\% \pm 0.02$, $p < 0.05$; number of adenomas, 4.1 ± 1.4 versus 0.6 ± 0.3, $p < 0.05$). No tumours or adenomas were found in CD-1 mice given NDEA alone or phenobarbital alone. The number per liver and volume per cent of hepato-cellular carcinomas in MT42 mice given NDEA only or NDEA plus phenobarbital were significantly higher than those in CD-1 mice at weeks 23 and 37. The proliferating cell nuclear antigen-labelling indices of the foci and adenomas in MT42 mice given NDEA alone or NDEA plus phenobarbital were significantly higher than those in CD-1 mice (Tamano *et al.*, 1994). [The Working Group noted the inadequate number of animals per group.]

3.3.2   *Promotion in rat liver*

(*a*)   *Effects of subsequent administration of phenobarbital*

Groups of (SD/Anl[Anl 66]) rats [initial number, sex and age not specified] were given diets containing 0.02% 2-acetylaminofluorene (AAF) for 11, 16, 21 or 26 days. At each of these intervals, 36 rats were transferred to the control diet and another 36 were transferred to a diet containing 0.05% phenobarbital. Four rats from each group were killed at 21-day intervals starting 91 days after the beginning of the experiment. The subsequent treatment with phenobarbital for up to 260 days increased the incidence of hepatomas at each of the four periods of AAF treatment (AAF 11 days, 2/105; AAF 11 days followed by phenobarbital, 17/106; AAF 16 days, 7/101; AAF 16 days followed by phenobarbital, 42/104; AAF 21 days, 18/103; AAF 21 days followed by phenobarbital, 64/102; AAF 26 days, 27/103; AAF 26 days followed by phenobarbital, 86/108; two-way analysis of variance for duration of AAF feeding, $p < 0.05$ and for phenobarbital treatment, $p < 0.01$). At each sacrifice interval, more rats given both AAF and phenobarbital had tumours. The hepatomas found at the early sacrifice intervals were seen only in the groups that had been fed AAF for the two longer periods (Peraino *et al.*, 1971).

To investigate the effects of varying the time of exposure to phenobarbital on enhancement of hepatocarcinogenesis, groups of 106–109 male Sprague-Dawley rats, 22 days of age, were given diets containing 0.02% AAF for 3 weeks and were then fed a diet containing 0.05% phenobarbital for various times: AAF diet for 18 days then phenobarbital diet; AAF diet for 18 days then phenobarbital diet for 5 days then control diet; AAF diet for 18 days then phenobarbital diet for 20 days then control diet; AAF diet for 18 days then control diet for 10 days then phenobarbital diet; AAF diet for 18 days then control diet for 30 days then phenobarbital diet. Beginning 101 days after the cessation of AAF feeding, 12 rats from each experimental group were killed at 3-week intervals and examined for tumours. Continuous treatment with phenobarbital, beginning immediately after 18 days of AAF feeding caused a threefold increase (73/109 versus 22/106) in the incidence of tumours of all sizes and an eightfold increase in that of larger ($\geq$ 10 mm) tumours (46/109 versus 5/106). Treatment with phenobarbital for only 5 days had no effect on the incidence of tumours but produced a 60% increase in the number of animals with larger tumours (8/106 versus 5/106). When administration of phenobarbital was increased to 20 days, it had a slightly greater effect (35/108 versus 22/106). In rats that received normal diet for 10 days and then phenobarbital, the effect on tumour incidence was similar to that in animals that received phenobarbital in the diet immediately after 18 days of AAF feeding (78/108 versus 73/109). When the treatment-free interval was increased to 30 days, a slight reduction was seen in the enhancing effect of phenobarbital (68/106 versus 73/109). When tumours of all sizes were taken into account, the rates of increase in the percentage of rats with tumours were parallel in the groups given AAF and AAF plus phenobarbital after 120 days, the tumour incidence in the latter group being threefold greater than that in the AAF group. The percentage of rats with larger tumours, however, increased at a higher rate in the group given AAF plus phenobarbital than in that given AAF. An increased rate of appearance of new tumour foci was also seen in rats given AAF plus phenobarbital, the largest increase occurring for tumours $\geq$ 10 mm (Peraino et al., 1973b). [The Working Group noted that no statistical analysis was provided.]

Groups of male Donryu rats [initial numbers not specified], 21 days old, were fed a basal diet containing 600 mg/kg 3'-methyl-4-(dimethylamino)azobenzene (3'-Me-DAB) for the first 3 weeks and then a diet containing 5–500 mg/kg phenobarbital. Groups of 5–10 animals were killed at 12 and 24 weeks of age. A dose-dependent effect of phenobarbital was clearly seen on both the number and size of enzyme-altered islands at concentrations > 10 mg/kg of diet. The increase in the total number of islands in these groups was significant (p < 0.05 or 0.01). The numbers of enzyme-altered islands in the largest size class (about 1000 μm) were significantly increased at 100 and 500 mg/kg of diet (p < 0.05 and < 0.01, respectively), while those in the next two lower size classes (500–999 and 250–499 μm) were significantly increased at the highest dietary concentration (p < 0.01) (Kitagawa et al., 1984). [The Working Group noted the small number of animals per group and the short duration of exposure.]

(b) *Effects of simultaneous administration of phenobarbital*

Six groups of 50 (SD/AnI[AnI66]) rats received either normal diet or a diet containing 0.05% phenobarbital, 0.01% AAF, 0.05% phenobarbital plus 0.01% AAF,

0.02% AAF or 0.05% phenobarbital plus 0.02% AAF. Three rats per group were killed at regular intervals over a 6-month period. Simultaneous feeding of AAF and pheno-barbital reduced the incidence of hepatic tumours when compared with that in rats given AAF only [incidences not given]. Highly differentiated hepatomas began to appear by day 72 in rats exposed to 0.02% AAF, and all rats in this group had multiple hepatomas after 120 days. Rats receiving both phenobarbital and 0.02% AAF did not develop hepatomas until 60 days after tumours appeared in rats receiving AAF alone. Furthermore, the livers of rats receiving phenobarbital and AAF were less cirrhotic than those receiving AAF alone [data for 0.01% AAF and phenobarbital not shown] (Peraino et al., 1971).

Groups of 5–10 male Donryu rats, 21 days of age, were given a diet containing 5–500 mg/kg phenobarbital simultaneously with 100 mg/kg 3'-Me-DAB. The animals were killed at 12 or 24 weeks of age. A concentration-dependent increase in the number of enzyme-altered islands was seen at 12 and 24 weeks of age (at 12 weeks, 20–500 mg/kg phenobarbital, 0.11 ± 0.09 to 0.32 ± 0.10 islands/cm^2; at 24 weeks, 20–500 mg/kg phenobarbital, 0.63 ± 0.12 to 0.97 ± 0.79 islands/cm^2; and 3'-Me-DAB alone, 0.04 ± 0.04 and 0.17 ± 0.13 islands/cm^2 at 12 and 24 weeks; $p < 0.01$ and < 0.05, respectively). Thus, phenobarbital given simultaneously with a low concentration of initiating carcinogen enhanced carcinogenesis at all the concentrations tested (Kitagawa et al., 1984). [The Working Group noted the small number of animals per group and the short duration of exposure.]

(c)   Time- and dose-related responses in phenobarbital promotion

Groups of male Sprague-Dawley rats [numbers and age not specified] received drinking-water containing 200 mg/L N-nitrosomorpholine (NMOR) or normal drinking-water for 3 weeks and 1 week later were placed on either basal diet or a diet containing 0.05% phenobarbital up to week 52. Some rats [number not stated] in both experimental and control groups were killed at week 4, and 7–13 animals per group were killed at weeks 16, 28, 40 and 52. The incidence of hepatocellular carcinomas in animals exposed to NMOR alone was 9.5% (2/21; data at 40 and 52 weeks combined), and subsequent administration of phenobarbital increased this incidence to 28.6% (6/21) [no p value given]. No hepatocellular carcinomas were found in rats exposed to phenobarbital alone or in those that were untreated. A time-related increase in the number and average size of altered hepatocellular foci was seen in groups receiving NMOR alone or NMOR plus phenobarbital. Subsequent administration of phenobarbital did not markedly increase the number of foci over that in the group treated with NMOR alone; however, phenobarbital increased the homogeneity of the histochemical reaction and increased the activity of glucose-6-phosphate dehydrogenase. This was associated with an increase in the acido-philic and mixed-cell character of the lesions (Ito et al., 1984).

Groups of male Wistar-derived rats [initial number not specified], weighing 80–120 g, were given a single intraperitoneal injection of 0, 1.1, 3.3, 10 or 30 mg/kg bw NDEA. One week later, some of these groups received sodium phenobarbital in the drinking-water at 0, 40, 100 or 1000 µg/mL for 12–18 months. Sodium pheno-barbital alone given for 12 months produced a few clear-cell foci, but NDEA at all doses caused both clear-cell foci and hyperplastic nodules. The number of lesions per animal showed a dose-related trend, those given 1.1 or 3.3 mg/kg bw NDEA having only one or two nodules per liver, while those given 30 mg/kg bw had > 20 nodules per liver. The incidence of basophilic foci showed a dose–response relationship: 0% at 1.1 mg/kg bw NDEA, 14% at 3.3 mg/kg bw, 50% at 10 mg/kg bw and 54% at 30 mg/kg bw. Among animals exposed to 30 mg/kg NDEA and no phenobarbital, 7/18 (36%) had hyperplastic nodules; the incidence of nodules increased to 22/28 (80%) with 1000 µg/mL phenobarbital. Since the dose of carcinogen used (30 mg/kg bw) induces clear-cell foci, basophilic foci and hyperplastic nodules in the absence of any promotion, no clear dose–response relationship for sodium phenobarbital promotion was discernible; however, the highest dose of sodium phenobarbital was essential for carcinoma development. Animals given sodium phenobarbital developed only clear-cell foci. Administration of the highest dose of sodium phenobarbital 43 weeks after the single dose of NDEA also resulted in carcinoma development in 38% of the animals, confirming the persistence of initiated cells. The authors concluded that baso-philic foci may be more important than hyperplastic nodules in carcinoma formation (Driver & McLean, 1986a).

Groups of male Wistar-derived rats [numbers not specified], weighing 60–100 g, were given protein-free diets for 3 days, then placed on a high-protein diet (50% casein) for 3 days and then returned to 41B stock pellet diet; 18 h after commencing the high-protein diet, groups of rats were given a single intraperitoneal injection of 15 mg/kg bw NDMA in saline. The total length of the experiment was 20 months. Two groups were fed 41B diet throughout and given NDMA. Beginning on day 10, some groups of animals received phenobarbital in the drinking-water at 40, 100 or 1000 µg/mL for the remainder of the 20 month-experiment. Rats given the protein-free or high-protein diet plus NDMA, followed by 40 or 100 µg/mL phenobarbital, showed no increase in the incidence of any lesions over that in the group given the diets and NDMA alone; however, when the phenobarbital concentration was increased to 1000 µg/mL, the numbers of animals with nodules (5/8) and of nodules per animal increased greatly, and half of the animals (4/8) developed hepatocellular carcinomas. None of eight animals given 41B diet, NDMA and the highest dose of phenobarbital developed hyperplastic nodules, but the incidence of carcinomas was similar (3/8). The effect of phenobarbital does not appear to be related to its ability to induce enzyme activity in the liver, as lower doses (40 or 100 µg/mL) given for 2 months did not promote liver tumour development in spite of being adequate for the induction of cytochrome P450 (CYP) enzymes and ethoxyresorufin deethylase (Driver & McLean, 1986b). [The Working Group noted the small number of animals per group and that ethoxyresorufin deethylase does not specifically represent the activity of pheno-barbital-specific CYPs.]

(d)   *Effect of age and sex on promotion by phenobarbital*

Groups of weanling, 6- and 12-month-old male and female Fischer 344 rats [initial number not specified] were subjected to a 70% partial hepatectomy and 24 h later were given NDEA by intubation in a single dose of 10 mg/kg bw. Two weeks later, the animals received 0.05% phenobarbital in the diet for 6 months. Although altered hepatic foci and neoplastic nodules were present in the livers of almost all animals that were initiated with NDEA and promoted with phenobarbital, the incidence of neoplastic nodules was much lower in rats initiated with NDEA at weaning (males, 4/17; females, 3/10) or at 6 months of age (males, 2/7; females, 3/6) than in those initiated at 12 months (males, 6/8; females, 8/8). The incidence of hepatocellular carcinomas was much lower in rats initiated with NDEA at 6 months (males, 2/9; females, 1/9) or 12 months (males, 0/8; females, 1/5) followed by phenobarbital promotion than in those initiated at weaning (males, 10/11; females, 4/10). The authors concluded that the stage of initiation and promotion at which phenobarbital acts in hepatocarcinogenesis in rats is altered by both the age and sex of the animal (Xu *et al.*, 1990). [The Working Group noted the small number of animals per group.]

(e)   *Promotion by phenobarbital after multi-organ (broad-spectrum) initiation*

Groups of 30 male Fischer 344 rats, 6 weeks of age, were given drinking-water containing 0.01% *N*-nitrosobutyl-*N*-(4-hydroxybutyl)amine (NBHBA) for 4 weeks and were then fed either a basal diet or a diet containing 0.05% phenobarbital for 32 weeks. Control groups of 30 rats each received either phenobarbital alone or remained untreated. Hyperplastic nodules developed in 8/30 rats that received the nitrosamine plus phenobarbital ($p < 0.01$ compared with the group given NBHBA) but in none of the other groups. Phenobarbital did not promote bladder tumours induced or initiated by NBHBA (Ito *et al.*, 1980). [The Working Group noted that size of the nodules and the numbers per rat were not given.]

Groups of 20–21 male Fischer 344 rats, 7 weeks of age, were given drinking-water containing 0.1% *N*-nitrosoethyl-*N*-hydroxyethylamine (NEHEA) for 2 weeks and were then placed either on a basal diet or a diet containing 0.05% phenobarbital for 32 weeks. A control group of 20 animals was given the diet containing phenobarbital. At the end of week 3, all rats were subjected to unilateral nephrectomy. The final weights of the rats given NEHEA plus phenobarbital or NEHEA alone were essentially similar to those of the controls [actual body weights not given]. All rats exposed to the nitrosamine with or without phenobarbital developed multiple hyperplastic hepatocellular nodules, although the incidence of hepatocellular carcinomas was significantly higher in the group given NEHEA plus phenobarbital than in the group given NEHEA only (14/17 versus 7/21, $p < 0.01$). No hepatocellular tumours were found in the group given phenobarbital only. Subsequent administration of phenobarbital had no significant effect on the incidence of kidney neoplastic nodules or renal-cell tumours induced by NEHEA (Hirose *et al.*, 1981).

Groups of male Fischer 344 rats [initial number not specified], weighing 100–120 g, were fed either a diet containing 0.02% AAF or given drinking-water containing 0.01% NBHBA for 4 weeks. They were then fed either basal diet or a diet containing 0.05% phenobarbital for 32 weeks. Subsequent administration of phenobarbital significantly increased the average number of hyperplastic nodules (5.5 versus $3.6/cm^2$, $p < 0.05$) and their area (3.5 mm^2 versus 1.9 mm^2/cm^2 of liver, $p < 0.05$) in AAF-treated rats. No hepatocellular carcinomas occurred in rats given AAF only but were found in 5/24 (21%) rats exposed to AAF followed by phenobarbital. Although NBHBA alone or phenobarbital alone induced no liver tumours, 8/30 (27%) rats exposed to NBHBA plus phenobarbital had hyperplastic nodules. Phenobarbital had no effect on bladder carcinogenesis initiated by AAF or NBHBA (Nakanishi *et al.*, 1982).

Groups of male and female Fischer 344 rats [initial numbers not specified], 4 weeks of age, received intravenous injections of *N*-methyl-*N*-nitrosourea (MNU) either as 0.05 mmol/kg bw once a week for 4 weeks (total dose, 0.2 mmol/kg bw) or as a single injection of 0.2 mmol/kg bw. Two weeks after the last injection, some groups of rats received drinking-water containing 0.05% phenobarbital until 52 or 80 weeks of age. Rats in one group received similar treatment with phenobarbital from the day of the first MNU injection. Between 53 and 80 weeks of age, subsequent exposure to phenobarbital promoted hepatocarcinogenesis, resulting in the development of hepatocellular adenomas and carcinomas in 50% of males and 40% of females exposed to multiple doses of MNU. Concurrent administration of phenobarbital with divided doses of MNU significantly enhanced the yield of hepatocellular $foci/cm^2$ but did not affect hepatic tumour development (MNU plus phenobarbital: 2/10 males and 1/10 females; MNU only: 0/10 males and females). Phenobarbital also promoted thyroid tumours initiated by MNU, but no other tumours initiated or induced by this nitrosourea were affected by phenobarbital (Diwan *et al.*, 1985).

Groups of male Fischer 344 rats [initial number not specified], 4 weeks of age, were given a single intraperitoneal injection of 0.05 nmol/kg bw *N*-nitrosomethyl(acetoxy-methyl)amine. Two weeks later, the rats were given either tap-water or water containing 500 mg/L phenobarbital for 78 weeks. None of the rats exposed to the nitrosamine alone developed liver tumours; however, subsequent phenobarbital treatment resulted in a significant increase in the incidence (5/15, $p < 0.05$) of hepatocellular tumours (three adenomas and two carcinomas). Phenobarbital promoted the development of thyroid tumours but not of any other tumours initiated by *N*-nitrosomethyl(acetoxymethyl)-amine (Diwan *et al.*, 1989c).

(f)   Effects of phenobarbital on promotion and progression stages of hepatocarcinogenesis

In a three-stage initiation–promotion–progression model, groups of 7–12 female Sprague-Dawley rats, 5 days of age, were initiated with a single intraperitoneal injection of 10 mg/kg bw NDEA, fed a diet containing phenobarbital at 0.05% at weaning for 6 months, subjected to partial hepatectomy at 6 months and given a putative progressor agent (100 mg/kg bw ENU 24 h later or 3 × 150 mg/kg bw hydroxyurea 20, 30 and 40 h later) intraperitoneally. Phenobarbital was discontinued after the progressor agent was given, and animals were killed 6 months after administration of the progressor. The number of promoter-independent altered hepatic foci in the group given NDEA plus phenobarbital (4900 ± 250 per liver) was increased to 18 500 ± 1500 per liver by the addition of ENU and 6600 ± 700 per liver by the addition of hydroxyurea. Hepatocytes isolated from animals exposed to ENU in this protocol showed a greater degree of chromosomal damage and aneuploidy than those from animals not given a second initiator. In a variation of the model in which the promoting agent was maintained after administration of the progressor agent, the number of heterogeneous altered hepatic foci (foci-in-foci) increased significantly after administration of either ENU or hydroxyurea. The incidence of hepatocellular carcinoma was 3/14 in rats given NDEA plus pheno-barbital, 1/12 in those given NDEA plus phenobarbital plus hydroxyurea and 2/17 in those given NDEA plus phenobarbital plus ENU. The incidence was increased when promotion was maintained until sacrifice, carcinomas being seen in 1/8 animals receiving NDEA plus phenobarbital, 6/9 given NDEA plus phenobarbital plus hydroxyurea and then phenobarbital and 8/9 in those given NDEA plus phenobarbital plus ENU and then phenobarbital (Dragan et al., 1993). [The Working Group noted the small number of animals per group.]

3.3.3   Promotion in hamster liver

Groups of male Syrian golden hamsters [initial numbers not specified], 5 weeks of age, received a single intraperitoneal injection of either 100 mg/kg bw NDEA or 20 mg/kg bw methylazoxymethanol acetate (MAMA) and 2 weeks later were given either tap-water or drinking-water containing 500 mg/L phenobarbital for 18, 45 or 62 weeks, and killed. Between 18 and 62 weeks, hepatocellular adenomas were induced by both NDEA (11/30, 37%) and MAMA (19/30, 63%), but carcinomas were seen only in MAMA-treated hamsters (2/18, 11%). Subsequent administration of pheno-barbital for up to 45–62 weeks had no significant effect either on the incidence (adenoma: NDEA plus phenobarbital, 27%; MAMA plus phenobarbital, 67%; carcinoma: MAMA plus phenobarbital, 11%) or on the histological appearance of pre-neoplastic or neoplastic hepatocellular lesions in either NDEA- or MAMA-initiated hamsters. Phenobarbital treatment alone did not induce hepatocellular lesions (Diwan et al., 1986b).

Groups of male Syrian golden hamsters, 5–6 weeks of age (initial number, 163), were given subcutaneous injections of 500 mg/kg bw N-nitrosobis(2-hydroxypropyl)-amine (NBHPA) once a week for 5 weeks, after which they were fed a basal diet alone or a diet containing 0.05% phenobarbital for 30 weeks. Control groups were given subcutaneous injections of saline once a week for 5 weeks followed by either a basal diet or diet containing 0.05% phenobarbital for 30 weeks. Phenobarbital treatment significantly decreased the final body weight of hamsters initiated with NBHPA (average, 135 g versus 145 g; $p < 0.05$). No significant effect was seen on the liver weights of animals exposed to phenobarbital or NBHPA plus phenobarbital. Hepatic hyperplastic nodules were found in 100% of animals exposed to the nitrosamine with or without phenobarbital. Hepatocellular carcinomas occurred in 13/24 (54%) hamsters given NBHPA plus phenobarbital but in only 2/15 (13%) given the nitrosamine alone ($p < 0.02$). Treatment with phenobarbital did not affect the development of bile-duct, gall-bladder or pancreatic lesions induced or initiated by NBHBA (Makino et al., 1986).

Groups of male Syrian golden hamsters, 6 weeks of age, received an intraperitoneal injection of 6 mg/kg bw NDMA and were then fed a basal diet (15 animals), the same dose of NDMA and 1 week later a diet containing 500 mg/kg diet phenobarbital for 30 weeks (11 animals), 1 week of basal diet and then the diet containing phenobarbital for 30 weeks (14 animals; controls), phenobarbital or basal diet continuously for 31 weeks (13 animals; untreated controls). All groups developed altered hepatic foci. The number (foci/cm^2) and size (mm$^2 \times 10^{-2}$) of foci induced by NDMA did not significantly change after subsequent treatment with phenobarbital (NDMA: number, 6.3 ± 3.4; size, 10.8 ± 8.9; NDMA plus phenobarbital: number, 7.3 ± 3.4, size 11.5 ± 9.0). Animals treated with phenobarbital alone developed significantly more foci than the untreated group (1.8 ± 0.8 versus 0.2 ± 0.3 foci/cm^2, $p < 0.01$). One hamster exposed to NDMA alone developed three adenomas, while three given NDMA plus phenobarbital developed one adenoma each. Treatment with phenobarbital alone did not result in tumour formation, but enlarged hepatocytes with abundant cytoplasm were observed. Thus, phenobarbital failed to promote liver carcinogenesis initiated by NDMA in hamsters (Tanaka et al., 1987).

3.3.4 *Promotion in monkey liver*

In a first study, nine pregnant patas monkeys (*Erythrocebus patas*) were injected intravenously twice weekly with NDEA to provide a cumulative dose of 0.6–3.2 mmol/kg bw. None of the nine mothers or six offspring developed tumours during 4 years of subsequent observation. At that time, three mothers and three offspring were given drinking-water containing phenobarbital at a concentration providing a dose of 15 mg/kg bw per day for the remainder of their lives or up to 43 months. Within less than 2 years, multiple hepatocellular neoplasms had developed in both offspring (5.6 adenomas and 0.3 carcinomas per animal) and mothers (11.6 adenomas per animal) given NDEA followed by phenobarbital, but none were found in those given NDEA alone. A few hepatocellular foci (0.3 foci/cm^2) were detected in monkeys treated with NDEA only. The authors concluded that, in patas monkeys, hepatocellular carcinogenesis could be initiated by prenatal exposure to NDEA and that the initiated cells could remain dormant for years. In a second study, young male and female patas monkeys [initial numbers not specified] received intra-peritoneal injections of 0.1–0.4 mmol/kg bw NDEA in phosphate-buffered saline at 14-day intervals for a total of 20 injections. Fifteen days later, four of the seven survivors were given drinking-water containing phenobarbital at a concentration providing a dose of 15 mg/kg bw per day for 9 months. A significant increase in the multiplicity of hepatocellular neoplasms was found among animals given NDEA plus phenobarbital (adenomas, 17.25 per animal; carcinomas, 2.0 per animal) when compared with those given NDEA alone (adenomas, 1.6 per animal; carcinomas, 0.3 per animal), and the increase in the incidence of adenomas was statistically significantly greater than that with NDEA plus phenobarbital [p value not given]. Animals exposed to phenobarbital alone had no tumours or foci. Thus, pheno-barbital is also an effective promoter of hepatocellular neoplasia in this non-rodent species (Rice *et al.*, 1989).

3.3.5   *Tumour promotion in the thyroid*

Table 4 summarizes studies of the promotion of tumours in the thyroid with phenobarbital.

Mouse: Pregnant B10.A mice were given a single intravenous injection of 0.5 mmol/kg bw ENU in citrate buffer on day 18 of gestation and were allowed to deliver normally. After sexing at 3 weeks of age, equal numbers of pups from each litter of dams treated with ENU were given ENU alone or ENU concomitantly with drinking-water containing 0.05% phenobarbital from 4 to 80 weeks of age. Postnatal administration of phenobarbital more than tripled the incidence of thyroid follicular-cell adenomas in ENU-treated offspring (ENU: males, 1/14; females, 1/14; ENU plus phenobarbital: males, 5/14; females, 2/14; 7% versus 25% in males and females combined, $p < 0.05$). Postnatal administration of phenobarbital had no effect on the development of intestinal or renal tumours induced or initiated by ENU (Diwan *et al.*, 1989d).

Rat: A total of 231 male Wistar rats, 6 weeks of age, were given a subcutaneous injection of 700 mg/kg bw NBHPA once a week for 4 or 6 weeks, and 1 week later were given either basal diet or a diet containing phenobarbital at 500 mg/kg during weeks 5–16 or weeks 7–18. Control groups received phenobarbital alone for similar durations. The experiment was terminated at 20 weeks. No significant effects were observed on the mean final body weights of rats given four injections of NBHPA, but those given six injections with or without phenobarbital weighed significantly less than the corresponding control groups ($p < 0.05$). The mean weights of the thyroid glands of rats exposed to phenobarbital alone or with NBHPA were higher than those of the corresponding control groups ($p < 0.05$). The incidence of thyroid tumours was 66% in the group exposed to phenobarbital after four injections of NBHPA, but no thyroid tumours were found in rats given four injections of NBHPA alone or phenobarbital alone. Thyroid tumours were found in 24% (5/21) of rats given six injections of

NBHPA and in 100% (21/21) given six injections of the nitrosamine followed by phenobarbital. Two rats given four doses of NBHPA followed by phenobarbital and 5/21 (24%) rats given six doses of NBHPA followed by phenobarbital developed malignant thyroid tumours. All rats given four or six doses of NBHPA followed by phenobarbital had multiple follicular adenomas (106 and 239, respectively) (Hiasa *et al.*, 1982).

Groups of male Wistar rats (total, 200), 6 weeks of age, received a single sub-cutaneous injection of 2800 mg/kg bw NBHPA, and 2 weeks later were given either a basal diet or a diet containing phenobarbital at 500 mg/kg for 6, 12 or 19 weeks. The study was terminated at 20 weeks. Of the rats given NBHPA, 21/24 (87%) developed thyroid follicular-cell adenomas when phenobarbital was given for 19 weeks, 19/24 (79%) when phenobarbital was given for 12 weeks and 10/24 (42%) when phenobarbital was given for 6 weeks. The incidences of thyroid adenomas in NBHPA-initiated rats exposed to phenobarbital for 19 and 12 weeks were significantly higher ($p < 0.05$) than that in rats given the nitrosamine alone (9/24, 37%). Ten, 5.2 and 2.6 thyroid tumours per rat were found after exposure to phenobarbital for 19, 12 and 6 weeks, respectively, and the total numbers of follicular-cell adenomas were 237, 124 and 62 in NBHPA-treated rats exposed to phenobarbital for 19, 12 and 6 weeks, respectively. Papillary adenomas occurred in three rats exposed to phenobarbital for 6 weeks and one each in those exposed for 19 and 12 weeks after initiation with NBHPA. Nine (37%) rats exposed to NBHPA only developed tumours, consisting of 23 follicular-cell adenomas. None of the rats exposed to phenobarbital only developed any thyroid tumours (Hiasa *et al.*, 1983).

Groups of 10 male and 10 female Fischer 344 rats, 4 weeks of age, received either a single intravenous injection of 0.2 mmol/kg bw MNU or four weekly injections of 0.05 mmol/kg bw MNU followed 2 weeks later by or concurrently with drinking-water containing 0.05% phenobarbital, which was continued until 52 or 80 weeks of age. At 52 weeks, phenobarbital given subsequent to MNU or concurrently with divided doses of MNU significantly enhanced the incidence of thyroid follicular-cell tumours only in males (MNU, 10–20%; MNU plus phenobarbital, 50%; MNU followed by pheno-barbital, 60–70%). Between 53 and 80 weeks of age, the thyroid tumour incidence was 70% in male rats exposed to MNU plus phenobarbital, 80–100% in male rats that received MNU followed by phenobarbital and about 30–40% in groups that received MNU only. The incidence of thyroid tumours in females exposed to MNU with or before phenobarbital (60–70%) was not significantly different from that in males, but a higher multiplicity of these tumours in males (average, 3.5 versus 2.1 per tumour-bearing rat) persisted in the groups given phenobarbital. Several animals developed both follicular-cell adenomas and carcinomas after treatment with MNU and pheno-barbital (Diwan *et al.*, 1985). [The Working Group noted the small number of animals per group.]

To investigate the effects of dose and sex on the development of thyroid tumours, groups of 24 male and 24 female Wistar rats, 6 weeks of age, received a single intraperitoneal injection of 2100 mg/kg bw (males) or 4200 mg/kg bw (females) NBHPA, and 1 week later were fed diets containing phenobarbital at a concentration of 20, 100, 500 or 2500 mg/kg for 19 weeks. Control groups received either NBHPA alone or various concentrations of phenobarbital in their diet. No significant differences were found in the body-weight gain of either male or female rats treated with NBHPA plus phenobarbital or phenobarbital alone, whereas rats exposed to NBHPA alone had lower body weights than controls. Thyroid follicular-cell tumours occurred only in groups that received NBHPA with or without phenobarbital. NBHPA treatment alone resulted in an 8% incidence of thyroid tumours in both male and female rats; with the addition of 500 mg/kg of diet phenobarbital, a threefold increase in tumour yield was found in male rats but no increase in females. At 2500 mg/kg of diet, a marked increase (about eightfold) in tumour yield was seen in male rats but a less than threefold increase in females. The incidences of follicular adenomas in rats given NBHPA followed by a concentration of 20, 100, 500 or 2500 mg/kg of diet phenobarbital were 8, 45, 70 and 66% for males and 12, 17, 50 and 58% for females, respectively. Papillary adenomas were seen in male rats only at 500 and 2500 mg/kg of diet phenobarbital (12% and 20%, respectively); only one female rat (4%) developed such a tumour when given 2500 mg/kg of diet. No thyroid tumours were found in control groups with or without phenobarbital treatment (Hiasa et $al.$, 1985).

A total of 120 male Wistar rats, 6 weeks of age, were given a single intraperitoneal injection of 2100 mg/kg bw NBHPA at the end of the first experimental week. Groups of 20 of these rats were castrated either at the beginning of the experiment or at the end of the second week and received the basal diet containing phenobarbital at 500 mg/kg from week 3 to week 40 of the experiment. The other groups were given the basal diet without phenobarbital. Significant differences in mean body weight were found between groups that received NBHPA only or NBHPA plus phenobarbital and those of castrated rats. The mean weights of the thyroid of rats that received phenobarbital after NBHPA initiation with or without castration at the end of the second week were (not significantly) higher than that in the group exposed to NBHPA alone, while the thyroids of rats that were castrated at the beginning of the experiment weighed significantly less than those of rats that were similarly castrated and given phenobarbital ($p < 0.05$). The incidence of thyroid follicular-cell adenomas was 20% in animals that received NBHPA only, 75% in those that received the nitrosamine plus phenobarbital, 30% in those that were castrated at the end of second week and received NBHPA plus phenobarbital and 0% in those that were castrated at the end of second week and received NBHPA only. The incidences of these tumours were 20% and 0% in rats castrated at the beginning of the first week, treated with NBHPA and given phenobarbital or basal diet, respectively. The incidence of thyroid carcinomas was 10% with NBHPA only, 40% with NBHPA plus phenobarbital and 15% in animals that were castrated at the end of the second week and given phenobarbital. No thyroid carcinomas occurred in any other groups. The serum concentration of thyroid-stimulating hormone (TSH) in the group given NBHPA plus phenobarbital was significantly higher than in groups that received NBHPA only or NBHPA plus phenobarbital with castration. Thus, castration inhibited the development of thyroid tumours in rats treated with NBHPA, and the inhibition was greater when the rats were castrated before receiving the nitrosamine (Hiasa *et al.*, 1987).

Groups of 20 male and 20 female CD(SD)BR rats (weighing 204 g and 143 g, respectively) were injected subcutaneously with 700 mg/kg bw NBHPA or saline once a week for 5 weeks and were then fed a control diet or a diet containing 500 mg/kg phenobarbital and/or L-thyroxine (T4) at a dose of 50 μg/kg bw per day from week 6 through week 20, when all animals were killed. The dose of T4 was required to maintain the normal thyroid gland weight in phenobarbital-treated rats and induced a slight increase in the serum concentration of T4 and a slight decrease in that of triiodothyronine (T3). The food consumption in all groups was comparable, but slightly decreased body weight was observed in all groups that received NBHPA. All rats treated with phenobarbital had increased liver weights, and NBHPA and T4 did not affect this increase. In male rats, phenobarbital increased the weight of the thyroid gland over that of controls ($p \leq 0.05$). NBHPA alone did not alter thyroid weights (~ 30 mg), but subsequent administration of phenobarbital resulted in a marked increase in thyroid weight (~ 55 mg). T4 reduced this response in groups given phenobarbital with or without NBHPA (~ 30 mg). No significant differences were seen in the weights of the thyroid gland in female rats. Six of 16 male rats exposed to NBHPA alone developed thyroid follicular-cell adenomas (20 tumour foci), and this incidence was significantly increased by treatment with phenobarbital (15/18, $p \leq 0.05$) (107 tumour foci). T4 reduced the incidences of both adenomas (5/20) and tumour foci (11). Only one female rat given NBHPA plus phenobarbital developed an adenoma. None of the rats exposed to phenobarbital alone developed thyroid tumours (McClain *et al.*, 1988). [The Working Group noted the short duration of exposure.]

Groups of 20 male Fischer 344 rats, 6 weeks of age, were given drinking-water containing 0.2% NBHPA for 1 week, and 1 week later were given either basal diet or a diet containing 0.05% phenobarbital, for 50 weeks. Controls received the diet containing 0.05% phenobarbital alone. The incidence of thyroid follicular-cell carcinomas in rats given NBHPA plus phenobarbital was significantly higher than that in rats given the nitrosamine alone (19/19 versus 14/20, $p < 0.05$). The mean number of tumours (adenomas and carcinomas) per rat given NBHPA plus phenobarbital was also significantly higher than in those given NBHPA only (2.63 ± 1.12 versus 1.56 ± 1.34, $p < 0.02$). One carcinoma in a rat given the combination metastasized to the lung. The difference in the incidence of thyroid adenomas in groups given NBHPA with and without phenobarbital (10/19 versus 7/20) was not statistically significant (Shirai *et al.*, 1988).

Pregnant Fischer 344/NCr rats were given a single intravenous injection of 0.2 mmol/kg bw MNU in citrate buffer on day 18 of gestation. After sexing, equal numbers of pups from each litter of dams treated with MNU were given MNU alone with a normal diet and tap-water or with drinking-water containing 0.05% phenobarbital from 4 to 80 weeks of age. Postnatal administration of phenobarbital had no effect on the incidence or latency of either neurogenic or renal tumours induced or initiated by MNU. However, phenobarbital given postnatally promoted the development of thyroid tumours of follicular cell origin (MNU: males, 1/19; females, 0/17; MNU plus phenobarbital: males, 13/17; females, 3/14), especially in male offspring exposed prenatally to MNU ($p < 0.01$). The multiplicity of thyroid tumours in the MNU plus phenobarbital group was 2.6 per rat in males and 1.3 per rat in females, while that with MNU only was 1 and 0 per rat, respectively. Thyroid follicular-cell carcinomas were found only in male rats exposed transplacentally to MNU and postnatally to pheno-barbital (6/17) (Diwan *et al.*, 1989d).

4. Other Data Relevant to an Evaluation of Carcinogenicity and its Mechanisms

4.1 Absorption, distribution, metabolism and excretion

4.1.1 *Humans*

Phenobarbital is readily absorbed from the gastrointestinal tract in humans (Lous, 1954) and is eliminated by hepatic extraction and renal excretion. In the liver, pheno-barbital is *para*-hydroxylated and subsequently conjugated (Butler, 1956). After oral administration of [^{14}C]phenobarbital (120 mg phenobarbital containing 31 μCi ^{14}C-label) to two healthy men, 78–87% of the dose was recovered in the urine over 16 days. Phenobarbital *N*-glucoside, *para*-hydroxyphenobarbital and unchanged phenobarbital accounted for approximately 27, 19 and 29% of the dose, respectively (average for the two subjects) (Tang *et al.*, 1979). Small amounts of the *O*-methylcatechol metabolite of phenobarbital were identified in the urine of a single individual given 300 mg orally (Treston *et al.*, 1987). In patients with epilepsy receiving long-term treatment, 57% of the daily dose was recovered in urine, 14% as the *N*-glucoside, 16% as *para*-hydroxy-phenobarbital and 27% as unchanged phenobarbital (Bernus *et al.*, 1994).

4.1.2 *Experimental systems*

After an intravenous injection of 50 mg/kg bw [^{14}C]phenobarbital to rats, the total amount of radiolabel in the liver was higher than that in other organs. Urinary elimi-nation of radiolabel associated with phenobarbital reached a peak after 6–8 h (Glasson *et al.*, 1959). The major pathways for biotransformation of phenobarbital in rodents appear to involve *para*-hydroxylation, with excretion in either the free form or as a glucuronide conjugate. The *N*-glucoside of phenobarbital was formed at < 1% and excreted in urine only in mice; it was not detected in the urine of rats, guinea-pigs, rabbits, cats, dogs, pigs or monkeys (Soine *et al.*, 1991). Less than 50% of a dose of phenobarbital administered to rodents was excreted in urine (Maynert, 1965). In addition to urinary excretion, 18% of a dose of 75 mg/kg bw phenobarbital was excreted in the bile of Sprague-Dawley rats within 6 h, the majority as conjugated metabolites (Klaassen, 1971). Very small amounts of *meta*-hydroxyphenobarbital, a 3,4-dihydrodiol and a 3,4-catechol derivative were also detected in the urine of rats and guinea-pigs given 110 and 56 mg/kg bw, respectively, by intraperitoneal injection (Harvey *et al.*, 1972). When phenobarbital was administered at a dose of 15 mg/kg bw to beagle pups at 4, 10, 20, 40 and 60 days of age, no difference in the elimination half-time was observed with age, and there was no apparent formation of the *para*-hydroxylated metabolite (Ecobichon *et al.*, 1988).

In male CFE rats and CF1 mice pretreated with phenobarbital, a total of 63% of phenobarbital and metabolites was excreted in 3 days in the urine and 30% with faeces in rats, and 72% and 11% in mice, respectively. After 2 weeks on a diet containing 0.1% (w/v) phenobarbital for rats and 0.05% (w/v) phenobarbital for mice, more phenobarbital and metabolites were excreted in the faeces of rats and less in those of mice than in animals that had not been pretreated. Most of the material excreted in urine was *para*-hydroxyphenobarbital and its conjugates, with lesser amounts of phenobarbital. The main effects of phenobarbital pretreatment on phenobarbital excretion in rats were increased urinary excretion of conjugated *para*-hydroxyphenobarbital, a similar decrease in the excretion of the free form of this metabolite and no change in total phenobarbital excretion. In mice, phenobarbital pretreatment caused a threefold increase in the urinary excretion of the free form of *para*-hydroxyphenobarbital, a small decrease in that of the conjugated form and about a twofold decrease in that of unchanged phenobarbital. The overall effect of phenobarbital pretreatment in mice appeared to be about a 50% increase in the amount of all forms of *para*-hydroxyphenobarbital, taking into account changes in urinary and faecal excretion. A minor urinary metabolite found in both species was not identified but was believed to be either the 3,4-dihydrodiol or the 3,4-catechol (Crayford & Hutson, 1980).

The half-time for clearance of phenobarbital was decreased to one-third by 70 weeks in C3H/He mice given phenobarbital at a dose of 85 mg/kg of diet for up to 90 weeks (Collins *et al.*, 1984).

4.1.3   *Comparison of animals and humans*

The *para*-hydroxylated metabolite of phenobarbital and its conjugates as well as unchanged phenobarbital have been identified in the urine of humans and rodents. The formation and urinary excretion of the *N*-glucoside of phenobarbital appears to occur selectively in humans, with minor amounts excreted in mice but not in other species examined.

4.2   Toxic effects

4.2.1   *Humans*

The most frequent side-effect of phenobarbital is sedation; however, tolerance develops after long-term treatment. Nystagmus and ataxia occur at excessive doses. Phenobarbital has produced irritability and hyperactivity in children and confusion in the elderly. Scarlatiniform or morbilliform rash, probably with other manifestations of drug allergy, occurred in 1–2% of patients (Hardman *et al.*, 1996).

Oppenheimer *et al.* (1968) showed increased T4 turnover in humans treated with phenobarbital. Ohnhaus and Studer (1983) determined that an induction sufficient to increase antipyrine clearance by at least 60% was required to change steady-state thyroid hormone levels in phenobarbital-treated patients. Induced patients had decreased concentrations of T4, but the concentrations of T3, TSH and the TSH response to thyrotropin-releasing hormone usually remained within normal limits. The concentrations of circulating free T3 and free T4 were reported to be reduced in children with epilepsy maintained on phenobarbital, although clinical hypothyroidism was not seen (Yüksel *et al.*, 1993).

4.2.2   *Experimental systems*

The intraperitoneal LD_{50} of phenobarbital was reported to be 340 mg/kg bw in mice (Collins & Horlington, 1969), and the oral LD_{50} was 162 mg/kg bw in rats (Goldenthal, 1971). The oral LD_{50} in rats for sodium phenobarbital was 660 mg/kg bw (Stecher, 1968).

(*a*)   *Cell proliferation and apoptosis*

Studies conducted during the 1960s suggested that phenobarbital causes liver enlargement by inducing both hyperplasia and hypertrophy of liver cells, mainly in the pericentral region of the liver (Ruttimann, 1972). Since that time, extensive studies have been conducted on the enhancement by phenobarbital of cell proliferation in the liver and in hepatocytes *in vitro*. The effects of the drug on cell proliferation after initiation by a carcinogen have also been investigated and the cell proliferation rates compared in hepatocytes in altered foci and in surrounding tissue.

(i)   *Studies in the absence of carcinogen initiation*

Peraino *et al.* (1971) measured the labelling index, which is the percentage of cells with intense labelling due to incorporation of radioactive precursors in DNA during semiconservative replication (i.e. not unscheduled DNA synthesis), after administration to male Sprague-Dawley rats of a diet containing 0.05% (w/v) phenobarbital for up to 8 weeks. The labelling indexes for hepatocytes and littoral cells (the lining cells of the sinusoids) measured at 2, 4 and 8 weeks were not significantly different in the phenobarbital-fed rats and the controls; however, when the labelling index was measured within about 3 days of phenobarbital administration, a marked increase was found in both hepatocytes and littoral cells, indicating that the stimulating effect of phenobarbital is relatively rapid and short-lived.

In another experiment, young male Sprague-Dawley rats were treated intraperitoneally with 83 mg/kg bw phenobarbital daily for up to 5 days, and the hepatocyte labelling index was measured 24 h after the last injection (Peraino et al., 1975). The labelling index peaked at four times the control level in rats exposed to phenobarbital for 3 days and returned to control values by 5 days, despite continued phenobarbital administration. The liver weight increased continuously throughout the 5-day period.

Ward and Ohshima (1985) investigated the cell proliferation (measured by [^{3}H]thymidine incorporation) accompanying promotion by phenobarbital of 'naturally occurring' foci in aged Fischer 344 rats. Rats aged 26 months were given drinking-water containing phenobarbital at 0.05% (w/v) for up to 27 weeks. Phenobarbital increased the number and volume of eosinophilic and γ-glutamyl transpeptidase-positive foci, but not of basophilic foci. The labelling indexes were increased in both the eosinophilic and basophilic foci in comparison with normal hepatocytes but were higher in the eosinophilic foci than in the basophilic foci. The index was not significantly increased in phenobarbital-exposed normal hepatocytes over that in controls. Of the phenobarbital-exposed rats, 30% developed eosinophilic adenomas; the controls had none.

Büsser and Lutz (1987) gave male SIV-50 SD rats a dose of 2.3 or 23 mg/kg bw phenobarbital orally and measured the labelling index in the liver 24 h later. The higher dose increased the index 2.5-fold, but the lower dose had no appreciable effect. Smith et al. (1991) fed a diet containing 0.1% (w/w) phenobarbital to male and female Sprague-Dawley rats and CD-1 mice for 1 or 5 weeks and assessed cell proliferation from the incorporation into DNA of bromodeoxyuridine released from osmotic minipumps during the entire 1-week administration of phenobarbital or during the last week for the 5-week experiment. The labelling index was increased several-fold in the livers of rats and mice of each sex at 1 week, but there were no increases at 5 weeks. However, the liver weight was increased by phenobarbital treatment at 1 and 5 weeks: in rats, the increase was 20–40% above control values, and in mice the increase was 50–75%.

The effects of administration of large doses of phenobarbital on liver cell proliferation were compared in 6–8-week-old male and female Fischer 344 rats and B6C3F$_1$ mice (Klaunig et al., 1991). The animals were treated with 500 mg/kg bw phenobarbital for 3, 7 and 14 days and evaluated for cell proliferation by measurement of radiolabelled thymidine. Phenobarbital enhanced cell proliferation in both species, with continued increases over the 14-day period. The effects were somewhat greater in males than in females.

Administration of 0.1% phenobarbital in the drinking-water of young male Fischer 344 rats increased the labelling index in hepatocytes from 0.1% to about 2.7% at 5 days, and the index remained elevated at 10 days. The plasma concentration of growth factor had increased about threefold by day 3 and remained elevated up to day 7. The investigators proposed that the increase in hepatocyte growth factor mediated phenobarbital-enhanced cell proliferation (Lindroos *et al.*, 1992).

The effect of phenobarbital on DNA synthesis was also examined in 8-week-old B6C3F$_1$ mice and Fischer 344 rats given a diet containing phenobarbital at 10, 50, 100 or 500 mg/kg for 7, 14, 21, 28 and 90 days. An increase in hepatic DNA synthesis — measured by [^{3}H]thymidine incorporation — was seen in both rat and mouse liver after 7 days at the two higher doses. The rates of DNA synthesis had returned to control values by 14 days in rats, whereas this effect was sustained throughout the 90 days of treatment in mouse liver (Kolaja *et al.*, 1995a, 1996b).

Loss of normal cellular regulation of apoptosis has been shown to be an important component of the carcinogenesis process. Cell growth may increase due to an increase in cell proliferation and/or a decrease in cell death (apoptosis). Less apoptosis was seen in non-focal hepatocytes of fasted rats given phenobarbital (0.05% in drinking-water) than in those of untreated fasted or non-fasted rats, all rats having been initiated with NDEA (10 mg/kg bw) after a 70% hepatectomy. Fasting increased apoptosis and decreased DNA synthesis in rat hepatic focal lesions, and phenobarbital treatment during fasting partially reversed these effects (Hikita *et al.*, 1998).

Phenobarbital (2 mmol/L) inhibited both transforming growth factor (TGF)β- and bleomycin-induced apoptosis in male mouse hepatocytes. In addition, the regulation of *p53*, *BCL-2* and *BAX* was modified in hepatocytes from male mice treated with phenobarbital (Christensen *et al.*, 1998).

BCL-2 plays an important role in the regulation of apoptosis. Treatment of male B6C3F$_1$ mice with phenobarbital (0.05% in the drinking-water for up to 30 days) increased the amount of BCL-2 protein and decreased that of the BAX protein. Greater expression of BCL-2 protein was observed in the 85% of basophilic hepatic foci and adenomas resulting from long-term treatment with phenobarbital than in surrounding normal cells. BCL-2 protein was expressed in only 12–14% of eosinophilic focal lesions and adenomas (Christensen *et al.*, 1999).

Phenobarbital increased DNA synthesis — measured by bromodeoxyuridine immunocytochemistry — in male Wistar rats treated orally at a dose of 80 mg/kg bw per day for 7 days, with significant increases in the labelling index in the liver, proximal tubule of the kidney and thyroid. The increased DNA synthesis reached a maximum in the liver after 3 days of treatment and increased steadily in the proximal tubule and thyroid over the 7 days of treatment. The labelling indexes in the testis, adrenal cortex and medulla, distal tubule of the kidney and exocrine pancreas were no different from those of controls. Significant decreases were observed in the labelling indexes in the pituitary and the endocrine pancreas (Jones & Clarke, 1993).

(ii)   *Administration after a carcinogen*

Mouse: B6C3F$_1$ mice, 15 days of age, were given a single intraperitoneal dose of NDEA at 5 mg/kg bw; at 24 weeks, some of the mice received drinking-water containing 0.05% (w/v) phenobarbital for 7 days. An osmotic minipump containing radiolabelled thymidine was implanted in all animals at 24 weeks of age. The labelling index in hepatocytes of altered foci in the NDEA-treated males and females was sixfold higher than in the surrounding hepatocytes. After exposure to phenobarbital, significantly increased labelling indexes were found in hepatocytes in foci and in surrounding hepatocytes in females, but in males the increase was observed only in the surrounding hepatocytes. The authors concluded that this difference explained the finding that phenobarbital promoted NDEA-initiated tumours in immature female mice and inhibited tumour formation in immature males (Weghorst & Klaunig, 1989).

The responsiveness of liver cells to mitogenic stimulation by phenobarbital in NDEA-initiated $B6C3F_1$ mice was investigated further. The mice were given feed containing NDEA at a concentration providing a dose of 5 mg/kg bw per day at 15 days or 24 weeks of age, after which they were given drinking-water containing 0.05% (w/v) phenobarbital for 2 weeks. Other groups received only NDEA or only phenobarbital. At days 7 and 14, but not at day 3, the DNA labelling indices were significantly increased by about fourfold in males and by about twofold in females given only phenobarbital. In males, phenobarbital given after initiation with NDEA produced a statistically significant decrease in the labelling of liver foci cells at 14 days but no change at 3 or 7 days. In females, increases of 1.5- and 1.3-fold were found at 7 and 14 days (Siglin et al., 1991).

Male $B6C3F_1$ mice, 30 days of age, were given a single intraperitoneal dose of 90 mg/kg bw of NDEA; after 36 weeks, they received drinking-water containing phenobarbital at 0.002, 0.01 or 0.05% (w/v) for up to 45 days. Phenobarbital increased the DNA labelling index in normal hepatocytes at concentrations of 0.01 and 0.05% but not at 0.002%, at 7 and 14 days. The values had returned to control levels by 28 and 45 days. Hepatocytes in liver foci showed increased DNA labelling indexes at 0.01 and 0.05% but not at 0.002%; the increased level persisted for at least 45 days. In contrast, adenomas were unresponsive to phenobarbital (Klaunig, 1973).

Female C3H and $C3B6F_1$ mice, 15 days of age, received a single dose of 16 mg/kg bw NDEA intraperitoneally; at 21 days of age, some groups were given drinking-water containing 0.05% phenobarbital for 140 days. C3H mice had 54.1 adenomas per mouse, while $C3B6F_1$ mice had 0.57 per animal, and in both strains the number was similar with and without phenobarbital. However, phenobarbital doubled the number of altered hepatic foci in C3H, but not in $C3B6F_1$ mice. Phenobarbital increased the labelling index of eosinophilic, but not basophilic, foci in C3H mice. The labelling index of cells in foci was similar in basophilic and eosinophilic adenomas in mice treated with NDEA with and without phenobarbital. The greatest effect of phenobarbital was to decrease the labelling index in normal hepatocytes compared with cells in altered foci in C3H mice, in which the ratio of the labelling index in cells in foci and in normal hepatocytes was 214 for basophilic and 82 for eosinophilic foci without phenobarbital, and 545 for basophilic and 455 for eosinophilic foci with phenobarbital. For $C3B6F_1$ mice, the ratios were 13.1 for basophilic and 11.4 for eosinophilic cells without phenobarbital, and 19.9 and 19.1 with phenobarbital. The author concluded that the relative effect of phenobarbital on proliferation in cells of altered foci and normal hepatocytes was the main determinant of strain sensitivity to carcinogenesis (Pereira, 1993).

Rat: Changes in cell proliferation were investigated in altered foci in the liver after initiation with AAF and promotion with phenobarbital in male Buffalo rats from 30 days of age. The rats were fed a diet containing 0.02% AAF for 4 weeks and then a diet containing 0.05% phenobarbital for 39 weeks, at which time the animals were killed. The labelling index and size were greatest for liver foci that were γ-GT-positive, ATPase-negative and glucose-6-phosphatase-negative. The average labelling index was 4.5 times that in representative 'background' areas which were γ-GT-negative, ATPase-positive and glucose-6-phosphatase-positive. All types of altered foci with γ-GT-positive phenotypic markers had an average labelling index ≥ 2.2 times background, whereas this was not the case for the other markers. Two solid hepatocellular carcinomas were found to have higher labelling indexes than the hyperplastic nodules from which they appeared to arise (Pugh & Goldfarb, 1978).

Altered foci were induced in female Wistar rats, 4–8 weeks old, by administration of a single dose of 75 or 150 mg/kg bw NDEA or 150 or 250 mg/kg bw NMOR. Other groups of animals were given drinking-water containing NDEA at a concentration providing a dose of 5 mg/kg bw per day for 40 days. Altered foci were identified by the presence of γ-GT-positive cells, and cell proliferation was measured by uptake of [³H]thymidine. The percentage of DNA-synthesizing cells 2–7.5 months after administration of the carcinogen was four- to 30-fold higher in hepatocytes of altered foci than in surrounding tissue. Administration of phenobarbital at 50 mg/kg bw by gavage 24–30 h before sacrifice stimulated DNA synthesis in γ-GT-positive foci to a greater extent than in surrounding normal hepatocytes (Schulte-Hermann *et al.*, 1981).

In NDEA-initiated male Wistar rats, phenobarbital increased the proliferation of preneoplastic cells over that of normal cells. Young rats were given drinking-water containing NDEA at a concentration providing a dose of 10 mg/kg bw per day for 2 or 4 weeks. One week after cessation of treatment with NDEA, the initiated animals were given drinking-water containing 0.07% (w/v) phenobarbital for various times; other groups were exposed to phenobarbital only. Labelling indexes were determined by the uptake of radiolabelled thymidine given as seven injections at 6-h intervals; this procedure ensured labelling of all cells entering DNA synthesis during the 36 h after the first injection. Administration of phenobarbital for 10 days increased the labelling index several-fold, but this effect was no longer evident after exposure for 1 month. Administration of NDEA alone for 2 weeks increased the labelling 4.5-fold in normal areas and 5.5-fold in foci, when measured after 12 months. Exposure to NDEA followed by 12 months of exposure to phenobarbital caused a 45% increase in the labelling index in normal hepatocytes as compared with exposure to NDEA alone and nearly a threefold increase in the number of altered foci. Similar findings were reported after 4 weeks of NDEA and 4 months of phenobarbital in the drinking-water, except that the labelling index in altered foci was increased by only 1.5-fold with phenobarbital as compared to NDEA only (Barbason *et al.*, 1983).

Seven-week-old female Wistar rats received NMOR at a single oral dose of 250 mg/kg bw and then received a diet containing phenobarbital providing a dose of 50 mg/kg bw per day for 10 or 28 weeks. The size of the liver and the DNA content increased during exposure to phenobarbital and returned to normal within a few weeks after cessation of exposure. The incidence of apoptotic bodies was very low in normal liver tissue but increased steeply when phenobarbital was withdrawn; resumption of phenobarbital somewhat inhibited the formation of apoptotic bodies. In eosinophilic altered foci, the number of apoptotic bodies was greater than in the surrounding liver tissue during exposure to phenobarbital and increased to much higher levels than in the surrounding liver after phenobarbital withdrawal. The number was significantly suppressed by re-administration of phenobarbital (Bursch *et al.*, 1984).

Female Wistar rats were given a single dose of 250 mg/kg bw NMOR by gavage at 5 weeks of age and 10 weeks later received phenobarbital in the diet at a concentration providing a dose of 50 mg/kg bw per day, or control diet. [^{3}H]Thymidine was infused continuously by means of osmotic minipumps during exposure to phenobarbital. Hepatocytes in altered foci were identified by histochemical staining for γ-GT or by reaction with anti-CYP2B antibodies which could be located by immunohistochemistry. After 14 days of exposure to phenobarbital, the liver mass had increased by 35%. The DNA labelling index increased steadily over the 14-day period, resulting in labelling of 12% of the cells compared with 3% in the controls. In normal hepatocytes, the phenobarbital-induced enhancement of DNA labelling was confined to the CYP2B-containing cells in the pericentral lobular region. In the absence of phenobarbital, the labelling index was approximately 10-fold higher in γ-GT-positive foci than in surrounding hepatocytes. Phenobarbital caused a further increase in the labelling index in foci, but only during the first 2 days of exposure (Schulte-Hermann *et al.*, 1986).

In a similar protocol, animals were fed a diet containing phenobarbital providing a dose of 50 mg/kg bw per day for 10, 28 or 49 weeks. The group treated for 10 weeks was not further treated for the subsequent 18 weeks, and that treated for 28 weeks was allowed an 11-week recovery period. Exposure to phenobarbital increased the liver weight by 20% during the first weeks of exposure and by 35% at the end of the experiment; the DNA content was also increased. The increase in liver weight was reversible within 2 weeks of phenobarbital withdrawal, while the increase in DNA content reversed more slowly. NMOR produced mostly basophilic foci, 50% of which were γ-GT-positive; after exposure to phenobarbital, however, most of the foci consisted of eosinophilic and diffusely basophilic hepatocytes, of which approximately 90% were γ-GT-positive. Phenobarbital increased the number of altered foci by fivefold. Throughout the experiment, the rate of cell proliferation, measured as the labelling index, was 10-fold higher within the foci than in surrounding hepatic tissue. On withdrawal of phenobarbital after 10 and 28 weeks of exposure, the number of foci declined rapidly, and the size remained constant rather than increasing progressively.

Phenobarbital increased the labelling index in the foci during the first 2 days of exposure, but this effect was no longer present after 2 weeks. No decrease in the labelling index was found with prolonged exposure to phenobarbital. Withdrawal of phenobarbital did not result in a significant decrease in the labelling index in normal hepatocytes or in the foci. The authors concluded that phenobarbital did not cause development of foci from single initiated cells. Instead, the γ-GT-positive altered foci appeared to derive from pre-existent foci of initiated cells. As had been seen in previous experiments, much less apoptosis was seen in liver foci during exposure to phenobarbital than in foci of controls, and more apoptosis occurred in the foci after cessation of phenobarbital exposure (Schulte-Hermann et al., 1990).

In a study of the longevity of hepatocytes during promotion by phenobarbital, measured as the loss of thymidine label, adult female Fischer 344 rats were given NDEA at a dose of 200 mg/kg bw intraperitoneally, followed 4 weeks later by partial hepatectomy and then 4 days later by administration of drinking-water containing 0.05% (w/v) phenobarbital for up to 28 weeks. Labelled thymidine (four doses over 18 h) was given after partial hepatectomy but before phenobarbital administration. The comparison group did not receive phenobarbital. There was no significant difference in the decrease in thymidine label in the liver measured at 9 and 28 weeks. It was concluded that the growth advantage of foci induced by phenobarbital was not due to enhanced destruction of normal hepatocytes (Hayes et al., 1987).

Comparison of mouse and rat: In NDEA-initiated mice and rats, phenobarbital at 100 or 500 mg/kg of diet increased DNA synthesis in hepatic foci in both species, but treatment with 10 mg/kg of diet failed to increase the growth of focal lesions. In addition, a significant decrease in apoptosis was observed in focal hepatocytes of both species. DNA synthesis in hepatic adenomas was unaffected by treatment with phenobarbital. The normal surrounding liver showed increased DNA synthesis at 7 days, which had returned to control levels by 28 and 45 days of treatment (Klaunig, 1993; Kolaja et al., 1995b, 1996c).

(b) *Biochemical events related to cell cycle growth factors and cell cycle regulation*

Administration of a diet containing 0.05% (w/w) phenobarbital to female Sprague-Dawley rats for 16 days decreased epidermal growth factor (EGF) receptor RNA by 65% and rat leukaemia virus RNA by 35% (Hsieh et al., 1988). No effects were found on the expression of c-*myc*, H-*ras* or 30S (an endogenous retrovirus-like sequence) RNAs. Gupta et al. (1988) found similar effects in male Sprague-Dawley rats given a semi-synthetic diet supplemented with choline and containing 0.06% (w/w) phenobarbital. EGF receptors were decreased by 12, 66 and 60% at 3, 10 and 28 days after the beginning of exposure to phenobarbital. Phenobarbital also decreased the EGF receptor–EGF dissociation constant. In another study, provision of drinking-water containing 0.1% (w/v) phenobarbital to female Fischer 344 rats decreased the EGF receptors by 33 and 73% at 2 and 8 weeks. Furthermore, phenobarbital diminished the inhibition of hepatocyte proliferation by extracellular Ca^{2+} (Eckl et al., 1988).

In female B6C3F$_1$ mice treated with NDEA followed by phenobarbital (500 mg/kg of diet for 4 months), the expression of TGFα, measured by immunohistochemistry, differed according to the type of foci. Treatment with phenobarbital modulated the relative number of basophilic and eosinophilic foci, but did not affect the staining pattern of the growth factor. In basophilic foci, TGFα staining was absent, in contrast to that seen in eosinophilic foci. Staining was also found in 20% of basophilic hepato-cellular adenomas and 60% of hepatocellular carcinomas. The presence of the EGF receptor followed the pattern of staining for TGFα (Moser et al., 1997).

Phenobarbital reduced the ability of normal hepatocytes (in contrast to NDEA-initiated hepatocytes) to respond to mitogenic stimuli. This decreased proliferative response was attributed to an increase in the concentrations of TGFβ1 and insulin-like growth factor receptor in the phenobarbital-treated hepatocytes. As this receptor activates the growth factor through proteolytic processes, the reduced mitogenic response may be due in part to the increased capacity of phenobarbital-treated hepa-tocytes to activate TGFβ1 (Jirtle et al., 1994). In male Fischer 344 rats, phenobarbital selectively promoted a subpopulation of NDEA-induced preneoplastic cells that expressed reduced concentrations of TGFβ receptor types I, II and III. The cells there-fore showed less ability to respond to negative growth signals mediated by this growth factor (Mansbach et al., 1996).

The expression of the WAF1/CIP1 gene product p21 was reduced by pheno-barbital in NDEA-initiated altered hepatic foci. Glutathione S-transferase (placental form)-positive eosinophilic altered foci showed decreased p21 expression, suggesting a role for altered signalling in the G$_1$–S phase check-point in liver carcinogenesis induced by phenobarbital (Martens et al., 1996).

Oncogene mutation and expression have been associated with several stages of carcinogenesis. Lafarge-Frayssinet and Frayssinet (1989) examined the expression of the protooncogenes ki-ras, fos and myc in one spontaneously transformed and one untransformed rat liver cell line derived from 10-day-old rats after treatment with phenobarbital. In the transformed cell line, strong expression of the three oncogenes was observed in the presence or absence of phenobarbital, but in the untransformed cells, phenobarbital caused overexpression of all three oncogenes. In primary rat hepatocyte cultures, phenobarbital induced a slight increase in c-fos expression but had no effect on c-myc expression. The authors suggested that this indicated a decrease in the G$_0$–G$_1$ cell-cycle shift (Duivenvoorden & Maier, 1994). Jenke et al. (1994) observed an increase in c-raf expression in NDEA-induced hepatic nodules and foci in female Sprague-Dawley rats after treatment with phenobarbital.

(c)   Effects related to oxidative damage

The possible involvement of arachidonic acid metabolism in promotion of tumours by phenobarbital was investigated in male Fischer 344 rats, 6–7 weeks of age, which were given a single intraperitoneal injection of 200 mg/kg bw NDEA; after 2 weeks, some animals were given a diet containing 0.05% (w/w) phenobarbital with varying amounts of inhibitors or antioxidants, for 10 weeks. Phenobarbital increased the number of γ-GT-positive foci by three- to 10-fold, depending on the experiment. Quercitin (an inhibitor of lipoxygenase), morin (a dual inhibitor of lipoxygenase and cyclooxygenase), acetylsalicylic acid (an inhibitor of cyclooxygenase) and *para*-bromophenacyl bromide (an inhibitor of phospholipase A_2) all partially inhibited this effect of phenobarbital, thereby indicating a role of lipoxygenase, cyclooxygenase and phospholipase A_2. The antioxidants *n*-propyl gallate and ethoxyquin also exerted dose-dependent inhibition of phenobarbital promotion (Denda *et al.*, 1989). Phenobarbital enhanced the formation of reactive oxygen in neoplastic rat liver nodules. Newborn Wistar rats were given a single injection of 0.15 µmol/kg bw [15.3 µg/kg bw] NDEA and, after weaning, were given a diet containing 0.05% (w/w) phenobarbital for 8–12 months. Some groups were removed from the phenobarbital diet 3–6 weeks before being killed. Reactive oxygen was measured by lucigenin chemiluminescence in liver microsomes isolated from nodules or from surrounding normal tissue. The level of reactive oxygen was about twofold greater in nodules than in surrounding tissue. Animals exposed to phenobarbital up to the time of death had twofold more reactive oxygen in both nodules and in surrounding tissue than did animals that had been withdrawn from the phenobarbital diet 3–6 weeks before. The generation of reactive oxygen was inhibited by 80–90% by SKF 525A, a specific inhibitor of CYP activity, indicating the involvement of the CYP enzyme systems. Accordingly, CYP content and CYP activity, measured as benzoxy-resorufin dealkylation rates, were greater in animals given phenobarbital up to time of death than in those withdrawn from phenobarbital 3–6 weeks before death, and there were no differences between nodules and surrounding tissue (Scholz *et al.*, 1990).

As prostaglandins have been implicated in tumour promotion, the expression of cyclooxygenase, an enzyme involved in prostaglandin synthesis, was examined in Kupffer cells of male Wistar rats *in vivo* and *in vitro* after treatment with pheno-barbital. Kupffer cells from rats given drinking-water containing phenobarbital at 0.075% (w/v) for 56 days or incubated *in vitro* with 1 mmol/L phenobarbital for 8 or 24 h showed an increase in cyclooxygenase-2 mRNA and protein and total cyclooxy-genase-2 activity, suggesting a role for paracrine activity involving Kupffer cells in the proliferative response of hepatocytes to phenobarbital (Kroll *et al.*, 1999).

Hepatocyte cell cultures have been used to investigate the possible mechanisms of the increased or inhibited cell proliferation found *in vivo*. Some investigators have studied the effects of various agents on cultured hepatocytes from pheno-barbital-exposed animals. Phenobarbital increased the incorporation of radiolabelled thymidine into the DNA of hepatocytes derived from adult male Wistar rats and maintained in a medium containing 30 nmol/L dexamethasone and 30 ng/mL EGF. The effect was related to the concentration of phenobarbital in the medium, 2 mmol/L producing a maximum increase of 30% (Edwards & Lucas, 1985). The continuous presence of 3 mmol/L phenobarbital permitted survival of hepatocytes isolated from the livers of 3-month-old Donryu male rats for at least 49 days. Phenobarbital also inhibited the proliferation of fibroblasts in the cultures. The hepatocytes continued to secrete relatively large amounts of albumin and maintained a high basal level of tyrosine aminotransferase activity, indicating that they had retained differentiated phenotypes (Miyazaki *et al.*, 1985).

Stimulation of DNA synthesis in hepatocytes isolated from male Sprague-Dawley rats by EGF was enhanced by 60–80% by the addition of 1 mmol/L phenobarbital to the medium 2 h after plating. EGF was added from the 12th to the 24th h. DNA synthesis was maximally stimulated between 44 and 46 h. EGF binding was increased by phenobarbital after 12 h as compared with controls. Phenobarbital was most effective in increasing DNA synthesis when added to hepatocytes in G_0 or G_1 phase (Sawada *et al.*, 1987). In contrast, phenobarbital had no effect on EGF binding to hepatocytes derived from female Fischer 344 rats, unless the hepatocytes were preincubated with phenobarbital for 1 h before addition of EGF, in which case, EGF binding was inhibited at phenobarbital concentrations in the millimolar range (Meyer *et al.*, 1989). Preincubation with phenobarbital inhibited the phorbol ester-induced redistribution of calcium and phospholipid-dependent protein kinase C in primary rat hepatocytes but reversibly inhibited phorbol ester-induced protein kinase C activation, suggesting that it alters a component of the signalling pathway other than protein kinase C isoenzymes (Brockenbrough *et al.*, 1991).

Hepatocytes isolated from animals given drinking-water containing 0.1% phenobarbital for up to 2 weeks showed greater rates of EGF-stimulated proliferation at physiological calcium concentrations (1.2–1.8 mmol/L) than with 0.2–0.4 mmol/L calcium, which is the optimal concentration for EGF-stimulated proliferation of hepatocytes from unexposed animals. Hepatocytes from animals exposed to phenobarbital for 3–28 days proliferated at two- to threefold greater rates than hepatocytes from unexposed animals. Hepatocytes from animals exposed to phenobarbital for more than 1 month proliferated slowly at all concentrations of calcium. The authors concluded that phenobarbital altered the cellular growth response to calcium, and that its effects on hepatocyte proliferation could therefore not be explained solely by changes in EGF receptors (Eckl *et al.*, 1988).

The effects of phenobarbital on EGF-induced DNA synthesis in normal hepatocytes was compared with those in hepatocytes derived from putative preneoplastic cells isolated from nodules induced in rats given drinking-water containing 0.005% NDEA for 2 months. Phenobarbital at up to 50 mmol/L was not mitogenic to normal hepatocytes cultured *in vitro*; at concentrations of 0.001–1.5 mmol/L, it stimulated EGF-induced DNA synthesis, as measured by [³H]thymidine incorporation. The greatest stimulation occurred with 0.001 and 0.01 mmol/L, whereas higher concentrations inhibited EGF-induced DNA synthesis. Less inhibition was seen in hepatocytes from foci induced by NDEA. Hepatocytes from animals given drinking-water containing 0.1% phenobarbital for 2 months required only 0.1 mmol/L phenobarbital to show reduced binding of EGF to its receptor, whereas > 1 mmol/L was required to produce a similar effect in control hepatocytes. Furthermore, EGF-stimulated DNA synthesis in hepatocytes from phenobarbital-exposed animals was more readily inhibited by TGFβ1. The authors concluded that phenobarbital down-regulated EGF receptors and that long-term exposure of rats to phenobarbital further sensitized the hepatocytes to down-regulation, by increasing the intracellular concentration of TGFβ1 (Jirtle & Meyer, 1991). Incubation of hepatocytes from normal male Fischer 344 rats with 3, 4, 5 or 6 mmol/L phenobarbital inhibited TGFα-induced DNA synthesis in a dose-dependent manner. Phenobarbital also inhibited DNA synthesis in hepatocytes derived from persistent hepatic nodules from rats initiated with 1,2-dimethylhydrazine and promoted with orotic acid (Manjeshwar et al., 1992).

Hepatocytes were isolated from both humans and rats and tested for the effects of phenobarbital on EGF-induced DNA synthesis. The labelling index of the rat hepatocytes was five- to 10-fold higher than that of the human hepatocytes. Whereas incubation with phenobarbital was found to increase EGF-induced DNA synthesis in rat hepatocytes, phenobarbital had no effect in human cells. However, initial differences between the human and rat hepatocytes with respect to viability and the relative biological ages of the donors may limit the significance of this comparison (Parzefall et al., 1991).

The mitogenic effects of phenobarbital were also examined in hepatocyte cultures from rats treated with N-nitrosomethyl(acetoxymethyl)amine. These initiated hepatocytes proliferated and formed colonies under conditions that induced senescence and death in hepatocytes from untreated rats. The colony-forming efficiency of the initiated cells isolated from liver 5 weeks after initiation was approximately 10% in the presence of 2 mmol/L phenobarbital in the medium and less than 0.2% in the absence of phenobarbital. A low rate of DNA synthesis was found in hepatocytes in the absence of phenobarbital; thus, proliferation of initiated hepatocytes in vivo appeared to depend on sustained exposure of the cells to phenobarbital (Kaufmann et al., 1988). Similarly, the propagation of a phenobarbital-dependent hepatocyte cell line (6/27/C1) was shown to be promoter-dependent, in that clonal expansion occurred only when phenobarbital was replaced by another liver tumour promoter in the culture medium (Kaufmann et al., 1997).

Treatment of rat and mouse hepatocytes with phenobarbital also resulted in induction of DNA synthesis and suppression of apoptosis. However, these effects appear to be species-specific, as hamster and guinea-pig cells showed no increase in DNA synthesis and no suppression of either spontaneous or TGFβ1-induced apoptosis (James & Roberts, 1996). Human hepatocytes were also refractory to these effects (Hasmall & Roberts, 1999).

In cultured rat hepatocytes, phenobarbital diminished spontaneous apoptosis and slightly suppressed TGFβ1-induced apoptosis. It increased endogenous and TGFβ-induced peroxide formation, significantly decreased superoxide dismutase formation and increased catalase by twofold (Díez-Fernández et al., 1998). Treatment of HepG2 cells with phenobarbital resulted in an increase in erythropoietin synthesis, which was related to a decrease in the intracellular concentration of hydroxyl free radicals involved in oxygen-regulated gene expression (Ehleben et al., 1998).

(d)   Effects on the thyroid

Reduced concentrations of T3 and T4 and resulting increases in the concentration of TSH have been shown to mediate the thyroid tumour promoting effects of hepatic microsomal enzyme inducers such as phenobarbital (McClain et al., 1989). Male Sprague-Dawley rats fed a diet containing 1200 mg/kg phenobarbital for 3, 7, 14, 21, 30, 45, 60 or 90 days showed a 25% reduction in T4 concentration and an 80% increase in thyroid weight. Thyroid cell proliferation was increased 2.6-fold after 7 days of treatment and returned to control levels only by day 45 of treatment (Hood et al., 1999). In another study, a mitogenic response was found in rat thyroid only after 8 weeks of treatment with phenobarbital at 0.1% (w/w) in drinking-water (Zbinden, 1988).

The effect of phenobarbital on thyroid function and biliary excretion of T4 was examined by giving male and female rats a diet containing phenobarbital to provide a target dose of 100 mg/kg bw per day for 2 weeks. Increased liver and thyroid gland weights, decreased circulating concentrations of T4 and T3 and increased TSH concentrations were found in both male and female rats. The effects on the hormones decreased after 3 months of treatment. Treatment of thyroidectomized rats with phenobarbital increased the plasma clearance of T4. Bile-duct cannulated phenobarbital-treated male rats showed a marked increase in hepatic uptake of $[^{125}I]$T4 and a 42% increase in its biliary excretion, due mainly to increased excretion of T4 glucuronide. This corresponded to an increase in the total hepatic activity of T4–UDP-glucuronosyl transferase (UGT). These effects were observed in both male and female rats, but the response was greater in males (McClain et al., 1989).

The effects of phenobarbital on hepatic microsomal T4–UGT and T3–UGT activities and thyroid function were examined in OF-1 male mice after 14 days' oral exposure to 80 mg/kg bw per day. Phenobarbital induced liver hypertrophy and increases in liver weight and microsomal protein and CYP content, but no significant change in T4–UGT or T3–UGT activity. No significant changes in serum T4 and T3 concentrations were observed, and the histological appearance of the thyroid was not affected. Thus, phenobarbital did not affect thyroid hormone metabolism or thyroid function in mice (Viollon-Abadie et al., 1999).

Treatment of male albino rats with a daily oral dose of 100 mg/kg bw phenobarbital for 2 weeks resulted in induction of CYP enzymes, had no effect on T4 concentrations but significantly decreased those of T3 on day 4, and increased TSH concentrations by 60% on day 16, although this increase was not statistically significant. The weight of the thyroid was significantly increased on day 16 and that of the liver on days 4 and 16. Mild to moderate thyroid follicular hypertrophy and moderate hepatocellular hypertrophy occurred in all phenobarbital-treated animals (Johnson et al., 1993).

The effect of phenobarbital on thyroid function and metabolism was also studied in thyroidectomized male Sprague-Dawley rats. The animals received thyroid hormone replacement via implanted osmotic minipumps, which resulted in T4 and T3 serum concentrations similar to those in controls, and were then given phenobarbital in the diet at 1200 mg/kg for 10 days. Phenobarbital reduced the total T4 concentration on days 3–10 and that of free T4 on days 7–10 after minipump implantation, and decreased the total T3 concentration on days 7–10. UGT activity towards T4 was increased 2.7-fold by phenobarbital and correlated with serum T4 concentrations (Barter & Klaassen, 1992). In a study in intact male Sprague-Dawley rats, administration of a diet containing phenobarbital at 1200 mg/kg for 21 days resulted in a 1.9-fold increase in UGT activity towards T4, a 30–40% reduction in T4 concentration and a concomitant increase (50%) in TSH concentration (Barter & Klaassen, 1994). Similar effects on thyroid hormone concentrations were observed in rats treated with an oral dose of 50–100 mg/kg bw phenobarbital daily for 7 or 14 days (de Sandro *et al.*, 1991) and in epileptic dogs treated with phenobarbital at a daily dose of 1.0–16.4 mg/kg bw for 1.3 weeks–8 years (Gaskill *et al.*, 1999). In contrast, treatment of euthyroid dogs with an oral dose of 1.8–3 mg/kg bw phenobarbital every 12 h for 1 week followed by 2.7–4.5 mg/kg bw every 12 h for 2 weeks did not change the serum concentrations of T4 (total and free) or TSH (Daminet *et al.*, 1999).

Feeding male Sprague-Dawley rats a diet containing 600–2400 mg/kg phenobarbital for 15 days resulted in dose-dependent induction of UGT activity towards T4 and a reduction in serum T4 concentrations (Liu *et al.*, 1995).

4.3   Reproductive and developmental effects

The potential teratogenic effect of phenobarbital has been reviewed (Friedman & Polifka, 1994). A classic pattern of minor dysmorphologies has been described in children born to mothers treated with phenobarbital for epilepsy during pregnancy. This syndrome includes nail hypoplasia and a typical appearance produced by midfacial hypoplasia, depressed nasal bridge, epicanthal folds and ocular hypertelorism. In an earlier review, Dansky and Finnell (1991) found evidence that phenobarbital monotherapy was associated with malformations similar to those reported with hydantoins, suggesting a common biochemical pathway. They also noted that the risks appeared to be greater after treatment of women with epilepsy than treatment of women without seizure disorders.

4.3.1   *Humans*

As reported in an abstract, 57 women receiving phenobarbital monotherapy during pregnancy were identified in a population of 61 090. When compared with a matched control group, the exposed infants showed significant increases in the frequency of major malformations or growth retardation (15.8% versus 6.7%), 'anticonvulsant face' (12.9% versus 2.5%) and fingernail hypoplasia (25.8% versus 4.5%) (Holmes *et al.*, 1990).

As reported in an abstract, pregnancy outcome was evaluated prospectively in 84 women given phenobarbital monotherapy who were identified through the California Teratogen Information Service (USA). Forty-six of 63 ascertained liveborn infants (seven cases were lost to follow-up and there were 12 spontaneous and one therapeutic abortions) were evaluated by a dysmorphologist. Of these, seven (15%) had facial features characteristic of anti-epileptic therapy and 11 (24%) had hypoplastic fingernails (Jones *et al.*, 1992a).

In a prospective cohort study of the pregnancy outcomes of women being treated for epilepsy with anti-convulsant therapy, 72 infants were born to mothers who had received phenobarbital monotherapy during the first trimester (Dravet *et al.*, 1992). This group comprised 12 infants with microcephaly, 44 who were not microcephalic and 16 unrecorded outcomes [odds ratio apparently not significant].

In a study of the risk of intrauterine growth delay in the offspring of mothers with epilepsy, prospective data on 870 newborn infants in Canada, Italy and Japan were pooled and analysed. A total of 88 infants were born to mothers who had received phenobarbital monotherapy. By logistic regression, the risk for small head circumference was shown to be higher (relative risk, 3.6; 95% CI, 1.4–9.4) among the infants of phenobarbital-exposed mothers (Battino *et al.*, 1999). Subsequent analysis showed statistically significant dose- and concentration-dependent effects of phenobarbital on small head circumference.

A study of the development of sexual identity was carried out among the offspring of mothers with epilepsy who had taken phenobarbital during the index pregnancy in the Amsterdam Academic Medical Centre between 1957 and 1972. Of 243 exposed subjects, 147 participated in the follow-up [age not indicated]. The controls were an equal number of persons from the original pool of 222, matched for birth date, sex and maternal age. Three tests of psychosexual development were used: the Gender Role Assessment Schedule, the Klein Sexual Orientation Grid and the Psychosexual Milestones in Puberty questionnaire. Exposed and control subjects did not differ with respect to 'gender' role behaviour, although greater numbers of persons exposed prenatally to anticonvulsants reported past or present cross-sexual behaviour and/or sexual dysphoria (Dessens *et al.*, 1999).

The intelligence scores of adult men whose mothers had received phenobarbital during pregnancy and who had no history of a central nervous system disorder were measured. The population was drawn from the Danish Perinatal Cohort that was assembled in 1959–61 (Reinisch *et al.*, 1995). A total of 114 exposed offspring and 153 controls were matched for a number of variables. Exposure to phenobarbital, especially during the last trimester, was associated with significantly lower verbal intelligence scores.

In a preliminary note on a prospective randomized double-blind trial on the efficacy of prenatal phenobarbital therapy in the prevention of neonatal hyperbilirubinaemia,

1522 exposed and 1553 control infants were studied (Yaffe & Dorn, 1991). The pheno-barbital treatment consisted of administration of a 100-mg tablet daily during weeks 34–36 of gestation. The frequency of neonatal hyperbilirubinaemia was reduced in those exposed to phenobarbital. In a follow-up of 36% (719) of the 2003 children in one of the two geographical study areas at the age of 5.1–6.8 years in three intelligence tests, the 415 children who had been exposed to phenobarbital tended to score higher than the controls, but the difference was significant only on the Visuo-Motor Integration Test. The observations were continued on 341 adolescents. Pubertal development appeared to be affected, in that there was a trend for the pubertal stage to be delayed in the treated group. The boys showed significantly higher cognitive function as assessed by the Wechler Intelligence Scale. [The Working Group could not locate a subsequent publi-cation on this cohort that contained a complete report.]

In a clinical intervention trial for infantile intracranial haemorrhage, 110 women in preterm labour were assigned to receive either placebo ($n = 60$) or phenobarbital (10 mg/kg bw intravenously followed by 100 mg/kg bw per day orally) until delivery (Shankaran et al., 1996a). There was a trend towards a decreased incidence of intra-cranial haemorrhage of any grade in the group given phenobarbital (22% versus 35%). The authors noted that the mode of action of this response is not clear but may be related to hypertensive peaks in the neonate. In a follow-up study, no adverse consequences on growth or in the McCarthy General Cognitive Index was seen in the phenobarbital-treated offspring up to 3 years of age (Shankaran et al., 1996b), but the study has been criticized for a low and potentially biased follow-up rate (Doyle, 1996).

The influence of prenatal exposure to phenobarbital on childhood IQ (measured by the Bayley Mental Development Index) at 2 years of age was studied in a double-blind, placebo-controlled trial in which the drug was given in utero for the prevention of intracranial haemorrhage to patients with an imminent risk of premature delivery (Thorp et al., 1999). The dose of phenobarbital was targeted to yield serum pheno-barbital concentrations in the mother and infant of 15–17 µg/mL. [The Working Group noted that the study group also received 10 mg vitamin K every 4 days until delivery.] The incidence of antenatal fetal or postnatal death did not differ between the groups. In the 121 (32%) of 375 children who participated in the 2-year follow-up, a significantly lower Bayley mental developmental index was found in the treated group compared with the controls (104 versus 113). Backward regression analysis indicated the presence of five other covariates that were statistically significant, including maternal education and patent ductus arteriosis.

A prospective study of 983 infants born to women with epilepsy in Canada, Italy and Japan indicated that the incidence of malformations in the infants of women who had not taken an anti-epileptic drug ($n = 98$) was 3.1%, whereas that in the infants of women on phenobarbital monotherapy ($n = 79$) was 5.1%; the resulting odds ratio was 1.7 [no CI provided]. No specific pattern of malformations was identified after pheno-barbital monotherapy. For any anti-epileptic therapy, the incidence of malformations was 9.0% (Kaneko et al., 1999).

In a review of exposure to anti-epileptic drugs and pregnancy outcome, it was noted that phenobarbital lowers folate concentrations in both humans and rats, which may contribute to its teratogenic potential (Lewis *et al.*, 1998).

4.3.2 *Experimental systems*

The teratogenic effects of phenobarbital in experimental animals have been reviewed (Finnell & Dansky, 1991). A paucity of work on the effects of exposure to phenobarbital *in utero* on pregnancy outcome was noted, the available evidence suggesting that the potency was less than that of other anti-convulsants, such as phenytoin and valproic acid.

In a review of the literature, the influences of route of administration and dose on the nature of the adverse pregnancy outcome were emphasized (Middaugh, 1986). Dietary exposure resulted in high blood concentrations (40–200 μg/mL), reduced food consumption and maternal weight gain and low birth weights and anatomical and bio-chemical abnormalities in the offspring. Studies in which injections were given that tended to result in plasma concentrations similar to those for therapeutic uses (5–20 μg/mL) showed smaller effects on pregnancy outcome, although effects on behavioural and biochemical end-points were sometimes apparent.

Long-Evans rats were given phenobarbital by oral gavage at a dose of 40 mg/kg bw per day during the first 7 days of lactation to investigate whether neonatal exposure altered the sensitivity to carcinogens later in life. Twenty-four hours after injection of 37-week-old male offspring with [^{3}H]aflatoxin B_1 at a dose of 1 mg/kg bw, more afla-toxin B_1–DNA adducts were found in the liver than in untreated controls. In other male offspring of the same age, neonatal exposure to phenobarbital caused a 2.6-fold increase in the activity of ethylmorphine-*N*-demethylase (Faris & Campbell, 1981).

(*a*) *Developmental toxicity*

(i) *Morphology*

Cleft palate was observed after exposure of groups of 2–28 A/J, C3H and CD1 mice to doses of 90–175 mg/kg bw phenobarbital by intramuscular injection at various deve-lopmental periods between days 11 and 14 of gestation. The A/J and CD1 strains were more sensitive than the C3H strain (Walker & Patterson, 1974).

The teratogenic effect of phenobarbital was studied in groups of 15–22 ICI mice given diets containing 0, 50 or 150 mg/kg on days 6–16 of gestation. One of 171 fetuses at the low dose, 6/155 at the high dose and none of the controls had cleft palate [not noted as significant unless pooled over all phenobarbital-treated litters]. No dose-related effects on maternal or fetal body weights or on fetal viability were observed (Sullivan & McElhatton, 1975).

The incidence of cleft palate after oral administration of phenobarbital at 0, 7.5, 20 or 40 mg/kg bw to NMRI-derived albino mice on days 6–15 of gestation was significantly elevated at the highest dose. The two higher doses caused sedation and dyspnoea in the treated females that lasted 1–3 h, but food intake and body-weight gain were not affected. There were no effects on fetal growth, viability or other malformations (Fritz *et al.*, 1976).

Thinning of the cerebral cortex was noted in the brains of neonates of does that received phenobarbital at 18.5 mg/kg bw per day by gavage during the last 10 days of gestation (Dydyk & Rutczynski, 1977).

Sodium phenobarbital was administered in the drinking-water to mice of three inbred strains (SWV, LM/Bc and C57BL/6J) for at least 20 days before mating and throughout gestation. The targeted doses were 0, 60, 120 and 240 mg/kg bw per day, but the actual plasma concentrations of phenobarbital were used to sort the dams into one of four groups (0, 1–10, 10.1–18 and >18.1 µg/mL). There were 5–11 females per group. Dose-related increases in the incidence of malformations were seen in all strains. While defects of the palate, heart, urogenital and skeletal systems were prominent in the SWV and Lm/Bc strains, no palate and only few heart defects were seen in the C57 strain (Finnell *et al.*, 1987a,b).

Concentrations of up to 800 µg/mL phenobarbital did not affect the ability of explants of day-12.5 ICR mouse secondary palates to grow medially and fuse in an organ culture system. The findings were in contrast to the inhibitory effects seen with two other anti-epileptic drugs (Mino *et al.*, 1994).

Phenobarbital was among seven anti-epileptic drugs evaluated for its effects on embryonic cardiac function in C57BL/6J mouse embryos. Day-10 embryos were exposed in whole-embryo culture to concentrations of up to 20 times the human therapeutic plasma concentration. Phenobarbital ranked third highest in potency to cause embryonic bradycardia, suggesting that the pharmacological effect of altered ion channels contributes to the teratogenic effects by affecting blood flow and pressure and subsequently contributing to hypoxia. It was postulated that the reoxygenation process also contributes to tissue damage (Azarbayjani & Danielsson, 1998).

Bradycardia and cardiovascular defects were also reported in 4-day-old white Leghorn chick embryos exposed *in situ* to phenobarbital at 1.75×10^{-5} mol (4.45 mg) by topical administration on eggs (Nishikawa *et al.*, 1987).

(ii)   *Perinatal effects on hepatic enzymes*

Behavioural effects were studied in the offspring of Sprague-Dawley rats given phenobarbital at a dose of 0, 5, 50 or 80 mg/kg bw per day on days 7–18 of gestation or 80 mg/kg bw per day on days 7–10, 11–14 or 15–18 of gestation by oral gavage. With the longer duration, the highest dose of phenobarbital increased the incidence of malformations and mortality in offspring, reduced fetal body weight, delayed the development of the mature swimming angle and induced trends towards delayed startle and reduced alternation behaviour. With the shorter durations, phenobarbital increased the mortality rate of offspring at all doses, but impaired growth only in those exposed on days 11–14. Swimming ability was delayed in those treated on days 7–10 and 11–14.

The author concluded that phenobarbital was a behavioural teratogen at high doses (Vorhees, 1983).

Sprague-Dawley rats [group size not specified] received a subcutaneous injection of 0 or 40 mg/kg bw per day phenobarbital on days 12–19 of gestation. At birth, the male offspring had a reduced anogenital distance, a marker of androgen action in the fetus, in the absence of an effect on body weight. [The Working Group noted that the individual and not the litter was used as the statistical unit.] In adulthood, the males showed a significant decrease in fertility, enlarged livers and reduced seminal vesicle weights (Gupta et al., 1980a). Exposure to phenobarbital at 40 mg/kg bw per day, beginning on gestation day 17, reduced the testosterone concentrations in fetal brain and in the serum of male offspring perinatally (Gupta & Yaffe, 1982). Evaluation of female offspring exposed to 40 mg/kg bw per day phenobarbital on days 12–19 of gestation (six dams per group) showed reduced body growth, a 2-day delay in puberty [not adjusted for reduced growth], altered estrous cycles and reduced fertility in adulthood (Gupta et al., 1980b). In a subsequent study, the same dose was given daily on gestation days 12–20, 14–20 and 17–20, and another group received 20 mg/kg bw per day on postnatal days 1–8 [group size not specified for any treatment] (Gupta & Yaffe, 1981). Litter size and birth weight were unaffected, but the growth of females was reduced between days 20 and 50 and the age at vaginal opening was delayed by 2–3 days in all phenobarbital-exposed groups [not adjusted for body weight]. Estrous cycles and fertility were also altered in all exposed groups. The researchers attributed the effects to androgen deficiency during a critical developmental period (Yaffe & Dom, 1991).

Administration of phenobarbital at a concentration of 500 mg/L in the drinking-water of Mongolian gerbils during gestation (intake, 60 mg/kg bw per day) and lactation (intake, 136 mg/kg bw per day) [group size appears to be 11, with four controls] reduced the proportion of animals bearing litters, decreased the pup weights at birth and delayed the development of early reflexes (Chapman & Cutler, 1988).

A series of experiments on brain development, behaviour and neurochemistry were conducted in HS/Ibg mice that received a diet containing phenobarbital (acid form) at 3 g/kg on days 9–18 of gestation. Postnatal growth and brain weights were reduced on day 22 but not on day 8, 15 or 50. Histological analysis of the brains from 50-day-old offspring indicated that, although the cerebellar and hippocampal layers were not affected, there were 30% fewer Purkinje cells and 15% fewer hippocampal pyramidal cells in treated offspring (Yanai et al., 1979). Beginning at 50 days of age, the offspring were tested in a radial-arm maze; significant decrements in performance were noted in the exposed offspring. No effects were found on brain acetylcholinesterase activity at this age (Kleinberger & Yanai, 1985). Impaired performance in the Morris water maze and greater calculated maximal binding of muscarinic receptors in the hippocampus were noted at 22 and 50 days of age (Yanai et al., 1989). In another study, basal protein kinase C activity was increased in the hippocampi of 50-day-old mice [sex not specified] that had been exposed prenatally to phenobarbital. In addition, the protein kinase C response to carbachol (a cholinergic agonist) was impaired, and there was increased hemicholinium binding, an indicator of the amount of choline transporters. There were no effects on maternal health, and the viability and growth of the offspring were not impaired. The results indicated behavioural effects related to learning and memory deficits (Steingart *et al.*, 1998).

Electroencephalograms were recorded in 90-day-old Sprague-Dawley rats born to dams that had received phenobarbital at 0, 20, 40 or 60 mg/kg bw per day by subcutaneous injection from 28 days before until the end of gestation. There were no statistically significant effects on the growth, viability or development of the offspring, although the average litter size was reduced from 11 pups in the control group to 7 pups per litter at the high dose. Because this reduction suggested that this dose was near the toxic level, electroencephalograms were not recorded for this group. The electroencephalographic spectra were averaged over a 24-h period before analysis as a percentage of the total spectral power. The results indicated suppression of phasic synchronization frequencies associated with learning and attention focus, particularly in female offspring (Livezey *et al.*, 1992).

Groups of 4–12 pregnant Sprague-Dawley rats received phenobarbital at 0, 20, 40 or 80 mg/kg bw per day by subcutaneous injection on days 5–20 of gestation. The offspring were evaluated for external abnormalities, growth, reproductive function and binding of spiroperidol (a dopamine agonist) in the hypothalamus. No malformations were seen, but early postnatal growth was reduced at the high dose. A significant decrease in spiroperidol-binding was noted in females at 22 days of age, but not at 2 months; no effects were noted in male offspring. Benzodiazepine-, muscarinic- and serotonin-binding sites in the frontal cortex were not altered in animals of either sex at either age. There was a dose-related reduction in the percentage of females with normal reproductive cycles at 8–9 weeks of age, but fertility and the litter size after successful mating were normal (Takagi *et al.*, 1986; Seth *et al.*, 1987).

Neonatal male Sprague-Dawley rats received phenobarbital at 30 mg/kg bw per day by subcutaneous injection on postnatal days 1, 3 and 5, and the controls received saline. When the animals were 24 weeks of age, testosterone metabolism was studied in microsomal preparations. Total CYP activity was not altered by exposure. In adult males, but not females, neonatal treatment with phenobarbital increased testosterone 16α- and 2α-hydroxylation and androstenedione formation. These products are formed primarily by the action of CYP2C11. Immunoblot analysis of hepatic protein kinase Cα activity indicated a 63% reduction in the livers of treated males. There were no effects on serum testosterone concentrations (Zangar *et al.*, 1995). A previous study by this group with the same protocol but western blot analysis indicated that phenobarbital increased the activity of CYP2B (Zangar *et al.*, 1993); however, the expected metabolites of testosterone resulting from the activity of this isozyme were not detected in the subsequent study, perhaps owing to low activity.

Neonatal male Sprague-Dawley rats received phenobarbital at 0 or 40 mg/kg bw per day by subcutaneous injection during the first 7 days of life. Body-weight gain was reduced throughout life. Serum testosterone concentrations were lowered between day 4 and 24 and were elevated in adulthood. Closer analysis indicated peaks of testosterone secretion in the adults (Wani *et al.*, 1996).

Growth hormone and monooxygenase activities were studied in adult Sprague-Dawley rats that received seven daily subcutaneous injections of phenobarbital at 0 or 40 mg/kg bw beginning on the first postnatal day. Neonatal exposure resulted in a long-term decrease in peak concentrations of growth hormone at 65 and 150 days of age in males and at 65 days in females. The body-weight gain of males was reduced by about 10% between days 5 and 30 and by 7% through 175 days of age. There was a 15-fold increase in microsomal hydroxylase activity in the livers of neonatal males and females. This effect was no longer observed at 25 or 45 days of age, but reappeared between 65 and 150 days of age, when the increase averaged 15–20% in males and 30–35% in females (Agrawal *et al.*, 1995).

Hepatic drug-metabolizing enzymes were studied in the offspring of Sprague-Dawley rats given phenobarbital by intraperitoneal injection at a dose of 80 mg/kg bw per day for 7 consecutive days before delivery. Pentoxyresorufin-*O*-deethylase activity and CYP2B expression were induced in 5-day-old, but not fetal or 10-day-old pups. Testosterone 6β hydroxylase was not affected. In groups that received drinking-water containing 0.1% phenobarbital from day 13 of gestation to 3 weeks after parturition (end of lactation), the activities of pentoxyresorufin-*O*-deethylase and CYP2B were increased at 3 but not 4 weeks of age in animals of each sex; no effects on testosterone 6β hydroxylase were observed. No effects on CYP3A expression were noted in any treated group (Asoh *et al.*, 1999).

(b)   Reproductive toxicity

Daily injections of 140 mg/kg bw phenobarbital to female hamsters slightly before, but not after, the period of pituitary gonadotropin (luteinizing hormone) release (14:00–15:00 h) blocked ovulation for up to 8 days. The authors speculated that the resistance arose from an alteration of the central mechanism controlling gonadotropin release (Alleva *et al.*, 1975).

4.4   Effects on enzyme induction or inhibition and gene expression

4.4.1   *Humans*

In healthy volunteers, oral administration of phenobarbital at 2–3 mg/kg bw per day for 3 weeks increased antipyrine clearance but not the liver size (Roberts *et al.*, 1976). Biopsy samples from the livers of patients treated for epilepsy with pheno-barbital and phenytoin were found to have elevated total CYP activity, and the livers of these patients were enlarged (Pirttiaho *et al.*, 1978).

4.4.2   *Experimental systems*

The ability of phenobarbital to induce the expression of CYP genes has been investigated and reviewed extensively (Conney, 1967; Okey, 1990; Waxman & Azaroff,
1992). The CYP types induced most effectively by phenobarbital in rat liver are
CYP2B1 and CYP2B2. Other members of the superfamily induced by phenobarbital
include CYP2A1, CYP2C6, CYP2C7, CYP2C11, CYP3A1 and CYP3A2. Relatively
high concentrations of phenobarbital (typically 80 mg/kg bw per day given by
intraperitoneal injection for 4 days) are required for this type of induction. Other
enzymes induced by phenobarbital include aldehyde dehydrogenase, epoxide
hydrolase, NADPH:cytochrome $P450$ reductase, UGT and several glutathione S-trans-
ferases. In addition, increased activities of γ-GT and catalase, but no change in
glutathione peroxidase, have been reported (Furukawa *et al.*, 1985). Phenobarbital at
0.05% (w/v) in drinking-water induced the activity of hepatic O^6-methyltransferase in
rats that had received a single dose of NDMA (O'Connor *et al.*, 1988). The induction
of detoxication enzymes may contribute to the observed inhibition of tumorigenesis by
phenobarbital administered before or concurrently with DNA-reactive carcinogens.

The levels of 4-aminobiphenyl adducts in bladder DNA of rats given this
carcinogen were decreased by phenobarbital at 0.1% (w/v) in drinking-water for 8 days
(Olsen *et al.*, 1993). This suggests that phenobarbital may induce drug-metabolizing
enzymes that deactivate carcinogens.

The dose–response relationship for the effects of phenobarbital on total CYP,
glucose-6-phosphatase and UGT activities was examined in male Sprague-Dawley
rats (age not specified) given intraperitoneal injections of phenobarbital at doses
ranging from 1 to 125 mg/kg bw per day on 6 consecutive days. The total CYP activity
was determined spectrophotometrically in microsomal preparations. Dose-related
increases in CYP activity were found: phenobarbital at 1 mg/kg bw per day had no
effect, at 3 mg/kg bw per day it caused a significant increase, and a maximal increase
(~ two-fold) was observed at 75 mg/kg bw per day. For UGT, a similar pattern was
seen: at 3 mg/kg bw per day, phenobarbital caused a significant increase, and a 2.8-
fold increase in activity was seen at 125 mg/kg bw per day. In contrast, the latter dose
caused a 50% decrease in the activity of glucose-6-phosphatase in liver microsomes
of these rats (Tavoloni *et al.*, 1983).

CYP and related enzymes were induced for up to 90 weeks in C3H mice by
exposing them to phenobarbital at 85 mg/kg bw per day. The concentration in the diet
was adjusted between 0.048% and 0.083% in order to maintain the dose. After 4 weeks
of exposure to phenobarbital, slight cellular and nuclear hypertrophy was seen in the
immediate vicinity of hepatic veins. After 4 weeks of age, hypertrophy of centrilobular
cells was evident. Between 25 and 40 weeks, focal proliferative lesions developed,
followed by large eosinophilic nodules. The activities of microsomal ethylmorphine
N-demethylase and 7-ethoxycoumarin O-deethylase were increased 8–11-fold and
three- to sixfold, respectively, during the exposure period. The activities of CYP and

NADPH-cytochrome c reductase were increased about twofold. Additionally, the activity of benzo[a]pyrene hydroxylase, which is associated with CYP1A1, was increased fivefold, and that of glutathione S-transferase was increased two-to-three fold (Collins $et\ al.$, 1984).

C57BL, C3H, B6C3F$_1$ (C57BL × C3H) and C3B6F$_1$ (C3H × C57BL) mice were compared with respect to their susceptibility to induction of liver enzyme activities by phenobarbital, as they differ markedly in their susceptibility to phenobarbital-induced carcinogenesis. Four-week-old mice were given drinking-water containing 0.05% phenobarbital for 4 or 28 days. The ratio of liver:body weight was increased in all strains and at both times. Similarly, increased activities of CYP isozymes, amino-pyrine-N-demethylase and 7-ethoxyresorufin-O-deethylase and an increased extent of testosterone oxidation were found in all strains. The authors concluded that the strain specificity of the cancer-promoting activity of phenobarbital was not due to any of these effects (Lin $et\ al.$, 1989).

The phenobarbital dose–response relationships for CYP2B-mediated enzymatic activities were investigated in male and female Fischer 344/Ncr rats. Rats aged 8 weeks were given diets containing phenobarbital at concentrations ranging from 0 to 0.15%. After 14 days, the animals were killed, and the enzyme activities were determined in liver homogenates. The maximal increases over control were: benzyloxy-resorufin O-dealkylation, 265-fold (female rats) and 54-fold (males); pentoxy-resorufin O-dealkylation, 197-fold and 58-fold; and testosterone 16β-hydroxylation, 1320-fold (females) and 118-fold (males) (Nims $et\ al.$, 1993).

The expression, inducibility and regulation of four CYP isozymes (PB$_1$, PB$_2$, MC$_1$ and MC$_2$) [CYP2C6, CYP2C11/12, CYP1A1, CYP1A2], glutathione transferases and microsomal epoxide hydrolase were studied in young female Wistar rats giving drinking-water containing 0.01% (w/v) NDEA for 10 days. One group of animals was not further exposed; a second group was given 3-methylcholanthrene by intraperitoneal injection at a dose of 40 mg/kg bw per day on 3 consecutive days before being killed, and a third group of animals was given NDEA and then a diet containing 0.05% (w/w) phenobarbital or an intraperitoneal injection at a dose of 80 mg/kg bw per day on 3 consecutive days before being killed. Frozen liver sections were analysed by immunohistochemistry for foci, nodules (adenomas) and carcinomas. Progressive loss of constitutive CYP expression was observed during tumorigenesis. Phenobarbital caused a heterogeneous pattern of response in preneoplastic and neoplastic lesions: some foci responded to the same degree as the surrounding normal liver, some were less, or not at all, inducible, and others were more inducible than the surrounding normal hepatocytes, particularly with regard to CYP2C11/12. The pattern of induction of this enzyme was closely linked to that of NADPH:cytochrome P450 reductase, suggesting that the regulation of these two enzymes is coordinated (Kunz $et\ al.$, 1987).

Incubation with 1.5 mmol/L phenobarbital caused a 2.5-fold increase in the activity of 7-ethoxycoumarin O-deethylase in cultured human hepatocytes, but had no effect on the activity of aryl hydrocarbon hydroxylase. The median effective dose (ED$_{50}$) for this increase was about 0.5 mmol/L (Donato *et al.*, 1990). In comparison, P450b, P450e and P450p [CYP2B1, CYP2B2 and CYP3A1] mRNA levels increased in primary cultures of adult rat hepatocytes exposed to various concentrations of phenobarbital. The concentrations that resulted in half-maximum increases in the activities of these three enzymes were 0.015, 0.0057 and 0.3 mmol/L, respectively, with maximal induction of 193-fold, 11-fold and 12.6-fold. Thus, there was only a threefold difference in ED_{50} between CYP2B1 and CYP2B2, whereas there was a 20-fold difference between CYP2B1 and CYP3A1. The authors concluded from the different ED_{50}s that the classes of CYP gene were induced by different pathways (Kocarek *et al.*, 1990).

Modification of gene expression is an important response to xenobiotic compounds, as changes in gene expression frequently modulate toxic response. In differential display approaches, the expression of over 7500 mRNAs was examined in the liver of chick embryos treated with phenobarbital *in vivo*. Twenty-nine cDNA fragments were significantly changed 48 h after treatment with phenobarbital *in ovo*. Of these, 18 were increased and 11 were decreased. The subcloning and sequencing of 20 of these fragments showed that CYP2H1, glutathione *S*-transferase, UGT, fibrinogen, glutamine synthetase and apolipoprotein B were up-regulated (Frueh *et al.*, 1997).

The aryl hydrocarbon (Ah) receptor mediates the transcriptional response to a number of hydrocarbons, resulting in the induction of CYP1A enzymes. Phenobarbital did not appear to bind strongly to the Ah receptor but did induce CYP1A in liver cells. In wild-type and Ah-receptor-knockout C57BL/6J mice, phenobarbital induced CYP1A2, but not CYP1A1, even in the absence of the Ah receptor (Corcos *et al.*, 1998).

A specific nuclear receptor (CAR) has now been identified that mediates induction by activation of the phenobarbital response element located in the 5′ flanking region of inducible CYP genes (Trottier *et al.*, 1995; Zelko & Negishi, 2000). Activation of nuclear factor κB modifies the expression of many genes, and Mejdoubi *et al.* (1999) reported that it participates in the expression of phenobarbital-responsive genes.

Altered hepatocyte foci in the livers of male rats given phenobarbital overexpressed two forms of CYP, CYP2B1,2 and CYP2C7 (Decloître *et al.*, 1990). In a study of the effects of phenobarbital on CYP2B1 and CYP2B2 in cultured rat hepatocytes, phenobarbital induced a concentration-dependent increase in benzyloxyresorufin *O*-deethylase activity up to 25-fold that of controls. Co-incubation with interleukin-6 or addition of interleukin-6 up to 12 h after phenobarbital inhibited this induction. The authors suggested that the inhibition is mediated by the early molecular events of the induction process (Clark *et al.*, 1996). In a study in C57BL/6 mice and in mouse hepatocytes in culture exposed to phenobarbital, the overall constitutive expression of CYP2B10 was greater in male than in female mice. Phenobarbital induced the expression of both CYP2B9 and CYP2B10 (Jarukamjorn *et al.*, 1999). The relationship between phenobarbital treatment, CYP gene expression and growth patterns in hepatic hyperplastic nodules induced by NDEA was studied in nodules from rats treated with phenobarbital. Phenobarbital increased the number of γ-GT-positive nodules, but it did not change the pattern of labelling indexes or the average labelling index. A slight but uniform increase in CYP1A2 expression was also seen. CYP2B1/2 was underexpressed in 53% of the γ-GT-positive nodules (Chen *et al.*, 1992).

The induction of CYP2B, CYP2C and CYP3A by phenobarbital was examined in male and female patas (*Erythrocebus patas*) and cynomologus (*Macaca fascicularis*) monkeys. Hydroxylation of testosterone associated with CYP3A was increased two- to fivefold in phenobarbital-treated animals. Testosterone-16β hydroxylation activity was induced up to 15-fold, and benzyloxyresorufin *O*-dealkylation was induced 10-fold by phenobarbital in both species of monkey. Induction of CYP2C was observed with phenobarbital and was more pronounced in the cynomologous monkeys than in the patas monkeys (Jones *et al.*, 1992b).

4.5 Genetic and related effects

4.5.1 *Humans*

The potential for phenobarbital to induce sister chromatid exchange in the peripheral lymphocytes of epilepsy patients on phenobarbital monotherapy was examined. Nine male patients (six smokers) of mean age 38.8 ± 1.25 (SE) years and nine male controls (six smokers) of mean age 38.4 ± 1.27 (SE) years were compared. The same exclusion criteria were applied to the two groups: age > 50 years, recent illness, use of medication other than phenobarbital, use of illicit drugs, alcoholism, surgery, anaesthesia, blood or blood product transfusions, chemotherapy, exposure to ionizing radiation and unusual exposure to ultraviolet radiation within 1 year of examination. The daily coffee consumption was 0–20 cups among the patients and 0–12 cups among the controls. The patients' serum phenobarbital concentrations were consistently in the range 10–40 μg/mL, except for two patients on maintenance doses resulting in concentrations of 5 and 6 μg/mL. The mean numbers of sister chromatid exchanges/cell were 6.82 ± 0.54 (SE) in the exposed group and 6.14 ± 0.51 (SE) in the controls (Schaumann *et al.*, 1989).

4.5.2 *Experimental systems* (see Table 6 for references)

In some studies, phenobarbital has been shown to be weakly mutagenic in *Salmonella typhimurium* TA1535 or TA100 in the absence, but not in the presence, of an exogenous metabolic activation system. The effect was observed in two of two studies with TA1535 and in two of five studies with TA100. Direct addition of phenobarbital enhanced the mutagenic effect in *S. typhimurium* TA1535 of sodium azide or 2-aminoanthracene, but not that of 4-nitroquinoline *N*-oxide or 2-nitrofluorene (Albertini & Gocke, 1992).

Phenobarbital induced aneuploidy, but not mutation or recombinational events in fungi; it did not induce sex-linked recessive lethal mutations, somatic cell mutations or mitotic recombination in *Drosophila melanogaster*.

Table 6. Genetic and related effects of phenobarbital

Test system	Result[a] Without exogenous metabolic system	Result[a] With exogenous metabolic system	Dose[b] (LED/HID)	Reference
Salmonella typhimurium TM677, forward mutation, 8-azaguanine resistance	–	–	500	Liber (1985)
Salmonella typhimurium TA100, TA1535, TA1537, TA98, reverse mutation	NT	–	5000 µg/plate	McCann et al. (1975)
Salmonella typhimurium TA100, TA1535, TA1538, TA98, reverse mutation	NT	–	2500 µg/plate	Anderson & Styles (1978)
Salmonella typhimurium TA100, reverse mutation[c]	(+)	–	4000 µg/plate	Baker & Bonin (1985)
Salmonella typhimurium TA100, TA98, TA97, TA102, reverse mutation	–	–	5000 µg/plate	Matsushima et al. (1985)
Salmonella typhimurium TA100, reverse mutation	(+)	NR	2000 µg/plate	McGregor & Prentice (1985)
Salmonella typhimurium TA100, TA1537, TA1538, TA98, reverse mutation	–	–	5000 µg/plate	Rexroat & Probst (1985)
Salmonella typhimurium TA100, TA98, TA97, reverse mutation	–	–	3333 µg/plate	Zeiger & Haworth (1985)
Salmonella typhimurium TA1535, reverse mutation	(+)	–	500 µg/plate	Rexroat & Probst (1985)
Salmonella typhimurium TA1535, reverse mutation	(+)	–	500 µg/plate	Zeiger & Haworth (1985)
Salmonella typhimurium TA100, TA98, reverse mutation	–	–	2000 µg/plate	Bruce & Heddle (1979)
Saccharomyces cerevisiae D7, gene conversion	–	–	10 000	Arni (1985)
Saccharomyces cerevisiae JD1, gene conversion	–	–	2000	Brooks et al. (1985)
Saccharomyces cerevisiae D7, mitotic recombination	–	–	10 000	Arni (1985)

Table 6 (contd)

Test system	Result[a]		Dose[b] (LED/HID)	Reference
	Without exogenous metabolic system	With exogenous metabolic system		
Aspergillus nidulans P1, genetic crossing-over	−	NT	500	Carere *et al.* (1985)
Saccharomyces cerevisiae D7, reverse mutation	−	−	10 000	Arni (1985)
Schizosaccharomyces pombe P1, forward mutation	−	−	40	Loprieno *et al.* (1985)
Saccharomyces cerevisiae D61.M, aneuploidy	+	NT	100	Albertini *et al.* (1985)
Drosophila melanogaster, mitotic recombination	−		185 (feed)	Vogel (1985)
Drosophila melanogaster, mitotic recombination	−		4640 (feed)	Würgler *et al.* (1985)
Drosophila melanogaster, somatic mutation	−		5000 (feed)	Fujikawa *et al.* (1985)
Drosophila melanogaster, somatic mutation	−		185 (feed)	Vogel (1985)
Drosophila melanogaster, somatic mutation	−		4640 (feed)	Würgler *et al.* (1985)
Drosophila melanogaster, sex–linked recessive lethal mutations	−		10 000 (feed)	Donner *et al.* (1979)
DNA strand breaks, cross-links or alkali-labile sites, Chinese hamster V79 cells *in vitro*	−	−	2320	Swenberg *et al.* (1976)
DNA strand breaks, cross-links or alkali-labile sites, rat hepatocytes *in vitro*	−	NT	765	Sina *et al.* (1983)
DNA strand breaks, cross-links or alkali-labile sites, rat hepatocytes *in vitro*	−	NT	581	Bradley (1985)
DNA strand breaks, cross-links or alkali-labile sites, Chinese hamster ovary cells *in vitro*	−	−	11 600	Douglas *et al.* (1985)
Unscheduled DNA synthesis, rat primary hepatocytes *in vitro*	−	NT	254	Probst & Hill (1985)

Table 6 (contd)

Test system	Result[a] Without exogenous metabolic system	Result[a] With exogenous metabolic system	Dose[b] (LED/HID)	Reference
Unscheduled DNA synthesis, rat primary hepatocytes *in vitro*	–	NT	10	Williams *et al.* (1985)
Gene mutation, Chinese hamster lung V79 cells, *Hprt* locus *in vitro*	(+)	NT	250	Kuroda *et al.* (1985)
Gene mutation, mouse lymphoma L5178Y cells, *Hprt* locus and ouabain resistance *in vitro*	–	–	200	Garner & Campbell (1985)
Gene mutation, mouse lymphoma L5178Y cells, ouabain resistance *in vitro*	(+)	?	1000	Styles *et al.* (1985)
Gene mutation, mouse lymphoma L5178Y cells, *Tk* locus *in vitro*	–	–	2500	Amacher & Turner (1980)
Gene mutation, mouse lymphoma L5178Y cells, *Tk* locus *in vitro*	–	NT	4126	Amacher *et al.* (1980)
Gene mutation, mouse lymphoma L5178Y cells, *Tk* locus *in vitro*	(+)	–	1000	Myhr *et al.* (1985)
Gene mutation, mouse lymphoma L5178Y cells, *Tk* locus *in vitro*	–	(+)	1500	Oberly *et al.* (1985)
Gene mutation, mouse lymphoma L5178Y cells, *Tk* locus *in vitro*	–	–	2000	Styles *et al.* (1985)
Gene mutation, BALB/c-3T3 cells *in vitro*, ouabain resistance	NT	–	6000	Matthews *et al.* (1985)
Sister chromatid exchange, Chinese hamster ovary cells *in vitro*	–	–	4000[d]	Gulati *et al.* (1985)
Sister chromatid exchange, Chinese hamster ovary cells *in vitro*	(+)	(+)	870	Natarajan *et al.* (1985)
Sister chromatid exchange, Chinese hamster V79 cells *in vitro*	+	NT	10	Ray-Chaudhuri *et al.* (1982)
Sister chromatid exchange, rat liver RL4 cells *in vitro*	–	NT	500	Priston & Dean (1985)
Micronucleus formation, Chinese hamster ovary cells *in vitro*	–	–	232	Douglas *et al.* (1985)
Chromosomal aberrations, Chinese hamster lung cells *in vitro*	–	–	2000	Ishidate *et al.* (1981)
Chromosomal aberrations, Chinese hamster liver cells *in vitro*	(+)	NT	100	Danford (1985)
Chromosomal aberrations, Chinese hamster ovary cells *in vitro*	(+)	(+)	500	Gulati *et al.* (1985)
Chromosomal aberrations, Chinese hamster lung cells *in vitro*	–	NT	2000	Ishidate & Sofuni (1985)

Table 6 (contd)

Test system	Result[a] Without exogenous metabolic system	Result[a] With exogenous metabolic system	Dose[b] (LED/HID)	Reference
Chromosomal aberrations, Chinese hamster ovary cells in vitro	–	+	3480	Natarajan et al. (1985)
Chromosomal aberrations, rat liver RL4 cells in vitro	–	NT	1000	Priston & Dean (1985)
Aneuploidy, Chinese hamster liver cells in vitro	–	NT	1000	Danford (1985)
Cell transformation, BALB/c 3T3 mouse cells	–	+	667	Matthews et al. (1985)
Cell transformation, C3H10T1/2 mouse cells	–	–	2000	Lawrence & McGregor (1985)
Cell transformation, Syrian hamster embryo cells, clonal assay	–	NT	100	Barrett & Lamb (1985)
Cell transformation, Syrian hamster embryo cells, clonal assay	+	NT	100	Sanner & Rivedal (1985)
Cell transformation, Syrian hamster embryo cells, clonal assay (pH 6.7)	+	NT	700	LeBoeuf et al. (1996)
Cell transformation, RLV/Fischer rat embryo cells	–	NT	30	Traul et al. (1981)
Inhibition of intercellular communication, Chinese hamster V79 cells in vitro	–	NT	500	Umeda et al. (1980)
Inhibition of intercellular communication, Chinese hamster V79 cells in vitro	+	NT	23	Williams (1980)
Inhibition of intercellular communication, Chinese hamster V79 cells in vitro	+	NT	150	Jone et al. (1985)
Inhibition of intercellular communication, Chinese hamster V79 cells in vitro	–	NT	1160	Umeda et al. (1985)
Inhibition of intercellular communication, Chinese hamster V79 cells in vitro (dye transfer)	+	NT	100	Zeilmaker & Yamasaki (1986)
Inhibition of intercellular communication, Djungarian hamster fibroblasts in vitro (dye transfer)	–[c]	NT	1000	Budunova et al. (1989)

Table 6 (contd)

Test system	Result[a]		Dose[b] (LED/HID)	Reference
	Without exogenous metabolic system	With exogenous metabolic system		
Inhibition of intercellular communication, male B6C3F$_1$ mouse primary hepatocytes *in vitro* (labelled nucleotide transfer)	+	NT	20	Klaunig & Ruch (1987a)
Inhibition of intercellular communication, male C3H and BALB/c mouse and Fischer 344 rat primary hepatocytes *in vitro* (labelled nucleotide transfer)	+	NT	100	Klaunig & Ruch (1987a)
Inhibition of intercellular communication, male C57BL mouse primary hepatocytes *in vitro* (labelled nucleotide transfer)	–	NT	500	Klaunig & Ruch (1987a)
Inhibition of intercellular communication, male B6C3F$_1$ mouse primary hepatocytes *in vitro* (labelled nucleotide transfer)	+[f]	NT	20, 8 h	Klaunig & Ruch (1987b)
Inhibition of intercellular communication, male B6C3F$_1$ mouse primary hepatocytes *in vitro* (labelled nucleotide transfer)	+	NT	20, 12 h	Ruch et al. (1987)
Inhibition of intercellular communication, male B6C3F$_1$ mouse primary hepatocytes *in vitro* (dye transfer)	+	NT	116, 2 h	Klaunig et al. (1990)
Inhibition of intercellular communication, rat kidney epithelial NRK-52E cells *in vitro* (dye transfer)	–	NT	1860, 24 h	Konishi et al. (1990)
Inhibition of intercellular communication, Wistar rat primary hepatocytes *in vitro* (dye transfer)	+	NT	116, 5 h	Leibold & Schwarz (1993a)
Inhibition of intercellular communication, BD VI rat primary hepatocytes co-cultured with BALB/c 3T3 A31-1-8 cells *in vitro* (dye transfer)	+	NT	100, 2 h	Mesnil et al. (1993)
Inhibition of intercellular communication, Fischer 344 rat and B6C3F$_1$ mouse primary hepatocytes *in vitro* (dye transfer)	+	NT	232, 4 h	Baker et al. (1995)

Table 6 (contd)

Test system	Result[a] Without exogenous metabolic system	Result[a] With exogenous metabolic system	Dose[b] (LED/HID)	Reference
Inhibition of intercellular communication, male and female rhesus monkey and (sex not given) human primary hepatocytes *in vitro* (dye transfer)	–	NT	696, 4 h	Baker *et al.* (1995)
Inhibition of intercellular communication, male Wistar rat primary hepatocytes *in vitro* (dye transfer)	+	NT	464, 4 h	Guppy *et al.* (1994)
Inhibition of intercellular communication, human urothelial carcinoma cell ine JTC-30 cells *in vitro* (dye transfer)	+	NT	375, 2 days[g]	Morimoto (1996)
Inhibition of intercellular communication, rat primary hepatocytes co-cultured with WB-F344 rat liver epithelial cells *in vitro* (dye transfer)	+	NT	23.2, 1 h	Ren & Ruch (1996)
Inhibition of intercellular communication, rat primary hepatocytes, primarily expressing Cx3 *in vitro* (dye transfer)	+	NT	232, 2 h	Ren *et al.* (1998)
Inhibition of intercellular communication, WB-F344 rat liver epithelial cells, expressing Cx43 and WB-a/32-10 cells, expressing Cx32 *in vitro* (dye transfer)	–	NT	696, 2 h	Ren *et al.* (1998)
Inhibition of intercellular communication, human hepatoma cells *in vitro* (labelled nucleotide transfer)	+	NT	10, 4 h	Rolin-Limbosch *et al.* (1986)
Gene mutation, human lymphoblast TK6 cells *in vitro*	–	–	1000	Crespi *et al.* (1985)
Gene mutation, human lymphoblast AHH-1 cells *in vitro*	(+)	NT	1000	Crespi *et al.* (1985)
Sister chromatid exchange, human lymphocytes *in vitro*	–	–	500	Obe *et al.* (1985)
Chromosomal aberrations, human lymphocytes *in vitro*	(+)	NT	22.4–111	Foerst (1972)
Chromosomal aberrations, human lymphocytes *in vitro*	+	NT	5	Nandan & Rao (1982a)

Table 6 (contd)

Test system	Result[a] Without exogenous metabolic system	Result[a] With exogenous metabolic system	Dose[b] (LED/HID)	Reference
DNA strand breaks and alkali-labile damage, male CD-1 mouse liver cells in vivo (single-cell gel electrophoresis assay)	+		140	Sasaki et al. (1997)
DNA strand breaks and alkali-labile damage, male CD-1 mouse lung, spleen, kidney and bone-marrow cells in vivo (single-cell gel electrophoresis assay)	–		140	Sasaki et al. (1997)
Gene mutation, transgenic female C57BL/6 mouse, lacI locus in liver cells in vivo	–		500 ppm diet, 120 days	Gunz et al. (1993)
Sister chromatid exchange, DBA/2 mouse bone-marrow cells in vivo	–		50 ip × 6	Tice et al. (1980)
Micronucleus formation, (C57BL/6 × C3H/He)F₁ mouse bone-marrow cells in vivo	–		500 ip × 5	Bruce & Heddle (1979)
Chromosomal aberrations, DBA/2 mouse bone-marrow cells in vivo	–		50 ip × 6	Tice et al. (1980)
Chromosomal aberrations, male Swiss mouse spermatogonial germ cells	+		42 po given over 5 or 60 days	Nandan & Rao (1982b)
Binding (covalent) to DNA (³²P-postlabelling), B3C6F₁/CrlBR mouse liver cells in vivo	–		200 po × 1	Whysner et al. (1998)
Binding (covalent) to DNA (³²P-postlabelling), B3C6F₁/CrlBR mouse liver cells in vivo	–		1000 ppm in diet; 2 weeks	Whysner et al. (1998)
Inhibition of intercellular communication, male ACI/N rat liver in vivo (freeze–fracture analysis of area occupied by gap junctions)	(+)		25 diet, 4–8 weeks	Sugie et al. (1987)

Table 6 (contd)

Test system	Result[a] Without exogenous metabolic system	Result[a] With exogenous metabolic system	Dose[b] (LED/HID)	Reference
Inhibition of intercellular communication, Wistar rat primary hepatocytes from γ-GT$^+$ and γ-GT$^-$ foci in vitro (dye transfer)	+		100 ip × 1, followed by 0.1% in drinking-water, 5 days	Leibold & Schwarz (1993b)
Inhibition of intercellular communication, male ACI/N rat liver in vivo (freeze–fracture analysis of area occupied by gap junctions)	−		0.05% diet, 2 weeks	Sugie et al. (1994)
Inhibition of intercellular communication, male Fischer 344 rat primary hepatocytes in vivo/in vitro (dye transfer)	+		400 po × 25	Krutovskikh et al. (1995)
Inhibition of intercellular communication, male Sprague-Dawley rat primary hepatocytes in vivo/in vitro (dye transfer)	+		50 po × 4 weeks	Ito et al. (1998)
Sperm morphology, (C57BL/6 × C3H/He)F$_1$ mouse in vivo	−		500 ip × 5	Bruce & Heddle (1979)
Sperm morphology, (CBA × BALB/c)F$_1$ mouse in vivo	−		100 ip × 5	Topham (1980)

γ-GT, γ-glutamyl transpeptidase

[a] +, positive; (+), weak positive; −, negative; NR, not reported; NT, not tested; ?, inconclusive

[b] LED, lowest effective dose; HID, highest ineffective dose; in-vitro tests, μg/mL; in-vivo tests, mg/kg bw per day; po, oral gavage; ip, intraperitoneal injection

[c] Negative with TA97, TA98, TA102

[d] Without metabolic activation, 1000 μg/mL was cytostatic.

[e] Dye transfer enhanced 1.5–2.0-fold

[f] Abolished by 0.1 mmol/L dibutyryl cAMP

[g] Toxic dose; a non-toxic dose (250 μg/mL, 4 days) gave negative results.

In cultured, non-human mammalian cells, no DNA strand breakage or induction of unscheduled DNA synthesis was observed. Although mutations were induced in some studies, the inconsistent positive results were weak and not clearly associated with a particular locus; both positive and negative results were obtained in experiments at the *Tk* and *Hprt* loci and tests for ouabain resistance. Similarly, results for the induction of both sister chromatid exchange and chromosomal aberrations were equally divided between positive and negative in different laboratories. Single studies in cultured mammalian cells for the induction of micronuclei and aneuploidy did not show any effect of phenobarbital treatment. Variable results were also obtained in assays for cell transformation conducted in different laboratories, but the differences may have been due partly to the different transformation assays used. Assays for gap-junctional inter-cellular communication, however, also gave variable results in different laboratories even when the same Chinese hamster lung V79 cell system was used in five of six studies. In a single study with Djungarian hamster fibroblasts, cell-to-cell communi-cation was actually enhanced. The negative result with NRK-52E cells, a rat kidney epithelial cell line, was interpreted by the authors as being consistent with the lack of effect of phenobarbital (which does not promote renal tumours) on the kidney, since barbital, a renal tumour promoter, did inhibit gap-junctional intercellular communi-cation in these cells (Konishi *et al.*, 1990).

In cultured human lymphoblastoid cells, no significant increase in the frequency of mutations was observed in one study, while, in cultured human lymphocytes, chromosomal aberrations were induced in two studies; sister chromatid exchange was not induced in another study.

In vivo, phenobarbital did not form adducts with DNA in mouse liver after either a single oral dose (200 mg/kg bw) or when given for 2 weeks in the diet (1000 mg/kg). A study of mutation induction in mice carrying the *Escherichia coli lacI* transgene as the target did not show any effect of phenobarbital. Studies of the bone-marrow cells of mice treated *in vivo* also did not show induction of sister chromatid exchange, micronuclei or chromosomal aberrations after treatment with phenobarbital alone. A significant response was observed in the single-cell gel electrophoresis assay with cells from the liver of mice given phenobarbital (140 mg/kg bw) by intraperitoneal injection 24 h before sacrifice, but not effect was seen with treatment 3 h before being killed; no effect was observed in a number of other organs. The frequency of morpho-logically abnormal sperm was not increased in mice treated with phenobarbital.

Phenobarbital was reported to induce chromosomal abnormalities, including trans-locations, in male mouse primary spermatocytes after oral administration for 5 or 60 days. [The Working Group noted that the level of the effects reported was little influenced by either the dose or the treatment regimen.]

A positive response was reported in a test for dominant lethal mutation in male Swiss mice (Nandan & Rao, 1983). [The Working Group noted that there was a significant response of all germ-cell stages, and a greater response in treated spermatogonial cells than in post-meiotic cells; this result is highly improbable and has not been reported previously with any chemical.]

In another study on mutation induction in the *lacI* transgene, transgenic mice were first given a single intraperitoneal injection of 50 mg/kg bw NDEA; 7 days later they were started on a diet containing 500 mg/kg sodium phenobarbital for 14 days, followed by a normal diet for 7 days. Increased liver weights were observed in the phenobarbital-treated mice, and the mutation frequencies in the *lacZ* gene recovered from liver were consistently higher than the values obtained from mice treated only with NDEA. Feeding a diet containing sodium phenobarbital at 500 mg/kg for 21 days did not affect the mutant frequency in the *lacZ* transgene in groups of mice given 100 mg/kg bw NDEA. The authors noted that no statistical analysis was performed, because of the small group sizes, which also limited interpretation of the data (Okada *et al.*, 1997). In female Sprague-Dawley rats that had undergone a 70% partial hepatectomy and then received NDEA by gavage (10 mg/kg bw), subsequent treatment with diets containing 0.05% (w/w) sodium phenobarbital for 12 months produced a significant increase in the number of hepatocytes containing chromosomal aberrations. Most of the damaged cells were seen in γ-GT-positive foci. Karyotypic analysis indicated that the most frequent aberrations in these foci were a trisomy of chromosome 1 or of its long arm and a monosomy of chromosome 3 or its short arm (Sargent *et al.*, 1992).

Klaunig and Ruch (1987a) found that phenobarbital inhibited gap-junctional inter-cellular communication most effectively in hepatocytes from B6C3F$_1$ mice, less so in primary hepatocytes from C3H and BALB/c mice and Fischer 344 rats and not at all in primary hepatocytes from C57BL mice. This finding was confirmed in part, and extended, in another study that showed that phenobarbital inhibited gap-junctional intercellular communication in primary hepatocytes from male Fischer 344 rats and B6C3F$_1$ mice, but did not do so in primary hepatocytes from male and female rhesus monkeys or from a human [sex unspecified] donor (Baker *et al.*, 1995).

In studies of the mechanism of inhibition of gap-junctional intercellular communication, it was shown that phenobarbital (20–500 μg/mL) reduced gap-junctional inter-cellular communication between B6C3F$_1$ mouse hepatocytes in culture. Phenobarbital (250 μg/mL) also reduced cAMP levels 1 h after treatment, but no effect was observed 2, 4 or 8 h after treatment. The addition of dibutyryl cAMP (0.1 mM) increased the cAMP levels approximately 50-fold in these mouse hepatocytes and completely abolished the inhibition of gap-junctional intercellular communication by pheno-barbital (Klaunig & Ruch, 1987b). Inhibition of protein synthesis by cycloheximide had no effect on the inhibition of gap-junctional intercellular communication by pheno-barbital in cultured rat hepatocytes, but inhibition was enhanced by treatment with diethylmaleate, to deplete intracellular glutathione, or by the addition of the CYP inhibitors, SKF 525A or metyrapone (Guppy *et al.*, 1994). It was later shown that phenobarbital-induced inhibition of gap-junctional intercellular communication is a complex phenomenon. Treatment with 2 mmol/L phenobarbital of primary rat hepa-tocytes co-cultured with WB-F344 rat liver epithelial cells for 1 h sharply reduced inter-hepatocyte dye-coupling from about 90% to 30%, but the cells fully recovered within 24 h, after which there was a more gradual reduction in dye-coupling to about 20% after 14 days. Dye-coupling between the WB-F344 cells was unaffected by pheno-barbital over the same period and, in co-cultures, there was no dye transfer between the two cell types. The connexin (Cx32) steady-state mRNA levels were unaffected by treatment of the primary rat hepatocytes with phenobarbital for 14 days, and there was no change in Cx32 protein levels (Ren & Ruch, 1996). A similar transient decrease in gap-junctional intercellular communication after a 1-h exposure to phenobarbital was observed by Mesnil *et al.* (1993) in rat hepatocytes co-cultured with BALB/c 3T3 mouse-embryo cells, but the decrease was maintained at 50% of control values during a 3-week treatment period. Later studies from this group indicated that the inhibitory action of phenobarbital on gap-junctional intercellular communication is cell-specific rather than connexin-specific. Thus, phenobarbital inhibited gap-junctional inter-cellular communication in hepatocytes, which express primarily *Cx32*, but not in WB-F344 rat epithelial cells, a highly communicating line that expresses *Cx43*, or in WB-aB1 cells, a gap-junctional intercellular communication-incompetent line derived from WB-F344 that still expresses *Cx43*, or in WB-a/32-10 cells, which are derived from WB-aB1 by stable transduction with a *Cx32* retroviral expression vector.

Cx32-deficient mice are resistant to liver tumour promotion by phenobarbital. Phenobarbital treatment led to an approximate fivefold increase in the volume fraction occupied by glucose-6-phosphatase-deficient liver lesions in $Cx32^{Y/+}$ mice, whereas there was no such increase in $Cx32^{Y/-}$ mice. Even more pronounced differences were observed with respect to tumour response, phenobarbital clearly promoting the occurrence of large hepatomas in Cx32-proficient but not in Cx32-deficient mice. These results demonstrate that functional Cx32 protein is required for tumour pro-motion with phenobarbital (Moennikes *et al.*, 2000).

After oral administration of phenobarbital (50 mg/kg bw per day for up to 6 weeks) to Sprague-Dawley rats, a direct microinjection dye-transfer assay was carried out on fresh liver slices (0.5–0.7 mm thick). The average area of dye spread decreased after 1 week and stayed at the same level up to week 6. The area and number of Cx32 spots per hepatocyte in the centrilobular zones of the liver also decreased between week 1 and week 6, whereas there was no change in the spots in the perilobular areas. No changes were observed in Cx26 (Ito *et al.*, 1998). Using a higher dose (400 mg/kg bw per day for 5 weeks), Krutovskikh *et al.* (1995) observed nearly total disappearance from the plasma membrane of cells in the centrilobular region of both the principal hepatocyte connexin Cx32 and Cx26, while Cx43 protein and the expression of its mRNA were stimulated.

DNA sequence analysis of the H-*ras* gene in liver tissue from male B6C3F$_1$ mice treated with phenobarbital (0.05% in the drinking-water for 1 year) revealed a point mutation (AAA) in codon 61 (normal sequence CAA) in one of nine hepatocellular adenomas and in none of five hepatocellular carcinomas. When 50 liver tumours found in the control group were analysed, an activated H-*ras* gene was found in 15/18 hepato-cellular adenomas and 10/14 hepatocellular carcinomas. The most frequent mutation in these tumours was a CG → AT transversion (59%), which is probably the result of a polymerase error (Fox *et al.*, 1990). During DNA synthesis on a non-instructional template, the most frequent polymerase error involves the preferential insertion of an adenine, the so-called 'A rule' (Strauss *et al.*, 1982).

In C3H/He mice, Ha-*ras* codon 61 mutations occurred in 6/21 (29%) liver tumours from untreated mice, but in 0/15 (0%) tumours from mice given a diet containing phenobarbital at a concentration of 0.04–0.07% providing a dose of 85 mg/kg bw per day. The absence of mutations in codon 61 (or in codon 12) in the phenobarbital-treated mice suggests a tumorigenic mechanism different from that of spontaneous tumours. In contrast, codon 61 mutations were found in 19/46 tumours from mice treated with NDEA (Rumsby *et al.*, 1991). In a similar study, two of eight CF1 mouse liver carcinomas that occurred after prolonged exposure to diets containing 1000 mg/kg phenobarbital were shown to carry a CG → AT transversion in the Ha-*ras* gene. One of eight tumours from control mice also carried a codon-61 mutation (Bauer-Hofmann *et al.*, 1990).

The same group analysed the pattern of codon 61 mutations in the Ha-*ras* gene of glucose-6-phosphatase-deficient hepatic lesions of male C3H/He mice given a diet containing 500 mg/kg sodium phenobarbital for 52 weeks. Ha-*ras* mutations were found in 12/21 lesions (57%) from untreated mice and in 4/16 (25%) in the phenobarbital-treated group ($p < 0.01$, Fisher's exact test). The commonest mutation was a CG → AT transversion (eight in untreated mice, three in treated mice). The wild-type sequence, CAA, was present in all the enzyme-deficient lesions, and, when a mutation was present, the signals for the wild-type and the mutant sequences were very similar. This result suggested that both normal and mutant alleles were present in each cell of the lesions (Bauer-Hofmann *et al.*, 1992).

Tumours from C3H/He mice were also screened for *p53* mutations in exons 5, 7 and 8, which contain nearly all the mutations so far described. No *p53* mutations were found in any of eight tumours recovered from mice treated with phenobarbital (Rumsby *et al.*, 1994).

4.6   Mechanistic considerations

4.6.1   *Liver tumours*

The available evidence indicates that phenobarbital is generally not genotoxic, and genotoxicity does not appear to play a role in its hepatocarcinogenicity. In particular, DNA adducts have not been detected with ^{32}P-postlabelling methods in animals given doses that produce liver tumours.

Phenobarbital is a microsomal enzyme inducer and has been studied extensively for its ability to promote hepatic tumours. There is evidence that the microsomal enzyme induction is correlated with hepatic tumour promotion by phenobarbital. Rats and mice that develop tumours after treatment with phenobarbital show expression of

CYP enzymes, CYP2B1 and CYP2B2 being the most important. The potency for CYP induction in mice and rats also correlates with the degree of tumour promotion. Phenobarbital does not induce these enzymes in hamsters and does not produce liver tumours in this species.

The enhancement of hepatic tumorigenesis by phenobarbital was shown to be due to tumour promotion rather than a syncarcinogenic effect. In an initiation–promotion model, phenobarbital administered before or with a carcinogen produced no tumours, whereas repeated exposure to phenobarbital after the carcinogen produced tumours.

Although the mechanisms of tumour promotion are not completely known, effects on the control of cell proliferation appear to play a role. Long-term exposure of rodents to phenobarbital produces hepatomegaly and hepatocellular hypertrophy and hyperplasia. Several studies have demonstrated a transient increase in DNA synthesis in normal hepatocytes. In initiation–promotion models, phenobarbital selectively increased the labelling index in foci as compared with normal surrounding liver. The foci progress to the stage of hepatocellular adenoma, in which cellular proliferation no longer depends on the presence of phenobarbital.

The mitogenic and tumour-promoting effects of phenobarbital appear to involve changes in growth factors, intracellular communication, gene expression and cell cycle signal transduction. These can mediate the effects of phenobarbital, including the transient increase in DNA synthesis, the selective mitogenic effects in foci and inhibition of apoptosis.

In addition, there are marked species and strain differences in susceptibility to hepatic tumour promotion by phenobarbital, which is genetically determined and heritable.

Overall, the experimental evidence supports the conclusion that the mode of action of phenobarbital in the production of hepatic tumours is non-genotoxic and involves tumour promotion.

4.6.2   *Thyroidal effects*

Although phenobarbital has not been shown to produce thyroid gland tumours in a bioassay for carcinogenicity, it has been shown to promote these tumours after administration of a carcinogen (NBHPA).

Phenobarbital is a microsomal enzyme inducer that increases the hepatic activity of thyroxin-UGT and alters thyroid function by enhancing the peripheral disposition of thyroid hormones. Phenobarbital-treated rats show decreased serum concentrations of thyroid hormones, increased concentrations of TSH, increased thyroid gland weights and follicular-cell hypertrophy and/or hyperplasia.

The tumour-promoting effects of phenobarbital have been shown to be mediated by increased pituitary secretion of TSH as a compensatory response to increased hepatic disposition of thyroid hormone, as opposed to a direct tumour-promoting or carcinogenic effect in the thyroid follicular epithelium.

5. Summary of Data Reported and Evaluation

5.1 Exposure data

Phenobarbital and its sodium salt have been very widely used as a mild sedative or hypnotic in the treatment of neuroses and in pre- or post-operative sedation, and as an anticonvulsant in the treatment of epilepsy. Phenobarbital was introduced in 1912. Its use has decreased since the 1960s, but it is still produced worldwide and used extensively.

5.2 Human carcinogenicity data

Three large follow-up studies of cancer, two of incidence and one of mortality, from Denmark, England and the USA of patients treated primarily with phenobarbital for epilepsy showed an occurrence of brain cancer higher than expected. However, in the two incidence studies, the excess numbers of cases of brain cancer occurred within 10 years of hospitalization and decreased significantly over time. This inverse relationship between excess risk and time since hospitalization for epilepsy suggests that the brain tumours of some of the patients were the cause of their seizure disorder and that the association between use of phenobarbital and brain cancer is not causal. The finding in a small case–control study from the USA of an increased risk for brain tumours after prenatal exposure to phenobarbital was not confirmed in a larger case–control study, also from the USA, or in a cohort study from Denmark of transplacental exposure to phenobarbital and other anti-convulsants.

Of the three cohort studies of epilepsy patients, two showed a significant increase in the relative risk for lung cancer, with no clear pattern of risk with length of follow-up. One showed a non-significant increase. Dose–response analyses in a nested case–control study of lung cancer in the largest of the cohort studies (in Denmark) revealed no consistent relationship between lung cancer and cumulative exposure to phenobarbital. A survey among the controls indicated a higher-than-average prevalence of smoking.

After exclusion from the largest of the cohorts of epilepsy patients known to have received radioactive Thorotrast during cerebral angiography, a slight, non-significant increase in risk for primary liver cancer was seen. However, a nested case–control study of liver cancer with adjustment for other anti-convulsant therapy revealed no association with phenobarbital treatment. No cases of liver cancer were seen in the other two cohort studies, from England and the USA.

In the cohort study in Denmark, the observed number of cases of thyroid cancer was close to that expected in the general Danish population. In the same study, a statistically significant deficit of urinary bladder cancer was noted, which was shown in an analysis of the dose–response relationship to be inversely related to use of phenobarbital.

Use of phenobarbital, mostly as a sedative, was associated with moderately increased risks for cancers of the lung, ovary and gall-bladder in a cohort study based on a prepaid medical care programme in the USA.

5.3   Animal carcinogenicity data

The carcinogenicity of phenobarbital was investigated by oral administration in multiple studies in mice and several studies in rats. Phenobarbital consistently produced hepatocellular adenomas and carcinomas in mice. Hepatocellular adenomas were produced in rats after lifetime exposure in one study. Oral administration of phenobarbital in combination with known carcinogens resulted in the enhancement or inhibition of effects, depending on the carcinogen and the time of administration. In several experiments in mice and rats, sequential exposure to phenobarbital with known carcinogens enhanced the incidences of hepatocellular preneoplastic foci, adenomas and carcinomas. In two studies each, phenobarbital was found to promote liver carcinogenesis in patas monkeys but not in hamsters. Phenobarbital promoted thyroid follicular-cell tumours in one study in mice and in several studies in rats.

5.4   Other relevant data

Most of an administered dose of phenobarbital in humans was excreted in urine. The major urinary excretion products include unmodified phenobarbital, *para*-hydroxy-phenobarbital, phenobarbital-*N*-glucoside and phenobarbital *para*-glucuronide. *para*-Hydroxyphenobarbital can be formed by direct hydroxylation of phenobarbital.

CYP2B1 and CYP2B2 are the primary members of the cytochrome P450 (CYP) superfamily of enzymes that are induced by phenobarbital *in vivo*. Although pheno-barbital causes large increases in the activity of these enzymes in liver, the metabolism of phenobarbital itself is not increased. Phenobarbital has also been found to induce the activities of other CYP enzymes, including benzo[*a*]pyrene hydroxylase, UDP-glucuro-nosyl transferase and several glutathione-*S*-transferases. 'Phenobarbital-like induction' describes the effect on liver hepatocyte CYP enzymes of various compounds, including sedatives, pesticides and other compounds that induce a similar spectrum of isozymes.

Cell proliferation is initially stimulated by phenobarbital in normal hepatocytes and lasts a few days. It may even be inhibited by down-regulation of epidermal growth factor receptors. Phenobarbital exerts a selective and sustained mitogenic effect in cells of altered foci that progress to adenomas that are no longer dependent on the mitogenic effects of phenobarbital.

The biochemical mechanisms underlying enhancement of cell proliferation and tumour promotion by phenobarbital may involve alterations in gene regulation. The dose–response relationship for microsomal enzyme induction is similar to that for tumour promotion. Consequently, changes in gene regulation that presumably lead to mitogenesis and up-regulation of growth factors parallel the induction of CYPs.

Phenobarbital has also been shown to inhibit intercellular communication in hepatocytes, which could impede the transmission of growth control signals between normal and altered hepatocytes.

Owing to its effects on the induction of microsomal enzymes, phenobarbital enhances the hepatic disposition of thyroid hormone. The promotion of thyroid gland tumours in rats by phenobarbital has been shown to be mediated by increased secretion of pituitary thyroid-stimulating hormone as a compensatory response to increased thyroid hormone glucuronidation and biliary excretion.

Phenobarbital is a teratogen and developmental neurotoxicant in humans and experimental animals. Exposure of rats *in utero* induces long-term effects on hepatic drug-metabolizing enzymes. Neuroendocrine effects on reproductive function have been noted in exposed adult male rats and female hamsters.

Phenobarbital did not induce sister chromatid exchange in patients with epilepsy receiving only this drug.

In studies in which rodents were exposed to phenobarbital *in vivo*, no covalent binding to mouse liver DNA was observed, but the frequency of alkali-labile damage in mouse liver cells was increased. Gene mutation was not induced in a transgenic mouse strain, and sister chromatid exchange, micronuclei and chromosomal aberrations were not induced in mouse bone-marrow cells. Phenobarbital did not increase the frequency of sperm-head abnormalities in mice, but spermatogonial germ-cell chromosomal aberrations were reported in male mice in one laboratory. Further increases in the frequency of chromosomal aberrations were found in liver foci cells of mice treated with phenobarbital after previous treatment with a genotoxic agent.

Chromosomal aberrations but not gene mutations were induced in cultured human lymphocytes.

Tests for the genetic effects of phenobarbital *in vitro* are numerous and include assays for DNA damage, DNA repair induction, gene mutation and chromosomal aberrations in mammalian cells, tests for gene mutation and mitotic recombination in insects and fungi and tests for gene mutation in bacteria. Although the majority of the test results were negative, the numerous positive results cannot be ignored, even though they do not present a consistent pattern of genetic toxicity. The inconsistency of the results, the absence of any direct evidence of an interaction with DNA and the generally negative in-vivo data lead to the conclusion that phenobarbital is not genotoxic.

Phenobarbital transformed hamster embryo cells. It inhibited gap-junctional intercellular communication in hepatocytes of rats treated *in vivo* and in primary cultures of hepatocytes from rats and mice but not (in a single study) in primary cultures of human or rhesus monkey hepatocytes.

5.5   Evaluation

There is *inadequate evidence* in humans for the carcinogenicity of phenobarbital. There is *sufficient evidence* in experimental animals for the carcinogenicity of phenobarbital.

Overall evaluation

Phenobarbital is *possibly carcinogenic to humans (Group 2B)*.

6.   References

Adenis, L., Vlaeminck, M.N. & Driessens, J. (1970) [Pulmonary adenoma in Swiss mice receiving urethane. VIII. Action of phenobarbital.] *C.R. Soc. Biol.*, **164**, 560–562 (in French)

Agrawal, A.K., Pampori, N.A. & Shapiro, B.H. (1995) Neonatal phenobarbital-induced defects in age- and sex-specific growth hormone profiles regulating monooxygenases. *J. Am. physiol. Soc.*, **31**, E439–E445

Albertini, S. & Gocke, E. (1992) Phenobarbital: Does the positive result in TA1535 indicate genotoxic properties? *Environ. mol. Mutag.*, **19**, 161–166

Albertini, S., Friederich, U., Gröschel-Stewart, U., Zimmermann, F.K. & Würgler, F.E. (1985) Phenobarbital induces aneuploidy in *Saccharomyces cerevisiae* and stimulates the assembly of porcine brain tubulin. *Mutat Res.*, **144**, 67–71

Alleva, J.J., Lipien, M.W., Alleva, F.R. & Balazs, T. (1975) Effect of daily injection of phenobarbital on ovulation in hamsters. *Toxicol. appl. Pharmacol.*, **34**, 491–498

Amacher, D.E. & Turner, G.N. (1985) Tests for gene mutational activity in the L5178Y/TK assay system. *Prog. Mutat. Res.*, **5**, 487–496

Amacher, D.E., Paillet, S.C., Turner, G.N., Ray, V.A. & Salsburg, D.S. (1980) Point mutations at the thymidine kinase locus in L5178Y mouse lymphoma cells. II. Test validation and interpretation. *Mutat Res.*, **72**, 447–474

Anderson, D. & Styles, J.A. (1978) An evaluation of six short-term tests for detecting organic chemical carcinogens. Appendix 2. The bacterial mutation test. *Br. J. Cancer*, **37**, 924–930

Annegers, J.F., Kurland, L.T. & Hauser, W.A. (1979) Brain tumours in children exposed to barbiturates [Letter to the Editor]. *J. natl Cancer Inst.*, **63**, 3

Anon. (2000) Top 200 generic drugs by prescription in 1999. *Drug Topics*, **144**, 70–71

Appel, K.E., Menden, M., Buchmann, A. & Schwarz, M. (1991) Effect of varying the concentration of phenobarbital and its duration of treatment on the evolution of carcinogen induced enzyme-altered foci in rat liver. *Cancer Lett.*, **57**, 75–82

Arni, P. (1985) Induction of various genetic effects in the yeast *Saccharomyces cerevisiae* strain D7. *Prog. Mutat. Res.*, **5**, 217–224

Asoh, M., Tateishi,T., Kumai,T. & Kobayashi, S. (1999) Induction of hepatic CYP2B in foetal and neonatal rats after maternal administration of phenobarbital. *Pharmacol. Toxicol.*, **84**, 18–23

Azarbayjani, F. & Danielsson, B.R. (1998) Pharmacologically induced embryonic dysrhythmia and episodes of hypoxia followed by reoxygenation: A common teratogenic mechanism for antiepileptic drugs? *Teratology*, **57**, 117–126

Baker, R.S.U. & Bonin, A.M. (1985) Tests with the *Salmonella* plate-incorporation assay. *Prog. Mutat. Res.*, **5**, 177–180

Baker, T.K., Bachowski, S., Stevenson, D.E., Walborg, E.F., Jr & Klaunig, J.E. (1995) Modulation of gap junctional intercellular communication in rodent, monkey and human hepatocyte by nongenotoxic compounds. *Prog. Clin. Biol. Res.*, **391**, 71–80

Barbason, H., Rassenfosse, C. & Betz, E.H. (1983) Promotion mechanism of phenobarbital and partial hepatectomy in DENA hepatocarcinogenesis cell kinetics effect. *Br. J. Cancer*, **47**, 517–525

Barbason, H., Mormont, C., Massart, S. & Bouzahzah, B. (1986) Anti-carcinogenic action of phenobarbital given simultaneously with diethylnitrosamine in the rat. *J. Cancer clin. Oncol.*, **22**, 1073–1078

Barrett, J.C. & Lamb, P.W. (1985) Tests with the Syrian hamster embryo cell transformation assay. *Prog. Mutat. Res.*, **5**, 623–628

Barter, R.A. & Klaassen, C.D. (1992) UDP-glucuronosyltransferase inducers reduce thyroid hormone levels in rats by an extrathyroidal mechanism. *Toxicol. appl. Pharmacol.*, **113**, 36–42

Barter, R.A. & Klaasen, C.D. (1994) Reduction of thyroid hormone levels and alteration of thyroid function by four representative UDP-glucuronosyltransferase inducers in rats. *Toxicol. appl. Pharmacol.*, **128**, 9–17

Battino, D., Kaneko, S., Andermann, E., Avanzini, G., Canevini, M.P., Canger, R., Croci, D., Fumarola, C., Guidolin, L., Mamoli, D., Molteni, F., Pardi, G., Vignoli, A., Fukushima, Y., Khan, R., Takeda A., Nakane,Y., Ogawa, Y., Dansky, L., Oguni, M., Lopez-Ciendas, I., Sherwin, A., Andermann, F., Seni, M.-H., Otani, K., Teranishi, T. & Goto, M (1999) Intra-uterine growth in the offspring of epileptic women: A prospective multicenter study. *Epilepsy Res.*, **36**, 53–60

Bauer-Hofmann, R., Buchmann, A., Wright, A.S. & Schwarz, M. (1990) Mutations in the Ha-ras proto-oncogene in spontaneous and chemically induced liver tumours of the CF1 mouse. *Carcinogenesis*, **11**, 1875–1877

Bauer-Hofmann, R., Buchmann, A., Mahr, J., Kress, S. & Schwarz, M. (1992) The tumour promoters dieldrin and phenobarbital increase the frequency of c-Ha-*ras* wild-type, but not of c-Ha-*ras* mutated focal liver lesions in male C3H/He mice. *Carcinogenesis*, **13**, 477–481

Bernus, I., Dickinson, R.G., Hooper, W.D. & Eadie, M.J. (1994) Urinary excretion of pheno-barbitone and its metabolites in chronically treated patients. *Eur. J. clin. Pharmacol.*, **46**, 473–475

Bertram, J.S. & Craig, A.W. (1972) Specific induction of bladder cancer in mice by butyl-(4-hydroxybutyl)-nitrosamine and the effects of hormonal modifications on the sex difference in response. *Eur. J. Cancer*, **8**, 587–594

Bradley, M.O. (1985) Measurement of DNA single-strand breaks by alkaline elution in rat hepatocytes. *Prog. Mutat. Res.*, **5**, 353–357

British Pharmacopoeia Commission (1993) *British Pharmacopoeia 1993*, Vols I & II, London, Her Majesty's Stationery Office, pp. 500–501, 1052–1053

Brockenbrough, J.S., Meyer, S.A., Li, C. & Jirtle, R.L. (1991) Reversible and phorbol ester-specific defect of protein kinase C translocation in hepatocytes isolated from phenobarbital-treated rats. *Cancer Res.*, **51**, 130–136

Brooks, T.M., Gonzalez, L.P., Calvert, R. & Parry, J.M. (1985) The induction of mitotic gene conversion in the yeast *Saccharomyces cerevisiae* strain JD1. *Prog. Mutat. Res.*, **5**, 225–228

Bruce, W.R. & Heddle, J.A. (1979) The mutagenic activity of 61 agents as determined by the micronucleus, *Salmonella*, and sperm abnormality assays. *Can. J. Genet. Cytol.*, **21**, 319–334

Budavari, S., ed. (2000) *The Merck Index*, 12th Ed., Version 12:3, Whitehouse Station, NJ, Merck & Co. & Boca Raton, FL, Chapman & Hall/CRC [CD-ROM]

Budunova, I.V., Mittelman, L.A. & Belitsky, G.A. (1989) Identification of tumor promoters by their inhibitory effect on intercellular transfer of lucifer yellow. *Cell Biol. Toxicol.*, **5**, 77–89

Bursch, W., Lauer, B., Timmermann-Trosiener, I., Barthel, G., Schuppler, J. & Schulte-Hermann, R. (1984) Controlled death (apoptosis) of normal and putative preneoplastic cells in rat liver following withdrawal of tumor promoters. *Carcinogenesis*, **5**, 453–458

Büsser, M.-T. & Lutz, W.K. (1987) Stimulation of DNA synthesis in rat and mouse liver by various tumor promoters. *Carcinogenesis*, **8**, 1433–1437

Butler, T.C. (1956) The metabolic hydroxylation of phenobarbital. *J. Pharmacol. exp. Ther.*, **116**, 326–336

Butler, W.H. (1978) Long-term effects of phenobarbitone-Na on male Fischer rats. *Br. J. Cancer*, **37**, 418–423

Carere, A., Conti, G., Conti, L. & Crebelli, R. (1985) Assays in *Aspergillus nidulans* for the induction of forward-mutation in haploid strain 35 and for mitotic nondisjunction, haploidization and crossing-over in diploid strain P1. *Prog. Mutat. Res.*, **5**, 307–312

Carthew, P., Martin, E.A., White, I.N.H., De Matteis, F., Edwards, R.E., Dorman, B.M., Heydon, R.T. & Smith, L.L. (1995) Tamoxifen induces short-term cumulative DNA damage and liver tumors in rats: Promotion by phenobarbital. *Cancer Res.*, **55**, 544–547

Cavaliere, A., Bacci, M. & Vitali, R. (1985) Lack of teratogenic and carcinogenic activity of phenobarbital sodium in the offspring of prepregnancy and pregnancy treated BALB/c/Cb/Se mice. *Pathologica*, **77**, 185–188

Cavaliere, A., Bufalari, A. & Vitali, R. (1986) Carcinogenicity and cocarcinogenicity test of phenobarbital sodium in adult BALB/c mice. *Tumori*, **72**, 125–128

Chao, M.K.C., Albert, K.S. & Fusari, S.A. (1978) Phenobarbital. *Anal. Profiles Drug Subst.*, **7**, 359–399

Chapman, J.B. & Cutler, M.G. (1988) Phenobarbitone:Adverse effects on reproductive performance and offspring development of the Mongolian gerbil (*Meriones unguiculatus*). *Psychopharmacology*, **94**, 365–370

Chen, Z.-Y., Farin, F., Omiecinski, C.J. & Eaton, D.L. (1992) Association between growth stimulation by phenobarbital and expression of cytochromes P450 1A1, 1A2, 2BI/2 and 3A1 in hepatic hyperplastic nodules in male F344 rats. *Carcinogenesis*, **13**, 675–682

Christensen, J.G., Gonzales, A.J., Cattley, R.C. & Goldsworthy, T.L. (1998) Regulation of apoptosis in mouse hepatocytes and alteration of apoptosis by nongenotoxic carcinogens. *Cell Growth Differ.*, **9**, 815–825

Christensen, J.G., Romach, E.H., Healy, L.N., Gonzales, A.J., Anderson, S.P., Malarkey, D.E., Corton, J.C., Fox, T.R., Cattley, R.C. & Goldsworthy, T.L. (1999) Altered bcl-2 family expression during non-genotoxic hepatocarcinogenesis in mice. *Carcinogenesis*, **20**, 1583–1590

CIS Information Services (2000a) *Directory of World Chemical Producers (Version 2000.1)*, Dallas, TX [CD-ROM]

CIS Information Services (2000b) *Worldwide Bulk Drug Users Directory (Version 2000)*, Dallas, TX [CD-ROM]

Clark, M.A., Williams, J.F., Gottschall, P.E. & Wecker, L. (1996) Effects of phenobarbital and interleukin-6 on cytochrome P450 2B1 and 2B2 in cultured rat hepatocytes. *Biochem. Pharmacol.*, **51**, 701–706

Clemmesen, J. & Hjalgrim-Jensen, S. (1977) On the absence of carcinogenicity to man of phenobarbital. *Acta pathol. microbiol. scand.*, **Suppl. 261**, 38–50

Clemmesen, J. & Hjalgrim-Jensen, S. (1981) Does phenobarbital cause intracranial tumors? A follow-up through 35 years. *Ecotox. Environ. Saf.*, **5**, 255–260

Clemmesen, J., Fuglsang-Frederiksen, V. & Plum, C.M. (1974) Are anticonvulsants oncogenic? *Lancet*, **i**, 705–707

Collins, A.J. & Horlington, M. (1969) A sequential screening test based on the running component of audiogenic seizures in mice, including reference compound PD50 values. *Br. J. Pharmacol.*, **37**, 140–150

Collins, M.A., Lake, B.G., Evans, J.G., Walker, R., Gangolli, S.D. & Conning, D.M. (1984) Sustained induction of hepatic xenobiotic metabolising enzyme activities by phenobarbitone in C3H/He mice: Relevance to nodule formation. *Toxicology*, **33**, 129–144

Conney, A.H. (1967) Pharmacological implications of microsomal enzyme induction. *Pharmacol. Rev.*, **19**, 317–366

Corcos, L., Marc, N., Wein, S., Fautrel, A., Guillouzo, A. & Pineau, T. (1998) Phenobarbital induces cytochrome P4501A2 hnRNA, mRNA and protein in the liver of C57BL/6J wild type and aryl hydrocarbon receptor knock-out mice. *FEBS Lett.*, **425**, 293–297

Council of Europe (1997) *European Pharmacopoeia*, 3rd Ed., Strasbourg, pp. 1311–1313

Crayford, J.V. & Hutson, D.H. (1980) Comparative metabolism of phenobarbitone in the rat (CFE) and mouse (CF1). *Fd Cosmet. Toxicol.*, **18**, 503–509

Crespi, C.L., Ryan, C.G., Seixas, G.M., Turner, T.R. & Penman, B.W. (1985) Tests for mutagenic activity using mutation assays at two loci in the human lymphoblast cell lines TK6 and AHH-1. *Prog. Mutat. Res.*, **5**, 497–516

Daminet, S., Paradis, M., Refsal, K.R. & Price, C. (1999) Short term influence of prednisone and phenobarbital on thyroid function in euthyroid dogs. *Can. vet. J.*, **40**, 411–415

Danford, N. (1985) Tests for chromosome aberrations and aneuploidy in the Chinese hamster fibroblast cell line CHl-L. *Prog. Mutat. Res.*, **5**, 397–411

Dansky, L.V. & Finnell, R.H. (1991). Parental epilepsy, anticonvulsant drugs, and reproductive outcome: Epidemiologic and experimental findings spanning three decades: 2. Human studies. *Reprod. Toxicol.*, **5**, 301–335

Decloître, F., Lafarge-Frayssinet, C., Barroso M., Lechner, M.C., Ouldelhkim, M. & Frayssinet, C. (1990) Effect of rat developmental stage at initation on the expression of biochemical markers during liver tumor promotion. *Tumor Biol.*, **11**, 295–305

Denda, A., Ura, H., Tsujiuchi, T., Tsutsumi, M., Eimoto, H., Takashima, Y., Kitazawa, S., Kinugasa, T. & Konishi, Y. (1989) Possible involvement of arachidonic acid metabolism in phenobarbital promotion of hepatocarcinogenesis. *Carcinogenesis*, **10**, 1929–1935

Dessens, A.B., Cohen-Kettenis, P.T., Mellenbergh, G.J., Van de Poll, N., Koppe, J.G. & Boer, K. (1999) Prenatal exposure to anticonvulsants and psychosexual development. *Arch. sexual Behav.*, **28**, 31–44

Díez-Fernández, C., Sanz, N., Alvarez, A.M., Wolf, A. & Cascales, M. (1998) The effect of non-genotoxic carcinogens, phenobarbital and clofibrate, on the relationship between reactive oxygen species, antioxidant enzyme expression and apoptosis. *Carcinogenesis*, **19**, 1715–1722

Diwan, B.A., Rice, J.M., Ward, J.M., Ohshima, M. & Lynch, P.H. (1984) Inhibition by pheno-barbital and lack of effect of amobarbital on the development of liver tumors induced by *N*-nitrosodiethylamine in juvenile B6C3F1 mice. *Cancer Lett.*, **23**, 223–234

Diwan, B.A., Palmer, A.E., Ohshima, M. & Rice, J.M. (1985) *N*-Nitroso-*N*-methylurea initiation in multiple tissues for organ-specific tumor promotion in rats by phenobarbital. *J. natl Cancer Inst.*, **75**, 1099–1105

Diwan, B.A., Rice, J.M., Ohshima, M. & Ward, J.M. (1986a) Interstrain differences in susceptibility to liver carcinogenesis initiated by *N*-nitrosodiethylamine and its promotion by phenobarbital in C57BL/6NCr, C3H/HeNCrMTV- and DBA/2NCr mice. *Carcinogenesis*, **7**, 215–220

Diwan, B.A., Ward, J.M., Anderson, L.M., Hagiwara, A. & Rice, J.M. (1986b) Lack of effect of phenobarbital on hepatocellular carcinogenesis initiated by *N*-nitrosodiethylamine or methylazoxymethanol acetate in male Syrian golden hamsters. *Toxicol. appl. Pharmacol.*, **86**, 298–307

Diwan, B.A., Rice, J.M., Nims, R.W., Lubet, R.A., Hu, H. & Ward, J.M. (1988) P-450 enzyme induction by 5-ethyl-5-phenylhydantoin and 5,5-diethylhydantoin analogues of barbiturate tumor promoters phenobarbital and barbital, and promotion of liver and thyroid carcinogenesis initiated by *N*-nitrosodiethylamine in rats. *Cancer Res.*, **48**, 2492–2497

Diwan, B.A., Hagiwara, A., Ward, J.M. & Rice, J.M. (1989a) Effects of sodium salts of phenobarbital and barbital on development of bladder tumors in male F344/NCr rats pretreated with either *N*-[4-(5-nitro-2-furyl)-2-thiazolyl]formamide or *N*-nitrosobutyl-4-hydroxybutylamine. *Toxicol. appl. Pharmacol.*, **98**, 269–277

Diwan, B.A., Ward, J.M. & Rice, J.M. (1989b) Promotion of malignant 'embryonal' liver tumors by phenobarbital: Increased incidence and shortened latency of hepatoblastomas in (DBA/2 x C57BL/6)F1 mice initiated with *N*-nitrosodiethylamine. *Carcinogenesis*, **10**, 1345–1348

Diwan, B.A., Ohshima, M. & Rice, J.M. (1989c) Promotion by sodium barbital of renal cortical and transitional cell tumors, but not intestinal tumors, in F344 rats given methyl-(acetoxymethyl)nitrosamine, and lack of effect of phenobarbital, amobarbital, or barbituric acid on development of either renal or intestinal tumors. *Carcinogenesis*, **10**, 183–188

Diwan, B.A., Ohshima, M. & Rice, J.M. (1989d) Effects of postnatal administration of tumor-promoting barbiturates on the development of tumors initiated by prenatal exposure to fetal rats and mice to *N*-alkylnitrosoureas. In: Napalkov, N.P., Rice, J.M., Tomatis, L. & Yamasaki, H., eds, *Perinatal and Multigeneration Carcinogenesis* (IARC Scientific Publication No. 96), Lyon, IARC, pp. 75–80

Diwan, B.A., Henneman, J.R. & Rice, J.M. (1995) Further evidence for promoter-dependent development of hepatoblastoma in the mouse. *Cancer Lett.*, **89**, 29–35

Donato, M.T., Gómez-Lechón, M.J. & Castell, J.V. (1990) Effect of xenobiotics on mono-oxygenase activities in cultured human hepatocytes. *Biochem. Pharmacol.*, **39**, 1321–1326

Donner, M., Sorsa, M. & Vainio, H. (1979) Recessive lethals induced by styrene and styrene oxide in *Drosophila melanogaster. Mutat. Res.*, **67**, 373–376

Douglas, G.R., Blakey, D.H., Liu-Lee, V.W., Bell, R.D.L. & Bayley, J.M. (1985) Alkaline sucrose sedimentation, sister-chromatid exchange and micronucleus assays in CHO cells. *Prog. Mutat. Res.*, **5**, 359–366

Doyle, L. (1996) Antenatal phenobarbitone and neonatal outcome. *Lancet*, **348**, 975–976

Dragan, Y.P., Sargent, L., Xu, Y.-D, Xu, Y.H. & Pitot, H.C. (1993) The initiation–promotion–progression model of rat hepatocarcinogenesis. *Proc. Soc. exp. Biol. Med.*, **202**, 16–34

Dragan, Y.P., Singh, J. & Pitot, H.C. (1996) Effect of the separate and combined administration of mestranol and phenobarbital on the development of altered hepatic foci expressing placental form of glutathione S-transferase in the rat. *Carcinogenesis*, 17, 2043–2052

Dravet, C., Julian, C., Legras, C., Magaudda, A., Guerrini, R., Genton, P., Soulayrol, S., Giraud, N., Mesdjian, E., Trentin, G., Roger, J. & Ayme, S. (1992) Epilepsy, antiepileptic drugs, and malformations in children of women with epilepsy: A French prospective cohort study. *Neurology*, **42** (Suppl. 5), 75–82

Driver, H.E. & McLean, A.E.M. (1986a) Dose–response relationship for phenobarbitone promotion of liver tumours initiated by single dose diethylnitrosamine. *Br. J. exp. Pathol.*, **67**, 131–139

Driver, H.E. & McLean, A.E.M. (1986b) Dose–response relationships for initiation of rat liver tumours by dimethylnitrosamine and promotion by phenobarbitone or alcohol. *Food chem. Toxicol.*, **24**, 241–245

Duivenvoorden, W.C.M. & Maier, P. (1994) Nongenotoxic carcinogens shift cultured rat hepatocytes into G1 cell cycle phase: Influence of tissue oxygen tension on cells with different ploidy. *Eur. J. Cell Biol.*, **64**, 368–375

Dydyk, L. & Rutczynski, M. (1977) Ultrastructure of the brain of newborn rabbit after trans-placental action of phenobarbital. *Neuropathol. Pol.*, **XV**, 545–554

Eckl, P.M., Meyer, S.A., Whitcombe, W.R. & Jirtle, R.L. (1988) Phenobarbital reduces EGF receptors and the ability of physiological concentrations of calcium to suppress hepatocyte proliferation. *Carcinogenesis*, **9**, 479–483

Ecobichon, D.J., D'Ver, A.S. & Ehrhart, W. (1988) Drug disposition and biotransformation in the developing beagle dog. *Fundam. appl. Toxicol.*, **11**, 29–37

Edwards, A.M. & Lucas, C.M. (1985) Phenobarbital and some other liver tumor promoters stimulate DNA synthesis in cultured rat hepatocytes. *Biochem. biophys. Res. Commun.*, **131**, 103–108

Ehleben, W., Porwol, T., Fandrey, J. & Acker, H. (1998) The influence of phenobarbital on cytochromes and reactive oxygen species in erythropoietin producing HepG2 cells. *FEBS Lett.*, **440**, 343–347

Evans, J.G., Collins, M.A., Lake, B.G. & Butler, W.H. (1992) The histology and development of hepatic nodules and carcinoma in C3H/He and C57BL/6 mice following chronic pheno-barbitone administration. *Toxicol. Pathol.*, **20**, 585–594

Faris, R.A. & Campbell, T.C. (1981) Exposure of newborn rats to pharmacologically active compounds may permanently alter carcinogen metabolism. *Science*, **211**, 719–720

Finnell, R.H. & Dansky, L.V (1991) Parental epilepsy, anticonvulsant drugs, and reproductive outcome: Epidemiologic and experimental findings spanning three decades: 1. Animal studies. *Reprod. Toxicol.*, **5**, 281–299

Finnell, R.,H. Shields, H.E. & Chernoff, G.F. (1987a) Variable patterns in anticonvulsant drug-induced malformations in mice: Comparisons of phenytoin and phenobarbital. *Teratog. Carcinog. Mutag.*, **7**, 541–549

Finnell, R.H., Shields, H.E., Taylor, S.M. & Chernoff, G.F. (1987b) Strain differences in pheno-barbital-induced teratogenesis in mice. *Teratology*, **35**, 177–185

Foerst, D. (1972) [Chromosome studies on the effect of primidone (mylepsinum®) and its meta-bolites phenobarbital and phenylethylmalondiamide in vitro.] *Acta genet. med. gemellol.*, **21**, 305–318 (in German)

Fox, T.R., Schumann, A.M., Watanabe, P.G., Yano, B.L., Maher, V.M. & McCormick, J.J. (1990) Mutational analysis of the H-*ras* oncogene in spontaneous C57BL/6 x C3H/He mouse liver tumors and tumors induced with genotoxic and nongenotoxic hepatocarcinogens. *Cancer Res.*, **50**, 4014–4019

Friedman, G.D. (1981) Barbiturates and lung cancer in humans. *J. natl Cancer Inst.*, **67**, 291–295

Friedman, G.D. & Habel, L.A. (1999) Barbiturates and lung cancer: A re-evaluation. *Int. J. Epidemiol.*, **28**, 375–379

Friedman, J. & Polifka, J. (1994) *Teratogenic Effects of Drugs: A Resource for Clinicians*, Baltimore, MD, The John's Hopkins University Press, pp. 490–494

Friedman, G.D. & Ury, H.K. (1980) Initial screening for carcinogenicity of commonly used drugs. *J. natl Cancer Inst.*, **65**, 723–733

Friedman, G.D. & Ury, H.K. (1983) Screening for possible drug carcinogenicity: Second report of findings. *J. natl Cancer Inst.*, **71**, 1165–1175

Fritz, H., Müller, D. & Hess, R. (1976) Comparative study of the teratogenicity of pheno-barbitone, diphenylhydantoin, and carbamazepine in mice. *Toxicology*, **6**, 323–330

Frueh, F.W., Zanger, U.M. & Meyer, U.A. (1997) Extent and character of phenobarbital-mediated changes in gene expression in the liver. *Mol. Pharmacol.*, **51**, 363–369

Fujikawa, K., Ryo, H. & Kondo, S. (1985) The *Drosophila* reversion assay using the unstable *zeste-white* somatic eye color system. *Prog. Mutat. Res.*, **5**, 319–324

Fullerton, F.R., Hoover, K., Mikol, Y.B., Creasia, D.A. & Poirier, L.A. (1990) The inhibition by methionine and choline of liver carcinoma formation in male C3H mice dosed with diethylnitrosamine and fed phenobarbital. *Carcinogenesis*, **11**, 1301–1305

Furukawa, K., Numoto, S., Furuya, K., Furukawa, N.T. & Williams, G.M. (1985) Effects of the hepatocarcinogen nafenopin, a peroxisome proliferator, on the activities of rat liver gluta-thione-requiring enzymes and catalase in comparison to the action of phenobarbital. *Cancer Res.*, **45**, 5011–5019

Garner, R.C. & Campbell, J. (1985) Tests for the induction of mutations to ouabain or 6-thio-guanine resistance in mouse lymphoma L5178Y cells. *Prog. Mutat. Res.*, **5**, 525–529

Gaskill, C.L., Burton, S.A., Gelens, H.C.J., Ihle, S.L., Miller, J.B., Shaw, D.H., Brimacombe, M.B. & Cribb, A.E. (1999) Effects of phenobarbital treatment on serum thyroxine and thyroid-stimulating hormone concentrations in epileptic dogs. *J. Am. vet. Med. Assoc.*, **215**, 489–496

Gennaro, A.R. (1995) *Remington: The Science and Practice of Pharmacy*, 19th Ed., Vol. II, Easton, PA, Mack Publishing Co., pp. 1164–1165

Glasson, B., Lerch, P. & Viret, J.P. (1959) [Study of radiolabelled phenobarbital in the rat.] *Helv. physiol. Acta*, **17**, 146–152 (in French)

Glauert, H.P., Schwarz, M. and Pitot, H.C. (1986) The phenotypic stability of altered hepatic foci: Effect of the short-term withdrawal of phenobarbital and of the long-term feeding of purified diets after the withdrawal of phenobarbital. *Carcinogenesis*, **7**, 117–121

Gold, E., Gordis, L., Tonascia, J. & Szklo, M. (1978) Increased risk of brain tumours in children exposed to barbiturates. *J. natl Cancer Inst.*, **61**, 1031–1034

Goldenthal, E.I. (1971) A compilation of LD_{50} values in newborn and adult animals. *Toxicol. appl. Pharmacol.*, **18**, 185–207

Goldhaber, M.K., Selby, J.V., Hiatt, R.A. & Quesenberry, C.P. (1990) Exposure to barbiturates *in utero* and during childhood and risk of intracranial and spinal cord tumours. *Cancer Res.*, **50**, 4600–4603

Goldsworthy, T., Campbell, H.A. & Pitot, H.C. (1984) The natural history and dose–response characteristics of enzyme-altered foci in rat liver following phenobarbital and dimethyl-nitrosamine administration. *Carcinogenesis*, **5**, 67–71

Gopalan, P., Tsuji, K., Lehmann, K., Kimura, M., Shinozuka, H., Sato, K. & Lotlikar, P.D. (1993) Modulation of aflatoxin B_1-induced glutathione *S*-transferase placental form positive hepatic foci by pretreatment of rats with phenobarbital and buthionine sulfoximine. *Carcinogenesis*, **14**, 1469–1470

Grasl-Kraupp, B., Waldhör, T., Huber, W. & Schulte-Hermann, R. (1993) Glutathione S-transferase isoenzyme patterns in different subtypes of enzyme-altered rat liver foci treated with the peroxisome proliferation nafenopin or with phenobarbital. *Carcinogenesis*, **14**, 2407–2412

Grube, D.D., Peraino, C. & Fry, R.J.M. (1975) The effect of dietary phenobarbital on the induction of skin tumors in hairless mice with 7,12-dimethylbenz[a]anthracene. *J. invest. Dermatol.*, **64**, 258–262

Gulati, D.K., Sabharwal, P.S. & Shelby, M.D. (1985) Tests for the induction of chromosomal aberrations and sister chromatid exchanges in cultured Chinese hamster ovary (CHO) cells. *Prog. Mutat. Res.*, **5**, 413–426

Gunz, D., Shephard, S.E. & Lutz, W.K. (1993) Can nongenotoxic carcinogens be detected with the *lacI* transgenic mouse mutation assay? *Environ. mol. Mutag.*, **21**, 209–211

Guppy, M.J., Wilton, J.C., Sharma, R., Coleman, R. & Chipman, J.K. (1994) Modulation of phenobarbitone-induced loss of gap junctional intercellular communication in hepatocyte couplets. *Carcinogenesis*, **15**, 1917–1921

Gupta, C. & Yaffe, S.J. (1981) Reproductive dysfunction in female offspring after prenatal exposure to phenobarbital: Critical period of action. *Pediatr. Res.*, **15**, 1488–1491

Gupta, C. & Yaffe, S.J. (1982) Prenatal exposure to phenobarbital permanently decreases testosterone and causes reproductive dysfunction. *Science*, **216**, 640–642

Gupta, C., Shapiro, B.H. & Yaffe, S.J. (1980a) Reproductive dysfunction in male rats following prenatal exposure to phenobarbital. *Pediatr. Pharmacol.*, **1**, 55–62

Gupta, C., Sonawane, B.R., Yaffe, S.J. & Shapiro, B.H. (1980b) Phenobarbital exposure in utero: Alterations in female reproductive function in rats. *Science*, **208**, 508–510

Gupta, C., Hattori, A., Betschart, J.M., Virji, M.A. & Shinozuka, H. (1988) Modulation of epidermal growth factor receptors in rat hepatocytes by two liver tumor-promoting regimens, a choline-deficient and a phenobarbital diet. *Cancer Res.*, **48**, 1161–1165

Habel, L.A., Bull, S.A. & Friedman, G.D. (1998) Barbiturates, smoking, and bladder cancer risk. *Cancer Epidemiol. Biomarkers Prev.*, **7**, 1049–1050

Hagiwara, A., Miyata, E., Tamano, S., Sano, M., Masuda, C., Funae, Y., Ito, N., Fukushima, S. & Shirai, T. (1999) Non-carcinogenicity, but dose-related increase in preneoplastic hepatocellular lesions, in a two-year feeding study of phenobarbital sodium in male F344 rats. *Food chem. Toxicol.*, **37**, 869–879

Hardman, J.G., Limbird, L.E., Molinoff, P.B. & Ruddon, R.W., eds (1996) *Goodman & Gilman's The Pharmacological Basis of Therapeutics*, 9th Ed., New York, McGraw-Hill, pp. 471–472

Harvey, D.J., Glazener, L., Stratton, C., Nowlin, J., Hill, R.M. & Horning, M.G. (1972) Detection of a 5-(3,4-dihydroxy-1,5-cyclohexadien-1-yl)-metabolite of phenobarbital and mephobarbital in rat, guinea pig and human. *Res. Commun. chem. Pathol. Pharmacol.*, **3**, 557–565

Hasmall, S.C. & Roberts, R.A. (1999) The perturbation of apoptosis and mitosis by drugs and xenobiotics. *Pharmacol. Ther.*, **82**, 63–70

Hayes, M.A., Lee, G., Tatematsu, M. & Farber, E. (1987) Influences of diethylnitrosamine on longevity of surrounding hepatocytes and progression of transplanted persistent nodules during phenobarbital promotion of hepatocarcinogenesis. *Int. J. Cancer*, **40**, 58–63

Hendrich, S., Glauert, H.P. & Pitot, H.C. (1986) The phenotypic stability of altered hepatic foci: Effects of withdrawal and subsequent readministration of phenobarbital. *Carcinogenesis*, **7**, 2041–2045

Hiasa, Y., Kitahori, Y., Ohshima, M., Fujita, T., Yuasa, T., Konishi, N. & Miyashiro, A. (1982) Promoting effects of phenobarbital and barbital on development of thyroid tumors in rats treated with N-bis(2-hydroxypropyl) nitrosamine. *Carcinogenesis*, **3**, 1187–1190

Hiasa, Y., Kitahori, Y., Konishi, N., Enoki, N. & Fujita, T. (1983) Effect of varying the duration of exposure to phenobarbital on its enhancement of N-bis(2-hydroxypropyl) nitrosamine-induced thyroid tumorigenesis in male Wistar rats. *Carcinogenesis*, **4**, 935–937

Hiasa, Y., Kitahori, Y., Konishi, N., Shimoyama, T. & Lin, J.-C. (1985) Sex differential and dose dependence of phenobarbital-promoting activity in *N*-bis(2-hydroxypropyl) nitrosamine-initiated thyroid tumorigenesis in rats. *Cancer Res.*, **45**, 4087–4090

Hiasa, Y., Kitahori, Y., Katoh, Y., Ohshima, M., Konishi, N., Shimoyama, T., Sakaguchi, Y., Hashimoto, H., Minami, S. & Murata, Y. (1987) Effects of castration before and after treatment with N-bis(2-hydroxypropyl) nitrosamine (DHPN) on the development of thyroid tumors in rats treated with DHPN followed by phenobarbital. *Jpn. J. Cancer Res.*, **78**, 1063–1067

Hikita, H., Nuwaysir, E.F., Vaughan, J., Babcock, K., Haas, M.J., Dragan, Y.P. & Pitot, H.C. (1998) The effect of short-term fasting, phenobarbital and refeeding on apoptotic loss, cell replication and gene expression in rat liver during the promotion stage. *Carcinogenesis*, **19**, 1417–1425

Hirose, M., Shirai, T., Tsuda, H., Fukushima, S., Ogiso, T. & Ito, N. (1981) Effect of phenobarbital, polychlorinated biphenyl and sodium saccharin on hepatic and renal carcinogenesis in unilaterally nephrectomized rats given N-ethyl-N-hydroxyethylnitrosamine orally. *Carcinogenesis*, **2**, 1299–1302

Holmes, L.B., Harvey, E.A., Hayes, A.M., Brown, K.S., Schoenfeld, D.A. & Khoshbin, S. (1990) The teratogenic effects of anticonvulsant monotherapy: Phenobarbital (Pb), carbamazepine (CBZ) and phenytoin (PHT) (Abstract). *Teratology*, **41**, 565

Hood, A., Liu, J. & Klaassen, C.D. (1999) Effects of phenobarbital, pregnenolone-16α-carbonitrile, and propylthiouracil on thyroid follicular cell proliferation. *Toxicol. Sci.*, **50**, 45–53

Hsieh, L.L., Peraino, C. & Weinstein, I.B. (1988) Expression of endogenous retrovirus-like sequences and cellular oncogenes during phenobarbital treatment and regeneration in rat liver. *Cancer Res.*, **48**, 265–269

IARC (1977) *IARC Monographs on the Evaluation of Carcinogenic Risk of Chemicals to Man*, Vol. 13, *Some Miscellaneous Pharmaceutical Substances*, Lyon, IARCPress, pp. 157–181

IARC (1987) *IARC Monographs on the Evaluation of Carcinogenic Risks to Humans*, Suppl. 7, *Overall Evaluations of Carcinogenicity: An Updating of* IARC Monographs *Volumes 1 to 42*, Lyon, IARCPress, pp. 313–316

Ida, K., Nakamura, S., Muro, H., Takai, M. & Kaneko, M. (1995) Promoting effects of phenobarbital on the enzyme-altered foci induced by intrahepatic γ-ray-irradiation in the rat liver. *Radiat. Oncol. Radiat. Med.*, **3**, 227–233

Imaida, K. & Wang, C.Y. (1986) Effect of sodium phenobarbital and sodium saccharin in AIN-76A diet on carcinogenesis initiated with *N*-[4-(5-nitro-2-furyl)-2-thiazolyl] formamide and *N,N*-dibutylnitrosamine in male F344 rats. *Cancer Res.*, **46**, 6160–6164

Irish Medicines Board (2000) Dublin

Ishidate, M., Jr & Sofuni, T. (1985) The in vitro chromosomal aberration test using Chinese hamster lung (CHL) fibroblast cells in culture. *Prog. Mutat. Res.*, **5**, 427–432

Ishidate, M., Jr, Sofuni, T. & Yoshikawa, K. (1981) Chromosomal aberration tests in vitro as a primary screening tool for environmental mutagens and/or carcinogens. *Gann Monogr. Cancer Res.*, **27**, 95–108

Ito, N., Nakanishi, K., Hagiwara, A., Shibata, M. & Fukushima, S. (1980) Induction of hyperplastic liver nodules by phenobarbital in rats initiated with *N*-butyl-*N*-(4-hydroxybutyl)-nitrosamine. *Gann*, **71**, 918–919

Ito, N., Moore, M.A. & Bannasch, P. (1984) Modifications of the development of N-nitrosomorpholine-induced hepatic lesions by 2-acetylaminofluorene, phenobarbital and 4,4′-diaminodiphenylmethane: A sequential histological and histochemical analysis. *Carcinogenesis*, **5**, 335–342

Ito, S., Tsuda, M., Yoshitake, A., Yanai, T. & Masegi, T. (1998) Effect of phenobarbital on hepatic gap junctional intercellular communication in rats. *Toxicol. Pathol.*, **26**, 253–259

James, N.H. & Roberts, R.A. (1996) Species differences in response to peroxisome proliferators correlate *in vitro* with induction of DNA synthesis rather than suppression of apoptosis. *Carcinogenesis*, **17**, 1623–1632

Jarukamjorn, K., Sakuma, T., Miyaura, J.-I. & Nemoto, N. (1999) Different regulation of the expression of mouse hepatic cytochrome P450 2B enzymes by glucocorticoid and phenobarbital. *Arch. Biochem. Biophys.*, **369**, 89–99

Jenke, H.S., Deml, E. & Oesterle, D. (1994) C-raf expression in early rat liver tumorigenesis after promotion with polychlorinated biphenyls or phenobarbital. *Xenobiotica*, **24**, 569–580

Jirtle, R.L. & Meyer, S.A. (1991) Liver tumor promotion: Effect of phenobarbital on EGF and protein kinase C signal transduction and transforming growth factor-β1 expression. *Dig. Dis. Sci.*, **36**, 659–668

Jirtle, R.L., Hankins, G.R., Reisenbichler, H. & Boyer, I.J. (1994) Regulation of mannose 6-phosphate/insulin-like growth factor-II receptors and transforming growth factor beta during liver tumor promotion with phenobarbital. *Carcinogenesis*, **15**, 1473–1478

Johnson, S., McKillop, D., Miller, J., Smith, I.K. (1993) The effects on rat thyroid function of a hepatic microsomal enzyme inducer. *Hum. exp. Toxicol.*, **12**, 153–158

Jone, C.M., Erickson, L.M., Trosko, J.E., Netzloff, M.L. & Chang, C.-C. (1985) Inhibition of metabolic cooperation by the anticonvulsants, diphenylhydantoin and phenobarbital. *Teratogen. Carcinog. Mutag.*, **5**, 379–391

Jones, H.B. & Clarke, N.A.B. (1993) Assessment of the influence of subacute phenobarbitone administration on multi-tissue cell proliferation in the rat using bromodeoxyuridine immunocytochemistry. *Arch. Toxicol.*, **67**, 622–628

Jones, K.L., Johnson, K.A. & Chambers, C.C. (1992a) Pregnancy outcome in women treated with phenobarbital monotherapy (Abstract). *Teratology*, **45**, 452–453

Jones, C.R., Guengerich, F.P., Rice, J.M. & Lubet, R.A. (1992b) Induction of various cytochromes CYP2B, CYP2C and CYP3A by phenobarbitone in non-human primates. *Pharmacogenetics*, **2**, 160–172

Kaneko, S., Battino, D., Andermann, E., Wada, K., Kan, R., Takeda, A., Nakane, Y., Ogawa, Y., Avanzini, G., Fumarola, C., Granata, T., Molteni, F., Pardi, G., Minotti, L., Canger, R., Dansky, L,. Oguni, M., Lopes-Cendas, I., Sherwin, A., Andermann, F., Seni, M.H., Okada, M. & Teranishi, T. (1999) Congenital malformations due to antiepileptic drugs. *Epilepsy Res.*, **33**, 145–158

Kanno, J., Matsuoka, C., Furuta, K., Onodera, H., Miyajima, H., Maekawa, A. & Hayashi, Y. (1990) Tumor promoting effect of goitrogens on the rat thyroid. *Toxicol. Pathol.*, **18**, 239–246

Kaufmann, W.K., Ririe, D.G. & Kaufman, D.G. (1988) Phenobarbital-dependent proliferation of putative initiated rat hepatocytes. *Carcinogenesis*, **9**, 779–782

Kaufmann, W.K., Byrd, L.L., Palmieri, D., Nims., R.W. & Rice, J.M. (1997) TGF-α sustains clonal expansion by promoter-dependent, chemically initiated rat hepatocytes. *Carcinogenesis*, **18**, 1381–1387

Kim, H.-C., Lee, Y.-S. & Nishikawa, A. (1997) Enhancing effects of phenobarbital and 3-methylcholanthrene on GST-P-positive liver foci development in a new medium-term rat liver bioassay using D-galactosamine. *J. Toxicol. environ. Health*, **50**, 519–528

Kitagawa, T., Hirakawa, T., Ishikawa, T., Nemoto, N. & Takayama, S. (1980) Induction of hepatocellular carcinoma in rat liver by initial treatment with benzo(a)pyrene after partial hepatectomy and promotion by phenobarbital. *Toxicol. Lett.*, **6**, 167–171

Kitagawa, T., Hino, O., Nomura, K. & Sugano, H. (1984) Dose–response studies in promoting and anticarcinogenic effects of phenobarbital and DDT in the rat hepatocarcinogenesis. *Carcinogenesis*, **5**, 1653–1656

Kitano, M., Ichihara, T., Matsuda, T., Wanibuchi, H., Tamano, S., Hagiwara, A., Imaoka, S., Funae, Y., Shirai, T. & Fukushima, S. (1998) Presence of a threshold for promoting effects of phenobarbital on diethylnitrosamine-induced hepatic foci in the rat. *Carcinogenesis*, **19**, 1475–1480

Klaassen, C.D. (1971) Bilary excretion of barbiturates. *Br. J. Pharmacol.*, **43**, 161–166

Klaunig, J.E. (1993) Selective induction of DNA synthesis in mouse preneoplastic and neoplastic hepatic lesions after exposure to phenobarbital. *Environ. Health Perspect.*, **101** (Suppl. 5), 235–240

Klaunig, J.E. & Ruch, R.J. (1987a) Strain and species effects on the inhibition of hepatocyte intercellular communication by liver tumor promoters. *Cancer Lett.*, **36**, 161–168

Klaunig, J.E. & Ruch, R.J. (1987b) Role of cyclic AMP in the inhibition of mouse hepatocyte intercellular communication by liver tumor promoters. *Toxicol. appl. Pharmacol.*, **91**, 159–170

Klaunig, J.E., Pereira, M.A., Ruch, R.J. & Weghorst, C.M. (1988a) Dose–response relationship of diethylnitrosamine-initiated tumors in neonatal Balb/c mice: Effect of phenobarbital promotion. *Toxicol. Pathol.*, **16**, 381–385

Klaunig, J.E., Weghorst, C.M. & Pereira, M.A. (1988b) Effect of phenobarbital on diethylnitrosamine and dimethylnitrosamine induced hepatocellular tumors in male B6C3F1 mice. *Cancer Lett.*, **42**, 133–139

Klaunig, J.E., Ruch, R.J. & Weghorst, C.M. (1990) Comparative effects of phenobarbital, DDT, and lindane on mouse hepatocyte gap junctional intercellular communication. *Toxicol. appl. Pharmacol.*, **102**, 553–563

Klaunig, J.E., Siglin, J.C., Schafer, L.D., Hartnett, J.A., Weghorst, C.M., Olson, M.J. & Hampton, J.A. (1991) Correlation between species and tissue sensitivity to chemical carcinogenesis in rodents and the induction of DNA synthesis. *Prog. clin. biol. Res.*, **369**, 185–194

Kleinberger, N. & Yanai, J. (1985) Early phenobarbital-induced alterations in hippocampal acetylcholinesterase activity and behavior. *Dev. Brain Res.*, **22**, 113–123

Kocarek, T.A., Schuetz, E.G. & Guzelian, P.S. (1990) Differentiated induction of cytochrome P450b/e and P450p mRNAs by dose of phenobarbital in primary cultures of adult rat hepatocytes. *Mol. Pharmacol.*, **38**, 440–444

Kolaja, K.I., Stevenson, D.E., Johnson, J.T., Walborg, E.F., Jr & Klaunig, J.E. (1995a) Hepatic effects of dieldrin and phenobarbital in male B6C3F1 mice and Fisher 344 rats: Selective induction of DNA synthesis. In: McClain, R.M., Slaga, T.J., Le Boeuf, R. & Pitot, H.C., eds, *Growth Factors and Tumor Promotion: Implications for Risk Assessment*, New York, Wiley-Liss, pp. 397–408

Kolaja, K.I., Stevenson, D.E., Walborg, E.F., Jr & Klaunig, J.E. (1995b) The effect of dieldrin and phenobarbital on preneoplastic hepatic lesion growth in male F344 rat and B6C3F1 mouse. In: McClain, R.M., Slaga, T.J., Le Boeuf, R. & Pitot, H.C., eds, *Growth Factors and Tumor Promotion: Implications for Risk Assessment*, New York, Wiley-Liss, pp. 409–423

Kolaja, K.L., Stevenson, D.E., Walborg, E.F. & Klaunig, J.E. (1996a) Reversibility of promoter induced hepatic focal lesion growth in mice. *Carcinogenesis*, **17**, 1403–1409

Kolaja, K.L., Stevenson, D.E., Johnson, J.T., Walborg, E.F., Jr & Klaunig, J.E. (1996b) Subchronic effects of dieldrin and phenobarbital on hepatic DNA synthesis in mice and rats. *Fundam. applied Toxicol.*, **29**, 219–228

Kolaja, K.L., Stevenson, D.E., Walborg, E.F., Jr & Klaunig, J.E. (1996c) Dose dependence of phenobarbital promotion of preneoplastic hepatic lesions in F344 rats and B6C3F1 mice: Effects on DNA synthesis and apoptosis. *Carcinogenesis*, **17**, 947–954

Konishi, N., Donovan, P.J. & Ward, J.M. (1990) Differential effects of renal carcinogens and tumor promoters on growth promotion and inhibition of gap junctional communication in two rat renal epithelial cell lines. *Carcinogenesis*, **11**, 903–908

Kramer, S., Ward, E., Meadows, A.T. & Malone, K.E. (1987) Medical and drug risk factors associated with neuroblastoma: A case–control study. *J. natl Cancer Inst.*, **78**, 797–804

Kroll, B., Kunz, S., Klein, T. & Schwarz, L.R. (1999) Effect of lindane and phenobarbital on cyclooxygenase-2 expression and prostanoid synthesis by Kupffer cells. *Carcinogenesis*, **20**, 1411–1416

Krutovskikh, V.A., Mesnil, M., Mazzoleni, G. & Yamasaki, H. (1995) Inhibition of rat liver gap junction intercellular communication by tumor-promoting agents *in vivo*. Association with aberrant localization of connexin proteins. *Lab. Invest.*, **72**, 571–577

Kunz, H.W., Buchmann, A., Schwarz, M., Schmitt, R., Kuhlmann, W.D., Wolf, C.R. & Oesch, F. (1987) Expression and inducibility of drug-metabolizing enzymes in preneoplastic and neoplastic lesions of rat liver during nitrosamine-induced hepatocarcinogenesis. *Arch Toxicol.*, **60**, 198–203

Kuroda, Y., Yokoiyama, A. & Kada, T. (1985) Assays for the induction of mutations to 6-thio-guanine resistance in Chinese hamster V79 cells in culture. *Prog. Mutat. Res.*, **5**, 537–542

Lafarge-Frayssinet, C. & Frayssinet, C. (1989) Over expression of proto-oncogenes: ki-ras, fos and myc in rat liver cells treated in vitro by two liver tumor promoters: phenobarbital and biliverdin. *Cancer Lett.*, **44**, 191–198

Lawrence, N. & McGregor, D.B. (1985) Assays for the induction of morphological transformation in C3H/10T1/2 cells in culture with and without S9-mediated metabolic activation. *Prog. Mutat. Res.*, **5**, 651–658

LeBoeuf, R.A., Kerckaert, G.A., Aardema, M.J., Gibson, D.P., Brauninger, R. & Isfort, R.J. (1996) The pH 6.7 Syrian hamster embryo cell transformation assay for assessing the carcinogenic potential of chemicals. *Mutat. Res.*, **356**, 85–127

Lee, G.-H., Nomura, K. & Kitagawa, T. (1989) Comparative study of diethylnitrosamine-initiated two-stage hepatocarcinogenesis in C3H, C57BL and BALB mice promoted by various hepatopromoters. *Carcinogenesis*, **10**, 2227–2230

Leibold, E. & Schwarz, L.R. (1993a) Inhibition of intercellular communication in rat hepatocytes by phenobarbital, 1,1,1-trichloro-2,2-bis(*p*-chlorophenyl)ethane (DDT) and γ-hexa-chlorocyclohexane (lindane): Modification by antioxidants and inhibitors of cyclo-oxygenase. *Carcinogenesis*, **14**, 2377–2382

Leibold, E. & Schwarz, L.R. (1993b) Intercellular communication in primary cultures of puta-tive preneoplastic and 'normal' hepatocytes. *Carcinogenesis*, **14**, 2127–2129

Lewis, D.P., Van Dyke, D.C., Stumbo, P.J. & Berg, M.J. (1998) Drug and environmental factors associated with adverse pregnancy outcomes. Part 1: Antiepileptic drugs, contraceptives, smoking and folate. *Ann. Pharmacother.*, **32**, 802–817

Liber, H. L. (1985) Mutation tests with *Salmonella* using 8-azaguanine resistance as the genetic marker. *Prog. Mutat. Res.*, **5**, 213–216

Lide, D.R. & Milne, G.W.A. (1996) *Properties of Organic Compounds*, Version 5.0, Boca Raton, FL, CRC Press [CD-ROM]

Lin, E.L.C., Klaunig, J.E., Mattox, J.K., Weghorst, C.M., McFarland, B.H. & Pereira, M.A. (1989) Comparison of the effects of acute and subacute treatment of phenobarbital in different strains of mice. *Cancer Lett.*, **48**, 43–51

Lindroos, P., Tsai, W.H., Zarnegar, R. & Michalopoulos, G.K. (1992) Plasma levels of HGF in rats treated with tumor promoters. *Carcinogenesis*, **13**, 139–141

Liu, J., Liu, Y., Barter, R.A. & Klaassen, C.D. (1995) Alteration of thyroid homeostasis by UDP-glucuronosyltransferase inducers in rats: A dose–response study. *J. Pharmacol. exp. Ther.*, **273**, 977–985

Livezey, G.T., Rayburn, W.F. & Smith, C.V. (1992) Prenatal exposure to phenobarbital and quantifiable alterations in the electroencephalogram of adult rat offspring. *Am. J. Obstet. Gynecol.*, **167**, 1611–1615

Loprieno, N., Boncristiani, G., Forster, R. & Goldstein, B. (1985) Assays for forward mutation in *Schizosaccharomyces pombe* strain P1. *Prog. Mutat. Res.*, **5**, 297–306

Lous, P. (1954) Plasma levels and urinary excretion of three barbituric acids after oral administration to man. *Acta pharmacol. toxicol.*, **10**, 147–165

Maekawa, A., Onodera, H., Ogasawara, H., Matsushima, Y., Mitsumori, K. & Hayashi, Y. (1992) Threshold dose dependence in phenobarbital promotion of rat hepatocarcinogenesis initiated by diethylnitrosamine. *Carcinogenesis*, **13**, 501–503

Makino, T., Obara, T., Ura, H., Kinugasa, T., Kobayashi, H., Takahashi, S. & Konishi, Y. (1986) Effects of phenobarbital and secondary bile acids on liver, gallbladder, and pancreas carcinogenesis initiated by *N*-nitrosobis(2-hydroxypropyl)amine in hamsters. *J. natl Cancer Inst.*, **76**, 967–975

Manjeshwar, S., Rao, P.M., Rajalakshmi, S. & Sarma, D.S.R. (1992) Inhibition of DNA synthesis by phenobarbital in primary cultures of hepatocytes from normal rat liver and form hepatic nodules. *Carcinogenesis*, **13**, 2287–2291

Mansbach, J.M., Mills, J.J., Boyer, I.J., De Souza, A.T., Hankins, G.R. & Jirtle, R.L. (1996) Phenobarbital selectively promotes initiated cells with reduced TGFβ receptor levels. *Carcinogenesis*, **17**, 171–174

Martens, U., Lennartsson, P., Högberg, J. & Stenius, U. (1996) Low expression of the WAF1/CIP1 gene product, p21, in enzyme-altered foci in rat liver by diethylnitrosamine or phenobarbital. *Cancer Lett.*, **104**, 21–26

Matsushima, T., Muramatsu, M. & Haresaku, M. (1985) Mutation tests on *Salmonella typhimurium* by the preincubation method. *Prog. Mutat. Res.*, **5**, 181–186

Matthews, E.J., DelBalzo, T. & Rundell, J.O. (1985) Assays for morphological transformation and mutation to ouabain resistance of Balb/c-3T3 cells in culture. *Prog. Mutat. Res.*, **5**, 639–650

Maynert, E.W. (1965) The alcoholic metabolites of pentobarbital and amobarbital in man. *J. pharmacol. exp. Ther.*, **150**, 118–121

McCann, J., Choi, E., Yamasaki, E. & Ames, B.N. (1975) Detection of carcinogens as mutagens in the *Salmonella*/microsome test: Assay of 300 chemicals. *Proc. natl Acad. Sci. USA*, **72**, 5135–5139

McClain, R.M., Posch, R.C., Bosakowski, T. & Armstrong, J.M. (1988) Studies on the mode of action for thyroid gland tumor promotion in rats by phenobarbital. *Toxicol. appl. Pharmacol.*, **94**, 254–265

McClain, R.M., Levin, A.A., Posch, R. & Downing, J.C. (1989) The effect of phenobarbital on the metabolism and excretion of thyroxine in rats. *Toxicol. appl. Pharmacol.*, **99**, 216–228

McGregor, D.B. & Prentice, R.D. (1985) Phenobarbital: Its mutagenicity and toxicity in the Ames' *Salmonella* test. *Prog. Mutat. Res.*, **5**, 741–743

Medical Products Agency (2000) Uppsala

Medicines Evaluation Board Agency (2000) The Hague

Mejdoubi, N., Henriques, C., Bui, E. & Porquet, D. (1999) NF-κB is involved in the induction of the rat hepatic α1-acid glycoprotein gene by phenobarbital. *Biochem. biophys. Res. Commun.*, **254**, 93–99

Mesnil, M., Piccoli, C. & Yamasaki, H. (1993) An improved long-term culture of rat hepatocytes to detect liver tumour-promoting agents: results with phenobarbital. *Eur. J. Pharmacol.*, **248**, 59–66

Meyer, S.A., Gibbs, T.A. & Jirtle, R.L. (1989) Independent mechanisms for tumor promoters phenobarbital and 12-*O*-tetradecanoylphorbol-13-acetate in reduction of epidermal growth factor binding by rat hepatocytes. *Cancer Res.*, **49**, 5907–5912

Middaugh, L. (1986) Phenobarbital during pregnancy in mouse and man. *Neurotoxicology*, **7**, 287–302

Mino, Y., Mizuswa, H. & Shiota, K. (1994) Effect of anticonvulsant drugs on fetal mouse palates cultured in vitro. *Reprod. Toxicol.*, **8**, 225–230

Miyazaki, M., Handa, Y., Oda, M., Yabe, T., Miyano, K. & Sato, J. (1985) Long-term survival of functional hepatocytes from adult rat in the presence of phenobarbital in primary culture. *Exp. cell. Res.*, **159**, 176–190

Mizutani, T. & Mitsuoka, T. (1988) Effect of dietary phenobarbital on spontaneous hepatic tumorigenesis in germfree C3H/He male mice. *Cancer Lett.*, **39**, 233–237

Moennikes, O., Buchmann, A., Romualdi, A., Ott, T., Werringloer, J., Willecke, K. & Schwarz, M. (2000) Lack of phenobarbital-mediated promotion of hepatocarcinogenesis in connexin32-null mice. *Cancer Res.*, **60**, 5087–5091

Moore, M.A., Hacker, H.-J., Kunz, H.W. & Bannasch, P. (1983) Enhancement of NNM-induced carcinogenesis in the rat liver by phenobarbital: A combined morphological and enzyme histochemical approach. *Carcinogenesis*, **4**, 473–479

Moore, M.A., Thamavit, W., Tsuda, H. & Ito, N. (1986) The influence of subsequent dehydro-epiandrosterone, diaminopropane, phenobarbital, butylated hydroxyanisole and butylated hydroxytoluene treatment on the development of preneoplastic and neoplastic lesions in the rat initiated with di-hydroxy-di-*N*-propyl nitrosamine. *Cancer Lett.*, **30**, 153–160

Morimoto, S. (1996) Alteration of intercellular communication in a human urothelial carcinoma cell-line by tumor-promoting agents. *Int. J. Urol.*, **3**, 212–217

Moser, G.J., Wolf, D.C. & Goldsworthy, T.J. (1997) Quantitative relationship between transforming growth factor-alpha and hepatic focal phenotype and progression in female mouse liver. *Toxicol. Pathol.*, **25**, 275–283

Myhr, B., Bowers, L. & Caspary, W. J. (1985) Assays for the induction of gene mutations at the thymidine kinase locus in L5178Y mouse lymphoma cells in culture. *Prog. Mutat. Res.*, **5**, 555–568

Nakanishi, K., Fukushima, S., Hagiwara, A., Tamano, S. & Ito, N. (1982) Organ-specific promoting effects of phenobarbital sodium and sodium saccharin in the induction of liver and urinary bladder tumors in male F344 rats. *J. natl Cancer Inst.*, **68**, 497–500

Nandan, S.D. & Rao, M.S. (1982a) Action of phenobarbitone on human chromosomes in vitro. *IRCS Med. Sci. Libr. Compend.*, **10**, 226–227

Nandan, S.D. & Rao, M.S. (1982b) Induction of chromosome aberrations by phenobarbitone in the germ cells of Swiss male mice. *Toxicol. Lett.*, **14**, 1–6

Nandan, S.D. & Rao, M.S. (1983) Evaluation of the mutagenic effects of phenobarbital by dominant lethal assay in Swiss mice. *Fd chem. Toxic*, **21**, 335–337

Narita, T., Watanabe, R. & Kitagawa, T. (1980) Mechanisms of inhibition by simultaneously administered phenobarbital of 3'-methyl-4-(dimethylamino) azobenzene-induced hepato-carcinogenesis in the rat. *Gann*, **71**, 755–758

Natarajan, A.T., Bussmann, C.J.M., van Kesteren-van Leeuwen, A.C., Meijers, M. & van Rijn, J.L.S. (1985) Tests for chromosome aberrations and sister-chromatid exchanges in Chinese hamster ovary (CHO) cells in culture. *Prog. Mutat. Res.*, **5**, 433–437

National Institute for Occupational Safety and Health (2000) *National Occupational Exposure Survey 1981–83*, Cincinnati, OH, Department of Health and Human Services, Public Health Service

Nims, R.W., Lubet, R.A., Jones, C.R. & Mellini, D.W. (1993) Comparative pharmaco-dynamics of CYP2B induction by phenobarbital in the male and female F344/NCr rat. *Biochem. Pharmacol.*, **45**, 521–526

Nishikawa, T., Bruyere, H.J., Takagi, Y., Matsuoka, R. & Gilbert, E.F. (1987) Experimentally induced cardiovascular malformations in the chick embryo. Part III. The teratogenic effect of phenobarbital on the embryonic chick heart. *Birth Defects: Orig. Art. Ser.*, **23**, 453–458

Norwegian Medicinal Depot (2000) Oslo

Obe, G., Hille, A., Jonas, R., Schmidt, S. & Thenhaus, U. (1985) Tests for the induction of sister-chromatid exchanges in human peripheral lymphocytes in culture. *Prog. Mutat. Res.*, **5**, 439–442

Oberly, T. J., Bewsey, B. J. & Probst, G.S. (1985) Tests for the induction of forward mutation at the thymidine kinase locus of L5178Y mouse lymphoma cells in culture. *Prog. Mutat. Res.*, **5**, 569–582

O'Connor, P.J., Fida, S., Fan, C.Y., Bromley, M. & Saffhill, R. (1988) Phenobarbital: A non-geno-toxic agent which induces the repair of O^6-methylguanine from hepatic DNA. *Carcino-genesis*, **9**, 2033–2038

Ohnhaus, E.E. & Studer, H. (1983) A link between liver microsomal enzyme activity and thyroid hormone metabolism in man. *Br. J. clin. Pharmacol.*, **15**, 71–76

Okada, N., Honda, A., Kawabata, M. & Yajima, N. (1997) Sodium phenobarbital-enhanced mutation frequency in the liver DNA of *lacZ* transgenic mice treated with diethyl-nitrosamine. *Mutagenesis*, **12**, 179–184

Okey, A.B. (1990) Enzyme induction in the cytochrome P-450 system. *Pharmacol. Ther.*, **45**, 241–298

Olsen, J.H., Boice, J.D., Jr, Jensen, P.A. & Fraumeni, J.F., Jr (1989) Cancer among epileptic patients exposed to anticonvulsant drugs. *J. natl Cancer Inst.*, **81**, 803–808

Olsen, J.H., Boice, J.D., Jr & Fraumeni, J.F., Jr (1990) Cancer in children of epileptic mothers and the possible relation to maternal anticonvulsant therapy. *Br. J. Cancer*, **62**, 996–999

Olsen, J.H., Walin, H., Boice, J.D., Jr, Rask, K., Schulgen, G. & Fraumeni, J.F., Jr (1993) Phenobarbital, drug metabolism, and human cancer. *Cancer Epidemiol. Biomarkers Prev.*, **2**, 449–452

Olsen, J.H., Schulgen, G., Boice, J.D., Jr, Whysner, J., Travis, L.B., Williams, G.M., Johnson, F.B. & McGee, J.O'D. (1995) Antiepileptic treatment and risk for hepatobiliary cancer and malignant lymphoma. *Cancer Res.*, **55**, 294–297

Oppenheimer, J.H., Bernstein, G. & Surks, M.I. (1968) Increased thyroxine turnover and thyroidal function after stimulation of hepatocellular binding of thyroxine by pheno-barbital. *J. clin. Invest.*, **47**, 1399–1406

Parzefall, W., Erber, E., Sedivy, R. & Schulte-Hermann, R. (1991) Testing for induction of DNA synthesis in human hepatocyte primary cultures by rat liver tumor promoters. *Cancer Res.*, **51**, 1143–1147

Peraino, C., Fry, R.J.M. & Staffeldt, E. (1971) Reduction and enhancement by phenobarbital of hepatocarcinogenesis induced in the rat by 2-acetylaminofluorene. *Cancer Res.*, **31**, 1506–1512

Peraino, C., Fry, R.J.M. & Staffeldt, E. (1973a) Enhancement of spontaneous hepatic tumori-genesis in C3H mice by dietary phenobarbital. *J. natl Cancer Inst.*, **51**, 1349–1350

Peraino, C., Fry, R.J.M., Staffeldt, E. & Kisieleski, W.E. (1973b) Effects of varying the expo-sure to phenobarbital on its enhancement of 2-acetylaminofluorene-induced hepatic tumorigenesis in the rat. *Cancer Res.*, **33**, 2701–2705

Peraino, C., Fry, R.J.M., Staffeldt, E. & Christopher, J.P. (1975) Comparative enhancing effects of phenobarbital, amobarbital, diphenylhydantoin, and dichlorodiphenyltrichloroethane on 2-acetylaminofluorene-induced hepatic tumorigenesis in the rat. *Cancer Res.*, **35**, 2884–2890

Peraino, C., Fry, R.J.M. & Staffeldt, E. (1977) Effects of varying the onset and duration of exposure to phenobarbital on its enhancement of 2-acetylaminofluorene-induced hepatic tumorigenesis. *Cancer Res.*, **37**, 3623–3627

Peraino, C., Staffeldt, E.F., Haugen D.A., Lombard, L.S., Stevens, F.J. & Fry, R.J.M. (1980) Effects of varying the dietary concentration of phenobarbital on its enhancement of 2-acetylaminofluorene-induced hepatic tumorigenesis. *Cancer Res.*, **40**, 3268–3273

Peraino, C., Haugen, D.A., Carnes, B.A., Reilly, C.A., Springer, D.L. & Mahlum, D.D. (1987) Phenotypically selective promotion of diethylnitrosamine-initiated altered hepatocyte foci by dietary phenobarbital or a topically applied coal-derived organic mixture in male and female rats. *Cancer Lett.*, **37**, 133–138

Pereira, M.A. (1993) Comparison in C3H and C3B6Fa mice of the sensitivity to diethyl-nitrosamine-initiation and phenobarbital-promotion to the extent of cell proliferation. *Carcinogenesis*, **14**, 299–302

Pereira, M.A., Knutsen, G.L. & Herren-Freund, S.L. (1985) Effect of subsequent treatment of chloroform or phenobarbital on the incidence of liver and lung tumors initiated by ethyl-nitrosourea in 15 day old mice. *Carcinogenesis*, **6**, 203–207

Pereira, M.A., Klaunig, J.E., Herren-Freund, S.L. & Ruch, R.J. (1986) Effect of phenobarbital on the development of liver tumors in juvenile and adult mice. *J. natl Cancer Inst.*, **77**, 449–452

Pirttiaho, H.I., Sotaniemi, E.A., Ahokas, J.T. & Pitkanen, U. (1978) Liver size and indices of drug metabolism in epileptics. *Br. J. Clin. Pharmacol.*, **6**, 273–278

Pitot, H.C., Goldsworthy, T.L., Moran, S., Kennan, W., Glauert, H.P., Maronpot, R. & Campbell, H.A. (1987) A method to quantitate the relative initiating and promoting potencies of hepatocarcinogenic agents in their dose–response relationship to altered hepatic foci. *Carcinogenesis*, **8**, 1491–1499

Pollard, M. & Luckert, P.H. (1997) Phenobarbital promotes multistage pulmonary carcino-genesis in MNU-inoculated L-W rats. *In Vivo*, **11**, 55–60

Pollard, M., Luckert, P.H. & Scheu, J. (1995) Phenobarbital promotes the development of adenocarcinomas in the accessory sex glands of MNU-inoculated LW rats. *Carcino-genesis*, **16**, 2419–2431

Ponomarkov, V., Tomatis, L. & Turusov, V, (1976) The effects of long-term administration of phenobarbital in CF-1 mice. *Cancer Lett.*, **1**, 165–172

Priston, R.A.J. & Dean, B.J. (1985) Tests for the induction of chromosome aberrations, polyploidy and sister-chromatic exchanges in rat liver RL$_4$ cells. *Prog. Mutat. Res.*, **5**, 387–395

Probst, G.S. & Hill, L.E. (1985) Tests for the induction of DNA-repair synthesis in primary cultures of adult rat hepatocytes. *Prog. Mutat. Res.*, **5**, 381–386

Pugh, T.D. & Goldfarb, S. (1978) Quantitative histochemical and autoradiographic studies of hepatocarcinogenesis in rats fed 2-acetylaminofluorene followed by phenobarbital. *Cancer Res.*, **38**, 4450–4457

Ray-Chaudhuri, R., Currens, M. & Iype, P.T. (1982) Enhancement of sister-chromatid exchanges by tumour promoters. *Br. J. Cancer*, **45**, 769–777

Reinisch, J.M., Sanders, S.A., Mortensen, E.L. & Rubin, D.B. (1995) In utero exposure to phenobarbital and intelligence deficits in adult men. *J. Am. med. Assoc.*, **274**, 1518–1525

Ren, P. & Ruch, R.J. (1996) Inhibition of gap junctional intercellular communication by barbiturates in long-term primary cultured rat hepatocytes is correlated with liver tumour promoting activity. *Carcinogenesis*, **17**, 2119–2124

Ren, P., Mehta, P.P. & Ruch, R.J. (1998) Inhibition of gap junctional intercellular communication by tumor promoters in connexin43 and connexin32-expressing liver cells: Cell specificity and role of protein kinase C. *Carcinogenesis*, **19**, 169–175

Rexroat, M. A. & Probst, G. S. (1985) Mutation tests with *Salmonella* using the plate-incorporation assay. *Prog. Mutat. Res.*, **5**, 201–212

Rice, J.M., Rehm, S., Donovan, P.J. & Perantoni, A.O. (1989) Comparative transplacental carcinogenesis by directly acting and metabolism-dependent alkylating agents in rodents and nonhuman primates. In: Napalkov, N.P., Rice, J.M., Tomatis, L. & Yamasaki, H. eds, *Perinatal and Multigeneration Carcinogenesis* (IARC Scientific Publications No. 96), Lyon, IARCPress, pp. 17–34

Roberts, C.J., Jackson, L., Halliwell, M. & Branch, R.A. (1976) The relationship between liver volume, antipyrine clearance and indocyanine green clearance before and after phenobarbitone administration in man. *Br. J. clin. Pharmacol.*, **3**, 907–913

Rolin-Limbosch, S., Moens, W. & Szpirer, C. (1986) Effects of tumour promoters on metabolic cooperation between human hepatoma cells. *Carcinogenesis*, **7**, 1235–1238

Rossi, L., Ravera, M., Repetti, G. & Santi, L. (1977) Long-term administration of DDT or phenobarbital-Na in Wistar rats. *Int. J. Cancer*, **19**, 179–185

Royal Pharmaceutical Society of Great Britain (2000) *Martindale, The Extra Pharmacopoeia*, 13th Ed., London, The Pharmaceutical Press [MicroMedex Online]

Ruch, R.J., Klaunig, J.E. & Pereira, M.A. (1987) Inhibition of intercellular communication between mouse hepatocytes by tumor promoters. *Toxicol. appl. Pharmacol.*, **87**, 111–120

Rumsby, P.C., Barrass, N.C., Phillimore, H.E. & Evans, J.G. (1991) Analysis of the Ha-*ras* oncogene in C3H/He mouse liver tumours derived spontaneously or induced with diethylnitrosamine or phenobarbitone. *Carcinogenesis*, **12**, 2331–2336

Rumsby, P.C., Davies, M.J. & Evans, J.G. (1994) Screening for *p53* mutations in C3H/He mouse liver tumors derived spontaneously or induced with diethylnitrosamine or phenobarbitone. *Mol. Carcinog.*, **9**, 71–75

Ruttiman, G. (1972) Effect of phenobarbital on hepatocyte proliferation in rats following partial hepatectomy. *Experientia*, **28**, 1196–1197

Sadtler Research Laboratories (1980) *Sadtler Standard Spectra, 1980 Cumulative Alphabetical Index*, Philadelphia, PA, p. 1030

Sagartz, J.E., Curtiss, S.W., Bunch, R.T., Davila, J.C., Morris, D.L. & Alden, C.L. (1998) Phenobarbital does not promote hepatic tumorigenesis in a twenty-six-week bioassay in *p53* heterozygous mice. *Toxicol. Pathol.*, **26**, 492–500

Sanders, B.M. & Draper, G.J. (1979) Childhood cancer and drugs in pregnancy. *Br. med. J.*, **1**, 717–718

de Sandro, V., Chevrier, M., Boddaert, A., Melcion, C., Cordier, A. & Richert, L. (1991) Comparison of the effects of propylthiouracil, amiodarone, diphenylhydantoin, phenobarbital, and 3-methylcholanthrene on hepatic and renal T4 metabolism and thyroid gland function in rats. *Toxicol. appl. Pharmacol.*, **111**, 263–278

Sanner, T. & Rivedal, E. (1985) Tests with the Syrian hamster embryo (SHE) cell transformation assay. *Prog. Mutat. Res.*, **5**, 665–671

Sargent, L.M., Sattler, G.L., Roloff, B., Xu, Y.-H., Sattler, C.A., Meisner, L. & Pitot, H.C. (1992) Ploidy and specific karyotypic changes during promotion with phenobarbital, 2,5,2',5'-tetrachlorobiphenyl, and/or 3,4,3',4'-tetrachlorobiphenyl in rat liver. *Cancer Res.*, **52**, 955–962

Sasaki, Y.F., Izumiyama, F., Nishidate, E., Matsusaka, N. & Tsuda, S. (1997) Detection of rodent liver carcinogen genotoxicity by the alkaline single-cell gel electrophoresis (Comet) assay in multiple mouse organs (liver, lung, spleen, kidney, and bone marrow). *Mutat. Res.*, **391**, 201–214

Sawada, N., Staecker, J.L. & Pitot, H.C. (1987) Effects of tumor-promoting agents 12-*O*-tetradecanoylphorbol-13-acetate and phenobarbital on DNA synthesis of rat hepatocytes in primary culture. *Cancer Res.*, **47**, 5665–5671

Schaumann, B.A., Winge, V.B. & Pederson, M. (1989) Genotoxicity evaluation in patients on phenobarbital monotherapy by sister chromatid exchange. *J. Toxicol. environ. Health*, **28**, 277–284

Scholz, W., Schütze, K., Kunz, W. & Schwarz, M. (1990) Phenobarbital enhances the formation of reactive oxygen in neoplastic rat liver nodules. *Cancer Res.*, **50**, 7015–7022

Schulte-Hermann, R., Ohde, G., Schuppler, J. & Timmermann-Trosiener, I. (1981) Enhanced proliferation of putative preneoplastic cells in rat liver following treatment with the tumor promoters phenobarbital, hexachlorocyclohexane, steroid compounds, and nafenopin. *Cancer Res.*, **41**, 2556–2562

Schulte-Hermann, R., Timmermann-Trosiener, I. & Schuppler, J. (1986) Facilitated expression of adaptive responses to phenobarbital in putative pre-stages of liver cancer. *Carcinogenesis*, **7**, 1651–1655

Schulte-Hermann, R., Timmermann-Trosiener, I., Barthel, G. & Bursch, W. (1990) DNA synthesis, apoptosis, and phenotypic expression as determinants of growth of altered foci in rat liver during phenobarbital promotion. *Cancer Res.*, **50**, 5127–5135

Schwarz, M., Bannasch, P. & Kunz, W. (1983) The effect of pre- and post-treatment with phenobarbital on the extent of γ-glutamyl transpeptidase positive foci induced in rat liver by *N*-nitrosomorpholine. *Cancer Lett.*, **21**, 17–21

Selby, J.V., Friedman, G.D. & Fireman, B.H. (1989) Screening prescription drugs for possible carcinogenicity: Eleven to fifteen years of follow-up. *Cancer Res.*, **49**, 5736–5747

Seth, P.K., Alleva, F.R., Takagi, S., Yen-Koo, H.C. & Balazs, T. (1987) Brain neurotransmitter receptor alterations in offspring of rats exposed to phenobarbital, phenytoin or their combination during pregnancy. *Neurotoxicology*, **8**, 45–53

Shankaran, S., Cepeda, E., Muran, G., Mariona, F., Johnson, S., Kazzi, S.M., Poland, R. & Bedard, M.P. (1996a) Antenatal phenobarbital therapy and neonatal outcome. I. Effect on intracranial hemorrhage. *Pediatrics*, **97**, 644–648

Shankaran, S., Woldt, E., Nelson, J., Bedard, M. & Black, V. (1996b) Antenatal phenobarbital therapy and neonatal outcome. II: Neurodevelopmental outcome at 36 months. *Pediatrics*, **97**, 649–652

Shibata, M.-A., Fukushima, S., Takahashi, S., Hasegawa, R. & Ito, N. (1990) Enhancing effects of sodium phenobarbital and *N,N*-dibutylnitrosamine on tumor development in a rat wide-spectrum organ carcinogenesis model. *Carcinogenesis*, **11**, 1027–1031

Shimo, T., Mitsumori, K., Onodera, H., Yasuhara, K., Kitaura, K., Takahashi, M., Kanno, J. & Hayashi, Y. (1994) Synergetic effects of phenobarbital and thiourea on proliferative lesions in the rat liver. *Cancer Lett.*, **81**, 45–52

Shinozuka, H., Lombardi, B. & Abanobi, S.E. (1982) A comparative study of the efficacy of four barbiturates as promoters of the development of γ-glutamyltranspeptidase-positive foci in the liver of carcinogen treated rats. *Carcinogenesis*, **3**, 1017–1020

Shirai, T., Lee, M.-S., Wang, C.Y. & King, C.M. (1981) Effects of partial hepatectomy and dietary phenobarbital on liver and mammary tumorigenesis by two *N*-hydroxy-*N*-acyl-aminobiphenyls in female CD rats. *Cancer Res.*, **41**, 2450–2456

Shirai, T., Imaida, K., Ohshima, M., Fukushima, S., Lee, M.-S., King, C.M. & Ito, N. (1985) Different responses to phenobarbital promotion in the development of γ-glutamyltrans-peptidase-positive foci in the liver of rats initiated with diethylnitrosamine, *N*-hydroxy-2-acetyl-aminofluorene and aflatoxin B1. *Jpn. J. Cancer Res. (Gann)*, **6**, 16–19

Shirai, T., Masuda, A., Imaida, K, M., Ogiso, T. & Ito, N. (1988) Effects of phenobarbital and carbazole on carcinogenesis of the lung, thyroid, kidney, and bladder of rats pretreated with N-bis(2-hydroxypropyl)nitrosamine. *Jpn. J. Cancer Res. (Gann)*, **79**, 460–465

Shirts, S.B., Annegers, J.F., Hauser, W.A. & Kurland, L.T. (1986) Cancer incidence in a cohort of patients with seizure disorders. *J. natl Cancer Inst.*, **77**, 83–87

Siglin, J.C., Weghorst, C.M. & Klaunig, J.E. (1991) Role of hepatocyte proliferation in alpha-hexachlorocyclohexane and phenobarbital tumor promotion in B6C3F1 mice. *Prog. Clin. Biol. Res.*, **369**, 407–416

Sills, R., Goldsworthy, T.L. & Sleight, S.D. (1994) Tumor-promoting effects of 2,3,7,8-tetra-chlorodibenzo-*p*-dioxin and phenobarbital in initiated weanling Sprague-Dawley rats: A quantitative, phenotypic, and *ras* p21 protein study. *Toxicol. Pathol.*, **22**, 270–281

Sina, J.F., Bean, C.L., Dysart, G.R., Taylor, V.I. & Bradley, M.O. (1983) Evaluation of the alkaline elution/rat hepatocyte assay as a predictor of carcinogenic/mutagenic potential. *Mutat. Res.*, **113**, 357–391

Smith, P.F., O'Brien, K.A. & Keenan, K.P. (1991) Evaluation of bromodeoxyuridine labeling in hepatomegaly produced by peroxisomal proliferation or P-450 induction in rodents. *Prog. clin biol. Res.*, **369**, 285–289

Society of Japanese Pharmacopoeia (1996) *The Japanese Pharmacopoeia JP XIII*, 13th Ed., Tokyo, pp. 561–562

Soine, W.H., Soine, P.J., England, T.M., Ferkany, J.W. & Agriesti, B.E. (1991) Identification of phenobarbital N-glucosides as urinary metabolites of phenobarbital in mice. *J. pharm. Sci.*, **80**, 99–103

Spanish Medicines Agency (2000) Madrid

Stecher, P.G., ed. (1968) *The Merck Index*, 8th Ed., Rahway, NJ, Merck & Co., pp.119, 809

Steingart, R.A., Barg, J., Maslaton, J., Nesher, M. & Yanai, J. (1998) Pre-and postsynaptic alterations in the septohippocampal cholinergic innervations after prenatal exposure to drugs. *Brain Res. Bull.*, **46**, 203–209

Strauss, B., Rabkin, F., Sagher, D. & Moore, P. (1982) The role of DNA polymerase in base substitution mutagenesis on noninstructional templates. *Biochimie*, **64**, 829–838

Styles, J.A., Clay, P. & Cross, M.F. (1985) Assays for the induction of gene mutations at the thymidine kinase and the $Na^{+/K+}$ ATPase loci in two different mouse lymphoma cell lines in culture. *Prog. Mutat. Res.*, **5**, 587–596

Sugie, S., Mori, H. & Takahashi, M. (1987) Effect of *in vivo* exposure to the liver tumor promoters phenobarbital or DDT on the gap junctions of rat hepatocytes: A quantitative freeze-fracture analysis. *Carcinogenesis*, **8**, 45–51

Sugie, S., Tanaka, T., Shima, H., Shinoda, T., Mori, H. & Muto, Y. (1994) Effects of a synthetic polyprenoic acid (E-5166) on the gap junction of rat hepatocytes treated with liver tumor promoters, phenobarbital, and *p,p'*-dichlorodiphenyltrichloroethane. *Toxicol. Pathol.*, **22**, 398–403

Sugie, S., Okamoto, K., Ohnishi, M., Makita, H., Kawamori, T., Watanabe, T., Tanaka, T., Nakamura, Y.K., Nakamura, Y., Tomita, I. & Mori, H. (1997) Suppressive effects of S-methyl methanethiosulfonate on promotion stage of diethylnitrosamine-initiated and phenobarbital-promoted hepatocarcinogenesis model. *Jpn. J. Cancer Res.*, **88**, 5–11

Sullivan, F. M. & McElhatton, P.R. (1975) Teratogenic activity of the antiepileptic drugs phenobarbital, phenytoin, and primidone in mice. *Toxicol. appl. Pharmacol.*, **34**, 271–282

Swenberg, J.A., Petzold, G.L. & Harbach, P.R. (1976) *In vitro* DNA damage/alkaline elution assay for predicting carcinogenic potential. *Biochem. biophys. Res. Commun.*, **72**, 732–738

Swiss Pharmaceutical Society, ed. (2000) *Index Nominum, International Drug Directory*, 16th Ed., Stuttgart, Medpharm Scientific Publishers [MicroMedex Online]

Takagi, S., Alleva, F.R., Seth, P.K. & Balazs, T. (1986) Delayed development of reproductive functions and alteration of dopamine receptor binding in hypothalamus of rats exposed prenatally to phenytoin and phenobarbital. *Toxicol. Lett.*, **34**, 107–113

Takagi, H., Sharp, R., Takayama, H., Anver, M.R., Ward, J.M. & Merlino, G. (1993) Collaboration between growth factors and diverse chemical carcinogens in hepatocarcinogenesis of transforming growth factor α transgenic mice. *Cancer Res.*, **53**, 4329–4336

Takahashi, M., Kokubo, T., Furukawa, F. & Kurokawa, Y. (1984) Effects of sodium chloride, saccharin, phenobarbital and aspirin on gastric carcinogenesis in rats after initiation with *N*-methyl-*N'*-nitro-*N*-nitrosoguanidine. *Gann*, **75**, 494–501

Tamano, S., Merlino, G.T. & Ward, J.M. (1994) Rapid development of hepatic tumors in transforming growth factor α transgenic mice associated with increased cell proliferation in precancerous hepatocellular lesions initiated by *N*-nitrosodiethylamine and promoted by phenobarbital. *Carcinogenesis*, **15**, 1791–1798

Tanaka, T., Mori, H. & Williams, G.M. (1987) Enhancement of dimethylnitrosamine-initiated hepatocarcinogenesis in hamsters by subsequent administration of carbon tetrachloride but not phenobarbital or p,p′-dichlorodiphenyltrichloroethane. *Carcinogenesis*, **8**, 1171–1178

Tang, B.K., Kalow, W. & Grey, A.A. (1979) Metabolic fate of phenobarbital in man. *N*-Glucoside formation. *Drug Metab. Disposition*, **7**, 315–318

Tavoloni, N., Jones, M.J.T. & Berk, P.D. (1983) Dose-related effects of phenobarbital on hepatic microsomal enzymes. *Proc. Soc. exp. Biol. Med.*, **174**, 20–27

Thorgeirsson, S.S. & Santoni-Rugiu, E. (1996) Transgenic mouse models in carcinogenesis: Interaction of c-*myc* with transforming growth factor α and hepatocyte growth factor in hepatocarcinogenesis. *Br. J. clin. Pharmacol.*, **42**, 43–52

Thorgeirsson, S.S., Santoni-Rugiu, E., Davis, C.D. & Snyderwine, E.G. (1997) Hepatic tumor induction in c-*myc* monotransgenic and TGF-α/c-*myc* double-transgenic mice. *Arch. Toxicol.*, **Suppl. 19**, 359–366

Thorp, J.A., O'Connor, M., Jones, A.M.H., Hoffman, E.L. & Belden, B. (1999) Dose perinatal phenobarbital exposure affect development outcome at age 2? *Am. J. Perinatol.*, **16**, 51–60

Thorpe, E. & Walker, A.I.T. (1973) The toxicology of dieldrin (HEOD). II. Comparative long-term oral toxicity studies in mice with dieldrin, DDT, phenobarbitone, β-BHC and γ-BHC. *Food Cosmet. Toxicol.*, **11**, 433–442

Tice, R.R., Costa, D.L. & Drew, R.T. (1980) Cytogenetic effects of inhaled benzene in murine bone marrow: Induction of sister chromatid exchanges, chromosomal aberrations, and cellular proliferation inhibition in DBA/2 mice. *Proc. natl Acad. Sci. USA*, **77**, 2148–2152

Topham, J.C. (1980) Do induced sperm-head abnormalities in mice specifically identify mammalian mutagens rather than carcinogens? *Mutat. Res.*, **74**, 379–387

Traul, K.A., Hink, R.J., Jr, Kachevsky, V. & Wolff, J.S., III (1981) Two-stage carcinogenesis in vitro: Transformation of 3-methylcholanthrene-initiated Rauscher murine leukemia virus-infected rat embryo cells by diverse tumor promoters. *J. natl Cancer Inst.*, **66**, 171–175

Treston, A.M., Philippides, A., Jacobsen, N.W., Eadie, M.J. & Hooper, W.D. (1987) Identification and synthesis of O-methylcatechol metabolites of phenobarbital and some *N*-alkyl derivatives. *J. pharm. Sci.*, **76**, 496–501

Trottier, E., Belzil, A., Stoltz, C. & Anderson, A. (1995) Localization of a phenobarbital-responsible element (PBRE) in the 5′-flanking region of the rat CYP2B2 gene. *Gene*, **158**, 263–268

Tsuchiya, E., Concetti, H.F., Sugano, H. & Kitagawa, T. (1984) Lack of promotion effect of phenobarbital on pulmonary tumorigenesis in DDY mice initiated by transplacental exposure to 1-ethyl-1-nitrosourea. *Gann*, **75**, 305–310

Tsuda, H., Asamoto, M., Ogiso, T., Inoue, T., Ito, N. & Nagano, M. (1988) Dose-dependent induction of liver and thyroid neoplastic lesions by short-term administration of 2-amino-3-methylimidazo[4,5-*f*]quinoline combined with partial hepatectomy followed by phenobarbital or low dose 3′-methyl-4-dimethylaminoazobenzene promotion. *Jpn. J. Cancer Res. (Gann)*, **79**, 691–697

Uchida, E. & Hirono, I. (1979) Effect of phenobarbital on induction of liver and lung tumors by dimethylnitrosamine in newborn mice. *Gann*, **70**, 639–644

Uchida, E. & Hirono, I. (1981) Effect of phenobarbital on the development of neoplastic lesions in the liver of cycasin-treated rats. *J. Cancer Res. clin. Oncol.*, **100**, 231–238

Umeda, M., Noda, K. & Ono, T. (1980) Inhibition of metabolic cooperation in Chinese hamster cells by various chemicals including tumor promoters. *Jpn. J. Cancer Res.*, **71**, 614–620

Umeda, M., Noda, K. & Tanaka, K. (1985) Assays for inhibition of metabolic cooperation by a microassay method. *Prog. Mutat. Res.*, **5**, 619–622

US Pharmacopeial Convention (1999) *The 2000 US Pharmacopeia*, 24th rev./*The National Formulary*, 19th rev., Rockville, MD, pp. 1305–1308, 2284

Uwagawa, S., Tsuda, H., Ozaki, K., Takahashi, S., Yamaguchi, S., Mutai, M., Aoki, T. & Ito, N. (1992) Modifying effects of various chemicals on tumor development in a rat wide-spectrum organ carcinogenesis model. *Jpn. J. Cancer Res.*, **83**, 812–820

Vidal (2000) *Le Dictionnaire*, Paris, Editions du Vidal

Viollon-Abadie, C., Lassere, D., Debruyne, E., Nicod, L., Carmichael, N. & Richert, L. (1999) Phenobarbital, β-naphthoflavone, clofibrate, and pregnenolone-16α-carbonitrile do not affect hepatic thyroid hormone UDP-glucuronosyl transferase activity, and thyroid gland function in mice. *Toxicol. appl. Pharmacol.*, **155**, 1–12

Vogel, E.W. (1985) The *Drosophila* somatic recombination and mutation assay (SRM) using the *white-coral* somatic eye color system. *Prog. Mutat. Res.*, **5**, 313–317

Vorhees, C.V. (1983) Fetal anticonvulsant syndrome in rats: Dose– and period–response relationships of prenatal diphenylhydantoin, trimethadione and phenobarbital exposure on the structural and functional development of the offspring. *J. Pharmacol. exp. Ther.*, **227**, 274–287

Walker, B.E. & Patterson, A. (1974) Induction of cleft palate in mice by tranquilizers and barbiturates. *Teratology*, **10**, 159–164

Walker, V.E. & Swenberg, J.A. (1989) Phenobarbital lacks promoting activity for neurogenic tumors in F344 rats transplacentally exposed to ethylnitrosourea. *J. Neuropathol. exp. Neurol.*, **48**, 263–269

Wang, C.Y., Garner, C.D. & Hirose, M. (1983) Effect of phenobarbital on the carcinogenesis of N-[4-(5-nitro-2-furyl)-2-thiazol]formamide in rats. *Cancer Lett.*, **19**, 305–310

Wani, J.H., Agrawal, A.K. & Sharpiro, B.H. (1996) Neonatal phenobarbital-induced persistent alterations in plasma testosterone profiles and testicular function. *Toxicol. appl. Pharmacol.*, **137**, 295–300

Ward, J.M. (1983) Increased susceptibility of livers of aged F344/NCr rats to the effects of phenobarbital on the incidence, morphology, and histochemistry of hepatocellular foci and neoplasms. *J. natl Cancer Inst.*, **71**, 815–823

Ward, J.M. & Ohshima, M. (1985) Evidence for lack of promotion of the growth of the common naturally occurring basophilic focal hepatocellular proliferative lesions in aged F344/NCr rats by phenobarbital. *Carcinogenesis*, **6**, 1255–1259

Watanabe, K. & Williams, G.M. (1978) Enhancement of rat hepatocellular-altered foci by the liver tumor promoter phenobarbital: Evidence that foci are precursors of neoplasms and that the promoter acts on carcinogen-induced lesions. *J. natl Cancer Inst.*, **61**, 1311–1314

Waxman, D.J. & Azaroff, L. (1992) Phenobarbital induction of cytochrome *P*-450 gene expression. *Biochem. J.*, **281**, 577–592

Weghorst, C.M. & Klaunig, J.E. (1989) Phenobarbital promotion in diethylnitrosamine-initiated infant B6C3F1 mice: Influence of gender. *Carcinogenesis*, **10**, 609–612

Weghorst, C.M., Pereira, M.A. & Klaunig, J.E. (1989) Strain differences in hepatic tumor promotion by phenobarbital in diethylnitrosamine- and dimethylnitrosamine-initiated infant male mice. *Carcinogenesis*, **10**, 1409–1412

Weghorst, C.M., Devor, D.E., Henneman, J.R. & Ward, J.M. (1994) Promotion of hepatocellular foci and adenomas by di(2-ethylhexyl)phthalate and phenobarbital in C3H/HeNCr mice following exposure to *N*-nitrosodiethylamine at 15 days of age. *Exp. Toxicol. Pathol.*, **45**, 423–431

White, S.J., McLean, A.E.M. & Howland, C. (1979) Anticonvulsant drugs and cancer: A cohort study in patients with severe epilepsy. *Lancet*, **ii**, 458–461

Whysner, J., Montandon, F., McClain, R.M., Downing, J., Verna, L.K., Steward, R.E., 3rd & Williams, G.M. (1998) Absence of DNA adduct formation by phenobarbital, polychlorinated biphenyls, and chlordane in mouse liver using the ^{32}P-postlabeling assay. *Toxicol. appl. Pharmacol.*, **148**, 14–23

Williams, G.M. (1980) Classification of genotoxic and epigenetic hepatocarcinogens using liver culture assays. *Ann. N.Y. Acad. Sci.*, **349**, 273–282

Williams, G.M. & Furuya, K. (1984) Distinction between liver neoplasm promoting and syncarcinogenic effects demonstrated by exposure to phenobarbital or diethylnitrosamine either before or after N-2-fluorenylacetamide. *Carcinogenesis*, **5**, 171–174

Williams, G.M., Tong, C. & Ved Brat, S. (1985) Tests with the rat hepatocyte primary culture/DNA-repair test. *Prog. Mutat. Res.*, **5**, 341–345

Wolff, G.L., Morrissey, R.L. & Chen, J.J. (1986) Amplified response to phenobarbital promotion of hepatocarcinogenesis in obese yellow $^{Any/}$A (C3H × VY) F1 hybrid mice. *Carcinogenesis*, **7**, 1895–1898

Würgler, F.E., Graf, U. & Frei, H. (1985) Somatic mutation and recombination test in wings of *Drosophila melanogaster*. *Prog. Mutat. Res.*, **5**, 325–340

Xu, Y.-H., Campbell, H.A., Sattler, G.L., Hendrich, S., Maronpot, R., Sato, K. & Pitot, H.C. (1990) Quantitative stereological analysis of the effects of age and sex on multistage hepatocarcinogenesis in the rat by use of four cytochemical markers. *Cancer Res.*, **50**, 472–479

Xu, Y.-D., Dragan, Y.P., Young, T. & Pitot, H.C. (1991) The effect of the format of administration and the total dose of phenobarbital on altered hepatic foci following initiation in female rats with diethylnitrosamine. *Carcinogenesis*, **12**, 1009–1016

Yaffe, S.J. & Dorn, L.D. (1991) Critical periods of neuroendocrine development: Effects of prenatal xenobiotics. *Adv. exp. Med. Biol.*, **296**, 81–89

Yanai, J., Rosselli-Austin, L. & Tabakoff, B. (1979) Neuronal deficits in mice following prenatal exposure to phenobarbital. *Exp. Neurol.*, **64**, 237–244

Yanai, J., Fares, F., Gavish, M., Greenfeld, Z., Katz, Y., Marcovici, B.G., Pick, C.G., Rogel-Fuchs, Y. & Weizman, A. (1989) Neural and behavioral alterations after early exposure to phenobarbital. *Neurotoxicology*, **10**, 543–554

Yüksel, A., Kartal, A., Cenani, A. & Yalçin, E. (1993) Serum thyroid hormones and pituitary response to thyrotropin-releasing hormone in epileptic children receiving anti-epileptic medication. *Acta paediat. Jpn.*, **35**, 108–112

Zangar, R.C., Springer, D.L. & Buhler, D.R. (1993) Alternations in cytochrome p-450 levels in adult rats following neonatal exposure to xenobiotics. *J. Toxicol. environ. Health*, **38**, 43–55

Zangar, R.C., Buhler, D.R. & Springer, D.L. (1995) Neonatal exposure to xenobiotics alters adult hepatic protein kinase c alpha levels and testosterone metabolism: Differential effects by diethylstilbestrol and phenobarbital. *J. Toxicol. environ. Health*, **45**, 47–58

Zbinden, G. (1988) Evaluation of thyroid gland activity by hormone assays and flow cytometry in rats. *Exp. Cell Biol.*, **56**, 196–200

Zeiger, E. & Haworth, S. (1985) Tests with a preincubation modification of the *Salmonella/* microsome assay. *Prog. Mutat. Res.*, **5**, 187–199

Zeilmaker, M.J. & Yamasaki, H. (1986) Inhibition of junctional intercellular communication as a possible short-term test to detect tumor-promoting agents: Results with nine chemicals tested by dye transfer assay in Chinese hamster V79 cells. *Cancer Res.*, **46**, 6180–6186

Zelko, I. & Negishi, M. (2000) Phenobarbital-elicited activation of nuclear receptor CAR in induction of cytochrome P450 genes. *Biochem. Biophys. Res. Commun.*, **277**, 1–6

ANTIFUNGAL AGENT

GRISEOFULVIN

This substance was considered by previous working groups, in 1975 (IARC, 1976) and 1987 (IARC, 1987). Since that time, new data have become available, and these have been incorporated into the monograph and taken into consideration in the present evaluation.

1. Exposure Data

1.1 Chemical and physical data

1.1.1 *Nomenclature*

Chem. Abstr. Serv. Reg. No.: 126-07-8
Deleted CAS Nos: 8027-03-0; 8055-10-5; 3426-54-8; 11103-62-1; 24659-79-8
Chem. Abstr. Name: (1'S,6'R)-7-Chloro-2',4,6-trimethoxy-6'-methylspiro[benzo-furan-2(3H),1'-[2]cyclohexene]-3,4'-dione
IUPAC Systematic Name: 7-Chloro-2',4,6-trimethoxy-6'β-methylspiro[benzo-furan-2(3H),1'-[2]cyclohexene]-3,4'-dione
Synonyms: (2S,4'R)-7-Chloro-2',4,6-trimethoxy-4'-methylspiro[benzofuran-2-(3H),3'-cyclohexene]-3,6'-dione; (1'S-trans)-7-chloro-2',4,6-trimethoxy-6'-methyl-spiro[benzofuran-2(3H),1'-[2]cyclohexene]-3,4'-dione; (+)-griseofulvin; (+)-7-chloro-4,6-dimethoxycoumaran-3-one-2-spiro-1'-(2'-methoxy-6'-methylcyclohex-2'-en-4'-one)

1.1.2 *Structural and molecular formulae and relative molecular mass*

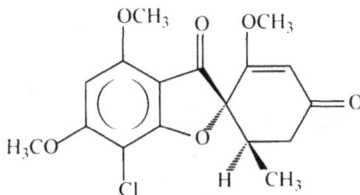

$C_{17}H_{17}ClO_6$ Relative molecular mass: 352.77

1.1.3   *Chemical and physical properties of the pure substance*

(*a*) *Description*: White to creamy- or yellowish-white, crystalline powder (Townley, 1979; Royal Pharmaceutical Society of Great Britain, 2000)

(*b*) *Melting-point*: 220 °C (Lide & Milne, 1996)

(*c*) *Spectroscopy data*: Infrared [prism/grating (72624)], ultraviolet (40309), nuclear magnetic resonance [proton (45536)] and mass spectral data have been reported (Sadtler Research Laboratories, 1995; Lide & Milne, 1996).

(*d*) *Solubility*: Very slightly soluble in water (0.2 g/L at 25 °C); sparingly soluble in ethanol and methanol; soluble in acetone, chloroform and dimethyl-formamide (Townley, 1979; Council of Europe, 1997; US Pharmacopeial Convention, 1999; Royal Pharmaceutical Society of Great Britain, 2000)

(*e*) *Optical rotation*: $[\alpha]_D^{17}$, +376 ° (Lide & Milne, 1996)

1.1.4   Technical products and impurities

To enhance its water solubility and bioavailability in pharmaceutical preparations, griseofulvin is mixed with a non-toxic, water-soluble polymer such as polyvinylpyrrolidone or hydroxypropyl cellulose and spray-dried before treatment with a wetting agent such as sodium lauryl sulfate on benzalkonium chloride. The resulting material is characterized as 'microsize' or 'ultramicrosize' crystals of griseofulvin (Martin & Tsuk, 1982).

The European Pharmacopoeia (Council of Europe, 1997) specifies that the particles of the powder are generally up to 5 μm in maximum dimension, although larger particles, which may occasionally exceed 30 μm, may be present; the *US Pharmacopeia* describes material with a predominance of particles of the order of 4 μm in diameter (US Pharmacopeial Convention, 1998).

Griseofulvin is commercially available as tablets containing 250 or 500 mg micro-size or 125, 165, 250 or 330 mg ultramicrosize crystals of griseofulvin, as capsules containing 250 mg microsize griseofulvin and as an oral suspension containing 125 mg/5 mL microsize griseofulvin (Medical Economics Co., 1999a,b; American Hospital Formulary Service, 2000).

The inactive ingredients in griseofulvin tablet formulations may also include calcium stearate, corn starch, colloidal silicon dioxide, lactose monohydrate, magnesium stearate, methylcellulose, methylparaben, polyethylene glycol, titanium dioxide, titanium oxide or wheat gluten. The suspension may also include 0.2% alcohol, dibasic calcium phosphate, docusate sodium, FD&C Red No. 40, FD&C Yellow No. 6, flavours, magnesium aluminium silicate, menthol, propylene glycol, propylparaben, saccharin sodium, simethicone emulsion, sodium alginate or sucrose (Medical Economics Co., 1999c).

Trade names for griseofulvin include Amudane, B-GF, Biogrisin, Curling factor, Delmofulvina, Dermogine, Fulcin, Fulcine, Fulsan, Fulvicin, Fulvicina, Fulviderm,

Fulvina, Fulvinil, Fulvistatin, Fungivin, Gefulvin, Greosin, Gricin, Grifulin, Grifulvin, Gris-PEG, Grisactin, Griséfuline, griseo von ct, Griseo, Griseoderm, Griseofort, Griseoful, Griseofulvin Capsules USP 23, Griseofulvin Leo, Griseofulvin Oral Suspension USP 23, Griseofulvin Tablets BP 1999, Griseofulvin Tablets USP 23, Griseofulvin Ultra, Griseofulvin Vetag, Griseofulvina, Griseomed, Griseostatin, Grisfulvin, Grisofulvin, Grisol, Grisomicon, Grisovin, Grisovina, Grivate, Grivin, Grizeofulvin, Grysio, Idifulvin, Lamoryl, Likuden, Microcidal, Neo-fulcin, Norofulvin, Polygris, Poncyl, Spirofulvin, Sporostatin, Sulvina, Ultragris, Ultramicrosize Griseofulvin Tablets USP 23, Vetmix Griseofulvin, Viro Griseo M and Walavin (Royal Pharmaceutical Society of Great Britain, 2000; Swiss Pharmaceutical Society, 2000)

1.1.5   *Analysis*

Several international pharmacopoeias specify infrared absorption spectrophotometry with comparison to standards and high-performance liquid chromatography (HPLC) with ultraviolet detection as the methods for identifying griseofulvin; ultraviolet absorption spectrophotometry and HPLC with ultraviolet detection are used to assay its purity. In pharmaceutical preparations, griseofulvin is identified by infrared and ultraviolet absorption spectrophotometry and HPLC with ultraviolet detection; ultraviolet absorption spectrophotometry and HPLC with ultraviolet detection are used to assay for griseofulvin content (British Pharmacopoeia Commission, 1993; Council of Europe, 1997; US Pharmacopeial Convention, 1999).

1.2   **Production**

Griseofulvin is an antifungal substance typically produced by the growth of certain strains of *Penicillium griseofulvum* (Royal Pharmaceutical Society of Great Britain, 2000). A method for the synthesis of griseofulvin from dimethoxyphenol has been reported (Pirrung *et al.*, 1991).

Information available in 2000 indicated that griseofulvin was manufactured by six companies in China, three in Japan and one each in India and the United Kingdom (CIS Information Services, 2000a) and that it was used in the formulation of pharmaceuticals by 44 companies in India, eight companies each in Germany and the United Kingdom, six companies each in Argentina, Japan and the USA, five companies each in Singapore, Switzerland, Taiwan and Thailand, four companies each in China, Indonesia, Italy and Malaysia; three companies each in Australia, Canada, Chile, Ecuador and the Netherlands, two companies each in Brazil, Egypt, Hong Kong, Mexico, New Zealand, Peru, the Philippines, Portugal, South Africa, Spain, Turkey and Viet Nam and one company each in Austria, Finland, Ireland, the Islamic Republic of Iran, Israel, Malta, Norway, Sweden and Venezuela (CIS Information Services, 2000b).

1.3   Use

Griseofulvin is an antibiotic fungistatic drug administered orally in the treatment of dermatophyte and ringworm infections. It is fungistatic against various species of *Microsporum*, *Epidermophyton* and *Trichophyton in vitro*. It is generally given for infections that involve the scalp, hair, nails and skin (e.g. tinea corporis (ringworm of the body), tinea pedis (athlete's foot), tinea cruris (ringworm of the groin or thigh), tinea barbae (barber's itch), tinea capitis (ringworm of the scalp), tinea unguium (onycho-mycosis; ringworm of the nails)) and which do not respond to topical treatments; infections of the soles of the feet, the palms of the hands and the nails respond slowly (Medical Economics Co., 1999a,b,c,d; Royal Pharmaceutical Society of Great Britain, 2000).

Because griseofulvin has some vasodilatatory activity, its use has resulted in some improvement in a small number of patients with Raynaud's disease and angina pectoris. Because it is structurally similar to colchicine and shares its activity as a metaphase inhibitor, griseofulvin has been used in the treatment of gout (American Hospital Formulary Service, 2000).

The dosage of griseofulvin varies depending on whether the drug is administered as a microsize or ultramicrosize preparation. In addition, the recommended doses of ultramicrosize griseofulvin vary slightly depending on the manufacturer and the formulation of the drug. Therapy with griseofulvin is generally maintained for at least 2–4 weeks for the treatment of tinea corporis; at least 4–12 weeks for the treatment of tinea capitis; 4–8 weeks for tinea pedis; and from 4–6 months to 1 year or longer for tinea unguium (American Hospital Formulary Service, 2000).

The usual adult dose of ultramicrosize griseofulvin for the treatment of tinea corporis, tinea cruris or tinea capitis is 330–375 mg/day in single or divided doses, depending on the manufacturer and formulation of the drug; the usual adult dose of ultramicrosize griseofulvin for the treatment of infections that are more difficult to era-dicate, such as tinea pedis and tinea unguium, is 660–750 mg/day, depending on the manufacturer and formulation. The usual adult dose of microsize griseofulvin for the treatment of tinea corporis, tinea cruris, or tinea capitis is 500 mg/day and 1 g daily for the treatment of infections that are more difficult to eradicate, such as tinea pedis and tinea unguium (Gennaro, 1995; American Hospital Formulary Service, 2000; Royal Pharmaceutical Society of Great Britain, 2000).

The usual dose of ultramicrosize griseofulvin for children > 2 years of age is approximately 7.3 mg/kg bw per day, although doses up to 10–15 mg/kg bw daily have been used. The manufacturers suggest that children weighing approximately 14–23 kg can receive 82.5–165 mg of ultramicrosize griseofulvin daily and those weighing > 23 kg can receive 165–330 mg/day. Alternatively, the manufacturers suggest that children weighing 16–27 kg can receive 125–187.5 mg of ultramicrosize griseofulvin daily and those weighing > 27 kg can receive 187.5–375 mg daily. For the treatment of tinea capitis and tinea corporis, the American Academy of Pediatrics recommends that children receive ultramicrosize griseofulvin at a single daily dose of 5–10 mg/kg bw (maximum dose, 750 mg). The usual paediatric dose of microsize griseofulvin is 10–11 mg/kg bw per day, although doses up to 20–25 mg/kg bw per day have been used. The manufacturers suggest that children weighing approximately 14–23 kg can receive 125–250 mg microsize griseofulvin daily and that children weighing > 23 kg can receive 250–500 mg daily. Alternatively, some clinicians suggest that children be given microsize griseofulvin at a dose of 300 mg/m^2 daily. The American Academy of Pediatrics recommends that children receive microsize griseofulvin at a daily dose of 10–20 mg/kg bw (maximum dose, 1 g) given in up to two divided doses (Gennaro, 1995; American Hospital Formulary Service, 2000; Royal Pharmaceutical Society of Great Britain, 2000).

When preparations, available in some countries, containing ultramicrocrystalline or ultramicrosize griseofulvin are used, the doses are reduced by one-third to one-half of the recommended doses of microcrystalline or microsize griseofulvin. Griseofulvin is probably best given with or after meals (Royal Pharmaceutical Society of Great Britain, 2000).

The duration of treatment depends on the thickness of the keratin layer: 2–6 weeks for infections of the hair and skin, up to 6 months for infections of the fingernails and 12 months or more for infections of the toenails (Royal Pharmaceutical Society of Great Britain, 2000).

Although griseofulvin is usually given systemically, beneficial responses in fungal skin infections have been reported with some topical formulations (Royal Pharmaceutical Society of Great Britain, 2000).

Griseofulvin is also used as a veterinary antifungal drug (US Pharmacopeial Convention, 1998; Budavari, 2000; Food and Drug Administration, 2000).

1.4 Occurrence

1.4.1 *Occupational exposure*

According to the 1981–83 National Occupational Exposure Survey (National Institute for Occupational Safety and Health, 2000), about 1700 pharmacists in the USA were potentially exposed to griseofulvin.

1.4.2 *Environmental occurrence*

No data were available to the Working Group.

1.5 Regulations and guidelines

Griseofulvin is listed in the pharmacopoeias of China, the Czech Republic, France, Germany, Italy, Japan, Poland, the United Kingdom and the USA and in the

European and International pharmacopoeias (British Pharmacopeia Convention, 1993; Society of Japanese Pharmacopoeia, 1996; Royal Pharmaceutical Society of Great Britain, 2000; Swiss Pharmaceutical Society, 2000; Vidal, 2000). It is also registered for human use in Ireland, Norway, Portugal, Spain and Sweden (Instituto Nacional de Farmacia e do Medicamento, 2000; Irish Medicines Board, 2000; Medical Products Agency, 2000; Norwegian Medicinal Depot, 2000; Spanish Medicines Agency, 2000).

2.   Studies of Cancer in Humans

2.1   Case report

A 48-year-old woman with a history of gastric ulcers was admitted to a dermatological clinic in Essen, Germany, with tinea affecting the skin and nails of the feet and left hand. She was treated orally with a total dose of 31 g of griseofulvin over a period of about 1.5 months. Analysis of the patient's peripheral blood did not show alterations suggestive of haematological disorders, and there was no apparent splenomegaly. Seven months later, when the woman was hospitalized after a minor traffic accident, analysis of the blood strongly suggested chronic granulocytic leukaemia. The patient was subsequently followed and treated for this condition (König *et al.*, 1969/70).

2.2   Cohort studies

Griseofulvin was included in a hypothesis-generating cohort study designed to screen a large number (215) of drugs for possible carcinogenicity, which covered more than 140 000 subscribers enrolled between July 1969 and August 1973 in a prepaid medical care programme in northern California (USA). Computer records of persons to whom at least one drug prescription has been dispensed were linked to the cancer records of hospitals covered by the medical care programme and the regional cancer registry. The observed numbers of cancers were compared with those expected, standardized for age and sex, for the entire cohort. Three publications summarized the findings for follow-up periods of up to 7 years (Friedman & Ury, 1980), 9 years (Friedman & Ury, 1983) and 15 years (Selby *et al.*, 1989). Griseofulvin was included only in the two most recent reports. In the 9-year follow-up, an excess of thyroid cancer was reported among 744 griseofulvin users (two observed cases versus 0.2 expected; $p < 0.05$), while no excess was seen for cancers at all sites (23 observed cases versus 22.7 expected). In the 15-year follow-up, no results were reported for griseofulvin, implying that no significant association was observed for any of the 56 cancer sites considered. [The Working Group noted, as did the authors, that, since some 12 000 comparisons were made in this hypothesis-generating study, the associations should be verified independently. Data on duration of use were not provided.]

3. Studies of Cancer in Experimental Animals

Griseofulvin has been evaluated previously (IARC, 1976). One new report has become available (Rustia & Shubik, 1978), and a selection of the most relevant studies from the previous monograph were re-analysed.

3.1 Oral administration

Mouse: Groups of male and female Charles River mice, 5–6 weeks of age, were fed diets containing 1% (w/w) griseofulvin of various particle sizes (regular, microcrystalline and milled) with specific surface areas of 0.41, 1.3 and 1.52 m²/g, respectively, for 12–16 months. 'Hepatomas' developed in 4/8 male and 0/9 female mice fed regular-size griseofulvin, 4/4 male and 4/5 female mice fed microcrystalline griseofulvin and 1/1 male and 3/3 female mice treated with milled griseofulvin. No tumours occurred in four male or four female controls (De Matteis *et al.*, 1966).

In the study published since the previous evaluation, groups of 30–40 male and 30–40 female Swiss mice, 7 weeks of age, were fed diets containing 0.1, 0.3, 1.5 or 3% (w/w) griseofulvin [purity unspecified] for life. The diets with the three higher concentrations were given daily for alternate 5-week periods (5 weeks on, 5 weeks off). A group of 100 male and 100 female controls received basal diet. The study was terminated at 120 weeks. A dose-related decrease in survival rate was seen in the treated groups, and 0/98, 1/38, 2/25, 20/29 and 15/18 males and 0/98, 0/38, 0/28, 15/28 and 20/23 females developed 'hepatomas' at the concentrations of 0 (control), 0.1, 0.3, 1.5 and 3%, respectively (Rustia & Shubik, 1978). [The Working Group noted that some of the tumours were described as 'less differentiated trabecular', which would be considered carcinomas under current histological criteria.]

Rat: In the study published since the previous evaluation, groups of 30 male and 30 female Wistar rats, 7 weeks of age, were fed diets containing 0.2, 1 or 2% (w/w) griseofulvin [purity unspecified] for life. Treatment was given daily for alternate 5-week periods (5 weeks on, 5 weeks off). A group of 100 male and 100 female controls received basal diet. The survival rate of treated animals was slightly higher than that of controls up to the end of the study of 160 weeks. Follicular-cell adenomas and carcinomas of the thyroid (both follicular and papillary) were found in 1/98, 4/30, 11/30 and 16/30 males and 2/99, 2/30, 8/30 and 7/30 females given the diets containing 0 (control), 0.2, 1 and 2% griseofulvin, respectively. The increases at the two higher doses were statistically significant (*p* < 0.001) (Rustia & Shubik, 1978).

Hamster: In the study published since the previous evaluation, groups of 30 male and 30 female Syrian hamsters, 7 weeks of age, were fed diets containing 0.3, 1.5 or 3% (w/w) griseofulvin [purity unspecified] for life. A group of 49 male and 49 female controls received basal diet. The study was terminated at 120 weeks, when the survival rate of treated animals was similar to that of controls. Most female hamsters had died by week 90. No increase in tumour incidence was observed (Rustia & Shubik, 1978).

3.2   Subcutaneous administration

Mouse: Random-bred infant Swiss (ICR/Ha) mice were injected subcutaneously with suspensions of griseofulvin. Doses of griseofulvin in excess of 0.25 mg on day 1 of life produced acute toxicity. After administration of 0.5, 0.5, 1.0 and 1.0 mg on days 1, 7, 14 and 21 of age, respectively (total dose, 3 mg), a higher incidence of 'hepatomas' was found in male mice alive at 49 weeks (7/16; 44%) than in solvent controls (4/48, 8%). No liver tumours were found in females (Epstein *et al.*, 1966). [The Working Group noted the inadequate survival in this study.]

3.3   Administration with known carcinogens

Mouse: Groups of female Swiss mice, 6 weeks of age, were given topical appli-cations of 240 µg benzo[*a*]pyrene followed by acetone, griseofulvin, croton oil or croton oil preceded 4 or 24 h earlier by griseofulvin. Griseofulvin had no promoting activity in skin carcinogenesis when given alone but reduced the skin tumour promoting activity of croton oil (Vesselinovitch & Mihailovich, 1968).

4.   Other Data Relevant to an Evaluation of Carcinogenicity and Its Mechanisms

4.1   Absorption, distribution, metabolism and excretion

4.1.1   *Humans*

The plasma–concentration time curve was bi-exponential in five male volunteers given 90–180 mg of griseofulvin intravenously, with a half-time of 0.7–1.7 h for the first exponent and 9.5–21 h for the second. Absorption was found to occur up to 30 h after oral ingestion of 500 mg griseofulvin, with 27–72.5% of the dose absorbed (Rowland *et al.*, 1968). Particle size, fat intake, dissolution rate, formulation and dosage all affected the degree of griseofulvin absorption (Lin & Symchowicz, 1975).

In humans, 6-desmethylgriseofulvin was the major urinary metabolite after oral administration of griseofulvin, with 48% of an oral dose recovered as the free form and 37.4% as the glucuronide conjugate. Very little was excreted as unmetabolized griseofulvin, and only 2% appeared as the glucuronide of 4-desmethylgriseofulvin (Lin *et al.*, 1973a).

4.1.2 *Experimental systems*

Oral administration of [³H]griseofulvin (9.2 μCi; dose not specified) to Sprague-Dawley rats [sex not specified] resulted in excretion of 18.2% of the radiolabel, 82% of which was during the first 48 h. A similar excretion pattern was seen after topical administration of griseofulvin, 17.6% appearing in the urine (Nimni *et al.*, 1990).

In bile-cannulated male CD rats, 77% of an intravenous dose of 7.5 mg/kg bw [¹⁴C]griseofulvin appeared in the bile and 12% in the urine. In contrast, in male New Zealand rabbits, only 11% of the dose was found in the bile and 78% in the urine. In the urine of intact and cannulated rats, two major metabolites were present, the 4- and 6-desmethyl derivatives of griseofulvin. Rabbit urine contained 6-desmethylgriseofulvin as the predominant metabolite. In rats, most of the 4-desmethylgriseofulvin appeared as the glucuronide conjugate, whereas 6-desmethylgriseofulvin occurred only in its free form (Symchowicz *et al.*, 1967).

In mice given griseofulvin orally, 34% appeared in the urine as 4-desmethylgriseofulvin and its glucuronide and 23% as free 6-desmethylgriseofulvin (Lin *et al.*, 1972).

4.1.3 *Comparison of animals and humans*

In mice and rats, 4-desmethylgriseofulvin glucuronide and unconjugated 6-desmethylgriseofulvin are the major metabolites of griseofulvin, but in humans (as in rabbits), 6-desmethylgriseofulvin, in both its conjugated and unconjugated forms, is the major metabolite.

4.2   Toxic effects

4.2.1 *Humans*

Griseofulvin therapy can disturb porphyrin metabolism in humans (Knasmüller *et al.*, 1997). A clear indication of a porphyrinogenic effect was found in a study of 84 patients, of whom 52 were receiving griseofulvin at a dose of 0.5 g three times daily for 1 month, followed by 0.5 g twice daily for 23 months. Forty-two of the patients had completed their course or were completing it during the study and had therefore been off treatment for 2–80 weeks. The total faecal porphyrin concentrations of patients currently receiving the drug were more than 2.5-fold higher than those of untreated controls, and those of patients who had finished their course were more than twofold higher (Rimington *et al.*, 1963).

4.2.2 *Experimental systems*

(*a*) *Effects on thyroid function*

Administration of griseofulvin by gavage at a dose of 100 or 2000 mg/kg bw per day to groups of 10 male and 10 female Wistar rats for 30 days resulted in a significant reduction in serum thyroxine concentrations in males at both doses. In females, a clear effect was restricted to the higher dose. Serum triiodothyronine concentrations were reduced only in the females at 2000 mg/kg bw per day. Serum thyroid-stimulating hormone concentrations were increased in both males and females at the highest dose, paralleled by a pronounced increase in thyroid gland weight (again only at the highest dose). Histopathological examination indicated the presence of follicles with high prismatic epithelial cells, but no hyperplastic changes (Sandow, J. & Rechberg, W. cited by Knasmüller *et al.*, 1997).

(*b*)   *Effects on liver*

Feeding mice a diet containing 1% griseofulvin for 5–8 days resulted in liver enlargement, porphyria and hypercholesterolaemia (De Matteis, 1966). The accumulation of protoporphyrin in mouse liver is due to decreased conversion of protoporphyrin to haem caused by inhibition of mitochondrial ferrochelatase. After feeding of 1% griseofulvin to mice, only 25% of the initial ferrochelatase activity in the liver was present after 3 days. Concomitantly, hepatic 5-aminolaevulinate synthetase activity was enhanced 6.6-fold. The effects seen in rats were much less pronounced (De Matteis & Gibbs, 1975). Griseofulvin-induced accumulation of porphyrins in mouse liver was followed by cell damage and necrotic and inflammatory processes (Gschnait *et al.*, 1975). A green pigment that inhibited ferrochelatase was isolated from the livers of mice treated with griseofulvin, which had chromatographic characteristics identical to those of *N*-methyl protoporphyrin (Holley *et al.*, 1990). In a detailed study of the dose–response relationship of the porphyrinogenic action of griseofulvin given to mice [strain not specified] at 0.1, 0.5 or 1.0% in the diet for 38–450 days, serum proto- and cycloprophyrins as well as liver protoporphyrin and liver weight were clearly increased at the two highest feed concentrations (Shimoyama & Nonaka, 1987).

Administration of a diet containing 2.5% griseofulvin to three random-bred albino mice [sex not specified] for up to 194 days resulted in accumulation of hyalin (Mallory) bodies in hepatocytes (Denk *et al.*, 1975).

Feeding a diet containing 0.5% griseofulvin for 10 days to partially hepatectomized male Sprague-Dawley rats resulted in a 26% stimulation of liver-weight gain over the regenerative response in hepatectomized controls (Gershbein & Pedroso, 1985).

Protoporphyria was also induced in CF1 mice by topical application of griseofulvin (dose not given) every other day for up to 52 days (Polo *et al.*, 1997).

(*c*)   *Other effects*

Griseofulvin has anti-mitotic properties, which were shown to be associated with binding to tubulin both in a cell-free system and in intact cells in culture. It was therefore concluded that it interfered with the normal polymerization of microtubule protein (Weber *et al.*, 1976; Wehland *et al.*, 1977). Griseofulvin was shown to interact directly with the tubulin dimer (Sloboda *et al.*, 1982). Microtubules have been suggested to play a role in thyroid secretion through an effect on colloid endocytosis

(Williams & Wolff, 1970). Contraction of microtubules is important in the process of fusion of colloid droplets and lysosomal bodies in follicular cells essential for thyroid-stimulating hormone-stimulated release of thyroxine and triiodothyronine from colloid and subsequent diffusion into the circulation (Capen, 2000).

4.3   Reproductive and prenatal effects

4.3.1   *Humans*

Fourteen volunteers were given 2 g of griseofulvin daily for 3 months. No changes in semen quality (motility or morphology) were detected. In eight men examined, no changes in the histological appearance of the testes were seen (MacLeod & Nelson, 1959).

Although there have been a few case reports, no adequate epidemiological studies on the teratogenic potential of griseofulvin in humans were available to the Working Group.

4.3.2   *Experimental systems*

High doses of griseofulvin (200–2000 mg/kg bw) given to mice simultaneously with human chorionic gonadotropin to induce ovulation caused mitotic arrest of the oocytes in metaphase I. The arrested cells could overcome the division block and form zygotes that were often polyploid. When griseofulvin was given 2 h after human chorionic gonadotropin, cell division was less affected, but the frequency of hyper-ploid cells was substantially increased. These effects were due to an action of the drug on the spindle apparatus (Knasmüller *et al.*, 1997).

High incidences of skeletal defects were reported in rats, mice, cats and dogs after administration of griseofulvin (summarized by Schardein, 1993). Some of these studies are reviewed below.

When female rats were given griseofulvin (microsize particles) orally at a dose of 125, 250, 750, 1250 or 1500 mg/kg bw per day on days 6–15 of gestation, mal-formations were observed in the offspring of dams at doses ≥ 250 mg/kg bw per day, and survival was decreased. The malformations included tail anomalies, anophthalmia, anal atresia and exencephaly (Klein & Beall, 1972). Slonitskaya (1969) made similar observations in rats given an oral dose of 50 or 500 mg/kg bw per day on days 11–14 of gestation.

Administration of micronized griseofulvin dissolved in polyethylene glycol 300 to rats at a dose of 50, 250 or 500 mg/kg bw per day [route not stated but probably oral] on days 6–15 of gestation caused a dose-related reduction in pup birth weight and in the number of live pups, while the incidence of resorptions was increased. A variety of severe vertebral and rib malformations were reported at the two higher doses [abstract only, numbers of malformations and of animals involved not specified] (Steelman & Kocsis, 1978).

A review of a number of case reports and a small study of four cats treated with griseofulvin for ring worm suggested that griseofulvin may be teratogenic in cats, causing a variety of defects in the central nervous system, the eye and soft tissue (Scott *et al.*, 1975).

4.4   Effects on enzyme induction/inhibition and gene expression

4.4.1   *Humans*

Griseofulvin affects microsomal enzymes in humans (Lapina *et al.*, 1989; Hammond & Strobel, 1990).

4.4.2   *Experimental systems*

Six mice [strain not specified] fed a diet containing 1% griseofulvin for 5–8 days had a hexobarbital sleeping time that was 55% that of 12 controls (De Matteis, 1966). Feeding of griseofulvin to mice led to hypertrophy of the endoplasmic reticulum, but no enhancement of the total cytochrome P450 (CYP) content, so that the CYP content per milligram of microsomal protein was decreased (Lin *et al.*, 1973b).

Administration of griseofulvin induced a 126-fold increase in CYP2A5 mRNA and a 10-fold increase in 7-hydroxylation of coumarin in the liver of DBA/2 mice; in C57BL/6 mice, the increases were ninefold and sevenfold, respectively (Salonpää *et al.*, 1995).

Feeding male BALB/c mice a diet containing 2% griseofulvin for 3 weeks resulted in a more than fourfold increase in liver cytosolic glutathione *S*-transferase activity (Vincent *et al.*, 1989).

Male Swiss albino mice given a diet containing 2.5% griseofulvin for 12 days showed a 50% reduction in total CYP content and a twofold increase in cytochrome b_5 (Denk *et al.*, 1977). When the same dose was given for 10 days to male CD_1 mice, similar effects were seen (Cantoni *et al.*, 1983). Denk *et al.* (1977) also showed that NADH and NADPH ferricyanide reductase activities (expressed per mg microsomal protein) were increased by 30% and 90%, as were NADH and NADPH cytochrome c reductase activities (by 150% and 275%). Decreases of 25–40% in CYP (expressed per mg microsomal protein) were seen in hepatic microsomal preparations of hyperplastic nodules that were induced by administration of a diet containing 2.5% griseofulvin for at least 6 months. These nodules also had increased activity of NADH and NADPH-cytochrome c reductase (4-fold and 1.4-fold, respectively), NADPH-ferricyanide reductase (1.5-fold) and stearoyl coenzyme A desaturase (nearly twofold). However, NADPH-supported lipid peroxidation was decreased (58%) (Denk *et al.*, 1980). Other studies in which male Swiss mice were given a diet containing 2.5% griseofulvin for 6–8 months followed by a standard diet for an additional 2 months showed induction of liver nodules, and the surrounding tissue had higher 5-aminolaevulinate synthase activity than the nodules (Denk *et al.*, 1981). The changes were more marked in control liver than in the nodules. The authors were further able to show that, with the same dose, route of administration and mouse strain, increased transglutaminase activity occurred from day 14 of treatment, continuing to day 79. The activity returned to normal when the griseofulvin-containing diet was replaced by a normal diet. Neoplastic nodules in the same livers showed similar increases in transglutaminase activity (Denk *et al.*, 1984).

Increased 5-aminolaevulinate synthetase (six- to sevenfold) was found when a diet containing 1% griseofulvin was given to mice [strain not specified] for 3 days. Rats receiving the same treatment had more than a twofold increase in the activity of this enzyme within 10 days (De Matteis & Gibbs, 1975).

Sprague-Dawley rats given a diet containing 2.5% griseofulvin for 12 days showed a 40% decrease in CYP, a twofold increase in NADPH-cytochrome *c* reductase, a 50% decrease in NADH-cytochrome *c* reductase, a 56% decrease in aryl hydroxylase and a 56% decrease in benzphetamine demethylase activity (NADPH and NADH), whereas the activity of glutathione *S*-transferase was increased twofold. Complexation of metyrapone with CYP was increased by 40% (Williams & Simonet, 1986). Rats also showed decreased activity of microsomal stearyl coenzyme A desaturase (75%) when given a diet containing 2.5% griseofulvin (Williams & Simonet, 1988).

When expression of multi-drug resistance genes was examined in male Swiss albino mice given griseofulvin at 2.5% in diet for up to 12 weeks, increased P-glycoprotein production was observed until 8 weeks. As treatment progressed, the expression began to decrease, and at 12 weeks complete loss of expression of P-glycoprotein was seen in affected cells. Northern blotting revealed increased expression of *mdr*2 (multi-drug resistant gene 2) and, to a lesser extent, increased *mdr*1*a* mRNA (Preisegger *et al.*, 1996).

Male Swiss albino mice 'intoxicated with griseofulvin' (given in feed, amount not specified) showed increased Tau (a microtubule-associated protein) mRNA expression in the liver. At 4.5 months, the expression was 30-fold higher than that in controls. The increased Tau mRNA expression was due to preferential splicing to yield isoform 1. Expression of isoforms 2 and 3 eventually became undetectable. The increase in liver Tau protein did not match the increased mRNA expression. Recovery of Tau splicing patterns occurred within 30 days of withdrawal (Kenner *et al.*, 1999).

A diet containing 0.5% griseofulvin was given to dd-Y mice for 2, 4, 6, 8 or 16 days, and the mRNA levels of selected liver, skin and peripheral blood cell enzymes were studied. In the liver, mRNA expression of δ-aminolaevulinic acid synthase and haem oxygenase-1 was increased. Similar increases were reported in peripheral blood cells. The changes in expression of these mRNAs in the skin were not significant. In liver, peripheral blood cells and skin ferrochelatase, mRNA expression remained less affected or unchanged, suggesting that inhibition of ferrochelatase by griseofulvin is post-transcriptional. The expression increased rapidly during the first 4 days, and when treament was stopped, expression began to decline to control levels. Erythrocyte protoporphyrin concentrations had increased by fivefold at 4 days and were 25-fold higher by 16 days of treatment. When treatment was stopped, the concentrations returned to control values (Inafuku *et al.*, 1999).

Genes thought to be important in hepatocellular proliferation were studied to determine their expression after exposure to griseofulvin. Male C3H mice given a diet containing 2.5% griseofulvin for 5 or 14 months had increased expression of c-*fos*, AP-1, NFκB, PPARβ, PPARγ, RARα, RARβ and RARγ. Expression of catalase, AOX, CYP4a1, the activated receptor α (PPARα) and the retinoid X receptor-α and γ (RXR) were down-regulated (Nagao *et al.*, 1998).

4.5   Genetic and related effects

The genotoxicity of griseofulvin has been reviewed (Knasmüller *et al.*, 1997).

4.5.1   *Humans*

No data were available to the Working Group.

4.5.2   *Experimental systems* (see Table 1 for references)

Griseofulvin did not induce SOS repair in *Escherichia coli* or a response in the *Bacillus subtilis rec* test, nor did it induce reverse mutation in various *Salmonella typhimurium* strains when tested either in the absence or in the presence of an endogenous metabolic system. Griseofulvin did not induce recombination or mutation in *Saccharomyces cerevisiae*, but induced DNA damage, somatic mutation and mitotic recombination in *Drosophila melanogaster*. It did not induce unscheduled DNA synthesis in primary rat hepatocytes *in vitro* or gene mutation in mouse lymphoma or Chinese hamster V79 cells. Griseofulvin induced micronucleus formation in a number of rodent cell lines and in human lymphocytes *in vitro*. In a study of micronucleus formation in isolated human lymphocytes, 99% of the micronuclei contained whole chromosomes (kinetochore-positive), indicating an aneuploidic event. In addition, griseofulvin altered the cell cycle of lymphocytes, thereby increasing the percentage of triploid cells. It induced aneuploidy in R3-5 cells *in vitro* and in mouse germ cells *in vivo*. Griseofulvin induced transformation of Syrian hamster embryo cells. It also induced sister chromatid exchange in bone-marrow cells and chromosomal aberrations in spermatocytes of mice treated *in vivo*, but it did not induce micronucleus formation in the bone-marrow cells of mice treated *in vivo*. Griseofulvin induced abnormal sperm morphology in one mouse strain but not in another.

Evidence has been obtained that griseofulvin interacts with the formation of microtubuli (Sloboda *et al.*, 1982) and can therefore disturb the correct distribution of chromosomes between daughter cells during cell division (colchicine-like effect) (Sehgal *et al.*, 1990).

Table 1. Genetic and related effects of griseofulvin

Test system	Result[a]		Dose[b] (LED/HID)	Reference
	Without exogenous metabolic system	With exogenous metabolic system		
Escherichia coli PQ37, SOS repair test	−	NT	1000 µg/test	Venier et al. (1989)
Bacillus subtilis H17/M45, rec test	−	NT	100 µg/disc	Ueno & Kubota (1976)
Bacillus subtilis H17/M45, HLL3g/HJ-15, rec test	NT	−	NR	Suter & Jaeger (1982)
Salmonella typhimurium TA100, TA1537, TA98, reverse mutation	−	−	500 µg/plate	Bruce & Heddle (1979)
Salmonella typhimurium TA100, TA1535, TA1537, TA98, reverse mutation	−	−	400 µg/plate	Wehner et al. (1978)
Salmonella typhimurium TA100, TA1530, TA1532, TA1535, TA1537, TA1538, TA98, TA1950, TA1975, TA1978, G46, reverse mutation	NT	−	500 µg/plate	Léonard et al. (1979)
Salmonella typhimurium TA100, TA1535, TA1937, TA98, TA97, reverse mutation	−	−	333 µg/plate	Zeiger et al. (1992)
Saccharomyces cerevisiae D61.M. recombination or mutation	−	NT	1600	Albertini et al. (1993)
Drosophila melanogaster, DNA damage	+		3000 in feed	Inoue et al. (1995)
Drosophila melanogaster, somatic mutation or mitotic recombination	+		3000 in feed	Inoue et al. (1995)
Drosophila melanogaster, eye, mitotic recombination	+		35.3 in feed	Rodriguez-Arnaiz & Aranda (1994)
Unscheduled DNA synthesis, primary Fischer 344 rat hepatocytes in vitro	−	NT	353	Williams et al. (1989)
Gene mutation, mouse lymphoma L5178Y cells, trifluorothymidine resistance in vitro	−	NT	150	Stopper et al. (1994)
Gene mutation, Chinese hamster V79 cells, 6-thioguanine resistance, forward mutation in vitro	−	NT	10	Kinsella (1982)
Sister chromatid exchange, Chinese hamster V79 cells in vitro	−	NT	10	Kinsella (1982)

Table 1 (contd)

Test system	Result[a] Without exogenous metabolic system	Result[a] With exogenous metabolic system	Dose[b] (LED/HID)	Reference
Micronucleus formation, Chinese hamster V79 cells in vitro	+	+	10	Seelbach et al. (1993)
Micronucleus formation, mouse lymphoma L5178 cells in vitro	+	NT	12.5	Stopper et al. (1994)
Micronucleus formation, Chinese hamster lung V79 cells in vitro	+	+	10	Kalweit et al. (1999)
Aneuploidy, R3-5 hybrid cell line in vitro	+	NT	15	Bourner et al. (1998)
Cell transformation, Syrian hamster embryo cells	−	NT	1	Amacher & Zelljadt (1983)
Cell transformation, Syrian hamster embryo cells	+	NT	8	Gibson et al. (1995)
Cell transformation, rat 3T3 cells	−[c]	NT	25	Seif (1980)
Micronucleus formation, human lymphocytes in vitro[d]	+	NT	5	Kolachana & Smith (1994)
Micronucleus formation, human lymphocytes in vitro[d]	+	NT	15.2	Migliore et al. (1996)
Gap junction intercellular communication, Chinese hamster V79 cells in vitro	−	NT	5.0	Kinsella (1982)
Sister chromatid exchange, Swiss albino mouse bone-marrow cells in vivo	+		100 ip × 1	Curry et al. (1984)
Micronucleus formation, (C57BL/6×C3H/He)F1 hybrid female mouse bone-marrow cells in vivo	−		8000 ip × 5	Bruce & Heddle (1979)
Micronucleus formation, BALB/c mouse bone-marrow cells in vivo	−		2000 ip × 1	Léonard et al. (1979)
Chromosomal aberrations, BALB/c mouse bone-marrow cells in vivo	−		2000 ip × 1	Léonard et al. (1979)
Chromosomal aberrations, Swiss mouse spermatocytes in vivo	+		500 po × 1	Fahmy & Hassan (1996)

Table 1 (contd)

Test system	Result[a]		Dose[b] (LED/HID)	Reference
	Without exogenous metabolic system	With exogenous metabolic system		
Aneuploidy, ICR mouse oocytes *in vivo*	+		1000 po × 1	Mailhes *et al.* (1993)
Aneuploidy, (102/El×C3H/E1)F₁ hybrid mouse sperm *in vivo*	+		1000 po × 1	Qinghua *et al.* (1999)
Sperm morphology, (C57BL/6×C3H/He)F₁ hybrid mice *in vivo*	+		8000 ip × 5	Bruce & Heddle (1979)
Sperm morphology, BALB/c mice *in vivo*	–		1500 ip × 1	Léonard *et al.* (1979)

NR, not reported

[a] +, positive; –, negative; NT, not tested

[b] LED, lowest effective dose; HID, highest ineffective dose; in-vitro tests, μg/mL; in-vivo tests, mg/kg bw per day; ip, intraperitoneal injection; po, oral gavage

[c] A 40-fold stimulation was reported of polyoma-virus A_2-induced cell transformation at a concentration of 2 ng/mL.

[d] Micronuclei were 94–99% kinetochore-positive in these assays.

4.6   Mechanistic considerations

Griseofulvin is reported to alter thyroid hormone homeostasis in rats. The under-lying mechanism for this effect is unknown, but it could be related to enzyme induction or to its anti-mitotic activity through tubulin binding. Chronic liver damage associated with porphyria, Mallory body formation, enhanced cell proliferation, liver enlargement and enzyme induction may all contribute to the hepatocarcinogenic effect of griseofulvin in mice.

Griseofulvin can be considered genotoxic by virtue of its ability to induce micro-nuclei and aneuploidy in rodent cells *in vitro* and *in vivo* and in human cells *in vitro*. It did not induce gene mutation in bacteria or cultured mammalian cells.

5.   Summary of Data Reported and Evaluation

5.1   Exposure data

Griseofulvin is an antifungal drug given orally for the treatment of dermatophyte and ringworm infections of the scalp, hair, nails and skin. It is also used as an anti-fungal agent in veterinary medicine.

5.2   Human carcinogenicity data

Griseofulvin was mentioned in the report of a cohort study designed to screen 215 drugs for carcinogenicity. Although an excess of thyroid cancer was reported among users of griseofulvin in a 9-year follow-up, no results for this drug were reported in a 15-year follow-up, implying that no significant association was observed for cancer at any site.

5.3   Animal carcinogenicity data

Griseofulvin was tested by oral administration in two studies in mice and in one study each in rats and hamsters. It produced hepatocellular adenomas and carcinomas in mice and thyroid follicular-cell adenomas and carcinomas in rats. The incidence of tumours was not increased in hamsters.

5.4   Other relevant data

Griseofulvin induces hepatic enlargement and accumulation of protoporphyrin in mice by inhibiting ferrochelatase. Hepatic porphyria is accompanied by cell damage, necrosis and inflammation. Administration of griseofulvin to mice increased P-glyco-protein in hepatic membranes and resulted in the formation of Mallory bodies. Griseofulvin induced the cytochrome P450 (CYP) 2A5 enzyme concentration in mouse liver. These effects may be related to its hepatocarcinogenic effects. Short-term treatment of rats by gavage caused thyroid gland enlargement, decreased serum thyroxine concentrations and increased serum concentrations of thyroid-stimulating hormone. Griseofulvin binds to tubulin, thereby interfering with the normal polymerization of micro-tubule protein.

Griseofulvin was teratogenic in rats and cats.

No data were available on the genetic and related effects of griseofulvin in humans. Griseofulvin induced sister chromatid exchange in bone-marrow cells and chromo-somal aberration in spermatocytes, but it did not cause micronucleus formation or chromosomal aberrations in bone-marrow cells of mice. It induced aneuploidy *in vivo* and *in vitro* and micronucleus formation in cells *in vitro*. Griseofulvin did not induce recombination or mutation in fungi, but it induced DNA damage and somatic mutation or mitotic recombination in insects. Griseofulvin was not mutagenic and did not induce DNA damage in bacteria.

5.5   Evaluation

There is *inadequate evidence* in humans for the carcinogenicity of griseofulvin.

There is *sufficient evidence* in experimental animals for the carcinogenicity of griseofulvin.

Overall evaluation

Griseofulvin is *possibly carcinogenic to humans (Group 2B).*

6.   References

Albertini, S., Brunner, M. & Würgler, F.E. (1993) Analysis of the six additional chemicals for in vitro assays of the European Economic Communities' EEC aneuploidy programme using *Saccharomyces cerevisiae* D61.M and in vitro porcine brain tubulin assembly assay. *Environ. mol. Mutag.*, **21**, 180–192

Amacher, D.E. & Zelljadt, I. (1983) The morphological transformation of Syrian hamster embryo cells by chemicals reportedly nonmutagenic to *Salmonella typhimurium*. *Carcinogenesis*, **4**, 291–295

American Hospital Formulary Service (2000) *AHFS Drug Information® 2000*, Bethesda, MD, American Society of Health-System Pharmacists [AHFSfirst CD-ROM]

Bourner, R.D.P., Parry, E.M. & Parry, J.M. (1998) Chemically induced aneuploidy: Investigations into chromosome specific effects in mitosis. *Mutat. Res.*, **404**, 191–197

British Pharmacopoeia Commission (1993) *British Pharmacopoeia 1993*, Vols I & II, London, Her Majesty's Stationery Office, pp. 316–317, 933–934

Bruce, R.W. & Heddle, J.A. (1979) The mutagenic activity of 61 agents as determined by the micronucleus, *Salmonella*, and sperm abnormality assay. *Can. J. Genet. Cytol.*, **21**, 319–334

Budavari, S., ed. (2000) *The Merck Index*, 12th Ed., version 12:3, Whitehouse Station, NJ, Merck & Co. & Boca Raton, FL, Chapman & Hall/CRC [CD-ROM]

Cantoni, L., di Padova, C., Rovagnati, P., Ruggieri, R., Dal Fiume, D. & Tritapepe, R. (1983) Bile secretion and liver microsomal mixed function oxidase system in mice with griseofulvin-induced hepatic protoporphyria. *Toxicology*, **27**, 27–29

Capen, C.C. (2000) Comparative anatomy and physiology. In: L.E. Braverman & Utiger, R.D., eds, *Werner and Inbars, The Thyroid. A Fundamental and Clinical Text*, 8th Ed., Lippincott Williams & Wilkins, Philadelphia, pp. 20–42

CIS Information Services (2000a) *Directory of World Chemical Producers (Version 2000.1)*, Dallas, TX [CD-ROM]

CIS Information Services (2000b) *Worldwide Bulk Drug Users Directory (Version 2000)*, Dallas, TX [CD-ROM]

Council of Europe (1997) *European Pharmacopoeia*, 3rd Ed., Strasbourg, pp. 916–917

Curry, P.T., Reed, R.N., Martino, R.M. & Kitchin, R.M. (1984) Induction of sister-chromatid exchanges *in vivo* in mice by the mycotoxins sterigmatocystin and griseofulvin. *Mutat. Res.*, **137**, 111–115

De Matteis, F. (1966) Hypercholesterolemia and liver enlargement in experimental hepatic porphyria. *Biochem. J.*, **98**, 23C–25C

De Matteis, F. & Gibbs, A.H. (1975) Stimulation of the pathway of porphyrin synthesis in the liver of rats and mice by griseofulvin, 3,5-diethoxycarbonyl-1,4-dihydrocollidine and related drugs: Evidence for two basically different mechanisms. *Biochem. J.*, **146**, 285–287

De Matteis, F., Donnelly, A.J. & Runge, W.J. (1966) The effect of prolonged administration of griseofulvin in mice with reference to sex differences. *Cancer Res.*, **26**, 721–726

Denk, H., Gschnait, F. & Wolff, K. (1975) Hepatocellular hyalin (Mallory bodies) in long term griseofulvin-treated mice: A new experimental model for the study of hyalin formation. *Lab. Invest.*, **32**, 773–776

Denk, H., Eckerstorfer, R., Talcott, R.E. & Schenkman, J.B. (1977) Alteration of hepatic micro-somal enzymes by griseofulvin treatment of mice. *Biochem. Pharmacol.*, **26**, 1125–1130

Denk, H., Abdelfattah-Gad, M., Eckerstorfer, R. & Talcott, R.E. (1980) Microsomal mixed-function oxidase and activities of some related enzymes in hyperplastic nodules induced by long-term griseofulvin administration in mouse liver. *Cancer Res.*, **40**, 2568–2573

Denk, H., Kalt, R., Abdelfattah-Gad, M. & Meyer, U.A. (1981) Effect of griseofulvin on 5-aminolevulinate synthase and on ferrochelatase in mouse liver neoplastic nodules. *Cancer Res.*, **41**, 1535–1538

Denk, H., Bernklau, G. & Krepler, R. (1984) Effect of griseofulvin treatment and neoplastic transformation on transglutaminase activity in mouse liver. *Liver*, **4**, 208–213

Esptein, S.S., Andrea, J., Joshi, S. & Mantel, N. (1966) Hepatocarcinogenicity of griseofulvin following parental administration to infant mice. *Cancer Res.*, **27**, 1900–1906

Fahmy, M.A. & Hassan, N.H.A. (1996) Cytogenetic effect of griseofulvin in mouse spermatocytes. *J. appl. Toxicol.*, **16**, 177–183

Food and Drug Administration (2000) *USFDA Greenbook of FDA Approved Animal Products*, Rockville, MD

Friedman, G.D. & Ury, H.K. (1980) Initial screening for carcinogenicity of commonly used drugs. *J. natl Cancer Inst.*, **65**, 723–733

Friedman, G.D. & Ury, H.K. (1983) Screening for possible drug carcinogenicity: Second report of findings. *J. natl Cancer Inst.*, **71**, 1165–1175

Gennaro, A.R. (1995) *Remington: The Science and Practice of Pharmacy*, 19th Ed., Vol. II, Easton, PA, Mack Publishing Co., p. 1329

Gershbein, L.L. & Pedroso, A.F. (1985) Action of drugs and chemical agents on rat liver regeneration. *Drug chem. Toxicol.*, **8**, 125–143

Gibson, D.P., Aardema, M.J., Kerckaert, G.A., Carr, G.J., Brauninger, R.M. & LeBoeuf, R.A. (1995) Detection of aneuploidy-inducing carcinogens in the Syrian hamster embryo (SHE) cell transformation assay. *Mutat. Res.*, **343**, 7–24

Gschnait, F., Konrad, K., Hönigsmann, H., Denk, H. & Wolff, K. (1975) Mouse model for protoporphyria. I. The liver and hepatic protoporphyrin crystals. *J. invest. Dermatol.*, **65**, 290–299

Hammond, D.K. & Strobel, H.W. (1990) Human colon tumor cell line LS174T drug metabolizing system. *Mol. Cell Biochem.*, **93**, 95–105

Holley, A., King, L.J., Gibbs, A.H. & De Matteis, F. (1990) Strain and sex differences in the response of mice to drugs that induce protoporphyria: Role of porphyrin biosynthesis and removal. *J. biochem. Toxicol.*, **5**, 175–182

IARC (1976) *IARC Monographs on the Evaluation of Carcinogenic Risk of Chemicals to Man*, Vol. 10, *Some Naturally Occurring Substances*, Lyon, IARC*Press*, pp. 153–161

IARC (1987) *IARC Monographs on the Evaluation of Carcinogenic Risks to Humans*, Suppl. 7, *Overall Evaluations of Carcinogenicity: An Updating of* IARC Monographs *Volumes 1 to 42*, Lyon, IARC*Press*, pp. 64, 391

IARC (1999) *IARC Monographs on the Evaluation of Carcinogenic Risks to Humans*, Vol. 71, *Re-evaluation of Some Organic Chemicals, Hydrazine and Hydrogen Peroxide*, Lyon, IARC*Press*, pp. 1181–1187

Inafuku, K., Takamiyagi, A., Oshiro, M., Kinjo, T., Nakashima, Y. & Nonaka S., (1999) Alteration of mRNA levels of δ-aminolevulinic acid syntase, ferrochelatase and heme oxygenase-1 in griseofulvin induced protoporphyria mice. *J. dermatol. Sci.*, **19**, 189–198

Inoue, H., Baba, H., Awano, K. & Yoshikawa, K. (1995) Genotoxic effect of griseofulvin in somatic cells of *Drosophila melanogaster*. *Mutat. Res.*, **343**, 229–234

Instituto Nacional de Farmacia e do Medicamento (2000) Lisbon

Irish Medicines Board (2000) Dublin

Kalweit, S., Utesch, D., von der Hude, W. & Madle, S. (1999) Chemically induced micronucleus formation in V79 cells — Comparison of three different test approaches. *Mutat. Res.*, **439**, 183–190

Kenner, L., Zatloukai, K., Stumptner, C., Eferl, R. & Denk, H. (1999) Altered microtubule-associated Tau messenger RNA isoform expression in livers of griseofulvin- and 3,5-diethoxy-carbonyl-1,4-dihydrocollidine-treated mice. *Hepatology*, **29**, 793–800

Kinsella, A.R. (1982) Elimination of metabolic co-operation and the induction of sister chromatid exchanges are not properties common to all promoting or co-carcinogenic agents. *Carcinogenesis*, **3**, 499–503

Klein, M.F. & Beall, J.R. (1972) Griseofulvin: A teratogenic study. *Science*, **175**, 1483–1484

Knasmüller, S., Parzefall, W., Helma, C., Kassie, F., Ecker, S. & Schulte-Hermann, R. (1997) Toxic effects of griseofulvin: Disease models, mechanisms, and risk assessment. *Crit. Rev. Toxicol.*, **27**, 495–537

Kolachana, P. & Smith, M.T. (1994) Induction of kinetochore-positive micronuclei in human lymphocytes by the anti-fungal drug griseofulvin. *Mutat. Res.*, **322**, 151–159

König, E., Berthold, K., Hienz, H.A. & Brittinger, G. (1969/70) Griseofulvin and chronic granulocytic leukaemia. *Helvet. med. Acta*, **35**, 103–107

Lapina, I.Z., Leshchenko, V.M., Bendikov, E.A. & Petrakov, A.V. (1989) [Detoxifying function of the liver in patients with rubromycosis during treatment with antimycotics.] *Vestn. Dermatol. Venerol.*, **4**, 51–54 (in Russian)

Léonard, A., Poncelet, F., Grutman, G., Carbonelle, E. & Fabry, L. (1979) Mutagenicity tests with griseofulvin. *Mutat. Res.*, **68**, 225–234

Lide, D.R. & Milne, G.W.A. (1996) *Properties of Organic Compounds*, Version 5.0, Boca Raton, FL, CRC Press, Inc. [CD-ROM]

Lin, C.-C. & Symchowicz, S. (1975) Absorption, distribution, metabolism and excretion of griseofulvin in man and animals. *Drug Metab. Rev.*, **4**, 75–95

Lin, C., Chang, R., Magat, J. & Symchowicz, S. (1972) Metabolism of [^{14}C]griseofulvin in the mouse. *J. Pharm. Pharmacol.*, **24**, 911–913

Lin, C.-C., Magat, J., Chang, R., McGlotten, J. & Symchowicz, S. (1973a) Absorption, metabolism and excretion of ^{14}C-griseofulvin in man. *J. Pharmacol. exp. Ther.*, **187**, 415–422

Lin, C.-C., Chang, R., Casmer, C. & Symchowicz, S. (1973b) Effects of phenobarbital, 3-methylcholanthrene and griseofulvin on the O-demethylation of griseofulvin by liver microsomes of rats and mice. *Drug Metab. Disposition*, **1**, 611–618

MacLeod, J. & Nelson, W.O. (1959) Griseofulvin and human spermatogenesis. *Proc. Soc. exp. Med. Biol.*, **102**, 259–260

Mailhes, J.B., Marchetti, F. & Aardema, M.J. (1993) Griseofulvin-induced aneuploidy and meiotic delay in mouse oocytes: Effect of dose and harvest time. *Mutat. Res.*, **300**, 155–163

Martin, F.H. & Tsuk, A.G. (1982) *Therapeutic Compositions with Enhanced Bioavailability (Patent No. 4,344,934)*. US Patent assignee: New York, American Home Products Corporation

Medical Economics Co. (1999a) Fulvicin P/G 165 & 330 tablets (Schering Corp.). In: *PDR®: Physicians' Desk Reference*, 53rd Ed., Montvale, NJ, Medical Economics Data Production Co. [MicroMedex Online]

Medical Economics Co. (1999b) Fulvicin P/G tablets (Schering Corp.). In: *PDR®: Physicians' Desk Reference*, 53rd Ed., Montvale, NJ, Medical Economics Data Production Co. [MicroMedex Online]

Medical Economics Co. (1999c) Grifulvin V tablets microsize and oral suspension microsize (ortho dermatological). In: *PDR®: Physicians' Desk Reference*, 53rd Ed., Montvale, NJ, Medical Economics Data Production Co. [MicroMedex Online]

Medical Economics Co. (1999d) Gris-PAG tablets (Allergan). In: *PDR®: Physicians' Desk Reference*, 53rd Ed., Montvale, NJ, Medical Economics Data Production Co. [MicroMedex Online]

Medical Products Agency (2000) Uppsala

Migliore, L., Cocchi, L. & Scarpato, R. (1996) Detection of the centromere in micronuclei by fluorescence *in situ* hybridisation: Its application to the human lymphocyte micronucleus assay after treatment with four suspected aneugens. *Mutagenesis*, **11**, 285–290

Nagao, Y., French, B.A., Cai, Y., French, S.W. & Wan, Y.-J.Y. (1998) Inhibition of PPARα/PXRα-mediated direct hyperplasia pathways during griseofulvin-induced hepato-carcinogenesis. *J. cell. Biochem.*, **69**, 189–200

National Institute for Occupational Safety and Health (2000) *National Occupational Exposure Survey 1981–83*, Cincinnati, OH, Department of Health and Human Services, Public Health Service

Nimni, M.E., Ertl, D. & Oakes, R.A. (1990) Distribution of griseofulvin in the rat: comparison of the oral and topical route of administration. *J. pharm. Pharmacol.*, **42**, 729–731

Norwegian Medicinal Depot (2000) Oslo

Pirrung, M.C., Brown, W.L., Rege, S. & Laughton, P. (1991) Total synthesis of (+)-griseo-fulvin. *J. Am. chem. Soc.*, **113**, 8561–8562

Polo, C.F., Buzaleh, A.M., Vazquez, E.S., Afonso, S.G., Navone, N.M. & Del Carmen Batlle, A.M. (1997) Griseofulvin-induced hepatopathy due to abnormalities in heme pathway. *Gen. Pharmacol.*, **29**, 207–210

Preisegger, K.H., Stumptner, C., Riegelnegg, D., Brown, P.C., Silverman, J.A., Thorgeirsson, S.S. & Denk, H. (1996) Experimental Mallory body formation is accompanied by modu-lation of the expression of multidrug-resistance genes and their products. *Hepatology*, **24**, 248–252

Qinghua, S., Schmid, T.E. & Adler, I.-D. (1999) Griseofulvin-induced aneuploidy and meiotic delay in male mouse germ cells: Detected by using conventional cytogenetics and three-color FISH. *Mutat. Res.*, **441**, 181–190

Rimington, C., Morgan, P.N., Nicholls, K., Everall, J.D. & Davies, R.R. (1963) Griseofulvin administration and porphyrin metabolism. A survey. *Lancet*, **13**, 318–322

Rodriguez-Arnaiz, R. & Aranda, J.H. (1994) Metabolic activation of four drugs in the eye mosaic assay measuring principally mitotic recombination in *Drosophila melanogaster*: Differences in strain susceptibility and route of exposure. *Mutat. Res.*, **305**, 157–163

Rowland, M., Riegelman, S. & Epstein, W.L. (1968) Absorption kinetics of griseofulvin in man. *J. pharm. Sci.*, **57**, 984–989

Royal Pharmaceutical Society of Great Britain (2000) *Martindale, The Extra Pharmacopoeia*, 13th Ed., London, The Pharmaceutical Press [MicroMedex Online]

Rustia, M. & Shubik, P. (1978) Thyroid tumours in rats and hepatomas in mice after griseo-fulvin treatment. *Br. J. Cancer*, **38**, 237–249

Sadtler Research Laboratories (1995) *Sadtler Standard Spectra, 1981–1995 Supplementary Alphabetical Index*, Philadelphia, PA, p. 388

Salonpää, P., Krause, K., Pelkonen, O. & Raunio, H. (1995) Up-regulation of CYP2A5 expression by porphyrinogenic agents in mouse liver. *Arch. Pharmacol.*, **351**, 446–452

Schardein, J.L. (1993) *Chemically Induced Birth Defects*, 2nd Ed., New York, Marcel Dekker, p. 374

Scott, F.W., De LaHunta, A., Schultz, R.D., Bistner, S.I. & Riis, R.C. (1975) Teratogenesis in cats associated with griseofulvin therapy. *Teratology*, **11**, 79–86

Seelbach, A., Fissler, B., Strohbusch, A. & Madle, S. (1993) Development of a modified micro-nucleus assay *in vitro* for detection of aneugenic effects. *Toxicol. In Vitro,* **7**, 185–193

Sehgal, A., Osgood, C. & Zimmering, S. (1990) Aneuploidy in *Drosophila*. III. Aneuploidogens inhibit in vitro assembly of Taxol-purified Drosophila microtubules. *Environ. Mol. Muta-genesis*, **16**, 217–224

Seif, R. (1980) Factors which disorganize microtubules or microfilaments increase the frequency of cell transformation by polyoma virus. *J. Virol.,* **36**, 421–428

Selby, J.V., Friedman, G.D. & Fireman, B.H. (1989) Screening prescription drugs for possible carcinogenicity: Eleven to fifteen years of follow-up. *Cancer Res.*, **49**, 5736–5747

Shimoyama, T. & Nonaka, S. (1987) Biochemical studies on griseofulvin induced proto-porphyria. *Ann. N.Y. Acad. Sci.*, **514**, 160–169

Sloboda, R.D., Van Blaricom, G., Creasey, W.A., Rosenbaum, J.L. & Malawista, S.E. (1982) Griseofulvin: Association with tubulin and inhibition of *in vitro* microtubule assembly. *Biochem. biophys. Res. Comm.*, **105**, 882–888

Slonitskaya, N.N. (1969) Teratogenic effect of griseofulvin-forte on rat foetus. *Antibiotiki*, **14**, 44–48

Society of Japanese Pharmacopoeia (1996) *The Japanese Pharmacopoeia JP XIII*, 13th Ed., Tokyo, p. 414

Spanish Medicines Agency (2000) Madrid

Steelman, R.L. & Kocsis, J.J. (1978) Determination of the teratogenic and mutagenic potential of griseofulvin (Abstract). *Toxicol. appl. Pharmacol.*, **45**, 343–344

Stopper, H., Eckert, I., Schiffmann, D., Spencer, D.L. & Caspary, W.J. (1994) Is micronucleus induction by aneugens an early event leading to mutagenesis? *Mutagenesis*, **9**, 411–416

Suter, W. & Jaeger, I. (1982) Comparative evaluation of different pairs of DNA repair-deficient and DNA repair-proficient bacterial tester strains for rapid detection of chemical mutagens and carcinogens. *Mutat. Res.*, **97**, 1–18

Swiss Pharmaceutical Society, ed. (2000) *Index Nominum, International Drug Directory*, 16th Ed., Stuttgart, Medpharm Scientific Publishers [MicroMedex Online]

Symchowicz, S., Staub, M.S. & Wong, K.K. (1967) A comparative study of griseofulvin-^{14}C metabolism in the rat and rabbit. *Biochem. Pharmacol.*, **16**, 2405–2411

Townley, E.R. (1979) Griseofulvin. *Anal. Profiles Drug Subst.*, **8**, 219–249

Ueno, Y. & Kubota, K. (1976) DNA-attacking ability of carcinogenic mycotoxins in recombi-nation-deficient mutant cells of *Bacillus subtilis*. *Cancer Res.*, **36**, 445–451

US Pharmacopeial Convention (1998) *USP Dictionary of USAN and International Drug Names, 1998*, Rockville, MD

US Pharmacopeial Convention (1999) *The 2000 US Pharmacopeia*, 24th Rev./*The National Formulary*, 19th Rev., Rockville, MD, pp. 788–791

Venier, P., Montini, R., Zordan, M., Clonfero, E., Paleologo, M. & Levis, A.G. (1989) Induction of SOS response in *Escherichia coli* strain PQ37 by 16 chemical compounds and human urine extracts. *Mutagenesis*, **4**, 51–57

Vesselinovitch, S.D. & Mihailovich, N. (1968) The inhibitory effect of griseofulvin on the 'promotion' of skin carcinogenesis. *Cancer Res.*, **28**, 2463–2465

Vidal (2000) *Le Dictionnaire*, 76th Ed., Paris, Editions du Vidal

Vincent, S.H., Smith, A.G. & Muller-Eberhard, U. (1989) Modulation of hepatic heme-binding Z protein in mice by the porphyrogenic carcinogens griseofulvin and hexachlorobenzene. *Cancer Lett.*, **45**, 109–114

Weber, K., Wehland, J. & Herzog, W. (1976) Griseofulvin interacts with microtubules both *in vivo* and *in vitro*. *J. mol. Biol.*, **102**, 817–829

Wehland, J., Herzog, W. & Weber, K. (1977) Interaction of griseofulvin with microtubules, microtubule protein and tubulin. *J. mol. Biol.*, **111**, 329–342

Wehner, F.C., Thiel, P.G., Van Rensburg, S.J. & Demasius, I.P.C. (1978) Mutagenicity to *Salmonella typhimurium* of some Aspergillus and Penicillium mycotoxins. *Mutat. Res.*, **58**, 193–203

Williams, M. & Simonet, L. (1986) Effects of griseofulvin on enzymes associated with phase I and II of drug metabolism. *Biochem. Pharmacol.*, **35**, 2630–2632

Williams, M. & Simonet, L. (1988) In vivo suppression of stearyl CoA desaturase activity by griseofulvin: Evidence against the involvement of lipid peroxidation. *Toxicol. appl. Pharmacol.*, **96**, 541–549

Williams, J.A. & Wolff, J. (1970) Possible role of microtubules in thyroid secretion. *Proc. natl Acad. Sci. USA*, **67**, 1901–1908

Williams, G.M., Mori, H. & McQueen, C.A. (1989) Structure–activity relationships in the rat hepatocyte DNA-repair test for 300 chemicals. *Mutat. Res.*, **221**, 263–286

Zeiger, E., Anderson, B., Haworth, S., Lawlor, T. & Mortelmans, K. (1992) *Salmonella* mutagenicity tests. V. Results from the testing of 311 chemicals. *Environ. mol. Mutag.*, **19** (Suppl. 21), 2–141

DIURETIC

SPIRONOLACTONE

This substance was considered by previous working groups, in 1980 (IARC, 1980) and 1987 (IARC, 1987). Since that time, new data have become available, and these have been incorporated into the monograph and taken into consideration in the present evaluation.

1. Exposure Data

1.1 Chemical and physical data

1.1.1 *Nomenclature*

Chem. Abstr. Serv. Reg. No.: 52-01-7
Chem. Abstr. Name: (7α,17α)-7-(Acetylthio)-17-hydroxy-3-oxopregn-4-ene-21-carboxylic acid, γ-lactone
IUPAC Systematic Name: 17-Hydroxy-7α-mercapto-3-oxo-17α-pregn-4-ene-21-carboxylic acid, γ-lactone, acetate
Synonym: 3-(3-Oxo-7α-acetylthio-17β-hydroxy-4-androsten-17α-yl)propionic acid, γ-lactone

1.1.2 *Structural and molecular formulae and relative molecular mass*

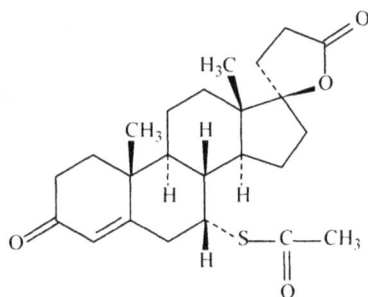

$C_{24}H_{32}O_4S$ Relative molecular mass: 416.58

1.1.3   *Chemical and physical properties of the pure substance*

   (*a*) *Description*: Light, cream-coloured to light-tan crystalline powder (Gennaro, 1995)
   (*b*) *Melting-point*: 198–207 °C, with decomposition; occasionally shows preliminary melting at about 135 °C, followed by resolidification (US Pharmacopeial Convention, 1999)
   (*c*) *Spectroscopy data*: Infrared, ultraviolet, nuclear magnetic resonance and mass spectral data have been reported (Sutter & Lau, 1975).
   (*d*) *Solubility*: Practically insoluble in water; soluble in chloroform, ethanol and most organic solvents; slightly soluble in fixed oils (Gennaro, 1995; Budavari, 2000)
   (*e*) *Optical rotation*: $[\alpha]_D^{20}$, –33.5° (chloroform) (Budavari, 1998)

1.1.4   *Technical products and impurities*

Spironolactone is available as 25-, 50- and 100-mg tablets (Gennaro, 1995).

Trade names for spironolactone include Aldace, Aldactone, Aldopur, Altex, Almatol, Aquareduct, Deverol, Diatensec, Dira, Duraspiron, Euteberol, Lacalmin, Lacdene, Laractone, Nefurofan, Osiren, Osyrol, Sagisal, SC-9420, Sincomen, Spiresis, Spiretic, Spiridon, Spiroctan, Spiroderm, Spirolactone, Spirolang, Spirolone, Spirone, Spiro-Tablinen, Supra-Puren, Suracton, Uractone, Urusonin, Verospiron, Verospirone and Xenalon.

1.1.5   *Analysis*

Several international pharmacopoeias specify infrared and ultraviolet absorption spectrophotometry with comparison to standards and thin-layer chromatography as the methods for identifying spironolactone; ultraviolet absorption spectrophotometry and high-pressure liquid chromatography (HPLC) with ultraviolet detection are used to assay its purity. In pharmaceutical preparations, spironolactone is identified by infrared absorption spectrophotometry and thin-layer chromatography; ultraviolet absorption spectrophotometry and HPLC with ultraviolet detection are used to assay for spironolactone content (British Pharmacopoeia Commission, 1993; Society of Japanese Pharmacopoeia, 1996; Council of Europe, 1997; US Pharmacopeial Convention, 1999).

1.2   Production

Spironolactone can be prepared by treating dehydroepiandrosterone (prepared from cholesterol or sitosterol) with acetylene to form the 17α-ethynyl-17β-hydroxy derivative, which is carbonated to the 17α-propiolic acid. Reduction of the unsaturated acid in alkaline solution yields the saturated acid, which cyclizes to the lactone on acidification. Bromination to the 5,6-dibromo compound, followed by oxidation of the

3-hydroxyl group to the ketone and dehydrobromination to the 7α-hydroxyl derivative, produces spironolactone when esterified with thiolacetic acid (Gennaro, 1995).

Information available in 2000 indicated that spironolactone was manufactured by two companies each in China and Germany and by one company each in France, Hong Kong, Hungary, Italy and the USA (CIS Information Services, 2000a).

Information available in 2000 indicated that spironolactone was manufactured and/or formulated as a pharmaceutical by 13 companies in Germany and Japan, nine companies in France, eight companies each in Austria, Italy and Switzerland, seven companies in the United Kingdom, six companies in India, five companies each in Spain, Sweden and the USA, three companies each in South Africa and Taiwan, two companies each in Argentina, Australia, Brazil, Chile, Colombia, Greece, the Islamic Republic of Iran, the Philippines, Poland, Portugal, Singapore and Thailand and one company each in Bulgaria, Canada, Denmark, Hungary, Indonesia, Ireland, Israel, Mexico, Norway, Peru, the Russian Federation, Turkey and Venezuela (CIS Information Services, 2000b).

1.3   Use

Spironolactone is a potassium-sparing diuretic used mainly in the treatment of oedema and hypertension. It is used in particular in the treatment of primary hyper-aldosteronism (e.g. associated with adrenal adenomas or bilateral adrenal hyperplasia) and in the treatment of refractory oedema associated with secondary aldosteronism (cardiac failure, hepatic cirrhosis, nephrotic syndrome, severe ascites).

Spironolactone is a synthetic steroid that acts as a competitive antagonist of the potent endogenous mineral–corticosteroid aldosterone. It has a slower onset of action than triamterene or amiloride, but its natriuretic effect is slightly greater during long-term therapy. By blocking the sodium-retaining effects of aldosterone on the distal convoluted tubule, it corrects one of the most important mechanisms responsible for the production of oedema, but spironolactone is effective only in the presence of aldosterone. It is a relatively weak diuretic and usually is used as an adjunct to other diuretics, such as the thiazides. When used in this combined manner, it enhances the excretion of sodium and decreases the excretion of potassium. Further increase in diuresis may be obtained by the use of a glucocorticoid with this drug in combination with another diuretic. Minor uses include the treatment of hirsutism in women with polycystic ovary syndrome or idiopathic hirsutism, and in controlling acne or other defects of familial precocious puberty (Gennaro, 1995; Hardman et al., 1996; American Hospital Formulary Service, 2000; Royal Pharmaceutical Society of Great Britain, 2000).

The usual adult oral dose of spironolactone is 25 mg four times a day; the usual range of doses is 25–200 mg/day. The usual paediatric oral dose of spironolactone is 3.3 mg/kg bw per day in divided doses. If a satisfactory diuretic effect is not achieved within 5 days, a thiazide diuretic is added to the regimen (Gennaro, 1995).

Spironolactone ranked 94th out of the 200 generic drugs most commonly sold by prescription in the USA in 1999 (Anon., 2000).

1.4   Occurrence

1.4.1   *Occupational exposure*

According to the 1981–83 National Occupational Exposure Survey (National Institute for Occupational Safety and Health, 2000), about 900 pharmacists in the USA were potentially exposed to spironolactone.

1.4.2   *Environmental occurrence*

No data were available to the Working Group.

1.5   Regulations and guidelines

Spironolactone is listed in the pharmacopoeias of China, the Czech Republic, France, Germany, Italy, Japan, Poland, the United Kingdom and the USA and in the European and International pharmacopoeias (Society of Japanese Pharmacopoeia, 1996; Royal Pharmaceutical Society of Great Britain, 2000; Swiss Pharmaceutical Society, 2000). It is registered for human use in Finland, Ireland, the Netherlands, Norway, Portugal, Spain and Sweden (Instituto Nacional de Farmacia e do Medicamento, 2000; Irish Medicines Board, 2000; Medical Products Agency, 2000; Medicines Evaluation Board Agency, 2000; National Agency for Medicines, 2000; Norwegian Medicinal Depot, 2000; Spanish Medicines Agency, 2000).

2.   Studies of Cancer in Humans

2.1   Case reports

Stierer *et al.* (1990) described 15 cases of cancer of the breast in men treated between 1972 and 1988 in Vienna, Austria. Seven of the patients (47%) had used spironolactone.

2.2   Cohort studies

Danielson *et al.* (1982) evaluated the relation between breast cancers and use of selected non-estrogenic drugs among 283 000 members of the Group Health Cooperative of Puget Sound in Washington State, USA. The information on the 302 new cases of breast cancer diagnosed between 1977 and 1980 in women aged 35–74 years was linked with an automated file of all drugs dispensed to individual members since July 1976. On the basis of 184 438 women–years of observation, the crude rate of breast cancer in non-users of spironolactone (1.6/1000) was compared with that in users (0/1000), to give an age-adjusted relative risk of 0.0 (90% confidence interval [CI], 0.0–3.0). There was a total of 634 women–years of exposure to spironolactone.

Three publications have summarized the findings at screening during follow-up periods of up to 7 years (Friedman & Ury, 1980), up to 9 years (Friedman & Ury, 1983) and up to 15 years (Selby et al., 1989) of a cohort of 143 574 members of the Kaiser Permanente Medical Care Program, whose computerized pharmacy records were available from 1969 to 1973. As of December 1984, 1 370 000 person–years of follow-up had been accumulated, and 68 695 persons (48% of the original cohort) remained active members of the Program (Selby et al., 1989). A total of 1475 users of spironolactone were identified, and 155 cancer cases were observed versus 127.4 expected (standardized morbidity ratio [SIR], 1.22; $p < 0.05$). Of the SIRs for 54 specific cancer sites and two combinations of sites examined, the only one that was significantly elevated was for 'pharynx unspecified' (20.5; $p < 0.01$; two cases observed, 0.1 expected).

2.3 Case–control studies

Ron et al. (1987) carried out a case–control study of 159 cases of thyroid cancer and 285 population controls between 1978 and 1980 in Connecticut, USA. Use of diuretics drugs was not associated with thyroid cancer. Use of spironolactone was reported by two patients and one control (relative risk, 4.3; 95% CI, 0.3–120).

Mellemgaard et al. (1994) conducted a study of 368 cases of renal-cell carcinoma and 396 population controls in Denmark between 1989 and 1992. The response rates were 76% among cases and 79% among controls. The relative risks for use of potassium-sparing diuretics (including agents such as spironolactone) were 2.2 (95% CI, 0.4–13) in men and 0.8 (95% CI, 0.3–2.2) in women, after adjustment for hypertension.

Another population-based case–control study on renal-cell cancer (Weinman et al., 1994) (206 cases and 292 controls) was carried out among members of the Kaiser Permanente Northwest Plan in the USA between 1980 and 1991 (men) or 1960 and 1991 (women). Data on potassium-sparing drugs were abstracted from medical records, and 46 users were identified among cases and 49 among control subjects, yielding a relative risk of 2.1 (95% CI, 1.3–3.6). There was no trend in risk with duration of use. According to the authors, it was impossible to disentangle the effect of potassium-sparing diuretics from that of other anti-hypertensive medications or from the effect of hypertension.

McLaughlin et al. (1995) studied 1732 patients with renal-cell cancer and 2309 non-hospital controls in five countries who were interviewed between 1989 and 1991. The response rates were 72% and 75% among cases and controls, respectively. The relative risks for use of potassium-sparing diuretics, after adjustment for hypertension, were 1.2 (95% CI, 0.7–1.8), 1.0 (95% CI, 0.6–1.6), 1.0 (95% CI, 0.6–1.7) and 0.6 (95% CI, 0.3–1.2) across four increasing levels of life-time consumption.

Yuan *et al.* (1998) conducted a case–control study on regular use of 58 diuretic and hypertensive drugs among 1204 cases of renal-cell carcinoma and 1204 neighbourhood controls in Los Angeles, USA, between 1986 and 1994 . There was no evidence that potassium-sparing diuretics were associated with renal-cell carcinoma among normotensive subjects (relative risk for heavy use versus no use, 1.1; 95% CI, 0.1–8.5). Hypertension was a strong risk factor, with a relative risk of 2.2 (95% CI, 1.8–2.6). Among subjects with hypertension, the relative risks for light and heavy use of potassium-sparing diuretics were 2.6 (1.5-4.3) and 1.8 (1.1-3.0) in comparison with subjects with no hypertension and no use of these drugs.

Shapiro *et al.* (1999) studied 238 cases of renal-cell carcinoma and 616 controls in Washington State, USA, between 1980 and 1995. The use of anti-hypertensive drugs was not associated with risk after adjustment for hypertension. Any use of potassium-sparing diuretics was associated with a relative risk of 2.0 (95% CI, 1.0-4.0) in men and 0.9 (0.4-1.7) in women, with no clear dose–response relationship. The relative risks after adjustment for hypertension were not presented.

3. Studies of Cancer in Experimental Animals

3.1   Oral administration

Rat: Groups of 36 male and 36 female Sprague-Dawley rats, 7 weeks of age, received diets providing a dose of 50, 150 or 500 mg/kg bw per day spironolactone for 78 weeks. Groups of 72 males and 72 females served as untreated controls. In a second experiment reported by the same authors, groups of 30 male and 30 female rats received diets providing a dose of 0 (control), 10, 30 or 100 mg/kg bw per day of spironolactone for 104 weeks. Both studies were terminated at the end of treatment. In the 78-week study, an excess of thyroid adenomas in both males and females and of interstitial-cell adenomas in the testis was observed at the two higher doses. The incidences of thyroid tumours in controls and at the three doses were 0/59, 4/33, 15/31 and 18/28 for males and 1/62, 1/31, 12/34 and 13/34 for females, respectively. Interstitial (Leydig-cell) tumours of the testis occurred in 0/72, 0/36, 5/36 and 12/36 males at the same doses, respectively. No increased tumour incidence was seen at these organ sites in the 104-week study at doses up to 100 mg/kg bw per day (Lumb *et al.*, 1978). [The Working Group noted inconsistencies in the effective numbers for different organ sites.]

3.2   Administration with known carcinogens

Rat: In an initial experiment, 70 female Sprague-Dawley rats, approximately 50 days of age (weight, 150–180 g), received a single dose of 40 mg 7,12-dimethylbenz[*a*]-anthracene (DMBA) dissolved in 2 mL of corn oil by oral gavage. Of these rats, 20 also received spironolactone (pharmaceutical-grade) at a dose of 100 mg/kg bw in 1 mL of distilled water by oral gavage twice daily for 7 days, starting 4 days before DMBA administration. The study was terminated 150 days after DMBA treatment, and the mammary tumour incidence determined by palpation. The incidence of palpable mammary tumours was reduced from 21/24 in the group receiving DMBA alone to 3/14 in that given DMBA plus spironolactone. In a second experiment, 80 female Sprague-Dawley rats received an intravenous injection into the jugular vein of 2 mg of DMBA in 0.4 mL of oil emulsion once daily on days 1, 4 and 7. Two days before the first DMBA injection, 40 of these rats received spironolactone (pharmaceutical-grade) at a dose of 100 mg/kg bw in 1 mL of distilled water by oral gavage twice daily for 12 consecutive days. On termination of the study 147 days after the start of DMBA treatment, mammary tumours were found at necropsy in 32/32 rats receiving DMBA alone and 23/36 rats receiving DMBA plus spironolactone ($p < 0.001$) (Kovacs & Somogyi, 1970).

4. Other Data Relevant to an Evaluation of Carcinogenicity and its Mechanisms

4.1 Absorption, distribution, metabolism and excretion

4.1.1 *Humans*

At the time spironolactone was introduced for clinical use, its bioavailability was inadequate, and this was improved by preparing the drug in finely powdered or micronized form. The absolute bioavailability was indirectly estimated at approximately 73%, which was enhanced in the presence of food. Nearly all absorbed spironolactone (> 90 %) is bound to plasma proteins and, with repeated dosing, a steady state is achieved within 8 days. After oral intake of a 100-mg dose, the plasma half-time of spironolactone was 1–2 h, the time to maximum plasma concentration was 2–3.2 h, the maximum blood concentration was 92–148 ng/mL, the area under the concentration–time (0–24 h) curve was 1430–1541 ng/mL per h and the elimination half-time was 18–20 h (Overdiek & Merkus, 1987).

Spironolactone is rapidly and extensively metabolized to compounds that are excreted in the urine and faeces. It undergoes enterohepatic recirculation, but no unchanged drug appears in urine or faeces (Sadée *et al.*, 1973, 1974a; Karim *et al.*, 1976a,b; Overdiek *et al.*, 1985; Overdiek & Merkus, 1987; Gardiner *et al.*, 1989).

The metabolites of spironolactone can be divided into two main groups: those in which the sulfur moiety is retained and those in which the sulfur is removed by dethioacetylation. For many years, it was thought that the dethioacetylated metabolite, canrenone, was the major metabolite; however, with more specific analytical methods such as HPLC, 7α-thiomethylspirolactone was recognized as the major metabolite of spironolactone (Overdiek *et al.*, 1985; Gardiner *et al.*, 1989). This metabolite is formed by hydrolysis of the thioacetate group to form 7α-thiospirolactone (as an inter-mediate), followed by S-methylation to 7α-thiomethylspirolactone. This can then be hydroxylated to form 6β-hydroxy-7α-thiomethylspirolactone and oxidized to form 7α-methylsulfinyl- and 7α-methylsulfonylspirolactone or via sulfoxidation to form 6β-hydroxy-7α-methylsulfinyl- and 6β-hydroxy-7α-methylsulfonylspirolactone.

For formation of the group of metabolites in which sulfur is removed, 7α-thio-methylspirolactone is also dethioacetylated to canrenone, which is further metabolized by three pathways: hydrolysis of the γ-lactone ring to form canrenoate, which is excreted in the urine as a glucuronic ester, and, next, hydroxylation to form 15α-hydroxy-canre-none or reduction to produce several di-, tetra- and hexa-hydro derivatives. Canrenone and canrenoate are in equilibrium with one another.

Not only spironolactone but several of its metabolites have biological activity; in decreasing order of potency, these are 7α-thiospirolactone, 7α-thiomethylspirolactone and canrenone.

4.1.2   Experimental systems

The disposition of [14C]spironolactone was studied in male rats, female dogs and female monkeys after intravenous or oral administration of 5 mg/kg bw. Gastro-intestinal absorption was estimated to be 82% in rats, 62% in dogs and 103% in monkeys. Spironolactone was extensively metabolized in all three species, and the metabolites were excreted primarily in the urine and faeces. The amount of radiolabel excreted in urine or faeces of all three species was similar after intravenous and after oral dosing. In monkeys, as in humans, the amounts excreted in urine and faeces were about equal, while faecal excretion predominated in rats and dogs as a result of biliary excretion. After the oral dose, the percentage of urinary excretion was 4.7% in rats, 18% in dogs and 46% in monkeys. The high excretion of radiolabel in the faeces of rats (90%) after intravenous administration shows the importance of biliary excretion for that species (Karim et al., 1976c). Species differences were also noted in the bio-transformation of spironolactone. Canrenone was a principal extractable metabolite in rat (Sadée et al., 1974b) and dog plasma, whereas in monkeys and humans, both canrenone and a very polar, unidentified metabolite were the major constituents. In the urine of all four species, canrenone was a principal constituent. Notable species differences in the metabolites of spironolactone in the faeces were found, the pattern of metabolites in dog faeces being markedly different from that in rats, monkeys or humans. Overall, it was concluded that the disposition and metabolism of spirono-lactone in monkeys, rather than that in rats or dogs, is closest to that in humans.

Spironolactone is metabolized by microsomal monooxygenases and is converted to a reactive metabolite that destroys microsomal cytochrome P450 (CYP) and decreases steroid hydroxylase activity. This effect is seen only in animals that produce cortisol rather than corticosterone and that have a high activity of adrenal steroid 17α-hydroxy-lase (Menard et al., 1974a,b, 1976, 1979). When spironolactone was incubated with guinea-pig hepatic, adrenal, renal or testicular microsomal preparations, 7α-thiospiro-lactone, a potent mineralocorticoid antagonist, was produced which destroyed adrenal and testicular CYP. In guinea-pig microsomes, the 7α-thiospirolactone metabolite was determined to be an obligatory intermediate in the action of spironolactone on adrenal monooxygenases, but required further metabolism for its toxicity. In contrast, hepatic microsomal CYP in guinea-pigs was not inhibited by spironolactone, apparently because 7α-thiospirolactone was not further metabolized (Sherry *et al.*, 1986). Further studies of the species difference in the effects of spironolactone on CYP showed inhibition in guinea-pigs and dogs but not in adrenal microsomes from rats or rabbits (Sherry *et al.*, 1988). Spironolactone was reported to inactivate dexamethasone-inducible rat hepatic CYP in a suicidal manner (Decker *et al.*, 1986, 1989). In adrenal glands, a good correlation was found between covalent binding and CYP destruction, consistent with the hypothesis that 7α-thiospirolactone is a suicide inhibitor of adrenal CYP and that covalent binding to protein is involved in the degradation of these isozymes (Colby *et al.*, 1991).

4.2 Toxic effects

4.2.1 *Humans*

Spironolactone is an aldosterone antagonist that acts on the mineralocorticoid receptor. It is a potassium-sparing diuretic, and hyperkalaemia is the most common and potentially serious complication of therapy. Impaired kidney function appears to increase this risk, as does supplementation with potassium chloride. Excessive diuresis can also lead to dehydration and hyponatraemia (Greenblatt & Koch-Weser, 1973). A number of endocrine effects have also been reported, the most common of which is gynaecomastia, with a dose-related incidence of 7–52%. This side-effect is reversible and disappears upon discontinuation of therapy (Jeunemaitre *et al.*, 1988; Nielsen, 1990; Thompson & Carter, 1993). Other endocrine effects include loss of sexual potency in men and menstrual irregularity, amenorrhoea, breast engorgement and chloasma in women. These effects are probably due to interaction of spirono-lactone with the antrogen receptor.

There are a few isolated case reports of idiosyncratic drug reactions, including one case of hepatitis (Shuck *et al.*, 1981) and several cases of agranulocytosis (Stricker & Oei, 1984; Jivraj *et al.*, 1987; Ferguson *et al.*, 1993; Whitling *et al.*, 1997; van der Klauw *et al.*, 1998). Approximately 10 cases have been reported of allergic contact dermatitis after topical application of spironolactone for various dermal indications involving its antiandrogen activity (Corazza *et al.*, 1996).

In an assessment of pituitary–thyroid function in spironolactone-treated hypertensive women, high doses for 4 weeks did not affect the basal serum concentrations of triiodothyronine (T3), thyroxine (T4) or thyroid-stimulating hormone (TSH) in six euthyroid, hypertensive women. It did augment the pituitary TSH and thyroid T3 response to thyrotropin-releasing hormone (Smals *et al.*, 1979). Spironolactone also had no consistent effect on basal serum concentrations of T3, T4 or TSH in healthy men who had taken similar doses of spironolactone for as long as 24 weeks (Caminos-Torres *et al.*, 1977).

4.2.2 *Experimental systems*

The acute toxicity of spironolactone was determined after administration via the oral and intraperitoneal routes in rats, mice and rabbits. The oral LD_{50} was > 1000 mg/kg bw in all species, and the intraperitoneal LD_{50} was 786 mg/kg bw, 356 mg/kg bw and 866 mg/kg bw in rats, mice and rabbits, respectively (Lumb *et al.*, 1978). Spironolactone can exert antiandrogenic effects by several mechanisms: it can destroy testicular CYP and decrease 17α-hydroxylase activity, resulting in decreased testosterone synthesis (Menard *et al.*, 1974b); and it can inhibit 5α-dihydrotestosterone binding to cytosolic androgen receptor in the prostate (Pita *et al.*, 1975; Rifka *et al.*, 1978).

Studies of toxicity were conducted in Sprague-Dawley-derived rats, beagle dogs and rhesus monkeys (*Macaca mulatta*). In a 26-week study, rats were given diets containing spironolactone at a concentration of 0, 120, 300 or 700 mg/kg for the first 3 weeks and 0, 150, 500 or 2000 mg/kg for the remaining 23 weeks. In a 78-week study, rats were given diets that provided a dose of 0, 50, 150 or 500 mg/kg bw per day; and in a 104-week study, the animals received a dose of 0, 10, 30 or 100 mg/kg bw per day. In dogs, a 13-week study was conducted, in which initial doses of 0, 12, 30 and 70 mg/kg bw per day were given in a capsule for 6 weeks and then increased to 100 mg/kg bw per day for weeks 7–9 and to 250 mg/kg bw per day for the last 4 weeks. In rhesus monkeys, a 26-week study was conducted in which the animals received a dose of 0 or 125 mg/kg bw per day in a banana sandwich, and a 52-week study was conducted with doses of 0, 20, 50 and 125 mg/kg bw per day for 9 weeks followed by 250 mg/kg bw per day for 43 weeks (Lumb *et al.*, 1978).

Rats treated for 78 weeks showed a dose-related increase in the weight of the liver at all doses, increased adrenal gland weights in males at the two higher doses and increased thyroid gland weights in males at the high dose and in all treated females. Dose-dependent decreases in prostate weights were seen in males at all doses. Similarly, in the 104-week study, liver weights were increased at all doses, and the thyroid gland weights were increased in males and females at the high dose. A slight arrest of maturation in the testis (an increased number of immature spermatozoal precursors) was noted in the 78-week study at the two higher doses. In monkeys, a slight decrease in testis weight and a slight depression of maturation was observed at the two higher doses. Although gynaecomastia occurs in male human patients treated with spironolactone, no mammary abnormalities were noted in rats or dogs, but male monkeys showed a treatment-related increase in cellular activity in the acini of the mammary gland (Lumb *et al.*, 1978).

These studies revealed marked species differences in effects on the thyroid gland. No changes were seen in dogs or monkeys treated for 3 months or up to 1 year, respectively. In rats, thyroid changes were seen as early as 13 weeks at the high dose. The thyroid gland weights were increased, and, histologically, the follicles were smaller than normal, with diminished colloid, and the epithelial cells were taller and in some cases swollen. Species differences were also noted in the liver. Rats showed increased liver weights with no histological changes, while dogs had no increase in organ weight or histological changes. In monkeys, no weight changes or histological findings were observed in females, but males had a slight increase in liver weight at the high dose with no associated histological changes (Lumb *et al.*, 1978).

Male rats were given diets containing spironolactone at concentrations that resulted in a dose of 0, 6, 50 or 200 mg/kg bw per day, for 13 weeks. Ten rats per group were killed after 2, 4 and 13 weeks of treatment for assessment of TSH, T4 and T3 concentrations, thyroid gland weights, histological appearance, thyroid iodine uptake and organification, and UDP glucuronosyltransferase (UGT) activity. After 13 weeks of treatment, the weights of the thyroid gland were significantly increased at all doses and the concentration of TSH was increased at the two higher doses. T3 and T4 concentrations were significantly decreased at the high dose at 2 and 4 weeks but had returned to normal by week 13. Thyroid iodine uptake and binding or organification were significantly increased at the high dose. Histologically, the follicular size patterns were altered in treated rats. The follicles were generally small to medium-sized, and the few remaining large follicles were lined with taller, wider follicular epithelial cells. In addition, the liver weights and *para*-nitrophenol UGT activity were significantly increased. The results of this study support the conclusion that spironolactone at high doses increases the hepatic clearance of T4 by inducing microsomal UGT activity. This causes a decrease in the serum concentrations of thyroid hormones, which activates a compensatory increase in pituitary TSH secretion resulting in increased thyroid gland weights and follicular-cell hypertrophy and hyperplasia (Semler *et al.*, 1989).

Marmosets (*Callithrix jacchus*) were given spironolactone at 30 or 100 mg/kg bw per day, phenobarbital (see monograph in this volume) at 50 mg/kg bw per day or methimazole (see monograph in this volume) at 10 or 30 mg/kg bw per day for 4 weeks. Spironolactone caused follicular-cell hypertrophy, but less severely than methimazole and with less reduction of T4 concentration. Spironolactone and phenobarbital, but not methimazole, increased hepatic CYP and T4-UGT activity (Kurata *et al.*, 2000).

4.3   Reproductive and prenatal effects

4.3.1   *Humans*

The anti-androgenic effects of spironolactone are discussed in section 4.2.

4.3.2 *Experimental systems*

No defects were produced in the offspring of rats and mice given intraperitoneal doses of up to 80 mg/kg bw per day potassium canrenoate, which is a metabolite of spironolactone in humans (Sadée *et al.*, 1973; Funder *et al.*, 1974) on days 8–14 (rats) or 7–13 (mice) of gestation, although at 80 mg/kg bw per day some resorptions occurred in mice (Miyakubo *et al.*, 1977). An increased resorption rate was found in rats that received 100 mg/kg bw per day for various periods before day 6 of gestation (Selye *et al.*, 1971).

Mature virgin female CD-1 mice were caged with fertile males for 2 weeks, during which time they were given an intraperitoneal injection of 100 mg/kg bw spironolactone daily. There was no effect on mating (8/15 treated versus 22/30 controls), but the number of mice that became pregnant was reduced (3/8 versus 19/22), and fewer embryos per pregnant mouse were observed (mean, 4.3 versus 13.3). Similar results were obtained when mice were injected intraperitoneally with 100 mg/kg bw spironolactone twice daily. It was shown that the anti-fertility effect of spironolactone was mediated by inhibition of both ovulation and implantation, since the number of implants in ovulating animals could be increased by injection of estradiol on day 3 after mating (Nagi & Virgo, 1982).

A group of Wistar rats with regular estrous cycles received daily intraperitoneal injections of 100 mg/kg bw spironolactone for 7 days. The time spent in diestrus was significantly increased from 2 to 4 days, and, during the 14 days after treatment, 12 days were spent in diestrus; none of the animals had a complete cycle. Absence of estrus was accompanied by a reduction in plasma estradiol of 48%. In a group of 15 female rats treated with spironolactone from day 21 to day 45 of age, the onset of puberty was prevented in 47% of the animals, whereas all controls were postpubertal by that time. When female rats were treated simultaneously with spironolactone (100 mg/kg bw per day) and estradiol (1 μg/kg bw per day) on days 21–45 of age, vaginal opening and uterine development were normal, showing that spironolactone did not inhibit the peripheral actions of estradiol (Nagi & Virgo, 1982).

Pregnant Wistar rats, weighing 130 g, were given daily subcutaneous injections of 10 or 20 mg spironolactone on days 14–20 of gestation and were then allowed to deliver their pups and rear them normally. At 70–80 days of age, some of the animals were killed while in the basal state or after injection of gonadotropin-releasing hormone plus thyrotropin-releasing hormone, and blood and tissue samples were taken for analysis. The offspring showed no changes in the external genitalia, body weight or testis weight after spironolactone treatment *in utero*, but males showed a dose-related decrease in ventral prostate and seminal vesicle weight. The basal and stimulated plasma concentrations of follicule-stimulating hormone, luteinizing hormone, testosterone and 5α-dihydrotestosterone were normal, but those of prolactin were decreased. In females, the estrus cycle was unaffected, but the weights of the ovaries and uterus were significantly increased in those given 20 mg spironolactone, and the plasma concentrations of follicle-stimulating hormone, prolactin, estradiol and progesterone were comparable to those of controls; however, the concentrations of luteinizing hormone were increased (Jaussan *et al.*, 1985).

4.4   Effects on enzyme induction or inhibition and gene expression

Spironolactone decreased the anaesthetic effects of pentobarbital and progesterone and a number of other compounds in female rats, and this was shown to be due to increase hepatic metabolism (Selye *et al.*, 1969). In male and female mice, spironolactone decreased hexobarbital sleeping time and increased substrate metabolism, liver weights and CYP content (Feller & Gerald, 1971). In spironolactone-pretreated rats, although substrate metabolism was increased, the content of CYP decreased, and the induction was sex-dependent, with greater induction of more substrates in female than male rats (Fujita *et al.*, 1982; Chung & Buhler, 1994).

In isolated hepatocytes from male Wistar rats pretreated with spironolactone, a dose-related increase in UGT activity was observed (Guibert *et al.*, 1983). Spironolactone increased *para*-nitrophenol UGT activity in male rats treated for 2 weeks at 200 mg/kg bw per day. It also induced bilirubin glucuronosyltransferase activity in rats and increased the plasma clearance and biliary excretion of bilirubin (Semler *et al.*, 1989). Spironolactone was found be a more specific and effective inducer of bilirubin UGT activity in rats than phenobarbital (Mottino *et al.*, 1989, 1991). The drug induced β-glucuronidase activity in the liver of female rats (Kourounakis & Tani, 1995) and glutathione *S*-transferase activity in the liver and jejunum, but not the colon, of male rats (Catania *et al.*, 1998).

4.5   Genetic and related effects

No data were available to the Working Group.

4.6   Mechanistic considerations

No data on the genotoxicity of spironolactone were available.

Spironolactone is a microsomal enzyme inducer and has been shown to increase UGT activity in rat liver. Studies on thyroid function in rats have shown decreased concentrations of thyroid hormones, increased concentrations of TSH, increased thyroid gland weight and follicular-cell hypertrophy and/or hyperplasia.

Increased pituitary secretion of TSH in response to increased thyroid hormone disposition is the likely mode of action for the production of thyroid neoplasms in rats. However, in view of the lack of data on genotoxicity, no definitive conclusion could be reached on the mechanism of spironolactone-induced carcinogenesis.

The increased incidence of Leydig-cell tumours of the testis may be related to the anti-androgenic effects of spironolactone.

5.   Summary of Data Reported and Evaluation

5.1   Exposure data

Spironolactone is a steroidal potassium-sparing diuretic used in the treatment of oedema, hypertension and hyperaldosteronism.

5.2   Human carcinogenicity data

Spironolactone was mentioned specifically in two cohort studies and one case–control study. In one cohort study carried out in the USA, an excess risk for pharyngeal cancer was found, which persisted with longer follow-up. No evidence for an association with breast cancer was found in the other cohort study, and use of spironolactone was not associated with thyroid cancer in one case–control study. All three studies were based on small numbers of cases.

In five case–control studies of renal-cell carcinoma, use of potassium-sparing diuretics was not clearly identified as a risk factor independently of hypertension.

5.3   Animal carcinogenicity data

Spironolactone was tested by oral administration in one study in rats. Increased incidences of thyroid follicular-cell adenomas and Leydig-cell tumours of the testis were reported. Spironolactone reduced the incidence of 7,12-dimethylbenz[a]-anthracene-induced mammary tumours in rats.

5.4   Other relevant data

No data were available on the genotoxicity of spironolactone.

The metabolic pathway of spironolactone is complex and can be divided into two main routes: those in which the sulfur moiety is retained and those in which the sulfur moiety is removed by dethioacetylation.

Hyperkalaemia is the most common side-effect of exposure to spironolactone in humans, and a number of endocrine effects have been observed, the most common of which is gynaecomastia in men.

Spironolactone is transformed to a reactive metabolite that can inactivate adrenal and testicular cytochrome P450 enzymes. It also has anti-androgenic activity.

Spironolactone is a microsomal enzyme inducer. Studies on thyroid function have shown increased hepatic activity of uridine diphosphate-glucuronosyl transferase, decreased plasma triiodothyronine and thyroxine concentrations, increased thyroid-stimulating hormone concentrations and increased thyroid weights and follicular-cell hypertrophy and/or hyperplasia.

At relatively high doses, spironolactone induced resorption of embryos in rats and mice when given during the second week of gestation. Spironolactone reduced fertility in mice and delayed the onset of puberty when administered to young female rats. Prenatal treatment of rats with spironolactone caused a reduction in the weight of the prostate and seminal vesicles in male offspring.

5.5   Evaluation

There is *inadequate evidence* in humans for the carcinogenicity of spironolactone. There is *limited evidence* in experimental animals for the carcinogenicity of spironolactone.

Overall evaluation

Spironolactone is *not classifiable as to its carcinogenicity to humans (Group 3)*.

6.   References

American Hospital Formulary Service (2000) *AHFS Drug Information® 2000*, Bethesda, MD, American Society of Health-System Pharmacists [AHFSfirst CD-ROM]

Anon. (2000) Top generic drugs by prescription in 1999. *Drug Topics*, **144**

British Pharmacopoeia Commission (1993) *British Pharmacopoeia 1993*, Vols I & II, London, Her Majesty's Stationery Office, pp. 627–628, 1111–1112

Budavari, S., ed. (2000) *The Merck Index*, 12th Ed., Version 12:3, Whitehouse Station, NJ, Merck & Co. & Boca Raton, FL, Chapman & Hall/CRC [CD-ROM]

Caminos-Torres, R., Ma, L. & Snyder, P.J. (1977) Gynecomastia and semen abnormalities induced by spironolactone in normal men. *J. clin. Endocrinol. Metab.*, **45**, 255–260

Catania, V.A., Luquita, M.G., Sánchez Pozzi, E.J. & Mottino, A.D. (1998) Differential induction of glutathione S-transferase subunits by spironolactone in rat liver, jejunum and colon. *Life Sci.*, **63**, 2285–2293

Chung, W.G. & Buhler, D.R. (1994) The effect of spironolactone treatment on the cytochrome P450-mediated metabolism of the pyrrolizidine alkaloid senecionine by hepatic microsomes from rats and guinea pigs. *Toxicol. appl. Pharmacol.*, **127**, 314–319

CIS Information Services (2000a) *Directory of World Chemical Producers (Version 2000.1)*, Dallas, TX [CD-ROM]

CIS Information Services (2000b) *Worldwide Bulk Drug Users Directory (Version 2000)*, Dallas, TX [CD-ROM]

Colby, H.D., O'Donnell, J.P., Flowers, N.L., Kossor, D.C., Johnson, P.B. & Levitt, M. (1991) Relationship between covalent binding to microsomal protein and the destruction of adrenal cytochrome *P*-450 by spironolactone. *Toxicology*, **67**, 143–154

Corazza, M., Strumìa, R., Lombardi, A.R. & Virgili, A. (1996) Allergic contact dermatitis from spironolactone. *Contact Derm.*, **35**, 365–366

Council of Europe (1997) *European Pharmacopoeia*, 3rd Ed., Strasbourg, pp. 1538–1539

Danielson, D.A., Jick, H., Hunter, J.R, Stergachis A. & Madsen, S. (1982) Nonestrogenic drugs and breast cancer. *Am. J. Epidemiol.*, **116**, 329–332

Decker, C., Sugiyama, K., Underwood, M. & Correia, M.A. (1986) Inactivation of rat hepatic cytochrome P-450 by spironolactone. *Biochem. biophys. Res. Commun.*, **136**, 1162–1169

Decker, C.J., Rashed, M.S., Baillie, T.A., Maltby, D. & Correia, M.A. (1989) Oxidative metabolism of spironolactone: evidence for the involvement of electrophilic thiosteroid species in drug-mediated destruction of rat hepatic cytochrome P450. *Biochemistry*, **28**, 5128–5136

Feller, D.R. & Gerald, M.C. (1971) Stimulation of liver microsomal drug metabolism in male and female mice by spironolactone and aldadiene. *Proc. Soc. exp. Biol. Med.*, **136**, 1347–1350

Ferguson, I., Fogg, C. & Baughan, P. (1993) Spironolactone induced agranulocytosis [Letter to the Editor]. *Med. J. Aust.*, **159**, 837

Friedman, G.D. & Ury, H.K. (1980) Initial screening for carcinogenicity of commonly used drugs. *J. natl Cancer Inst.*, **65**, 723–733

Friedman, G.D. & Ury, H.K. (1983) Screening for possible drug carcinogenicity: second report of findings. *J. natl Cancer Inst.*, **71**, 1165–1175

Fujita, S., Uesugi, T., Ohta, M. & Kitani, K. (1982) Effect of spironolactone on hepatic microsomal monooxygenase and azoreductase activities. *Res. Commun. chem. Pathol. Pharmacol.*, **36**, 87–103

Funder, J.W., Feldman, D., Highland, E. & Edelman, I.S. (1974) Molecular modifications of anti-aldosterone compounds: Effects on affinity of spirolactones for renal aldosterone receptors. *Biochem. Pharmacol.*, **23**, 1493–1501

Gardiner, P., Schrode, K., Quinlan, D., Martin, B.K., Boreham, D.R., Rogers, M.S., Stubbs, K., Smith, M. & Karim, A. (1989) Spironolactone metabolism: Steady-state serum levels of the sulfur-containing metabolites. *J. clin. Pharmacol.*, **29**, 342–347

Gennaro, A.R. (1995) *Remington: The Science and Practice of Pharmacy*, 19th Ed., Vol. II, Easton, PA, Mack Publishing Co., p. 1048

Greenblatt, D.J. & Koch-Weser, J. (1973) Adverse reactions to spironolactone. A report from the Boston Collaborative Drug Surveillance Program. *J. Am. med. Assoc.*, **225**, 40–43

Guibert, E.E., Morisoli, L.S., Monti, J.A. & Rodríguez Garay, E.A. (1983) Effect of spironolactone on *p*-nitrophenol glucuronidation in isolated rat hepatocytes. *Experientia*, **39**, 527–528

Hardman, J.G., Limbird, L.E., Molinoff, P.B., Ruddon, R.W. & Gillman, A.G., eds (1996) *Goodman & Gilman's, The Pharmacological Basis of Therapeutics*, 9th Ed., New York, McGraw-Hill, pp. 707–709

IARC (1980) *IARC Monographs on the Evaluation of the Carcinogenic Risk of Chemicals to Humans, Vol. 24, Some Pharmaceutical Drugs,* Lyon, IARCPress, pp. 259-273

IARC (1987) *IARC Monographs on the Evaluation of Carcinogenic Risks to Humans,* Suppl. 7, *Overall Evaluations of Carcinogenicity: An Updating of* IARC Monographs Volumes 1 to 42, Lyon, IARCPress, p. 344

Instituto Nacional de Farmacia e do Medicamento (2000) Lisbon

Irish Medicines Board (2000) Dublin

Jaussan, V., Lamarchand-Béraud, T. & Gómez, F. (1985) Modifications of the gonadal function in the adult rat after fetal exposure to spironolactone. *Biol. Reprod.*, **32**, 1051–1061

Jeunemaitre, X., Kreft-Jais, C., Chatellier, G., Julien, J., Degoulet, P., Plouin, P.-F., Ménard, J. & Corvol, P. (1988) Long-term experience of spironolactone in essential hypertension. *Kidney int.*, **34**, Suppl. 26, S14–S17

Jivraj, K.T., Noseworthy, T.W., Friesen, E.G., Shustack, A.S., Konopad, E.M. & Johnston, R.G. (1987) Spironolactone-induced agranulocytosis. *Drug Intell. clin. Pharm.*, **21**, 974–975

Karim, A., Zagarella, J., Hribar, J. & Dooley, M. (1976a) Spironolactone. I. Disposition and metabolism. *Clin. Pharmacol. Ther.*, **19**, 158–169

Karim, A., Zagarella, J., Hutsell, T.C., Chao, A. & Baltes, B.J. (1976b) Spironolactone. II. Bio-availability. *Clin. Pharmacol. Ther.*, **19**, 170–176

Karim, A., Kook, C., Zitzewitz, D.J., Zagarella, J., Doherty, M. & Campion, J. (1976c) Species differences in the metabolism and disposition of spironolactone. *Drug Metab. Disposition*, **4**, 547–555

van der Klauw, M.M., Wilson, J.H. & Stricker, B.H. (1998) Drug-associated agranulocytosis: 20 years of reporting in the Netherlands (1974–1994). *Am. J. Hematol.*, **57**, 206–211

Kourounakis, P.N. & Tani, E. (1995) Effect of phenobarbital, spironolactone and pregnenolone-16 α-carbonitrile on rat hepatic β-glucuronidase. *Res. Commun. mol. Pathol. Pharmacol.*, **88**, 119–122

Kovacs, K. & Somogyi, A. (1970) Suppression by spironolactone of 7,12-dimethylbenz(a)-anthracene-induced mammary tumors. *Eur. J. Cancer*, **6**, 195–201

Kurata, Y., Wako, Y., Tanaka, K., Inoue, Y. & Makinodan, F. (2000) Thyroid hyperactivity induced by methimazole, spironolactone and phenobarbital in marmosets (*Callithrix jacchus*): Histopathology, plasma thyroid hormone levels and hepatic T_4 metabolism. *J. vet. Med. Sci.*, **62**, 606–614

Lumb, G., Newberne, P., Rust, J.H. & Wagner, B. (1978) Effects in animals of chronic administration of spironolactone — A review. *J. environ. Pathol. Toxicol.*, **1**, 641–660

McLaughlin, J.K., Chow, W.H., Mandel, J.S., Mellemgaard, A., McCredie, M., Lindblad, P., Schlehofer, B., Pommer, W., Niwa, S. & Adami, H.-O. (1995) International renal-cell cancer study. VIII. Role of diuretics, other anti-hypertensive medications and hypertension. *Int. J. Cancer*, **63**, 216–221

Medical Products Agency (2000) Uppsala

Medicines Evaluation Board Agency (2000) The Hague

Mellemgaard, A., Niwa, S., Mehl, E.S., Engholm, G., McLaughlin, J.K. & Olsen, J.H. (1994) Risk factors for renal cell carcinoma in Denmark: Role of medication and medical history. *Int. J. Epidemiol.*, **23**, 923–930

Menard, R.H., Martin, H.F., Stripp, B., Gillette, J.R. & Bartter, F.C. (1974a) Spironolactone and cytochrome P-450: Impairment of steroid hydroxylation in the adrenal cortex. *Life Sci.*, **15**, 1639–1648

Menard, R.H., Stripp, B. & Gillette, J.R. (1974b) Spironolactone and testicular cytochrome P-450: Decreased testosterone formation in several species and changes in hepatic drug metabolism. *Endocrinol.*, **94**, 1628–1636

Menard, R.H., Bartter, F.C. & Gillette, J.R. (1976) Spironolactone and cytochrome *P*-450: Impairment of steroid 21-hydroxylation in the adrenal cortex. *Arch. Biochem. Biophys.*, **173**, 395–402

Menard, R.H., Guenthner, T.M., Kon, H. & Gillette, J.R. (1979) Studies on the destruction of adrenal and testicular cytochrome P-450 by spironolactone. Requirement for the 7α-thio group and evidence for the loss of the heme and apoproteins of cytochrome P-450. *J. biol. Chem.*, **254**, 1726–1733

Miyakubo, H., Saito, S., Tokunaga, Y., Ando, H. & Nanba, H. (1977) [SC-14266 was administered intraperitoneally to pregnant rats and mice for the examination of pre- and post-natal development in their offspring.] *Nichidai Igaku Zasshi*, **36**, 261–282 (in Japanese)

Mottino, A.D., Guibert, E.E. & Rodríguez Garay, E.A. (1989) Additive effect of combined spironolactone and phenobarbital treatment on hepatic bilirubin UDP-glucuronyl-transferase. *Biochem. Pharmacol.*, **38**, 851–853

Mottino, A.D., Guibert, E.E. & Rodríguez Garay, E.A. (1991) Effect of spironolactone and phenobarbital administration on bilirubin glucuronidation in hepatic and extrahepatic rat microsomes. *Biochem. Pharmacol.*, **41**, 1075–1077

Nagi, S. & Virgo, B.B. (1982) The effects of spironolactone on reproductive functions in female rats and mice. *Toxicol. appl. Pharmacol.*, **66**, 221–228

National Agency for Medicines (2000) Helsinki

National Institute for Occupational Safety and Health (2000) *National Occupational Exposure Survey 1981–83*, Cincinnati, OH, Department of Health and Human Services, Public Health Service

Nielsen, B.B. (1990) Fibroadenomatoid hyperplasia of the male breast. *Am. J. Surg. Pathol.*, **14**, 774–777

Norwegian Medicinal Depot (2000) Oslo

Overdiek, H.W.P.M. & Merkus, F.W.H.M. (1987) The metabolism and biopharmaceutics of spironolactone in man. *Rev. Drug Metab. Drug Interactions*, **5**, 273–302

Overdiek, H.W.P.M., Hermens, W.A. & Merkus, F.W.H.M. (1985) New insights into the pharmacokinetics of spironolactone. *Clin. Pharmacol. Ther.*, **38**, 469–474

Pita, J.C., Jr, Lippman, M.E., Thompson, E.B. & Loriaux, D.L. (1975) Interaction of spironolactone and digitalis with the 5 alpha-dihydrotestosterone (DHT) receptor of rat ventral prostate. *Endocrinology*, **97**, 1521–1527

Rifka, S.M., Pita, J.C., Vigersky, R.A., Wilson, Y.A. & Loriaux, D.L. (1978) Interaction of digitalis and spironolactone with human sex steroid receptors. *J. clin. Endocrinol. Metab.*, **46**, 338–344

Ron, E., Kleinerman, R.A., Boice, J.D., Jr, LiVolsi, V.A., Flannery, J.T. & Fraumeni, J.F., Jr (1987) A population-based case–control study of thyroid cancer. *J. natl Cancer Inst.*, **79**, 1–12

Royal Pharmaceutical Society of Great Britain (2000) *Martindale, The Extra Pharmacopoeia*, 13th Ed., London, The Pharmaceutical Press [MicroMedex Online]

Sadée, W., Dagcioglu, M. & Schröder, R. (1973) Pharmacokinetics of spironolactone, canrenone and canrenoate-K in humans. *J. Pharmacol. exp. Ther.*, **185**, 686–695

Sadée, W., Schröder, R., Leitner, E.V. & Dagcioglu, M. (1974a) Multiple dose kinetics of spironolactone and canrenoate-potassium and cardiac and hepatic failrue. *Eur. J. clin. Pharmacol.*, **7**, 195–200

Sadée, W., Abshagen, U., Finn, C. & Rietbrock, N. (1974b) Conversion of spironolactone to canrenone and disposition kinetics of spironolactone and canrenoate-potassium in rats. *Arch. Pharmacol.*, **283**, 303–318

Selby, J.V., Friedman, G.D. & Fireman, B.H. (1989) Screening prescription drugs for possible carcinogenicity: Eleven to fifteen years of follow-up. *Cancer Res.*, **49**, 5736-5747

Selye, H., Mécs, I. & Savoie, L. (1969) Inhibition of anesthetics and sedative actions by spironolactone. *Anesthesiology*, **31**, 261–264

Selye, H., Taché, Y. & Szabo, S. (1971) Interruption of pregnancy by various steriods. *Fertil. Steril.*, **22**, 735–740

Semler, D.E., Chengelis, C.P. & Radzialowski, F.M. (1989) The effects of chronic ingestion of spironolactone on serum thyrotropin and thyroid hormones in the male rat. *Toxicol. appl. Pharmacol.*, **98**, 263–268

Shapiro, J.A., Williams, M.A., Weiss, N.S., Stergachis, A., LaCroix, A.Z. & Barlow, W.E. (1999) Hypertension, antihypertensive medication use, and risk of renal cell carcinoma. *Am. J. Epidemiol.*, **149**, 521–530

Sherry, J.H., O'Donnell, J.P., Flowers, L., LaCagnin, L.B. & Colby, H.D. (1986) Metabolism of spironolactone by adrenocortical and hepatic microsomes: Relationship to cytochrome P-450 destruction. *J. Pharmacol. exp. Ther.*, **236**, 675–680

Sherry, J.H., Johnson, P.B. & Colby, H.D. (1988) Species differences in adrenal spironolactone metabolism: Relationship to cytochrome P-450 destruction. *Biochem. Pharmacol.*, **37**, 355–357

Shuck, J., Shen, S., Owensby, L., Leftik, M. & Cucinell, S. (1981) Spironolactone hepatitis in primary hyperaldosteronism. *Ann. intern. Med.*, **95**, 708–710

Smals, A.G.H., Kloppenborg, P.W.C., Hoefnagels, W.H.L. & Drayer, J.I.M. (1979) Pituitary–thyroid function in spironolactone treated hypertensive women. *Acta endocrinol.*, **90**, 577–584

Society of Japanese Pharmacopoeia (1996) *The Japanese Pharmacopoeia JP XIII*, 13th Ed., Tokyo, pp. 639–640

Spanish Medicines Agency (2000) Madrid

Stierer, M., Spoula, H. & Rosen, H.R. (1990) [Breast cancer in the male — A retrospective analysis of 15 cases.] *Onkologie*, **13**, 128–131 (in German)

Stricker, B.H.Ch. & Oei, T.T. (1984) Agranulocytosis caused by spironolactone. *Br. med. J.*, **289**, 731

Sutter, J.L. & Lau, E.P.K. (1975) Spironolactone. *Anal. Profiles Drug Subst.*, **4**, 431–451

Swiss Pharmaceutical Society, ed. (2000) *Index Nominum, International Drug Directory*, 16th Ed., Stuttgart, Medpharm Scientific Publishers [MicroMedex Online]

Thompson, D.F. & Carter, J.R. (1993) Drug-induced gynecomastia. *Pharmacotherapy*, **13**, 37–45

US Pharmacopeial Convention (1999) *The 2000 US Pharmacopeia*, 24th Rev./*The National Formulary*, 19th Rev., Rockville, MD, pp. 1546–1547

Weinman, S., Glass, A.G., Weiss, N.S., Psaty, B.M., Siscovick, D.S. & White, E. (1994) Use of diuretics and other antihypertensive medications in relation to the risk of renal cell cancer. *Am. J. Epidemiol.*, **140**, 792–804

Whitling, A.M., Pérgola, P.E., Sang, J.L. & Talbert, R.L. (1997) Spironolactone-induced agranulocytosis. *Ann. Pharmacother.*, **31**, 582–585

Yuan, J.-M., Castelao, J.E., Gago-Dominguez, M., Ross, R.K. & Yu, M.C. (1998) Hypertension, obesity and their medications in relation to renal cell carcinoma. *Cancer*, **77**, 1508–1513

ANTIBACTERIAL AGENTS

SULFAMETHAZINE AND ITS SODIUM SALT

1. Exposure Data

1.1 Chemical and physical data

1.1.1 *Nomenclature*

Sulfamethazine

Chem. Abstr. Serv. Reg. No.: 57-68-1
Chem. Abstr. Name: 4-Amino-*N*-(4,6-dimethyl-2-pyrimidinyl)benzenesulfonamide
IUPAC Systematic Name: N^1-(4,6-dimethyl-2-pyrimidinyl)sulfanilamide
Synonyms: 2-(4-Aminobenzenesulfonamido)-4,6-dimethylpyrimidine; 2-(*para*-aminobenzenesulfonamido)-4,6-dimethylpyrimidine; 4-amino-*N*-(2,6-dimethyl-4-pyrimidinyl)benzenesulfonamide; 4,6-dimethyl-2-sulfanilamidopyrimidine; sulfa-dimethylpyridine; 2-sulfanilamido-4,6-dimethylpyrimidine; sulfadimidine; sulfa-midine; sulphadimethylpyrimidine; sulphadimidine

Sodium sulfamethazine

Chem. Abstr. Serv. Reg. No.: 1981-58-4
Chem. Abstr. Name: 4-Amino-*N*-(4,6-dimethyl-2-pyrimidinyl)benzenesulfonamide, monosodium salt
IUPAC Systematic Name: N^1-(4,6-dimethyl-2-pyrimidinyl)sulfanilamide, mono-sodium salt
Synonyms: Sodium sulfadimidine; sulfadimidine sodium; sulfamethazine sodium; sulfamethazine sodium salt

1.1.2 *Structural and molecular formulae and relative molecular mass*

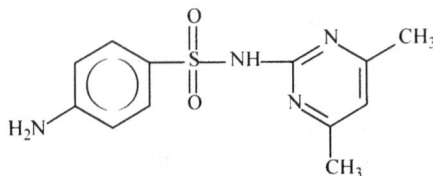

$C_{12}H_{14}N_4O_2S$ Relative molecular mass: 278.33

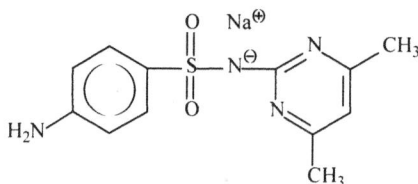

$C_{12}H_{13}NaN_4O_2S$ Relative molecular mass: 300.31

1.1.3   Chemical and physical properties of the pure substance (sulfamethazine)

(a) *Description*: Pale-yellow crystals (Lide & Milne, 1996)

(b) *Melting-point*: 198.5 °C (Lide & Milne, 1996)

(c) *Spectroscopy data*: Infrared [prism (423), grating (15044)], ultraviolet, nuclear magnetic resonance [proton (6671), C-13 (4417)] and mass spectral data have been reported (Sadtler Research Laboratories, 1980; Lide & Milne, 1996).

(d) *Solubility*: Slightly soluble in water (1.5 g/L at 29 °C), acids and alkali; solubility increases rapidly with an increase in pH (Lide & Milne, 1996; Budavari, 2000)

(e) *Dissociation constants*: pK_1, 7.4, pK_2, 2.7 (Papapstephanou & Frantz, 1978)

1.1.4   Technical products and impurities

Trade names for sulfamethazine include A 502, Azolmetazin, BN 2409, Calfspan, Cremomethazine, Diazil, Diazyl, Dimezathine, Kelametazine, Mermeth, Neasina, Neazina, Pirmazin, S-Dimidine, Spanbolet, Sulfadimerazine, Sulfadimesin, Sulfadimesine, Sulfadimethyldiazine, Sulfadimethylpyrimidine, Sulfadimezin, Sulfadimezine, Sulfadimidin, Sulfadimidine, Sulfadine, Sulfamethiazine, Sulfodimesin, Sulfodimezine, Sulmet, Sulphadimethylpyrimidine, Sulphadimidine, Sulphamethasine, Sulphamethazine, Sulphamezathine, Sulphamidine, Sulphodimezine, Superseptil, Superseptyl and Vertolan.

Trade names for sulfamethazine sodium include Bovibol, Sulmet and Vesadin.

1.1.5   Analysis

Several international pharmacopoeias specify infrared absorption spectrophotometry with comparison to standards and thin-layer chromatography as the methods for identifying sulfamethazine; electrometric titration with sodium nitrite is used to assay its purity. In pharmaceutical preparations, sulfamethazine is identified by infrared absorption spectrophotometry and high-performance liquid chromatography (HPLC) with ultraviolet detection; HPLC with ultraviolet detection and electrometric titration with sodium nitrite are used to assay for sulfamethazine content (British Pharmacopoeia Commission, 1993; Council of Europe, 1997; US Pharmacopeial Convention,, 1999).

The British Pharmacopoeia specifies infrared absorption spectrophotometry with comparison to standards as the method for identifying sodium sulfamethazine; electrometric titration with sodium nitrite is used to assay its purity (British Pharmacopoeia Commission, 1993).

Methods for the analysis of sulfamethazine in animal fluids (milk, plasma, urine) and tissues (muscle, organs), eggs, bee honey, animal feeds, meat-based baby food and animal wastewater have been reported. The methods include colorimetry, biosensor immunoassay, enzyme-linked immunosorbent assay, microbiological diffusion assay, microtitre plate assay, gas chromatography with positive chemical-ionization mass spectrometry, atomic emission, electron-capture or flame-ionization detection, thin-layer chromatography, high-performance thin-layer chromatography with spectro-densitometric detection, liquid chromatography with tandem mass or thermospray spectrometry or fluorimetric detection, reverse-phase liquid chromatography, gas–liquid chromatography, HPLC with chemiluminescence, fluorescence, fluorimetric, photo-diode array or ultraviolet detection (Cieri, 1976; Belliardo, 1981; Holder *et al.*, 1981; Munns & Roybal, 1982; Schwartz, 1982; Jonas *et al.*, 1983; Petz, 1983; Stout *et al.*, 1984; McGary, 1986; Smallidge *et al.*, 1988; Weber & Smedley, 1989; Agarwal, 1990; Kruzik *et al.*, 1990; Larocque *et al.*, 1990; Park & Lee, 1990; Takatsuki & Kikuchi, 1990; Carignan & Carrier, 1991; Diserens *et al.*, 1991; Hoffmeister *et al.*, 1991; Van Poucke *et al.*, 1991; Mineo *et al.*, 1992; Weber & Smedley, 1993; Sekiguchi *et al.*, 1994; Boison & Keng, 1995; Strebel & Schneider, 1995; Tsai *et al.*, 1995; Casetta et al., 1996; Martínez García & Holzwarth, 1996; Nishimura *et al.*, 1996; Edder *et al.*, 1997; Le Boulaire *et al.*, 1997; Chiavarino *et al.*, 1998; Jen *et al.*, 1998; Lynas *et al.*, 1998; Martínez García *et al.*, 1998; Nishimura *et al.*, 1998; Petkov & Gechev, 1998a,b; Tsai *et al.*, 1998; Watanabe *et al.*, 1998; Baxter *et al.*, 1999; Fránek *et al.*, 1999; Gaudin & Pavy, 1999; Park, 1999; Reeves, 1999; Shaikh *et al.*, 1999; Sugama *et al.*, 1999; Yang, 1999; Bartolucci *et al.*, 2000; Buick *et al.*, 2000; Stoev & Michailova, 2000).

1.2   Production

Sulfamethazine can be prepared by reacting acetylsulfanilyl chloride with 2-amino-4,6-dimethylpyrimidine suspended in dry pyridine or in acetone and pyridine, followed by alkaline hydrolysis of the 2-(N^4-acetylsulfanilamido)-4,6-dimethylpyrimidine; the resulting salt is neutralized with SO_2. The 2-amino-4,6-dimethylpyrimidine is prepared by condensing acetylacetone with guanidine carbonate in toluene. It can also be prepared by condensation of equimolar amounts of sulfanilylguanidine and acetyl-acetone directly. It is precipitated in the presence of water in the form of very pale-yellow crystals (Papastephanou & Frantz, 1978; Gennaro, 1995).

Information available in 2000 indicated that sulfamethazine was manufactured by 23 companies in China, two companies in India and one company each Egypt, Mexico and Spain, while sulfamethazine sodium was manufactured by four companies in

China and one company each in Egypt, Mexico and Spain (CIS Information Services, 2000a).

Information available in 2000 indicated that sulfamethazine was formulated as a pharmaceutical by 26 companies in Italy, 20 companies in India, 13 companies in Canada, 12 companies in the USA, 11 companies in Mexico, seven companies each in Argentina and the United Kingdom, five companies in South Africa, four companies in China, three companies each in Australia, Egypt and New Zealand, two companies each in Colombia and Spain and one company each in the Czech Republic, Germany, Greece, Hungary, Ireland, the Islamic Republic of Iran, Malta, Peru, Poland, Taiwan and Thailand. The same source indicated that sulfamethazine sodium was formulated as a pharmaceutical by 14 companies in Canada, eight companies in Mexico, five companies each in Colombia, the United Kingdom and the USA, four companies each in Italy and South Africa, three companies each in Australia, Austria and the Netherlands, two companies in Argentina and one company each in Belgium, France, India, Ireland, the Islamic Republic of Iran, Peru, Spain, Switzerland and Turkey (CIS Information Services, 2000b).

1.3   Use

Sulfamethazine is a sulfonamide used to treat a variety of bacterial diseases in humans and other species. It has been used since the late 1950s to treat respiratory disease and promote growth in food-producing animals (cattle, sheep, pigs and poultry). It is a short-acting sulfonamide drug with similar properties to those of sulfamethoxazole (see monograph in this volume). There is currently no single-entity dosage form of sulfa-methazine, and it is used only in combinations. It has been used with trimethoprim and with other sulfa drugs, particularly sulfadiazine and sulfamerazine. The sulfamethazine sodium salt may be given orally (2 g initial dose followed by 0.1–1.0 g every 6–8 h) or parenterally. The usual adult dose of a combination with equal amounts of sulfadiazine and sulfamerazine (trisulfapyrimidines) has been 6–8 g/day (Gennaro, 1995; WHO, 1995; American Hospital Formulary Service, 1997; Food & Drug Administration, 1988; Royal Pharmaceutical Society of Great Britain, 2000).

1.4   Occurrence

1.4.1   *Occupational exposure*

According to the 1981–83 National Occupational Exposure Survey (National Institute for Occupational Safety and Health, 2000), about 17 000 workers, including 12 400 food production workers, 4000 agricultural service workers (2000 veteri-narians) and 700 health service workers, were potentially exposed to sulfamethazine in the USA.

1.4.2   *Environmental occurrence*

No data were available to the Working Group.

1.5   Regulations and guidelines

Sulfamethazine is listed in the pharmacopoeias of China, the Czech Republic, France, Germany and the USA and in the European and International pharmacopoeias (Council of Europe, 1997; US Pharmacopeial Convention, 1999; Royal Pharmaceutical Society of Great Britain, 2000; Swiss Pharmaceutical Society, 2000), and sodium sulfamethazine is listed in the pharmacopoeias of Austria, the Czech Republic and the United Kingdom and in the International Pharmacopoeia (Royal Pharmaceutical Society of Great Britain, 2000; Swiss Pharmaceutical Society, 2000).

In 1994, the Joint FAO/WHO Expert Committee on Food Additives (JECFA) established an acceptable daily intake (ADI) of 0–50 µg/kg bw. The Codex Committee on Food Additives and Contaminants recommended maximum residue limits (MRLs) for sulfamethazine of 100 µg/kg in muscle, liver, kidney and fat of cattle, sheep, pigs and poultry; and 25 µg/L in milk. Sulfamethazine should not be used in laying hens, and an MRL was not recommended for eggs (WHO, 1995).

2.   Studies of Cancer in Humans

No data were available to the Working Group.

3.   Studies of Cancer in Experimental Animals

3.1   Oral administration

Mouse: Groups of 96 male and 96 female $B6C3F_1$ mice, 3–4 weeks of age, were fed diets containing sulfamethazine (purity, 97–99%) at 300, 600, 1200, 2400 or 4800 mg/kg for 24 months, while 192 males and 192 female controls received basal diet. Additional groups of 24 male and 24 female mice were included for necropsy at 12 and 18 months. No deaths occurred. A statistically significant ($p < 0.001$) increase in the incidence of follicular-cell adenomas of the thyroid gland was observed in mice at the highest dietary concentration killed after 24 months. The incidences were 2/184, 0/95, 1/92, 4/88, 4/94 and 31/93 for males, and 5/180, 1/91, 1/93, 0/95, 2/94 and 23/89 for females in the controls and at the five concentrations, respectively. One male at 2400 mg/kg of diet and one female each at 600 and 4800 mg/kg had one follicular-cell carcinoma. Diffuse and focal thyroid follicular-cell hyperplasia was also observed at the three highest concentrations in males and at the two highest concentrations in females.

Marginally significant but inconsistent, non-dose-related increases in the incidence of hepatocellular tumours were also reported in female mice (Littlefield *et al.*, 1989). [The Working Group analysed the data for liver tumours by Fisher's exact test for differences between groups and a Cochrane-Armitage test for trend and found no statistically significant increase in liver tumour incidence.]

Rat: Groups of 90 male and 90 female Fischer 344 rats were fed diets containing sulfamethazine (purity > 99%) at a concentration of 10, 40, 600, 1200 or 2400 mg/kg from weaning for 24 months. The rats were derived from parents fed diets containing the same concentration of sulfamethazine for at least 80 days before mating. At weaning, the offspring were allocated to different groups so that littermates were housed separately. A group of 180 male and 180 female controls received basal diet, and additional groups of 15 males and 15 females were included for necropsy at 3, 12 and 18 months. After 2 years on the study, the mortality rate of the female controls was approximately 41%, while the rates were 36, 35, 26, 19 and 19% at the five concentrations of sulfamethazine, respectively. The corresponding figures in males were 37% for controls and 24–28% for the treated groups. One male at 1200 mg/kg and one at 2400 mg/kg that were killed at 12 months had a follicular-cell adenoma of the thyroid gland. The incidences of combined thyroid gland follicular-cell adenomas and adenocarcinomas at 24 months were 0, 2, 0, 5, 5 and 11% (0/180, 2/87, 0/90, 4/88, 4/83 and 10/87) in males and 4, 0, 1, 5, 10 and 9% (6/170, 0/90, 1/85, 4/84, 9/87 and 8/88) in females in controls and at the five dietary concentrations, respectively. The corresponding incidences of follicular-cell adenocarcinomas were 0/180, 2/87, 0/90, 2/88, 2/83 and 7/87 for males and 1/170, 0/90, 0/85, 0/84, 6/87 and 6/88 for females. The differences in the incidence of thyroid neoplasia were statistically significant at the two higher doses in both males and females when compared with controls ($p < 0.05$). There were no other treatment-related neoplasms. Thyroid follicular-cell hyperplasia, described as focal, multifocal or diffuse, was observed at the three higher doses (Littlefield *et al.*, 1990).

4.   Other Data Relevant to an Evaluation of Carcinogenicity and Its Mechanisms

4.1   Absorption, distribution, metabolism and excretion

4.1.1   *Humans*

Sulfamethazine acetylation phenotypes were determined in 19 healthy adults (aged 17–46 years; 15 men, four women; nine white, nine oriental, one black) given a single oral dose of 20 mg/kg bw sulfamethazine in 200 mL of water. The results showed a well-defined trimodal pattern for acetylation clearance and for overall elimination or metabolic rate constants and confirmed that the fast acetylator phenotype can be subdivided into intermediate and rapid acetylator groups. The average acetylation clearance rate for rapid acetylators (1.34 mL/min per kg bw) was 8.8 times the estimated clearance for slow acetylators (0.15 mL/min per kg bw) and 1.8 times that for intermediate acetylators (0.75 mL/min per kg bw). The average percentage of an absorbed dose excreted as acetylsulfamethazine in 72-h urine was 93.7 for rapid acetylators, 87.7 for intermediate acetylators and 65.6 for slow acetylators (Chapron *et al.*, 1980). A trimodal distribution of sulfamethazine acetylator phenotypes was also indicated by measurements of the percentage acetylation of sulfamethazine in plasma samples obtained from 49 persons in South India 6 h after ingestion of a single dose of 10 mg/kg bw (51% slow, 12% intermediate, 37% rapid acetylators) (Peters *et al.*, 1975).

After 10 male and two female healthy volunteers were given oral doses of sulfamethazine of 12–17 mg/kg bw, 10–20% of the dose was excreted in the urine as free and conjugated hydroxylated metabolites and 61–81% as N^4-acetylsulfamethazine. Six of the individuals were considered to be fast acetylators and six slow acetylators. The plasma concentration–time curve for sulfamethazine in the fast acetylators was biphasic, with half-times of 1.7 and 5.4 h, respectively, whereas in the slow acetylators it was monophasic, with a half-time of 7.6 h (Vree *et al.*, 1986).

Five healthy men received an oral dose of 10 or 40 mg/kg bw sulfamethazine approximately 14 days apart in a non-randomized cross-over study. Non-linear kinetics was determined at the high dose, as a dose-dependent decrease in absorption rate was observed in some subjects, whereas apparent metabolic clearance decreased with increasing dose in all subjects (Du Souich *et al.*, 1979).

4.1.2 *Experimental systems*

Suspensions of parenchymal, but not non-parenchymal cells, isolated from male Wistar rats metabolized sulfamethazine by acetylation and other pathways (Mørland & Olsen, 1977; Olsen & Mørland, 1981). Hydroxylation of sulfamethazine in isolated hepatocytes from male Wistar rats was significantly greater than in hepatocytes from female or castrated male rats. Acetylation activity was higher in females than males (Van't Klooster *et al.*, 1993).

After a single intravenous administration of 20 mg/kg bw sulfamethazine to seven male and eight female Wistar rats, male rats showed faster clearance from the plasma than females and excreted larger amounts of the hydroxy metabolites and smaller amounts of its N^4-acetylated metabolite (Witkamp *et al.*, 1992). Two phenotypes of sulfamethazine acetylation in rats — a high and a low percentage of acetylsulfamethazine in urine — were described in females, but not males, of five inbred strains and two random-bred stocks (Zídek & Janku, 1976).

4.1.3   *Comparison of animals and humans*

Sulfamethazine is metabolized similarly in animals and humans, with N^4-acetylation dominating. A trimodal pattern of sulfamethazine acetylation is seen in humans. Differences in acetylation rates were observed between male and female rats and among females of different strains.

4.2   Toxic effects

4.2.1   *Humans*

The toxic side-effects of sulfamethazine are expected to be similar to those of other sulfonamides, which include disorders of the haematopoietic system and hypersensitivity reactions.

4.2.2   *Experimental systems*

Sulfamethazine inhibited the iodination of tyrosine catalysed by porcine thyroid peroxidase in a reversible manner; the approximate median inhibitory concentration was 0.5 mmol/L, and the K_i was 0.42 mmol/L (Doerge & Decker, 1994).

Groups of 12 male and female $B6C3F_1$ mice and Fischer 344 rats were fed either a control diet or a diet containing 300, 600, 1200, 2400 or 3600 mg/kg sulfamethazine for 90 days. In the mice, no treatment-related lesions were seen grossly or by light microscopy. Thyroid gland enlargement was seen in one of 24 rats fed the diet containing 2400 mg/kg and in 12 of 24 rats at the highest dietary concentration. Thyroid gland hyperplasia was evident in all treated rats but was more pronounced and occurred at a higher incidence in rats at the higher concentrations (Heath & Littlefield, 1984a,b).

In $B6C3F_1$ mice that received diets containing sulfamethazine at a concentration of 0, 300, 600, 1200, 2400 or 4800 mg/kg for 24 months, non-neoplastic dose-related lesions were observed in both males and females, including follicular-cell hyperplasia (diffuse and focal) of the thyroid gland (Littlefield *et al.*, 1989).

Fischer 344 rats received diets containing sulfamethazine at a concentration of 0, 10, 40, 600, 1200 or 2400 mg/kg for 24 months, and interim sacrifices were carried out after 3, 12 and 18 months. The incidences of non-neoplastic lesions of the thyroid gland were significantly higher among treated animals than among controls and included follicular-cell hyperplasia, follicular cellular change and multilocular cysts (Littlefield *et al.*, 1990).

Groups of 120 male and 120 female Fischer 344 rats were fed diets containing 10, 40, 600, 1200 or 2400 mg/kg sulfamethazine. The control group consisted of 210 males and 210 females. Serum samples were analysed for concentrations of thyroid-stimulating hormone (TSH), total thyroxine, total triiodothyronine and triiodothyronine uptake after 12, 18 or 24 months of continuous exposure. There was no statistically significant difference in triiodothyronine concentration or percentage uptake in animals of either sex after any length of exposure. Serum TSH concentrations were not statistically significantly altered, although there was a trend for increasing concentrations in animals receiving 600 mg/kg of diet or more (703 ± 206 ng/100 mL with 2400 mg/kg, 575 ± 133 ng/100 mL in controls at 12 months; 420 ± 184 ng/100 mL with 2400 mg/kg, 217 ± 81 ng/100 mL in controls at 18 months). At each sacrifice time, rats at 1200 and 2400 mg/kg of diet had significantly heavier thyroid glands than controls (Fullerton *et al.*, 1987). [The Working Group noted that any change in thyroid hormone homeostasis occurring before 12 months would not have been revealed in this study. The high, dose-related increase in the variance of the values for TSH was also noted.]

Groups of 15 Sprague-Dawley CR/CD rats [sex not specified] were fed diets containing 0, 20, 40, 80, 160, 400, 800, 1600, 3300, 8000 or 12 000 mg/kg sulfamethazine for 4 weeks. This range of concentrations spanned the doses that induced thyroid tumours in rodents. A characteristic log dose–response relationship was observed in thyroid weight increases, decreased serum thyroxine concentration, decreased serum triiodothyronine concentration and increased serum TSH concentration. There were no significant effects at low concentrations, but a sharp, relatively linear rise was seen at higher concentrations: thyroid weights increased and serum thyroxine and triiodothyronine concentrations decreased at ≥ 3300 mg/kg of diet, and the serum TSH concentration increased at ≥ 1600 mg/kg of diet. All the morphological changes seen in the thyroid gland were reversible after withdrawal of sulfamethazine treatment. Supplemental dietary administration of thyroid hormone completely inhibited the functional and morphological changes observed with sulfamethazine at concentrations that normalized but did not suppress TSH. Further, no detectable effects on the thyroid gland were observed in hypophysectomized rats treated with sulfamethazine [experimental details not given]. *In vitro*, sulfamethazine did not increase cell proliferation in FRTL-5 cells in the absence of TSH [experimental details not given]. No effect on thyroid gland function was observed in cynomolgus monkeys (*Macaca fascicularis*) at doses of up to 300 mg/kg bw per day for 13 weeks [no further experimental details given] (McClain, 1995).

4.3 Reproductive and prenatal effects

4.3.1 *Humans*

Heinonen *et al.* (1977) reported no increase in malformation rates in the offspring of 47 women treated with sulfamethazine during the first four lunar months of pregnancy.

4.3.2 *Experimental systems*

The effect of sulfamethazine on fertility was assessed in three groups of 20 male and 20 female Swiss CD-1 mice given diets containing the drug at 0.25, 0.5 or 1.0% (equivalent to 0, 313, 625 and 1250 mg/kg bw per day) and compared with a control group of 38 males and 38 females. The mice were exposed to sulfamethazine continuously during the 7-day pre-mating and 98-day co-habitation periods. At the conclusion of this phase of the study, cross-over matings were performed with the parental mice, consisting of control male × control female; high-dose (1% sulfamethazine) male × control female; control male × high-dose female. The effects observed in the F_0 group receiving 1% sulfamethazine included significant decreases in the number of litters produced and in the number of live pups per litter and a significant increase in the proportion of live male pups per total live pups per litter. No significant difference was found in the percentage of motile sperm, sperm concentration or percentage of abnormal sperm in the cauda epididymis in the group fed 1% sulfamethazine versus the control group. The cross-over part of the study showed that fertility was affected in animals of each sex, the average number of live pups per litter being significantly decreased. No treatment-related histopathological effects were observed in the pituitary or reproductive organs of male or female mice in the group fed 1% sulfamethazine. Exposure of mice to 0.25 or 0.5% sulfamethazine in the diet during the continuous breeding phase of the study had no effect on fertility or reproductive performance (Reel *et al.*, 1992).

4.4   Effects on enzyme induction or inhibition and gene expression

4.4.1   *Humans*

No data were available to the Working Group.

4.4.2   *Experimental systems*

Intraperitoneal administration of various doses of sulfamethazine to adult male Wistar rats for 3 or 5 days and to Hubbard chickens for 3 days significantly increased the electron transport components (rats only) and the activities of aminopyrine *N*-de-methylase and aniline hydroxylase at a dose of 150 mg/kg bw. A dose of 300 mg/kg bw produced a significant decrease in cytochrome P450 content and in the activity of amino-pyrine *N*-demethylase in the rats and of aniline hydroxylase in the chickens. Admi-nistration of sulfamethazine to young male rats resulted in significant induction of electron transport components and drug-metabolizing enzymes at both 150 and 300 mg/kg bw. However, treatment of old rats produced significant decreases in electron transport components and aminopyrine *N*-demethylase activity at both doses. A signifi-cant increase in electron transport components was observed with 150 mg/kg bw sulfa-methazine in female rats. These studies suggest that sulfamethazine is a substrate of the mixed-function oxidase system, and induction is dependent on the dose and on the age and sex of the animals. Intraperitoneal administration of a single dose of 300 mg/kg bw sulfamethazine to rats pretreated with intraperitoneal doses of 80 mg/kg bw per day phenobarbital for 3 days decreased microsomal protein, electron transport components and drug-metabolizing enzyme activities to a greater extent than phenobarbital alone (Kodam & Govindwar, 1995; Kodam *et al.*, 1996; Kodam & Govindwar, 1997).

4.5   Genetic and related effects

4.5.1   *Humans*

No data were available to the Working Group.

4.5.2   *Experimental systems* (see Table 1 for references)

Sulfamethazine did not induce mutations in *Salmonella typhimurium* and it did not induce unscheduled DNA synthesis in human fibroblasts in culture. [The Working Group was aware of data from three different laboratoires, showing that sulfamethazine (*a*) did not induce gene mutation at the *Hprt* locus (at concentrations up to 7 μg/mL) or chromosomal aberrations (at up to 5000 μg/mL) in Chinese hamster ovary cells in the absence or presence of exogenous metabolic activation, (*b*) gave rise to sister chromatid exchange in these cells (at concentrations up to 1500 μg/mL) in the absence but not in the presence of an exogenous metabolic activation systems, and (*c*) did not induce chromosomal aberrations in bone-marrow cells of rats treated with a single oral dose of 3000 mg/kg bw (WHO, 1994).]

4.6   Mechanistic considerations

Sulfamethazine is considered not to be genotoxic, since it did not induce mutagenicity in bacterial or mammalian cells *in vitro* and was not clastogenic in mammalian cells *in vitro* or *in vivo*.

The available data indicate that thyroid hormone imbalance plays a role in the development of follicular-cell neoplasia caused by sulfamethazine in rats and mice. The drug altered thyroid hormone homeostasis in rats treated with doses spanning the range that induced thyroid tumours in this species, and it produced thyroid gland enlargement (goitre) in rats and follicular-cell hypertrophy and hyperplasia in rats and mice. The mechanism is based on reversible inhibition of thyroid peroxidase, as with other sulfonamides.

On the basis of this information, which meets the criteria laid out in the IARC consensus report (Capen *et al.*, 1999), sulfamethazine would be expected not to be carcinogenic to humans exposed to concentrations that do not lead to alterations in thyroid hormone homeostasis. In addition, no effects on thyroid gland function were found in cynomolgus monkeys treated with sulfamethazine.

The hyperplasia induced by sulfamethazine in the thyroid gland is diffuse, in analogy with the morphological changes induced by TSH stimulation, rather than only multifocal, as would be induced by a genotoxic thyroid carcinogen (Hard, 1998). Further support for the absence of an effect of sulfamethazine in primates comes from a study by Takayama *et al.* (1986), who examined species differences between male Sprague-Dawley rats and male squirrel monkeys (*Saimiri sciureus*) treated with sulfa-monomethoxine, a prototype goitrogenic sulfonamide. Whereas sulfamonomethoxine

Table 1. Genetic and related effects of sulfamethazine

Test system	Result[a]		Dose[b] (LED/HID)	Reference
	Without exogenous metabolic system	With exogenous metabolic system		
Salmonella thyphimurium TA100, TA1535, TA1537, TA98, reverse mutation	–	–	333 µg/plate	Mortelmans *et al.* (1986)
Unscheduled DNA synthesis, human fibroblasts	–	NT	100	Allred *et al.* (1982)

[a] –, negative; NT, not tested
[b] LED, lowest effective dose; HID, highest ineffective dose; in-vitro tests, µg/mL

decreased the serum triiodothyronine concentration, increased the serum TSH concentration and caused thyroid follicular-cell hypertrophy and hyperplasia with accompanying thyroid enlargement in the rats, no such changes were seen in the monkeys. The median inhibitory concentration for sulfamethazine on thyroid peroxidase isolated from rats was 2.2×10^{-7} mol/L, whereas that for monkeys was $> 10^{-4}$ mol/L.

5.   Summary of Data Reported and Evaluation

5.1   Exposure data

Sulfamethazine is a sulfonamide drug that has been used to treat bacterial diseases in human and veterinary medicine and to promote growth in cattle, sheep, pigs and poultry.

5.2   Human carcinogenicity data

No data were available to the Working Group.

5.3   Animal carcinogenicity data

Sulfamethazine was tested by oral administration in one study in mice and in one study in rats that included exposure *in utero*. It produced thyroid follicular-cell adenomas in mice and follicular-cell adenomas and carcinomas in rats. No statistically significant increase was seen in the incidence of tumours at other sites in mice or rats.

5.4   Other relevant data

Sulfamethazine shows a trimodal pattern of polymorphic acetylation in humans. It caused thyroid gland enlargement (goitre) in rats and diffuse hypertrophy and hyperplasia in rats and mice. Administration of sulfamethazine to rats under bioassay conditions that caused tumours resulted in alteration of thyroid hormone homeostasis, including increased secretion of thyroid-stimulating hormone and morphological changes in the thyroid consistent with this increase. The underlying mechanism for these changes is reversible inhibition of thyroid peroxidase activity. A study in which cynomolgus monkeys were given sulfamethazine did not result in alterations in thyroid gland function.

In a continuous breeding study in mice, sulfamethazine reduced fertility in both males and females but did not change sperm parameters.

No data were available on the genetic and related effects of sulfamethazine in humans. The compound did not induce chromosomal aberrations in bone-marrow cells of rats treated *in vivo* or in Chinese hamster cells. It did induce sister chromatid

exchange in Chinese hamster cells in the absence but not in the presence of an exogenous metabolic system in one experiment. It did not induce DNA damage or mutations in mammalian cells *in vitro* or in bacteria. Sulfamethazine is considered not to
be genotoxic *in vitro* or *in vivo*.

5.5   Evaluation

There is *inadequate evidence* in humans for the carcinogenicity of sulfamethazine.
There is *sufficient evidence* in experimental animals for the carcinogenicity of
sulfamethazine.

Overall evaluation

Sulfamethazine is *not classifiable as to its carcinogenicity to humans (Group 3)*.
Sulfamethazine produces thyroid tumours in mice and rats by a non-genotoxic
mechanism, which involves inhibition of thyroid peroxidase resulting in alterations in
thyroid hormone concentrations and increased secretion of thyroid-stimulating
hormone. Consequently, sulfamethazine would be expected not to be carcinogenic to
humans exposed to doses that do not alter thyroid hormone homeostasis.
Evidence from epidemiological studies and from toxicological studies in experimental animals provide compelling evidence that rodents are substantially more sensitive than humans to the development of thyroid tumours in response to thyroid hormone
imbalance.

6.   References

Agarwal, V.K. (1990) Detection of sulfamethazine residues in milk by high-performance liquid
      chromatography. *J. Liq. Chromatogr.*, **13**, 3531–3539
Allred, L.E., Oldham, J.W., Milo, G.E., Kindig, O. & Capen, C.C. (1982) Multiparametric
      evaluation of the toxic responses of normal human cells treated *in vitro* with different
      classes of environmental toxicants. *J. Toxicol. environ. Health*, **10**, 143–156
American Hospital Formulary Service (1997) *AHFS Drug Information® 97*, Bethesda, MD,
      American Society of Health-System Pharmacists
Bartolucci, G., Pieraccini, G., Villanelli, F., Moneti, G. & Triolo, A. (2000) Liquid chromato-
      graphy tandem mass spectrometric quantitation of sulfamethazine and its metabolites:
      Direct analysis of swine urine by triple quadrupole and by ion trap mass spectrometry.
      Rapid Commun. mass Spectrom., **14**, 967–973
Baxter, G.A., O'Connor, M.C., Haughey, S.A., Crooks, S.R.H. & Elliott, C.T. (1999) Evaluation
      of an immunobiosensor for the on-site testing of veterinary drug residues at an abattoir.
      Screening for sulfamethazine in pigs. *Analyst*, **124**, 1315–1318
Belliardo, F. (1981) Determination of sulfonamide residues in honeys by high-pressure liquid
      chromatography. *J. apic. Res.*, **20**, 44–48

Boison, J.O. & Keng, L.J.-Y. (1995) Determination of sulfadimethoxine and sulfamethazine residues in animal tissues by liquid chromatography and thermospray mass spectrometry. *J. Assoc. off. anal. Chem. int.*, **78**, 651–658

British Pharmacopoeia Commission (1993) *British Pharmacopoiea 1993*, Vols I & II, London, Her Majesty's Stationery Office, pp. 641–642; 1116–1117

Budavari, S., ed. (2000) *The Merck Index*, 12th Ed., Version 12:3, Whitehouse Station, NJ, Merck & Co. & Boca Raton, FL, Chapman & Hall/CRC [CD-ROM]

Buick, R.K., Greer, N.M. & Elliott, C.T. (2000) A microtitre plate assay for the detection of antibiotics in porcine urine. *Analyst*, **125**, 395–396

Capen, C.C., Dybing, E., Rice, J.M. & Wilbourn, J.D., eds (1999) *Species Differences in Thyroid, Kidney and Urinary Bladder Carcinogenesis* (IARC Scientific Publications No. 147), Lyon, IARCPress

Carignan, G. & Carrier, K. (1991) Quantitation and confirmation of sulfamethazine residues in swine muscle and liver by LC and GC/MS. *J. Assoc. off. anal. Chem.*, **74**, 479–482

Casetta, B., Cozzani, R., Cinquina, A.L. & di Marzio, S. (1996) Sulfamethazine, sulfothiazole and albendazole residue dosage in food products determined by liquid chromatography/tandem mass spectrometry. *Rapid Commun. mass Spectrom.*, **10**, 1497–1503

Chapron, D.J., Kramer, P.A. & Mercik, S.A. (1980) Kinetic discrimination of three sulfamethazine acetylation phenotypes. *Clin. Pharmacol. Ther.*, **27**, 104–113

Chiavarino, B., Crestoni, M.E., Di Marzio, A. & Fornarini, S. (1998) Determination of sulfonamide antibiotics by gas chromatography coupled with atomic emission detection. *J. Chromatogr. B. Biomed. Sci. Appl.*, **706**, 269–277

Cieri, U.R. (1976) Detection of sulfonamides in animal feeds. *J. Assoc. off. anal. Chem.*, **59**, 56–59

CIS Information Services (2000a) *Directory of World Chemical Producers (Version 2000.1)*, Dallas, TX [CD-ROM]

CIS Information Services (2000b) *Worldwide Bulk Drug Users Directory (Version 2000)*, Dallas, TX [CD-ROM]

Council of Europe (1997) *European Pharmacopoeia*, 3rd Ed., Strasbourg, pp. 1552–1553

Diserens, J.M., Renaud-Bezot, C. & Savoy-Perroud, M.-C. (1991) Simplified determination of sulfonamide residues in milk, meat, and eggs. *Dtsch. Lebensm.-Rundsch.*, **87**, 205–211

Doerge, D.R. & Decker, C.J. (1994) Inhibition of peroxidase-catalyzed reactions by arylamines: Mechanism for the anti-thyroid action of sulfamethazine. *Chem. Res. Toxicol.*, **7**, 164–169

Du Souich, P., Lalka, D., Slaughter, R., Elvin, A.T. & McLean, A.J. (1979) Mechanisms of nonlinear disposition kinetics of sulfamethazine. *Clin. Pharmacol. Ther.*, **25**, 172–183

Edder, P., Cominoli, A. & Corvi, C. (1997) [Analysis of residues of sulfonamides in foods of animal origin (liver, kidney, meat, fish, eggs, milk) by liquid chromatography with prederivatization and fluorimetric detection.] *Trav. chim. aliment. hyg.*, **88**, 554–569 (in French)

Food & Drug Administration (1988) Sulfamethazine review. *FDA Consumer*, March 28

Fránek, M., Kolár, V., Deng, A. & Crooks, S. (1999) Determination of sulphadimidine (sulfamethazine) residues in milk, plasma, urine and edible tissues by sensitive ELISA. *Food agric. Immunol.*, **11**, 339–349

Fullerton, F.R., Kushmaul, R.J., Suber, R.L. & Littlefield, N.A. (1987) Influence of oral administration of sulfamethazine on thyroid hormone levels in Fischer 344 rats. *J. Toxicol. environ. Health*, **22**, 175–185

Gaudin, V. & Pavy, M.-L. (1999) Determination of sulfamethazine in milk by biosensor immuno-assay. *J. Assoc. off. anal. Chem. int.*, **82**, 1316–1320

Gennaro, A.R. (1995) *Remington: The Science and Practice of Pharmacy*, 19th Ed., Vol. II, Easton, PA, Mack Publishing Co., p. 1276

Hard, G.C. (1998) Recent developments in the investigation of thyroid regulation and thyroid carcinogenesis. *Environ. Health Perspect.*, **106**, 427–436

Heath, J.E. & Littlefield, N.A. (1984a) Effect of subchronic oral sulfamethazine administration on Fischer 344 rats and B6C3F$_1$ mice. *J. exp. Pathol. Toxicol.*, **5**, 201–214

Heath, J.E. & Littlefield, N.A. (1984b) Morphological effects of subchronic oral sulfa-methazine administration on Fischer 344 rats and B6C3F$_1$ mice. *Toxicol. Pathol.*, **12**, 3–9

Heinonen, O.P., Slone, D. & Shapiro, S. (1977) *Birth Defects and Drugs in Pregnancy*, Littleton, MA, Publishing Sciences Group, pp. 298, 301

Hoffmeister, A., Suhren, G. & Heeschen, W. (1991) High-pressure liquid chromatographic determination of sulfadimidine residues in milk — Incidence in consumer milk from various European countries. *Milchwissenschaft*, **46**, 770–774

Holder, C.L., Thompson, H.C., Jr & Bowman, M.C. (1981) Trace analysis of sulfamethazine in animal feed, human urine, and wastewater by electron capture gas chromatography. *J. chromatogr. Sci.*, **19**, 625–633

Jen, J.-F., Lee, H.-L. & Lee, B.-N. (1998) Simultaneous determination of seven sulfonamide residues in swine wastewater by high-performance liquid chromatography. *J. Chromatogr.*, **A793**, 378–382

Jonas, D., Knupp, G. & Pollmann, H. (1983) [Rapid identification of 18 sulfonamides in animal tissues by a bacteriological method in combination with high-performance thin layer chro-matography.] *Arch. Lebensmittelhyg.*, **34**, 138–141 (in German)

Kodam, K.M. & Govindwar, S.P. (1995) Effect of sulfamethazine on mixed function oxidase in chickens. *Vet. hum. Toxicol.*, **37**, 340–342

Kodam, K.M. & Govindwar, S.P. (1997) In vivo and in vitro effect of sulfamethazine on hepatic mixed function oxidases in rats. *Vet. hum. Toxicol.*, **39**, 141–146

Kodam, K.M., Adav, S.S. & Govindwar, S.P. (1996) Effect of sulfamethazine on phenobarbital and benzo[*a*]pyrene induced hepatic microsomal mixed function oxidase system in rats. *Toxicol. Lett.*, **87**, 25–30

Kruzik, P., Weiser, M., Damoser, J. & Helsberg, I. (1990) [Determination of antibiotic drug residues in food of animal origin: Sulfonamides, nitrofurans, nicarbazin, tetracyclines, tylosin, and chloramphenicol.] *Wien. Tieraerztl. Monatsschr.*, **77**, 141–146 (in German)

Larocque, L., Carignan, G. & Sved, S. (1990) Sulfamethazine (sulfadimidine) residues in Canadian consumer milk. *J. Assoc. off. anal. Chem.*, **73**, 365-367

Le Boulaire, S., Bauduret, J.-C. & Andre, F. (1997) Veterinary drug residues survey in meat: An HPLC method with a matrix solid phase dispersion extraction. *J. agric. Food Chem.*, **45**, 2134–2142

Lide, D.R. & Milne, G.W.A. (1996) *Properties of Organic Compounds*, Version 5.0, Boca Raton, FL, CRC Press [CD-ROM]

Littlefield, N.A., Gaylor, D.W., Blackwell, B.-N. & Allen, R.R. (1989) Chronic toxi-city/carcinogenicity studies of sulphamethazine in B6C3F$_1$ mice. *Food chem. Toxicol.*, **27**, 455–463

Littlefield, N.A., Sheldon, W.G., Allen, R. & Gaylor, D.W. (1990) Chronic toxicity/carcino-genicity studies of sulphamethazine in Fischer 344/N rats: Two-generation exposure. *Food chem. Toxicol.*, **28**, 157–167

Lynas, L., Currie, D., McCaughey, W.J., McEvoy, J.D.G. & Kennedy, D.G. (1998) Contamination of animal feedingstuffs with undeclared antimicrobial additives. *Food Addit. Contam.*, **15**, 162–170

Martínez García, E. & Holzwarth, F. (1996) [Determination of sulfonamide residues in meat samples by high-performance thin-layer chromatography.] *Quim. ind.*, **43**, 32–34, 36–37 (in Spanish)

Martínez García, E., Marín Camaches, M.D., Pacheco Martínez, F. & Martínez Gambín, R. (1998) [Comparative thin layer chromatographic (TLC) and high performance liquid chromatographic study for the sulfamethazine.] *Alimentaria*, **297**, 77–81 (in Spanish)

McClain, R.M. (1995) Mechanistic considerations for the relevance of animal data on thyroid neoplasia to human risk assessment. *Mutat. Res.*, **333**, 131–142

McGary, E.D. (1986) Quantitative determination of sulfamethazine and carbadox in animal feeds by paired ion high-performance liquid chromatography. *Analyst*, **111**, 1341–1342

Mineo, H., Kaneko, S., Koizumi, I., Asida, K. & Akahori, F. (1992) An analytical study of anti-bacterial residues in meat: The simultaneous determination of 23 antibiotics and 13 drugs using gas chromatography. *Vet. hum. Toxicol.*, **34**, 393–397

Mørland, J. & Olsen, H. (1977) Metabolism of sulfadimidine, sulfanilamide, *p*-aminobenzoic acid, and isoniazid in suspensions of parenchymal and nonparencymal rat liver cells. *Drug Metab. Disposition*, **5**, 511–517

Mortelmans, K., Haworth, S., Lawlor, T., Speck, W., Tainer, B. & Zeiger, E. (1986) Salmonella mutagenicity tests. II. Results from the testing of 270 chemicals. *Environ. Mutag.*, **8** (Suppl. 7), 1–119

Munns, R.K. & Roybal, J.E. (1982) Rapid gas–liquid chromatographic method for determi-nation of sulfamethazine in swine feed. *J. Assoc. off. anal. Chem.*, **65**, 1048–1053

National Institute for Occupational Safety and Health (2000) *National Occupational Exposure Survey 1981–83*, Cincinnati, OH, Department of Health and Human Services, Public Health Service

Nishimura, K., Hirama, Y. & Nakano, M. (1996) [Simultaneous determination of residual sulfa drugs and their metabolites in meat by high performance liquid chromatography with photodiode array detection.] *Hokkaidoritsu Eisei Kenkyushoho*, **46**, 63–65 (in Japanese)

Nishimura, K., Chonan, T. & Hirama, Y. (1998) [Simultaneous determination of 10 kinds of veterinary drugs by high performance liquid chromatography.] *Hokkaidoritsu Eisei Kenkyushoho*, **48**, 81–84 (in Japanese)

Olsen, H. & Mørland, J. (1981) Sulfonamide acetylation in isolated rat liver cells. *Acta pharmacol. toxicol.*, **49**, 102–109

Papapstephanou, C. & Frantz, M. (1978) Sulfamethazine. *Anal. Profiles Drug Subst.*, **7**, 401–422

Park, J.H. (1999) Immunochemical detection of sulfamethazine residues in pork tissue. *Kor. J. Anim. Sci.*, **41**, 129–134

Park, J.H. & Lee, M.H. (1990) [Screening for sulfamethazine residue in pork.] *Han'guk Ch'uksan Hakhoechi*, **32**, 715–717 (in Korean)

Peters, J.H., Gordon, G.R. & Karat, A.B.A. (1975) Polymorphic acetylation of the antibacterials, sulfamethazine and dapsone, in South Indian subjects. *Am. J. trop. Med. Hyg.*, **24**, 641–648

Petkov, R. & Gechev, I. (1998a) [Methods for detection of residual antibiotics and sulfonamides in bee honey.] *Vet. Med.*, **4**, 193–196 (in Bulgarian)

Petkov, R. & Gechev, I. (1998b) [Antibiotic and sulfonamide residues in bee honey.] *Vet. Med.*, **4**, 197–199 (in Bulgarian)

Petz, M. (1983) [High-pressure liquid chromatographic method for the determination of residual chloramphenicol, furazolidone and five sulfonamides in eggs, meat and milk.] *Z. Lebensm.- Unters. Forsch.*, **176**, 289–293 (in German)

Reel, J.R., Tyl, R.W., Lawton, A.D. & Lamb, J.C. IV (1992) Reproductive toxicity of sulfamethazine in Swiss CD-1 mice during continuous breeding. *Fundam. appl. Toxicol.*, **18**, 609–615

Reeves, V.B. (1999) Confirmation of multiple sulfonamide residues in bovine milk by gas chromatography–positive chemical ionization mass spectrometry. *J. Chromatogr.*, **B723**, 127–137

Royal Pharmaceutical Society of Great Britain (2000) *Martindale, The Extra Pharmacopoeia*, 13th Ed., London, The Pharmaceutical Press [MicroMedex Online]

Sadtler Research Laboratories (1980) *Sadtler Standard Spectra, 1980 Cumulative Alphabetical Index*, Philadelphia, PA, p. 1412

Schwartz, D.P. (1982) Rapid screening test for sulfamethazine in swine feeds. *J. Assoc. off. anal. Chem.*, **65**, 701–705

Sekiguchi, Y., Koiguchi, S., Hasegawa, M., Kamakura, K., Yamana, T. & Tonogai, Y. (1994) [Simultaneous determination and identification of synthetic antibacterials in cattle muscles and internal organs.] *Kankyo Kagaku*, **4**, 452–453 (in Japanese)

Shaikh, B., Rummel, N. & Donoghue, D. (1999) Determination of sulfamethazine and its major metabolites in egg albumin and egg yolk by high performance liquid chromatography. *J. liq. Chromatogr. relat. Technol.*, **22**, 2651–2662

Smallidge, R.L., Kentzer, E.J., Stringham, K.R., Kim, E.H., Lehe, C., Stringham, R.W. & Mundell, E.C. (1988) Sulfamethazine and sulfathiazole determination at residue levels in swine feeds by reverse-phase liquid chromatography with post-column derivatization. *J. Assoc. off. anal. Chem.*, **71**, 710–717

Stoev, G. & Michailova, A. (2000) Quantitative determination of sulfonamide residues in foods of animal origin by high-performance liquid chromatography with fluorescence detection. *J. Chromatogr.*, **A871**, 37–42

Stout, S.J., Steller, W.A., Manuel, A.J., Poeppel, M.O. & daCunha, A.R. (1984) Confirmatory method for sulfamethazine residues in cattle and swine tissues, using gas chromatography–chemical ionization mass spectrometry. *J. Assoc. off. anal. Chem.*, **67**, 142–144

Strebel, K. & Schneider, N. (1995) [Official control of meat, milk, and eggs on chloramphenicol and sulfonamide by adapted enzyme immunoassays.] *Mitt. Geb. Lebensmittelunters. Hyg.*, **86**, 191–212 (in German)

Sugama, Y., Tomita, R. & Yotoriyama, M. (1999) [Screening of 11 animal pharmaceuticals including flubendazole in chicken and egg.] *Tochigi-ken Hoken Kankyo Senta Nenpo* (volume date 1998), **4**, 68–70 (in Japanese)

Swiss Pharmaceutical Society, ed. (2000) *Index Nominum, International Drug Directory*, 16th Ed., Stuttgart, Medpharm Scientific Publishers [MicroMedex Online]

Takatsuki, K. & Kikuchi, T. (1990) Gas chromatographic–mass spectrometric determination of six sulfonamide residues in egg and animal tissues. *J. Assoc. off. anal. Chem.*, **73**, 886–892

Takayama, S., Ahihara, K., Onodera, T. & Akimoto, T. (1986) Antithyroid effects of propyl-thiouracil and sulfamonomethoxine in rats and monkeys. *Toxicol. appl. Pharmacol.*, **82**, 191–199

Tsai, C.-E., Kondo, F., Ueyama, Y. & Azama, J. (1995) Determination of sulfamethazine residue in chicken serum and egg by high-performance liquid chromatography with chemilumi-nescence detection. *J. chromatogr. Sci.*, **33**, 365–369

Tsai, S.-C., Rau, Y.-H., Hsu, S.-C., Chou, C.-C. & Fu, W. (1998) [Development of a high perfor-mance liquid chromatographic method for detection of sulfonamide residues in egg.] *Yaowu Shipin Fenxi*, **6**, 505–510 (in Chinese)

US Pharmacopeial Convention (1999) *The 2000 US Pharmacopeia*, 24th Rev./*The National Formulary*, 19th Rev., Rockville, MD, pp. 1569–1570; 2293

Van Poucke, L.S.G., Depourcq, G.C.I. & Van Peteghem, C.H. (1991) A quantitative method for the detection of sulfonamide residues in meat and milk samples with a high-performance thin-layer chromatographic method. *J. Chromatogr. Sci.*, **29**, 423–427

Van't Klooster, G.A.E., Woutersen-Van Nijnanten, F.M.A., Blaauboer, B.J., Noordhoek, J. & Van Miert, A.S.J.P.A.M. (1993) Sulphadimidine metabolism *in vitro*: I. Sex differences in acetylation and hydroxylation in cultured rat hepatocytes. *J. vet. Pharmacol. Ther.*, **16**, 343–349

Vree, T.B., Hekster, Y.A., Nouws, J.F.M. & Baakman, M. (1986) Pharmacokinetics, meta-bolism, and renal excretion of sulfadimidine and its N_4-acetyl and hydroxy metabolites in humans. *Ther. Drug Monit.*, **8**, 434–439

Watanabe, K., Osawa, T., Takahata, J. & Hori, M. (1998) [Screening method for the remaining veterinary medicines from flesh.] *Sendai-shi Eisei Kenkyushoho*, **28**, 145–149 (in Japanese)

Weber, J.D. & Smedley, M.D. (1989) Liquid chromatographic determination of sulfamethazine in milk. *J. Assoc. off. anal. Chem.*, **72**, 445–447

Weber, J.D. & Smedley, M.D. (1993) Liquid chromatographic method for determination of sulfa-methazine residues in milk: Collaborative study. *J. Assoc. off. anal. Chem. int.*, **76**, 725–729

Witkamp, R.F., Yun, H.-I., Van't Klooster, G.A.E., van Mosel, J.F., van Mosel, M., Ensink, J.M., Noordhoek, J. & Van Miert, A.S.J.P.A.M. (1992) Comparative aspects and sex differentiation of plasma sulfamethazine elimination and metabolite formation in rats, rabbits, dwarf goats, and cattle. *Am. J. vet. Res.*, **53**, 1830–1835

WHO (1994) *Toxicological Evaluation of Certain Veterinary Drug Residues in Food* (WHO Food Additives Series 33), Geneva, International Programme on Chemical Safety, pp. 91–103

WHO (1995) *Evaluation of Certain Veterinary Drug Residues in Food* (Technical Report Series 851), Geneva

Yang, H. (1999) Determination of sulphadimidine residues in milk, swine plasma and swine urine by ELISA.] *Huaxi Yaoxue Zazhi*, **14**, 238–241 (in Chinese)

Zídek, Z. & Janku, I. (1976) Sex and genetic differences in the elimination of sulphadimidine in rats. *Pharmacology*, **14**, 556–562

SULFAMETHOXAZOLE

This substance was considered by previous working groups, in 1980 (IARC, 1980) and 1987 (IARC, 1987). Since that time, new data have become available, and these have been incorporated into the monograph and taken into consideration in the present evaluation.

1. Exposure Data

1.1   Chemical and physical data

1.1.1   *Nomenclature*

Chem. Abstr. Serv. Reg. No.: 723-46-6
Deleted CAS Reg. No.: 129378-89-8
Chem. Abstr. Name: 4-Amino-*N*-(5-methyl-3-isoxazolyl)benzenesulfonamide
IUPAC Systematic Name: N^1-(5-Methyl-3-isoxazolyl)sulfanilamide
Synonyms: 3-(*para*-Aminophenylsulfonamido)-5-methylisoxazole; 5-methyl-3-sulfanilamidoisoxazole; sulfamethylisoxazole; sulfamethoxazol; 3-sulfanilamido-5-methylisoxazole; sulfisomezole; sulphamethoxazole

1.1.2   *Structural and molecular formulae and relative molecular mass*

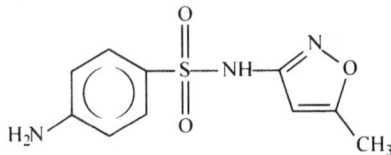

$C_{10}H_{11}N_3O_3S$ Relative molecular mass: 253.28

1.1.3   *Chemical and physical properties of the pure substance*

(*a*) *Description*: White to slightly off-white crystalline powder (Gennaro, 1995)
(*b*) *Melting-point*: 167 °C (Budavari, 2000)

(c) *Spectroscopy data*: Infrared [prism/grating (80313)], ultraviolet (46353), nuclear magnetic resonance [proton (53244), C-13 (32650)] and mass spectral data have been reported (Rudy & Senkowski, 1973; Sadtler Research Laboratories, 1995; Lide & Milne, 1996).

(d) *Solubility*: Slightly soluble in water (0.5 g/L) and benzene; slightly soluble in chloroform, diethyl ether and isopropanol; soluble in ethanol and methanol (Rudy & Senkowski, 1973; Gennaro, 1995)

1.1.4   *Technical products and impurities*

Sulfamethoxazole is available as 500-mg and 1-g tablets and as a 500-mg/5 mL oral suspension (Gennaro, 1995).

Trade names for sulfamethoxazole include Gantanol, MS-53, Radonil, Ro 4-2130 and Sinomin.

1.1.5   *Analysis*

Several international pharmacopoeias specify infrared and ultraviolet absorption spectrophotometry with comparison to standards as the methods for identifying sulfamethoxazole; potentiometric or electrometric titration with sodium nitrite is used to assay its purity. In pharmaceutical preparations, sulfamethoxazole is identified by infrared absorption spectrophotometry and thin-layer chromatography; visible absorption spectrophotometry and potentiometric or electrometric titration with sodium nitrite are used to assay for sulfamethoxazole content (British Pharmacopoeia Commission, 1993; Society of Japanese Pharmacopoeia, 1996; US Pharmacopeial Convention, 1999).

Methods for the analysis of sulfamethoxazole in human and animal fluids (milk, plasma, serum, urine) and tissues (muscle, organs), eggs, bee honey, meat-based baby food, animal wastewater, effluents and river water and drugs have been reported. The methods include enzyme immunoassay, gas chromatography with atomic emission, flame ionization or nitrogen–phosphorus detection, gas chromatography with mass spectrometry or pulsed positive ion–negative ion–chemical ionization mass spectrometry, thin-layer chromatography, high-performance thin-layer chromatography, liquid chromatography with fluorescence or fluorimetric detection, high-performance liquid chromatography (HPLC) with electrospray tandem mass spectrometry, fluorescence, photodiode array, spectrofluorimetric, or ultraviolet detection, and reversed-phase HPLC with ultraviolet detection (Ascalone, 1978; Schlatterer & Weise, 1982; Petz, 1983; Siegert, 1985; Van der Steuijt & Sonneveld, 1987; Aerts *et al.*, 1988; Van Poucke *et al.*, 1989; Kruzik *et al.*, 1990; Rychener *et al.*, 1990; Takatsuki & Kikuchi, 1990; Diserens *et al.*, 1991; Mineo *et al.*, 1992; Nie *et al.*, 1992; Takeda & Akiyama, 1992; Guggisberg *et al.*, 1993; Martin *et al.*, 1993; Mengelers *et al.*, 1993; Mooser & Koch, 1993; Shao *et al.*, 1993; Tsai & Kondo, 1993; Endoh *et al.*, 1994; Horie *et al.*, 1994; Tachibana *et al.*, 1994; Takahashi *et al.*, 1994; Lin *et al.*, 1995; Tsai & Kondo, 1995a,b; Nishimura *et al.*,

1996; Edder *et al.*, 1997; Gehring *et al.*, 1997; Le Boulaire *et al.*, 1997; Chiavarino *et al.*, 1998; Jen *et al.*, 1998; Petkov & Gechev, 1998; Hirsch *et al.*, 1999; Stoev & Michailova, 2000).

1.2   Production

Sulfamethoxazole can be prepared by reacting 3-amino-5-methylisoxazole with *para*-acetamidobenzenesulfonyl chloride (made by treating acetanilide with chloro-sulfonic acid). The acetyl group is then cleaved to yield sulfamethoxazole (Rudy & Senkowski, 1973; Gennaro, 1995).

Information available in 2000 indicated that sulfamethoxazole was manufactured by 29 companies in China, 26 companies in India, three companies each in Brazil and Turkey, two companies in Taiwan and 1 company each in Croatia, Egypt, Hungary, Israel, Japan, Mexico, the Republic of Korea, Spain, Switzerland and the USA (CIS Information Services, 2000a).

Information available in 2000 indicated that sulfamethoxazole was formulated as a pharmaceutical by 194 companies in India, 41 companies in Brazil, 38 companies in Mexico, 29 companies in Germany, 26 companies in Spain, 24 in the Philippines, 20 companies in Argentina, 19 companies in South Africa, 18 in China, 17 in Indonesia, 15 companies in Colombia, 14 companies in Turkey, 13 companies each in Ecuador, Peru, Switzerland and the USA, 12 companies in Taiwan, 11 companies in Chile, 10 companies in Italy, 9 each in Greece and Thailand, eight companies in the Islamic Republic of Iran, seven companies each in Austria, Singapore and the United Kingdom (sodium salt), six companies each in Canada, Japan, Malaysia and the Netherlands, five companies each in Egypt, Poland and Portugal, four companies each in Australia, France and Viet Nam, three companies each in Belgium, Israel, the United Kingdom and Venezuela, two companies each in Bulgaria, Sri Lanka, Sweden, Hong Kong, Hungary and Ireland and one company each in Denmark, Ireland, Latvia, Malta, New Zealand, Pakistan, the Republic of Korea, the Russian Federation, Saudi Arabia, the Slovak Republic and Yugoslavia (CIS Information Services, 2000b).

1.3   Use

Sulfamethoxazole is an antibacterial drug which has been used since the 1960s in the treatment of various systemic infections in humans and other species. The main use has been in the treatment of acute urinary tract infections. It has also been used against gonorrhoea, meningitis and serious respiratory tract infections (*Pneumocystis carinii*) and prophylactically against susceptible meningococci. Despite its relatively unfavourable pattern of tissue distribution, it is the sulfonamide most commonly used around the world in combination with trimethoprim or pyrimethamine for the treatment of various systemic infections. The combination with trimethoprim is used mainly for the treatment of urinary tract infections; with pyrimethamine, it is used in the treatment of chloroquine-resistant *Plasmodium falciparum* malaria (IARC, 1980; Gennaro, 1995; Budavari, 2000).

The usual adult oral dose of sulfamethoxazole is initially 2 g, followed by 1 g twice a day. The usual paediatric (> 1 month of age) oral dose is initially 50–60 mg/kg bw, followed by 25–30 mg/kg bw every 12 h; the total dose should not exceed 75 mg/kg bw per day (Gennaro, 1995).

1.4   Occurrence

1.4.1   *Occupational exposure*

According to the 1981–83 National Occupational Exposure Survey (National Institute for Occupational Safety and Health, 2000), about 21 200 workers, including 11 500 nurses, 4200 pharmacists, 2100 health aides and 1500 veterinarians, were potentially exposed to sulfamethoxazole in the USA.

1.4.2   *Environmental occurrence*

No data were available to the Working Group.

1.5   Regulations and guidelines

Sulfamethoxazole is listed in the pharmacopoeias of China, the Czech Republic, European, France, Germany, Italy, Japan, Poland, the United Kingdom and the USA and in the European and International pharmacopoeias (Royal Pharmaceutical Society of Great Britain, 2000; Society of Japanese Pharmacopoeia, 1996; Swiss Pharmaceutical Society, 1999; US Pharmacopeial Convention, 1999; Vidal, 2000). It is registered for human use in Finland, Ireland, the Netherlands, Norway, Portugal, Spain and Sweden (Instituto Nacional de Farmacia e do Medicamento, 2000; Irish Medicines Board, 2000; Medical Products Agency, 2000; Medicines Evaluation Board Agency, 2000; National Agency for Medicines, 2000; Norwegian Medicinal Depot, 2000; Spanish Medicines Agency, 2000).

2.   Studies of Cancer in Humans

Sulfamethoxazole was included in a hypothesis-generating cohort study designed to screen a large number (215) of drugs for possible carcinogenicity, which covered more than 140 000 subscribers enrolled between July 1969 and August 1973 in a prepaid medical care programme in northern California (USA). Computer records of persons to whom at least one drug prescription has been dispensed were linked to the cancer records of hospitals covered by the medical care programme and the regional cancer registry. The observed numbers of cancers were compared with those expected, standardized for age and sex, for the entire cohort. Three publications summarized the findings for follow-up periods of up to 7 years (Friedman & Ury, 1980), 9 years (Friedman & Ury, 1983) and 15 years (Selby *et al.*, 1989). In the 7-year report, among the 1709 persons who had used sulfamethoxazole, significant excesses were noted of nasopharyngeal cancer (three cases observed versus 0.1 expected; $p < 0.002$) and of cervical cancer after a 2-year lag time allowance (seven cases observed versus 2.2 expected; $p < 0.05$), while a significant deficit of colon cancers was reported (no cases observed versus 4.7 expected; $p < 0.05$). No changes in the significance of the observed associations was noted in the 9-year follow-up report. In the 15-year follow-up report, positive associations with p values between 0.01 and 0.05 were observed for cancers of the lung (23 observed versus 14.5 expected), uterine cervix (12 observed versus 5.9 expected), multiple myeloma (five observed versus 1.3 expected) and lymphomas and leukaemias combined (16 observed versus 7.6 expected). [The Working Group noted, as did the authors, that, since some 12 000 comparisons were made in this hypothesis-generating study, the associations should be verified independently. Data on duration of use were not provided.]

3. Studies of Cancer in Experimental Animals

3.1   Oral administration

Rat: Groups of 25–26 male and 24–25 female Charles River CD rats [age unspecified] were fed diets providing a dose of 0 (control), 25, 50, 150, 300 or 600 mg/kg bw per day sulfamethoxazole for 60 weeks, at which time the animals were killed. Thyroid follicular-cell tumours were observed in 0/28, 7/30, 20/29, 19/27, 23/23 treated males and females combined, at the five doses, respectively. No thyroid tumours were observed in two control groups of 28 and 26 rats. Lung metastases were observed in four rats at the three higher doses (Swarm *et al.*, 1973). [The Working Group interpreted the tumours as adenomas and carcinomas from illustrations in the report.]

4. Other Data Relevant to an Evaluation of Carcinogenicity and Its Mechanisms

4.1   Absorption, distribution, metabolism and excretion

4.1.1   *Humans*

The acetylation pattern of sulfamethoxazole was examined in six male and 16 female healthy volunteers selected according to their acetylation phenotype by analysis of the acetylation pattern of sulfadimidine. They were given a single oral dose of 10 mg/kg bw sulfamethoxazole, and blood (at 6 h) and urine (0–6 h) were analysed for the presence of total and free sulfamethoxazole (total minus free was considered to be the acetylated form). Sulfamethoxazole did not appear to undergo polymorphic acetylation (Bozkurt *et al.*, 1990).

Acetylation of sulfamethoxazole by human hepatic monomorphic (NAT1) and polymorphic (NAT2) arylamine *N*-acetyltransferase showed a higher affinity for the monomorphic enzyme (K_{max}, 1.2 mmol/L and approximately 5 mmol/L for NAT1 and NAT2, respectively). The higher affinity for NAT1 indicated that acetylation by this enzyme predominates at therapeutic plasma concentrations, in agreement with the observed monomorphic acetylation of sulfamethoxazole *in vivo* (Cribb *et al.*, 1993). There were no differences in affinity between human recombinant NAT1 and NAT2 enzymes in converting sulfamethoxazole hydroxylamine to the reactive *N*-acetoxy-sulfamethoxazole (Nakamura *et al.*, 1995).

Sulfamethoxazole was oxidized to its hydroxylamine metabolite in an NADPH-dependent process by liver microsomes prepared from two human livers. Three healthy volunteers ingested 1000 mg of sulfamethoxazole, and their urine was collected for 24 h. Sulfamethoxazole hydroxylamine constituted 3.1 ± 0.7% of the drug excreted in the urine, and 54% of the ingested dose was excreted during the same period (Cribb & Spielberg, 1992). In four male and two female volunteers given a single dose of 800 mg of sulfamethoxazole, 16.5 ± 5.5% was recovered as the parent compound, 46.2 ± 6.6% as N^4-acetylsulfamethoxazole and 2.4 ± 0.8% as the hydroxylamine in the urine after 96 h. The mean residence time of the hydroxylamine metabolite was 5.5 ± 1.5 h, and its renal clearance time was 4.4 ± 0.9 h (Van der Ven *et al.*, 1994).

4.1.2 *Experimental systems*

An oral dose of 1.0 g/kg bw sulfamethoxazole was absorbed rapidly by mice, and a peak plasma concentration of approximately 1.0 mg/mL was achieved 1 h after administration. The plasma elimination half-time was approximately 6 h. In rats, high concentrations of sulfamethoxazole were found in kidney, lung, liver, spleen and brain. The rate of elimination of the drug from these tissues paralleled that from blood (Nishimura *et al.*, 1958).

Murine hepatic microsomes oxidized sulfamethoxazole at the N^4-position to form the hydroxylamine in a cytochrome P450-catalysed reaction (Cribb & Spielberg, 1990).

4.1.3 *Comparison of animals and humans*

Sulfamethoxazole did not show evidence of polymorphic acetylation in humans. Both mice and humans oxidized sulfamethoxazole to the potentially toxic hydroxylamine metabolite.

4.2   Toxic effects

4.2.1   *Humans*

Sulfamethoxazole is associated with a variety of idiosyncratic toxic effects, including hepatotoxicity and systemic hypersensitivity reactions (reviewed by Mandell & Petri, 1996). Of hospitalized patients who were monitored during 359 courses of therapy with sulfamethoxazole, 3.0% experienced allergic reactions. Skin rashes, eosinophilia and drug fever were the commonest manifestations, and serious reactions were rare (Koch-Weser *et al,*. 1971).

Human monocytes and neutrophils activated by phorbol myristate acetate *in vitro* metabolized sulfamethoxazole to its hydroxylamine and to nitrosulfamethoxazole, whereas the presumed nitroso intermediate was not detected (Cribb *et al.*, 1990). Purification of human peripheral blood mononuclear cells showed that the $CD8^+$ population was highly susceptible to the cytotoxic effects of sulfamethoxazole hydroxylamine (Hess *et al.*, 1999). Covalent binding of sulfamethoxazole to human liver microsomal protein was NADPH-dependent. The pattern of protein targets was similar in human and rat liver microsomes (Cribb *et al.*, 1996).

In two separate double-blind cross-over studies with human volunteers, one with 10 men and the other one with 10 women, half the subjects were given co-trimoxazole (80 mg trimethoprim and 400 mg sulfamethoxazole per tablet) as two tablets daily for 10 days and, after 3 weeks, co-trifamole (80 mg trimethoprim and 400 mg sulfa-moxole per tablet) as two tablets immediately, then one tablet twice a day for 10 days. The remaining volunteers received these treatments in reverse order. Administration of co-trimoxazole resulted in a significant but moderate lowering of serum concentrations of thyroxine and triiodothyronine and of the free thyroxine index, whereas the serum thyroid-stimulating hormone (TSH) concentrations were not altered (Cohen *et al.*, 1980).

The plasma concentrations of thyroxine, triiodothyronine and TSH were measured in 49 subjects, six of whom were boys aged 2–19 years, who had received co-trimoxazole (10 mg sulfamethoxazole and 2 mg trimethoprim per kg bw per day) for up to 11 years (mean, 4.7 years). All the TSH values were within the normal range. An analysis of variance showed no significant difference in mean thyroxine or triiodo-thyronine concentrations with duration of prophylaxis or the age of the patients (Smellie *et al.*, 1982).

4.2.2   *Experimental systems*

Rat liver microsomes activated sulfamethoxazole *in vitro* to products that covalently bound to microsomal protein in the presence of NADPH, as detected by a polyclonal antibody. Sulfamethoxazole and sulfamethoxazole hydroxylamine elicited similar patterns of covalent binding targets. No covalent binding was detected *in vivo* after administration of sulfamethoxazole to rats (Cribb *et al.*, 1996).

Sulfamethoxazole hydroxylamine, but not sulfamethoxazole, was toxic to the immortal rat thyroid cell line FRTL5, which lacks active thyroid peroxidase. Both sulfamethoxazole and sulfamethoxazole hydroxylamine were toxic to primary sheep thyroid cells with active thyroid peroxidase (Gupta *et al.*, 1992).

Groups of four male Wistar rats were given a weekly intraperitoneal injection of 10, 50 or 250 mg/kg bw sulfamethoxazole, 10 mg/kg bw sulfamethoxazole hydroxylamine, 10 mg/kg bw nitroso sulfamethoxazole or vehicle, for 4 weeks. The immunogenic potential of sulfamethoxazole and its reactive metabolites was assessed by analysing serum samples from these rats for the presence of anti-sulfamethoxazole immuno-globulin G antibodies. A high titre of antibodies was present in sera from rats given nitroso sulfamethoxazole, whereas no antibodies were detected in sulfamethoxazole-treated or control rats. Sulfamethoxazole hydroxylamine resulted in only a weak immunogenic response after 3 weeks of dosing (Gill *et al.*, 1997).

Groups of 10 male and 10 female Sprague-Dawley rats were given 25 mg/kg bw sulfamethoxazole by gavage daily for 10 consecutive days. There was no clear indication that sulfamethoxazole had altered thyroid hormone synthesis, even though the serum TSH concentration was significantly elevated in male rats. When sulfamethoxazole was administered with trimethoprim (co-trimoxazole) at 600 mg/kg bw per day for 10 days, marked changes in hormone concentrations consistent with altered thyroid hormone homeostasis were produced. Significant increases in thyroid gland weight and follicular-cell hyperplasia were also demonstrated (Cohen *et al.*, 1981). [The Working Group noted that this dose was equivalent to the lowest dose used in the bioassay of carcinogenicity.]

Groups of 25 male and 25 female CD rats were given diets containing sulfamethoxazole at concentrations providing an intake of 0, 25, 50, 150, 300 or 600 mg/kg bw per day for up to 60 weeks. Autopsies and histological examinations were performed on five rats per sex per group at the end of 13 and 52 weeks and on all surviving animals at the end of the experiment. At 13, 52 and 60 weeks, dose-dependent increases in the weights of the thyroid glands were observed, and dose-dependent thyroid hyperplasia was seen in all treated animals. In groups of four male and four female rhesus monkeys given sulfamethoxazole by gavage at a dose of 0, 50, 150 or 300 mg/kg bw per day on 6 days per week for 52 weeks, no thyroid hyperplasia was observed (Swarm *et al.*, 1973).

In a comparison of species differences in the anti-thyroid effects of the sulfonamide prototype drug sulfamonomethoxine, groups of six to seven male Sprague-Dawley rats were given an oral dose of 30 or 270 mg/kg bw per day, while groups of three to four male squirrel monkeys (*Saimiri sciureus*) were given an oral dose of 270 mg/kg bw per day through the nose for 5 weeks. Rats at the highest dose showed a decrease in serum thyroxine concentration and in ^{131}I incorporation into thyroid hormone precursors, with an increased serum concentration of TSH, increased thyroid weight and hyperplasia of the follicular epithelium of the thyroid gland. No change was found in monkey thyroids. The concentration of sulfamonomethoxine required for 50% inhibition *in vitro* of peroxidase isolated from rat thyroid was 2.2×10^{-7} mol/L. For the enzyme isolated from monkey thyroid this value was $> 10^{-4}$ mol/L (Takayama *et al.*, 1986).

4.3 Reproductive and prenatal effects

4.3.1 *Humans*

Although sulfamethoxazole can be used alone, it is usually administered in the form of co-trimoxazole, a combination with the folic acid antagonist trimethoprim.

Sulfamethoxazole crossed the human placenta and reached a peak concentration at 10 h. After several gestational weeks, the concentration of sulfamethoxazole was lower in amniotic fluid and in the fetus than in maternal serum (Reid *et al.*, 1975). No increase in the incidence of defects was found in the offspring of 120 pregnant women who had been treated with sulfamethoxazole for bacteriuria, but only 10 of the women had been treated before the 16th week of pregnancy (Williams *et al.*, 1969). Heinonen *et al.* (1977) reported no increase in the rate of malformations in the offspring of 46 women treated with sulfamethoxazole during the first four lunar months of pregnancy.

In a case–control study in Hungary of use of co-trimoxazole during 1980–84, 1.25% (124/9893) of mothers of healthy babies had used co-trimoxazole compared with 2.31% (144/6228) ($p < 0.001$) of mothers of babies with congenital anomalies. Most of the mothers had used the drug during the third trimester of pregnancy, however, and analysis of the association between exposure during the critical periods and a range of nine specific malformations showed no increased risk in the exposed group. Nevertheless, the total rate of malformations was significantly raised (odds ratio, 2.3; 95% confidence interval, 1.2–4.0), and a teratogenic risk cannot be excluded (Czeizel, 1990). [The Working Group noted that the contribution of trimethoprim cannot be assessed.]

4.3.2 *Experimental systems*

Sulfamethoxazole given daily at 600 mg/kg bw on days 8–16 of gestation to Wistar rats caused cleft palate in the fetuses (Udall, 1969). It had no adverse effect on fetal development of rabbits (Medical Economics Co., 2000).

4.4 Effects on enzyme induction or inhibition and gene expression

No data were available to the Working Group.

4.5 Genetic and related effects

4.5.1 *Humans*

Administration to patients of sulfamethoxazole in combination with trimethoprim at therapeutic doses (800 mg sulfamethoxazole and 80 mg trimethoprim twice a day for 10 days) did not increase the frequency of chromosomal aberrations in peripheral lymphocytes (Stevenson *et al.*, 1973) or in bone-marrow (Sørensen & Krogh Jensen, 1981). However, an increased number of micronuclei was observed in the bone marrow (Sørensen & Krogh Jensen, 1981).

4.5.2   *Experimental systems* (see Table 1 for references)

Sulfamethoxazole did not induce mutations in *Salmonella typhimurium.* [The Working Group noted that the bacterial toxicity of the compound limited the doses that could be used.] No chromosomal aberrations were observed in human lymphocytes treated with sulfamethoxazole *in vitro*.

Sulfamethoxazole in combination with trimethoprim (250 μg/mL) did not increase the frequency of chromosomal breaks in human fibroblasts *in vitro* (Byarugaba *et al.*, 1975).

4.6   Mechanistic considerations

Insufficient data were available to evaluate the genotoxicity of sulfamethoxazole.

Sulfamethoxazole induced thyroid enlargement and hyperplasia in rats but not in monkeys. It was toxic to thyroid cells *in vitro* in the presence but not in the absence of thyroid peroxidase. There is no clear evidence that sulfamethoxazole alters thyroid homeostasis in rats. A prototype sulfonamide, sulfamonomethoxine, acted as an anti-thyroid substance in rats, but not in monkeys. Sulfamethoxazole is metabolized to a hydroxylamine metabolite in both humans and experimental animals.

5.   Summary of Data Reported and Evaluation

5.1   Exposure data

Sulfamethoxazole is a sulfonamide drug. It is used worldwide in the treatment of bacterial and protozoal infections, particularly in combination with other drugs in treating acute urinary tract infections and malaria.

5.2   Human carcinogenicity data

In one hypothesis-seeking epidemiological study, statistically significant positive associations were noted between sulfamethoxazole use and the risks for cancers of the lung and cervix and multiple myeloma and the combination of lymphomas and leukaemias.

Table 1. Genetic and related effects of sulfamethoxazole

Test system	Result[a] Without exogenous metabolic system	Result[a] With exogenous metabolic system	Dose[b] (LED/HID)	Reference
Salmonella typhimurium TA100, TA1535, TA1537, TA98, reverse mutation	–	–	10 µg/plate	Mortelmans et al. (1986)
Chromosomal aberrations, human lymphocytes *in vitro*	–	NT	150 µg/mL	Stevenson et al. (1973)

[a] –, negative; NT, not tested
[b] LED, lowest effective dose; HID, highest ineffective dose

5.3 Animal carcinogenicity data

Sulfamethoxazole was tested by oral administration in one study in rats. It produced follicular-cell adenomas and carcinomas of the thyroid.

5.4 Other relevant data

Sulfamethoxazole does not appear to be polymorphically acetylated in humans. Sulfamethoxazole is metabolized to its potentially toxic hydroxylamine in both humans and experimental animals. This metabolite has been associated with idiosyncratic toxicity, such as systemic hypersensitivity reactions, in humans. Sulfamethoxazole induced thyroid enlargement and hyperplasia in rats but not in monkeys. There is no convincing evidence that sulfamethoxazole alters thyroid hormone homeostasis in rats.

Administration of sulfamethoxazole to patients at therapeutic doses in combination with trimethoprim increased the number of micronuclei in their bone-marrow cells but did not increase the frequency of chromosomal aberrations. Sulfamethoxazole did not induce chromosomal aberrations in human lymphocytes *in vitro* or mutations in bacteria. Insufficient data were available to reach a conclusion about the genotoxicity of the agent.

5.5 Evaluation

There is *inadequate evidence* in humans for the carcinogenicity of sulfamethoxazole.

There is *limited evidence* in experimental animals for the carcinogenicity of sulfamethoxazole.

Overall evaluation

Sulfamethoxazole is *not classifiable as to its carcinogenicity to humans (Group 3)*.

6. References

Aerts, M.M.L., Beek, W.M.J. & Brinkman, U.A.T. (1988) Monitoring of veterinary drug residues by a combination of continuous flow techniques and column-switching high-performance liquid chromatography. I. Sulfonamides in egg, meat and milk using post-column derivatization with dimethylaminobenzaldehyde. *J. Chromatogr.*, **435**, 97–112

Ascalone, V. (1978) [Specific gas-chromatographic determination of trimethoprim, sulfamethoxazole, and its N⁴-acetylated metabolite in human body fluids, at therapeutic and subtherapeutic concentrations, using a new nitrogen detector.] *Boll. chim. Farm.*, **117**, 176–86 (in Italian)

Bozkurt, A., Basci, N.E., Isimer, A., Tuncer, M., Erdal, R. & Kayaalp, S.O. (1990) Sulpha-methoxazole acetylation in fast and slow acetylators. *Int. J. clin. Pharmacol. Ther. Toxicol.*, **28**, 164–166

British Pharmacopoeia Commission (1993) *British Pharmacopoeia 1993*, Vols I & II, London, Her Majesty's Stationery Office, pp. 644, 856–859

Budavari, S., ed. (2000) *The Merck Index*, 12th Ed., Version 12:3, Whitehouse Station, NJ, Merck & Co. & Boca Raton, FL, Chapman & Hall/CRC [CD-ROM]

Byarugaba, W., Rüdiger, H.W., Koske-Westphal, T., Wöhler, W. & Passarge, E. (1975) Toxi-city of antibiotics on cultured human skin fibroblasts. *Humangenetik*, **28**, 263–267

Chiavarino, B., Crestoni, M.E., Di Marzio, A. & Fornarini, S. (1998) Determination of sulfo-namide antibiotics by gas chromatography coupled with atomic emission detection. *J. Chromatogr. B. Biomed. Sci. Appl.*, **706**, 269–277

CIS Information Services (2000a) *Directory of World Chemical Producers (Version 2000.1)*, Dallas, TX [CD-ROM]

CIS Information Services (2000b) *Worldwide Bulk Drug Users Directory (Version 2000)*, Dallas, TX [CD-ROM]

Cohen, H.N., Beastall, G.H., Ratcliffe, W.A., Gray, C., Watson, I.D. & Thomson, J.A. (1980) Effects on human thyroid function of sulphonamide and trimethoprim combination drugs. *Br. med. J.*, **281**, 646–647

Cohen, H.N., Fyffe, J.A., Ratcliffe, W.A., McNicol, A.M., McIntyre, H., Kennedy, J.S. & Thomson, J.A. (1981) Effects of trimethoprim and sulphonamide preparations on the pituitary–thyroid axis of rodents. *J. Endocrinol.*, **91**, 299–303

Cribb, A.E. & Spielberg, S.P. (1990) Hepatic microsomal metabolism of sulfamethoxazole to the hydroxylamine. *Drug Metab. Dispos.*, **18**, 784–787

Cribb, A.E. & Spielberg, S.P. (1992) Sulfamethoxazole is metabolized to the hydroxylamine in humans. *Clin. Pharmacol. Ther.*, **51**, 522–526

Cribb, A.E., Miller, M., Tesoro, A. & Spielberg, S.P. (1990) Peroxidase-dependent oxidation of sulfonamides by monocytes and neutrophils from humans and dogs. *Mol. Pharmacol.*, **38**, 744–751

Cribb, A.J., Nakamura, H., Grant, D.M., Miller, M.A. & Spielberg, S.P. (1993) Role of poly-morphic and monomorphic human arhylamine *N*-acetyltransferases in determining sulfa-methoxazole metabolism. *Biochem. Pharmacol.*, **45**, 1277–1282

Cribb, A.E., Nuss, C.E., Alberts, D.W., Lamphere, D.B., Grant, D.M., Grossman, S.J. & Spielberg, S.P. (1996) Covalent binding of sulfamethoxazole reactive metabolites to human and rat liver subcellular fractions assessed by immunochemical detection. *Chem. Res. Toxicol.*, **9**, 500–507

Czeizel, A. (1990) A case–control analysis of the teratogenic effects of co-trimoxazole. *Reprod. Toxicol.*, **4**, 305–313

Diserens, J.M., Renaud-Bezot, C. & Savoy-Perroud, M.C. (1991) Simplified determination of sulfonamide residues in milk, meat, and eggs. *Dtsch. Lebensm.-Rundsch.*, **87**, 205–211

Edder, P., Cominoli, A. & Corvi, C. (1997) Analysis of residues of sulfonamides in foods of animal origin (liver, kidney, meat, fish, eggs, milk) by liquid chromatography with prederi-vatization and fluorimetric detection. *Mitt. Geb. Lebensmittelunters. Hyg.*, **88**, 554–569

Endoh, Y.S., Takahashi, Y., Hamamoto, S., Ishihara, Y., Nishikawa, M. & Nogawa, H. (1994) [Usefulness of enzyme immunoassay (EIA) as an analytical method of sulfamethoxazole residues in animal tissues.] *Shokuhin Eiseigaku Zasshi*, **35**, 292–298 (in Japanese)

Friedman, G.D. & Ury, H.K. (1980) Initial screening for carcinogenicity of commonly used drugs. *J. natl Cancer Inst.*, **65**, 723–733

Friedman, G.D. & Ury, H.K. (1983) Screening for possible drug carcinogenicity: Second report of findings. *J. natl Cancer Inst.*, **71**, 1165–1175

Gehring, T.A., Rushing, L.G. & Thompson, H.C., Jr (1997) Determination of sulfonamides in edible salmon tissue by liquid chromatography with postcolumn derivatization and fluorescence detection. *J. Assoc. off. anal. Chem. int.*, **80**, 751–755

Gennaro, A.R. (1995) *Remington: The Science and Practice of Pharmacy*, 19th Ed., Vol. II, Easton, PA, Mack Publishing Co., pp. 1276–1277

Gill, H.J., Hough, S.J., Naisbitt, D.J., Maggs, J.L, Kitteringham, N.R., Pirmohamed, M. & Park, B.K. (1997) The relationship between the disposition and immunogenicity of sulfamethoxazole in the rat. *J. Pharmacol. exp. Ther.*, **282**, 795–801

Guggisberg, D., Mooser, A.E. & Koch, H. (1993) [Screening method for the quantitative determination of twelve sulfonamides in meat, liver, and kidney by HPLC with online postcolumn derivatization.] *Mitt. Geb. Lebensmittelunters. Hyg.*, **84**, 263–273 (in German)

Gupta, A., Eggo, M.C., Uetrecht, J.P., Cribb, A.E., Daneman, D., Rieder, M.J., Shear, N.H., Cannon, M. & Spielberg, S.P. (1992) Drug-induced hypothyroidism: The thyroid as a target organ in hypersensitivity reactions to anticonvulsants and sulfonamides. *Clin. Pharmacol. Ther.*, **51**, 56–67

Heinonen, O.P., Slone, D. & Shapiro, S. (1977) *Birth Defects and Drugs in Pregnancy*, Littleton, MA, Publishing Sciences Group, pp. 298, 301

Hess, D.A., Sisson, M.E., Suria, H., Wijsman, J., Puvanesasingham, R., Madrenas, J. & Rieder, M.J. (1999) Cytotoxicity of sulfonamide reactive metabolites: Apoptosis and selective toxicity of $CD8^+$ cells by the hydroxylamine of sulfamethoxazole. *FASEB J.*, **13**, 1688–1698

Hirsch, R., Ternes, T., Haberer, K. & Kratz, K.-L. (1999) Occurrence of antibiotics in the aquatic environment. *Sci. total Environ.*, **225**, 109–118

Horie, M., Saito, K., Nose, N. & Nakazawa, H. (1994) [Simultaneous determination of sulfonamides and their N4-acetylated metabolites in meat by semi-micro high performance liquid chromatography.] *Kuromatogurafi*, **15**, 147–152 (in Japanese)

IARC (1977) *IARC Monographs on the Evaluation of the Carcinogenic Risk of Chemicals to Man*, Vol. 13, *Some Miscellaneous Pharmaceutical Substances*, pp. 233–242

IARC (1980) *IARC Monographs on the Evaluation of the Carcinogenic Risk of Chemicals to Man*, Vol. 24, *Some Pharmaceutical Drugs*, Lyon, IARCPress, pp. 285–295

IARC (1987) *IARC Monographs on the Evaluation of Carcinogenic Risks to Humans*, Suppl. 7, *Overall Evaluations of Carcinogenicity: An Updating of* IARC Monographs *Volumes 1 to 42*, Lyon, IARCPress, p. 348

Instituto Nacional de Farmacia e do Medicamento (2000) Lisbon

Irish Medicines Board (2000) Dublin

Jen, J.F., Lee, H.L. & Lee, B.N. (1998) Simultaneous determination of seven sulfonamide residues in swine wastewater by high-performance liquid chromatography. *J. Chromatogr.*, **A793**, 378–382

Koch-Weser, J., Sidel, V.W., Dexter, M., Parish C., Finer, D.C. & Kanarek, P. (1971) Adverse reactions to sulfisoxazole, sulfamethoxazole, and nitrofurantoin. *Arch. intern. Med.*, **128**, 399–404

Kruzik, P., Weiser, M., Damoser, J. & Helsberg, I. (1990) [Determination of antibiotic drug residues in food of animal origin: Sulfonamides, nitrofurans, nicarbazin, tetracyclines, tylosin, and chloramphenicol.] *Wien. Tieraerztl. Monatsschr.*, **77**, 141–146 (in German)

Le Boulaire, S., Bauduret, J.-C. & Andre, F. (1997) Veterinary drug residues survey in meat: An HPLC method with a matrix solid phase dispersion extraction. *J. agric. Food Chem.*, **45**, 2134–2142

Lide, D.R. & Milne, G.W.A. (1996) *Properties of Organic Compounds*, Version 5.0, Boca Raton, FL, CRC Press, Inc. [CD-ROM]

Lin, C.-L., Hong, C.-C. & Kondo, F. (1995) Simultaneous determination of residual sulfonamides in the presence and absence of *p*-aminobenzoic acid by high-performance liquid chromatography. *Microbios*, **83**, 175–183

Mandell, G.L. & Petri, W.A., Jr (1996) Sulfonamides, trimethoprim-sulfamethoxazole, quinolones and agents for urinary tract infections. In: Hardman, J.G., Limbird, L.E., Molinoff, P.B., Ruddon, R.W. & Gilman, A.G., eds, *Goodman & Gilman's The Pharmacological Basis of Therapeutics*, 9th Ed., New York, McGraw-Hill, pp. 1057–1072

Martin, E., Duret, M. & Vogel, J. (1993) [Determination of sulfonamide residues in eggs.] *Trav. chim. aliment. Hyg.*, **84**, 274–280 (in French)

Medical Economics Co. (2000) Sulfamethoxazole. In: *PDR®: Physicians' Desk Reference*, 53rd Ed., Montvale, Medical Economics Data Production Co. [MicroMedex Online]

Medical Products Agency (2000) Uppsala

Medicines Evaluation Board Agency (2000) The Hague

Mengelers, M.J.B., Polman, A.M.M., Aerts, M.M.L., Kuiper, H.A. & Van Miert, A.S.J. P.A.M. (1993) Determination of sulfadimethoxine, sulfamethoxazole, trimethoprim and their main metabolites in lung and edible tissues from pigs by multi-dimensional liquid chromatography. *J. liq. Chromatogr.*, **16**, 257–278

Mineo, H., Kaneko, S., Koizumi, I., Asida, K. & Akahori, F. (1992) An analytical study of antibacterial residues in meat: The simultaneous determination of 23 antibiotics and 13 drugs using gas chromatography. *Vet. hum. Toxicol.*, **34**, 393–397

Mooser, A.E. & Koch, H. (1993) Confirmatory method for sulfonamide residues in animal tissues by gas chromatography and pulsed positive ion–negative ion–chemical ionization mass spectrometry. *J. Assoc. off. anal. Chem. int.*, **76**, 976–982

Mortelmans, K., Haworth, S., Lawlor, T., Speck, W., Tainer, B. & Zeiger, E. (1986) Salmonella mutagenicity tests: II. Results from the testing of 270 chemicals. *Environ. Mutag.*, **8**, 1–119

Nakamura, H., Uetrecht, J., Cribb, A.E., Miller, M.A., Zahid, N., Hill, J., Josephy, P.D., Grant, D.M. & Spielberg, S.P. (1995) *In vitro* formation, disposition and toxicity of *N*-acetoxy-sulfamethoxazole, a potential mediator of sulfamethoxazole toxicity. *J. Pharmacol. exp. Ther.*, **274**, 1099–1104

National Agency for Medicines (2000) Helsinki

National Institute for Occupational Safety and Health (2000) *National Occupational Exposure Survey 1981–83*, Cincinnati, OH, Department of Health and Human Services, Public Health Service

Nie, H., Arnold, D., Balizs, G. & Somogyi, A. (1992) [Rapid HPLC determination of sulfonamide residues in pork.] *Fenxi Ceshi Tongbao*, **11**, 56–59 (in Chinese)

Nishimura, H., Nakajima, K., Okamoto, S., Shimaoka, N. & Sasaki, K. (1958) Part II. Comparative evaluation of MS-53 and sulfisoxazole: Therapeutic effectiveness, excretion and tissue distribution. *Ann. Rep. Shionogi Res. Lab.*, **8**, 770–790

Nishimura, K., Hirama, Y. & Nakano, M. (1996) [Simultaneous determination of residual sulfa drugs and their metabolites in meat by high performance liquid chromatography with photodiode array detection.] *Hokkaidoritsu Eisei Kenkyushoho*, **46**, 63–65 (in Japanese)

Norwegian Medicinal Depot (2000) Oslo

Petkov, R. & Gechev, I. (1998) [Methods for detection of residual antibiotics and sulfonamides in bee honey.] *Vet. Med.*, **4**, 193–196 (in Bulgarian)

Petz, M. (1983) [High-pressure liquid chromatographic method for the determination of residual chloramphenicol, furazolidone and five sulfonamides in eggs, meat and milk.] *Z. Lebensm.-Unters. Forsch.*, **176**, 289–293 (in German)

Reid, D.W.J., Caillé, G. & Kaufmann, N.R. (1975) Maternal and transplacental kinetics of trimethoprim and sulfamethoxazole, separately and in combination. *Can. med. Assoc. J.*, **112**, 67S–72S

Royal Pharmaceutical Society of Great Britain (2000) *Martindale, The Extra Pharmacopoeia*, 13th Ed., London, The Pharmaceutical Press [MicroMedex Online]

Rudy, B.C. & Senkowski, B.Z. (1973) Sulfamethoxazole. *Anal. Profiles Drug Subst.*, **2**, 467–486

Rychener, M., Mooser, A.E. & Koch, H. (1990) [Residue determination of sulfonamides and their N^4-metabolites in meat, liver, and kidney by HPLC.] *Mitt. Geb. Lebensmittelunters. Hyg.*, **81**, 522–543 (in German)

Sadtler Research Laboratories (1995) *Sadtler Standard Spectra, 1981–1995 Supplementary Molecular Formula Index*, Philadelphia, PA, p. 162

Schlatterer, B. & Weise, E. (1982) [Analysis of sulfonamides in tissues of slaughtered animals. Comparison of results from a microbiological test and from thin-layer chromatographic analysis after derivatization with fluorescamine.] *Z. Lebensm.-Unters. Forsch.*, **175**, 392–398 (in German)

Selby, J.V., Friedman, G.D. & Fireman, B.H. (1989) Screening prescription drugs for possible carcinogenicity: Eleven to fifteen years of follow-up. *Cancer Res.*, **49**, 5736–5747

Shao, J., Yuan, Z., Nie, H. & Zhang, J. (1993) [Simultaneous determination of the veterinary drug residues of 10 sulfonamides in meat by high performance liquid chromatography.] *Sepu*, **11**, 373–375 (in Chinese)

Siegert, K. (1985) [Detection of sulfonamides and antibiotics by gas chromatography combined with mass spectrometry.] *Fleischwirtschaft*, **65**, 1496–1497 (in German)

Smellie, J.M., Bantock, H.M. & Thompson, B.D. (1982) Co-trimoxazole and the thyroid (Letter to the Editor). *Lancet*, **ii**, 96

Society of Japanese Pharmacopoeia (1996) *The Japanese Pharmacopoeia JP XIII*, 13th Ed., Tokyo, pp. 644–645

Sørensen, P.J. & Krogh Jensen, M. (1981) Cytogenetic studies in patients treated with trimethoprim–sulfamethoxazole. *Mutat. Res.*, **89**, 91–94

Spanish Medicines Agency (2000) Madrid

Stevenson, A.C., Clarke, G., Patel, C.R. & Hughes, D.T.D. (1973) Chromosomal studies *in vivo* and *in vitro* of trimethoprim and sulfamethoxazole (co-trimoxazole). *Mutat Res.*, **17**, 255–260

Stoev, G. & Michailova, A. (2000) Quantitative determination of sulfonamide residues in foods of animal origin by high-performance liquid chromatography with fluorescence detection. *J. Chromatogr.*, **A871**, 37–42

Swarm, R.L, Roberts, G.K.S., Levy, A.C. & Hines, L.R. (1973) Observations on the thyroid gland in rats following the administration of sulfamethoxazole and trimethoprim. *Toxicol. appl. Pharmacol.*, **24**, 351–363

Swiss Pharmaceutical Society, ed. (2000) *Index Nominum, International Drug Directory*, 16th Ed., Stuttgart, Medpharm Scientific Publishers [MicroMedex Online]

Tachibana, M., Aoyama, M., Taniguchi, R., Anabuki, K. & Kumagai, K. (1994) [Simultaneous determination of residual synthetic antibacterials in chicken by HPLC.] *Tokyo-to Suginami-ku Eisei Shikensho Nenpo*, **12**, 86–89 (in Japanese)

Takahashi, Y., Endoh, Y.S., Hamamoto, S., Ishihara, Y., Nishikawa, M. & Nogawa, H. (1994) Enzyme immunoassay of sulfamethoxazole in chicken tissues: Interlaboratory study. *J. vet. Med. Sci.*, **56**, 1207–1208

Takatsuki, K. & Kikuchi, T. (1990) Gas chromatographic–mass spectrometric determination of six sulfonamide residues in egg and animal tissues. *J. Assoc. off. anal. Chem.*, **73**, 886–892

Takayama, S., Aihara, K., Onodera, T. & Akimoto, T. (1986) Antithyroid effects of propyl-thiouracil and sulfamonomethoxine in rats and monkeys. *Toxicol. appl. Pharmacol.*, **82**, 191–199

Takeda, N. & Akiyama, Y. (1992) Rapid determination of sulfonamides in milk using liquid chromatographic separation and fluorescamine derivatization. *J. Chromatogr.*, **607**, 31–35

Tsai, C.E. & Kondo, F. (1993) Simple continuous and simultaneous determination of multiple sulfonamide residues. *J. Food Prot.*, **56**, 1067–1072

Tsai, C.E. & Kondo, F. (1995a) A sensitive high-performance liquid chromatography method for detecting sulfonamide residues in swine and tissues after fluorescamine derivatization. *J. Liq. Chromatogr.*, **18**, 965–976

Tsai, C.E. & Kondo, F. (1995b) Liquid chromatographic determination of fluorescent derivatives of six sulfonamides in bovine serum and milk. *J. Assoc. off. anal. Chem. Int.*, **78**, 674–678

Udall, V. (1969) Toxicology of sulphonamide–trimethoprim combinations. *Postgrad. med. J.*, **45** (Suppl.), 42–45

US Pharmacopeial Convention (1999) *The 2000 US Pharmacopeia*, 24th rev./*The National Formulary*, 19th rev., Rockville, MD, pp. 1571–1575, 2293

Van der Steuijt, K. & Sonneveld, P. (1987) Concurrent analysis of methotrexate, trimethoprim, sulfamethoxazole and their major metabolites in plasma by high-performance liquid chromatography. *J. Chromatogr.*, **422**, 328–333

Van der Ven, A.J., Mantel, M.A., Vree, T.B., Koopmans, P.P. & Van der Meer, J.W. (1994) Formation and elimination of sulphamethoxazole hydroxylamine after oral administration of sulphamethoxazole. *Br. J. clin. Pharmacol.*, **38**, 147–150

Van Poucke, L., Rousseau, D., De Spiegeleer, B. & Van Peteghem, C. (1989) A rapid high-performance thin-layer chromatographic screening method for sulfonamides residues in animal muscle tissues. In: *Agriculture Food Chemistry Consumption, Proceedings of the Fifth European Conference on Food Chemistry,* Vol. 2, Paris, National Institute for Agronomic Research, pp. 438–442

Vidal (2000) *Le Dictionnaire*, Paris, Editions du Vidal

Williams, J.D., Brumfitt, W., Condie, A.P. & Reeves, D.S. (1969) The treatment of bacteriuria in pregnant women with sulphamethoxazole and trimethoprim. A microbiological, clinical and toxicological study. *Postgrad. med. J.*, **45** (Suppl.), 71–76

PESTICIDES

AMITROLE

This substance was considered by previous working groups, in 1974 (IARC, 1974), 1986 (IARC, 1986a) and 1987 (IARC, 1987). Since that time, new data have become available, and these have been incorporated into the monograph and taken into consideration in the present evaluation.

1. Exposure Data

1.1 Chemical and physical data

1.1.1 *Nomenclature*

Chem. Abstr. Serv. Reg. No.: 61-82-5
Deleted CAS Reg. Nos: 155-25-9; 6051-75-8; 11121-00-9; 16681-74-6; 29212-82-6; 30922-30-6
Chem. Abstr. Name: 1*H*-1,2,4-Triazol-3-amine
IUPAC Systematic Name: 3-Amino-*s*-triazole; 1*H*-1,2,4-triazol-3-ylamine
Synonyms: Aminotriazole; 2-amino-1,3,4-triazole; 3-aminotriazole; 3-amino-1,2,4-triazole; 3-amino-1*H*-1,2,4-triazole; 5-amino-1,2,4-triazole; 5-amino-1*H*-1,2,4-triazole; AT; 3,A-T; ATA; ENT 25 445

1.1.2 *Structural and molecular formulae and relative molecular mass*

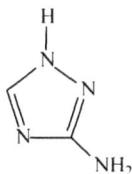

$C_2H_4N_4$ Relative molecular mass: 84.08

1.1.3   *Chemical and physical properties of the pure substance*

    (*a*) *Description*: White to yellowish crystalline powder (FAO/WHO, 1999)

    (*b*) *Melting-point*: 159 °C (Lide & Milne, 1996)

    (*c*) *Spectroscopy data*: Infrared [prism (8667), grating (21258)], nuclear magnetic resonance [proton (9499), C-13 (6254)] and mass spectral data have been reported (Sadtler Research Laboratories, 1980; Lide & Milne, 1996).

    (*d*) *Solubility*: Soluble in water (280 g/L at 25 °C), chloroform, ethanol, and methanol; sparingly soluble in ethyl acetate; insoluble in acetone and diethyl ether (WHO, 1994; Lide & Milne, 1996; Budavari, 2000)

    (*e*) *Volatility*: Vapour pressure, < 1 mPa at 20 °C (FAO/WHO, 1999; Tomlin, 1999)

    (*f*) *Ionization constant*: pK_a = 4.0 (FAO/WHO, 1999)

    (*g*) *Octanol/water partition coefficient (P)*: log P, –0.77 at pH 7.1 (FAO/WHO, 1999)

    (*h*) *Conversion factor*[1]: mg/m^3 = 3.44 × ppm

1.1.4   *Technical products and impurities*

    As of 1990, two types of product were commercially available: soluble concentrates containing 200–500 g/L amitrole and water-soluble powders containing 50–90% amitrole. A water-soluble granule containing 86% amitrole is in the process of registration in many countries worldwide (FAO/WHO, 1999)

    Impurities that have been identified in commercial formulations of amitrole include 3-(*N*-formylamino)-1,2,4-triazole, 4*H*-1,2,4-triazole-3,4-diamine and 4*H*-1,2,4-triazole-3,5-diamine (WHO, 1994; FAO/WHO, 1999).

    Trade names for amitrole include Amizol, Amitrol, Amitrol 90, ATA (amine), Azaplant, Cytrol, Cytrole, Herbidal total and Weedazol.

1.1.5   *Analysis*

    Selected methods for the analysis of amitrole in air, water, soil, plant materials and foods are presented in Table 1.

1.2   Production

    The synthesis of amitrole was first reported by J. Thiele and W. Manchot in 1898, involving the reaction of aminoguanidine with formic acid (Carter, 1976). The industrial process, described by Allen and Bell (1946) and patented in 1954 by Allen, involves the

---

[1] Calculated from: mg/m^3 = (molecular weight/24.45) × ppm, assuming standard temperature (25 °C) and pressure (760 mm Hg [101.3 kPa])

Table 1. Methods for the analysis of amitrole

Sample matrix	Sample preparation	Assay procedure	Limit of detection	Reference
Air	Draw air through impinger containing water	HPLC/UV	0.004 mg/m³	Occupational Safety and Health Administration (1998)
Fruit, crops, wine, soil	Extract with ethanol:water (2:1) or rotary evaporate; acetylate with acetic anhydride; partition into dichloromethane; clean-up	GLC/NPD	0.01 mg/kg	H.J. Jarczyk & E. Möllhoff (1991), cited in FAO/WHO (1999)
Blackberries	Extract with ethanol:water; treat with H_2O_2; clean-up with ion exchange; convert to a complex with fluorescamine	HPLC/FD	0.02 mg/kg	FAO/WHO (1999)
Grapes[a]	Extract with acetone:water; partition into dichloromethane; acidify; clean-up; evaporate to dryness; resuspend in pyridine; derivatize	GC/MS	Method validated over the range 0.005–0.5 mg/kg	C.H. McGuire (1997), cited in FAO/WHO (1999)
Water	Apply sample to cation exchange column; elute with ammonia; clean-up with column chromatography	HPLC/ECD	0.1 µg/L	E. Weber (1988), cited in FAO/WHO (1999)
Crops, soil, milk, eggs, muscle	Extract with acetone:water (1:3); partition into dichloromethane; clean-up	HPLC/ECD	0.005 mg/kg	E. Weber (1997), cited in FAO/WHO (1999)

HPLC/UV, high-performance liquid chromatography/ultraviolet detection; HPLC/FD, high performance liquid chromatography/fluorescence detection; GC/MS, gas chromatography/mass spectrometry; GLC/NPD, gas–liquid chromatography/nitrogen–phosphorus detection; HPLC/ECD, high-performance liquid chromatography/electrochemical detection
[a] This method is now being validated for must and wine, barley, wheat, peas and canola seeds.

same reaction, in which an aminoguanidine salt is heated to 100–120 °C with formic acid in an inert solvent (Carter, 1976; Sittig, 1980).

Information available in 2000 indicated that 3-aminotriazole was manufactured by two companies each in China, France and Japan and one company each in Armenia, Belgium, Canada, India, Switzerland and the USA (CIS Information Services, 2000).

1.3   Use

Amitrole was introduced in the USA in the mid-1950s as a herbicide and plant-growth regulator (Carter, 1976). Registrations for use in food crop production were cancelled in 1971, but it remains an important specialty herbicide (Carter, 1976; Environmental Protection Agency, 1984).

Amitrole is a fast acting herbicide which is taken up predominantly through the leaves of plants. It is used on industrial land, roadsides, railways and ditches and is also used worldwide as a herbicide in vineyards and orchards against all kinds of weeds (grasses and dicotyledons, annual, biannual and perennial) and as a total weed killer after harvest and before the next annual sowing (FAO/WHO, 1999).

1.4   Occurrence

1.4.1   *Occupational exposure*

According to the 1981–83 National Occupational Exposure Survey (National Institute for Occupational Safety and Health, 2000), about 700 workers in the USA were potentially exposed to amitrole, including assemblers and technicians in the manufacture of transport equipment. Farmers were not included in the survey. According to the Finnish Register of Employees Exposed to Carcinogens, about 100 chemical process workers and laboratory workers were exposed in Finland in 1997 (Savela *et al.*, 1999).

Amitrole was reported to be released during dry crushing, and to a lesser extent from bagging, in a plant where the chemical was manufactured, but the concentrations of amitrole in the workroom air were not reported (Alary *et al.*, 1984). No data on levels of exposure to amitrole during its application were available.

1.4.2   *Environmental occurrence*

Amitrole undergoes rapid degradation in the environment, and no systematic measurements of environmental concentrations have been reported. A review (WHO, 1994) presented some anecdotal data on environmental concentrations of this chemical. Air concentrations as high as 100 $\mu g/m^3$ were reported in the vicinity of a facility where amitrole was produced (Alary *et al.*, 1984). The concentration in pond-water immediately after application for aquatic weed control was reported to be 1340 $\mu g/L$ initially, decreasing to 80 $\mu g/L$ after 27 weeks. Similar spraying of a larger watershed in Oregon, USA, showed an initial concentration of 155 $\mu g/L$ within 30 min after spraying, which decreased to below detectable (2 $\mu g/L$) within 6 days (WHO, 1994). Measurements in an aeration pond treated with amitrole showed concentrations up to 200 mg/L, but downstream, rapid degradation and dilution reduced the concentration to 0.5 mg/L (Alary *et al.*, 1984). A series of studies carried out in Japan in 1984 and in France in 1991 indicated no detectable (< 4 μg/L and < 0.1 μg/L, respectively) amounts in typical ponds. Amitrole is readily degraded in soil or attaches irreversibly to soil particles (WHO, 1994).

1.5   Regulations and guidelines

Occupational exposure limits and guidelines for amitrole have been established in several countries (see Table 2).

Amitrole was first considered by the Joint FAO/WHO Meeting on Pesticide Residues (JMPR) in 1974 and given a conditional acceptable daily intake (ADI) of 0–0.00003 mg/kg bw. In 1993, the Codex Committee on Pesticide Residues set a temporary ADI of 0–0.0005 mg/kg bw. A full ADI (0–0.002 mg/kg bw) was allocated in 1997. The 1998 JMPR recommended a maximum residue limit (MRL) of 0.05 mg/kg in grapes and 0.05 mg/kg (limit of detection) in pome fruits and stone fruits (FAO/WHO, 1999; WHO, 1999).

Table 2. Occupational exposure limits and guidelines for amitrole

Country	Year	Concentration (mg/m^3)	Interpretation
Australia	1993	0.2	TWA
Austria	1993	0.2	TWA
Belgium	1993	0.2	TWA
Denmark	1993	0.2 (Ca)	TWA
Finland	1993	(Ca)	TWA
Germany	2000	0.2 (IF) (3B)	TWA
Ireland	1997	0.2	TWA
Netherlands	1999	0.2	TWA
Switzerland	1993	0.2	TWA
USA			
ACGIH (TLV)	2000	0.2 (A3)	TWA
NIOSH (REL)	1999	0.2 (Ca)	TWA

From American Conference of Governmental Industrial Hygienists (ACGIH) (2000); Deutsche Forschungsgemeinschaft (2000)
TWA, time-weighted average; TLV, threshold limit value; NIOSH, National Institute for Occupational Safety and Health; REL, recommended exposure limit; Ca, carcinogen; IF, inhalable fraction of the aerosol; A3, confirmed animal carcinogen of unknown relevance to humans; 3B, substances for which in-vitro or animal studies have yielded evidence of carcinogenic effects that is not sufficient for classification of the substance in one of the other categories; further studies are required before a final decision can be made. A maximum acceptable concentration (MAC) value can be established provided no genotoxic effects have been detected.

2. Studies of Cancer in Humans

2.1   Cohort study

In a study of mortality in Sweden, a cohort of 348 male railroad workers who had been exposed for 45 days or more to amitrole and/or chlorophenoxy herbicides (see IARC, 1986b) was followed up from 1957 to 1972 and again in 1978 (Axelson & Sundell, 1974; Axelson *et al*., 1980). There was a deficit of deaths from all causes (45 observed, 49 expected) but an excess of deaths from malignant neoplasms (17 observed, 11.9 expected). In a subcohort exposed to amitrole but not chlorophenoxy herbicides, there were five deaths from cancer (two lung cancers, one pancreatic cancer, one reticulum-cell sarcoma and one maxillary sinus cancer), with 3.3 expected (not significant); three of the deaths (with 2.0 expected) occurred in workers first exposed 10 years or more before death. In a subcohort of men exposed to both amitrole and chlorophenoxy herbicides, there were six deaths from cancer with 2.9 expected. All six (with 1.8 expected; $p < 0.005$) occurred in workers first exposed 10 years or more before death. The men were also exposed to other organic (e.g., monuron and diuron) and inorganic chemicals (e.g., potassium chlorate). The results obtained during the extended follow-up period (1972–78), in which the exposure assessment would not have been influenced by knowledge of the disease, are similar to the results for the whole period 1957–78 reported above, i.e. a statistically significant excess of deaths from cancers at all sites in the subcohort exposed to both amitrole and chlorophenoxy herbicides but not in the subcohort exposed to amitrole alone. No thyroid tumours were reported.

3. Studies of Cancer in Experimental Animals

3.1   Oral administration

Mouse: In a preliminary report of a screening study, groups of 18 male and 18 female (C57BL/6×C3H/Anf)F_1 and (C57BL/6×AKR)F_1 mice, 7 days of age, were given 0 (control) or 1000 mg/kg bw (maximum tolerated dose) amitrole [purity unspecified] in distilled water daily by stomach tube until 4 weeks of age. Subsequently, the animals were fed diets containing 0 (control) or 2192 mg/kg amitrole (maximum tolerated dose) until the end of the observation period (53–60 weeks). Thyroid follicular-cell tumours (carcinomas) were reported in 64/72 treated males and females of both strains combined. 'Hepatomas' were observed in 34/36 pooled treated male and female (C57BL/6×C3H/Anf)F_1 mice and in 33/36 pooled treated male and female (C57BL/6×AKR)F_1 mice. In pooled control groups, 8/166 (C57BL/6×CeH/Anf)F_1 mice and 6/172 (C57BL/6×AKR)F_1 mice had 'hepatomas' (National Cancer Institute,

1968; Innes *et al.*, 1969). [The Working Group noted the lack of a published final report that would have provided more details on the study.]

Groups of C3H female mice were treated at weaning with neutron irradiation or fed a diet containing amitrole [purity unspecified], or both. Amitrole was mixed into the diet at a concentration of 1% (10 000 mg/kg) during the first 4 weeks of a 5-week cycle, and this cycle was repeated continuously for life. The groups that received amitrole alone or after neutron irradiation had a 100% incidence of liver tumours (29/29 and 33/33, respectively), whereas in the group treated with neutrons but not fed amitrole in the diet, 2/37 (5%) mice had liver tumours (Feinstein *et al.*, 1978a). [The Working Group noted the lack of an untreated control group and that the liver tumours were not specified as adenomas or carcinomas.]

Groups of 75 male and 75 female NMRI mice, 6 weeks of age, were fed diets containing 0 (control), 1, 10 or 100 mg/kg amitrole (technical grade, 97% pure) for life. There was no difference in body weights or survival rate (average survival time, 637–734 days) between amitrole-treated and control mice. No indication of a carcinogenic effect was seen (Steinhoff *et al.*, 1983). [The Working Group noted the low range of doses administered.]

Groups of male and female B6C3F$_1$ mice were fed diets containing 0 (control) or 500 mg/kg amitrole [purity unspecified] continuously from weaning until 90 weeks. In the 55 males, nine hepatocellular adenomas and 11 hepatocellular carcinomas were observed; in the 49 females, there were five hepatocellular adenomas and four hepatocellular carcinomas. In control mice, held for 90 weeks only, one hepatocellular adenoma was observed among 98 males and 96 females (Vesselinovitch, 1983). [The Working Group noted that the increased tumour incidences were statistically significant, as calculated by a previous working group (IARC, 1986a).]

Groups of 6-week-old stocks and strains of female DS, ICR (Crj:CD-1®) and NOD (derived from ICR) mice were given amitrole [purity not specified] in the drinking-water at 1% for up to 6 months in two experiments. The mice were treated for 3 months in the first experiment and for 6 months in the second experiment, killed and evaluated for the presence of hyperplastic nodules and neoplastic lesions in the liver. The incidences of hyperplastic nodules were 15/19 in NOD, 3/5 in DS and 0/5 in ICR mice in the first experiment and 19/19 in NOD, 18/18 in DS and 17/19 in ICR mice in the second experiment. One hepatocellular carcinoma was also observed in a NOD mouse treated for 6 months. The hyperplastic nodules were larger in NOD mice than in either DS or ICR mice (Mori *et al.*, 1985). [The Working Group noted the lack of a matched untreated control group for each strain and experiment.]

Rat: Groups of rats [initial numbers, sex, strain and age unspecified] were fed diets containing 0 (control), 10, 50 or 100 mg/kg amitrole [purity unspecified] for 104 weeks. Thyroid follicular-cell adenomas were observed in 1/10, 2/15 (one 'adenocarcinomatous') and 17/26 (four 'adenocarcinomatous') rats at the three concentrations, respectively. No thyroid tumour was found in the five controls examined (Jukes & Shaffer,

1960). [The Working Group noted the small number of control rats and the lack of detail in this report.]

Groups of 27–32 male and female random-bred white rats (weighing 100–120 g) were either given drinking-water containing amitrole to provide a dose of 20–25 mg/rat per day, or were fed diets providing a dose of 250 or 500 mg/rat per day for life (5–23 months). Of the group receiving amitrole in the drinking-water, eight were alive at the time of appearance of the first thyroid follicular-cell tumour, and three thyroid and six hepatocellular tumours were observed. Of the groups receiving amitrole in the diet, 10 and 11 rats were alive at the time of appearance of the first tumour in the groups given 250 and 500 mg/rat, respectively; two thyroid and eight liver tumours were observed in the group fed 250 mg amitrole; five thyroid and 10 liver tumours were seen in the group receiving 500 mg amitrole (Napalkov, 1962). [The Working Group noted the lack of matching control groups.]

Groups of rats [initial numbers, sex, strain and age unspecified] were fed diets containing 0, 10, 50 or 100 mg/kg amitrole [purity unspecified] for 104 weeks. Thyroid follicular-cell adenomas were observed in 15/27 rats at the highest concentration and in 1–3/27 in the other two treated groups (Hodge et al., 1966). [The Working Group noted that the experiment was inadequately reported and that control data were not included.]

Six groups of female Wistar rats, weighing approximately 200 g, received the following treatments: group 1 (40 rats) received drinking-water containing 2500 mg/L amitrole [purity unspecified] for 70 weeks; group 2 (30 rats) received a partial thyroidectomy and then, 2 weeks later, amitrole in the drinking-water; group 3 (30 rats) received a partial thyroidectomy followed by re-implantation of the autochthonous thyroid tissue and, 2 weeks later, amitrole in the drinking-water; group 4 (10 rats) served as untreated controls; group 5 (10 rats) received a partial thyroidectomy with no further treatment; and group 6 (10 rats) received a partial thyroidectomy followed by re-implantation of the autochthonous thyroid tissue with no further treatment. Rats that lived longer than 30 weeks comprised the effective animals. Premature deaths were largely a result of infection; the survival rate at 30 weeks was 70–80% for rats not receiving amitrole and 47–65% for amitrole-treated rats. Papillary follicular-cell adenomas were observed in the thyroid in 3/26, 1/14 and 1/10 rats in groups 1, 2 and 3, respectively, and invasive follicular-cell tumours of the thyroid were found in 19/26, 14/14 and 10/10 rats in groups 1, 2 and 3, respectively. These results were significantly different ($p < 0.001$) from those in the matching control groups (0/7, 0/7 and 0/8 in groups 4, 5 and 6, respectively) (Tsuda et al., 1976).

Groups of female Wistar rats weighing approximately 200 g received one of the following treatments: 20 rats received drinking-water containing 2500 mg/L amitrole [purity unspecified] and a standard diet (containing 5 mg/kg iodine); 20 rats were fed a low-iodine (0.25 mg/kg) diet; and 20 rats were fed a standard diet (containing 5 mg/kg iodine) and served as untreated controls. The experiment was terminated at 60 weeks; rats that lived 30 weeks or more were considered to be the effective animals. Follicular-cell carcinomas of the thyroid were observed in 9/13 rats treated with amitrole alone, in 4/9 rats fed the low-iodine diet and in 0/16 untreated controls (Tsuda *et al.*, 1978).

Groups of 75 male and 75 female Wistar rats, 6 weeks of age, were fed diets containing 0 (control), 1, 10 or 100 mg/kg amitrole (technical grade, 97% pure) for life. No difference was observed in body-weight gain, and the average survival exceeded 900 days in all groups. Increased incidences of thyroid follicular-cell tumours were observed in the group at the high dietary concentration. The incidences of benign thyroid tumours in the four groups were 5/36, 9/41, 4/44 and 45/53 for males and 7/59, 12/67, 8/60 and 44/71 for females, and the incidences of malignant thyroid tumours were 3/36, 0/41, 3/44 and 18/53 for males and 0/59, 1/67, 4/60 and 28/71 for females. The incidences of benign pituitary tumours (adenomas) were marginally increased in females, being 4/36, 9/41, 10/44 and 10/53 for males and 14/59, 20/67, 15/60 and 36/41 for females (Steinhoff *et al.*, 1983).

Hamster: Groups of 76 male and 76 female golden hamsters, 6 weeks of age, were fed diets containing 0 (control), 1, 10 or 100 mg/kg amitrole (technical grade, 97% pure) for life. No difference was observed in the body-weight gains or survival of controls and animals at the two lower dietary concentrations. Reduced body-weight gain and a significant reduction in survival were observed at the high concentration. There was no indication of a carcinogenic effect (Steinhoff *et al.*, 1983).

3.2   Dermal application

Mouse: Groups of 50 male and 50 female C3H/Anf mice, 2–4 months old, received weekly applications to the skin of 0.1 or 10 mg analytical-grade amitrole in 0.2 mL acetone:methanol (65:35) for life. The median length of survival ranged from 44 to 57 weeks. No skin tumour was observed (Hodge *et al.*, 1966).

3.3   Subcutaneous administration

Rat: A group of 19 male and female random-bred white rats, weighing 100–120 g, received twice-weekly subcutaneous injections of 125 mg amitrole [purity unspecified] in water for 11 months and were observed up to 23 months. Of the seven rats alive at the appearance of the first tumour, five had liver tumours and five had thyroid follicular-cell tumours (Napalkov, 1962). [The Working Group noted the lack of a matching control group.]

3.4   Perinatal exposure

Mouse: Pregnant C57BL/6 mice (mated with C3H males) were fed a diet containing 500 mg/kg amitrole [purity unspecified] from day 12 of gestation until delivery, and the B6C3F$_1$ offspring were maintained on a standard diet without amitrole for 90 weeks. Four hepatocellular adenomas and two hepatocellular carcinomas were observed in 74 male B6C3F$_1$ offspring, but there were no liver tumours in the 83 females. In unexposed B6C3F$_1$ mice held for 90 weeks, only one hepatocellular adenoma was observed in 98 males, and there were no liver tumours in 96 females (Vesselinovitch, 1983).

Groups of B6C3F$_1$ mice were exposed to amitrole perinatally, being nursed by dams fed diets containing 500 mg/kg amitrole [purity unspecified] from birth until weaning. The offspring were then maintained on a standard diet until the end of the study at 90 weeks. In 45 males, six hepatocellular adenomas and four hepatocellular carcinomas were observed; no liver tumours occurred in 55 females. In untreated controls observed for 90 weeks, one hepatocellular adenoma was observed in a group of 98 males; none was observed among 96 females (Vesselinovitch, 1983). [The Working Group noted that the increased tumour incidences were statistically significant as calculated by a previous working group (IARC, 1986).]

3.5   Administration with known carcinogens or modifying factors

Rat: Two groups of 30 male albino rats, 2–3 months of age, were fed a diet containing 0.06% 4-dimethylaminoazobenzene (DAB), and one of the groups also received an intraperitoneal injection of amitrole [purity unspecified] every 2 days as a 10% solution in water until the end of the study to provide a dose of 1000 mg/kg bw. The surviving 16 DAB-treated and 19 DAB plus amitrole-treated rats were killed at 21 weeks. The incidences of liver tumours were 12/16 in the group receiving DAB alone and 4/19 in the group that received DAB plus amitrole ($p < 0.01$). The liver tumours produced by DAB alone were mostly hepatocellular carcinomas, whereas those in the group treated with DAB plus amitrole were hepatocellular carcinomas and cholangio-carcinomas (Hoshino, 1960).

Groups of 12 male Wistar rats, 6 weeks of age, received the following treatments: group 1 received four weekly subcutaneous injections to provide a dose of 700 mg/kg bw *N*-nitrosobis(2-hydroxypropyl)amine (NBHPA), followed by a diet containing 2000 mg/kg amitrole [purity unspecified] for a total of 12 weeks; group 2 received four weekly injections of NBHPA only; group 3 was fed a diet containing 2000 mg/kg amitrole beginning at week 4 for 12 weeks; group 4 received eight weekly injections of NBHPA followed by a diet containing 2000 mg/kg amitrole for 12 weeks; group 5 received eight weekly injections of NBHPA only; group 6 was fed a diet containing 2000 mg/kg diet amitrole beginning at week 8; and group 7 was fed a standard diet and served as untreated controls. All animals were killed after 20 weeks. No thyroid tumours were found in group 2, 3, 6 or 7, but thyroid tumours were observed in 7/12 rats in group 5. A significantly increased incidence ($p < 0.05$) of thyroid follicular-cell tumours was observed in rats in group 1 (9/11) when compared with groups 7 and 2. A significant increase in tumour incidence ($p < 0.05$) was also observed in rats in group 4 (12/12) when compared with groups 7 and 5. The tumours found in groups 1, 4 and 5 were mainly thyroid follicular-cell tumours. Thus, amitrole promoted NBHPA-induced thyroid neoplasia (Hiasa *et al.*, 1982).

A group of 75 male Wistar-Furth rats, castrated at 40 days of age, were divided into six groups: group 1 (five rats) received no further treatment and served as untreated controls; group 2 (10 rats) was given drinking-water containing 1500 mg/L amitrole [purity unspecified] starting 7 days after castration; group 3 (10 rats) received a subcutaneous implant of a pellet on the back containing 5 mg diethylstilbestrol and 45 mg cholesterol, which was replaced every 2 months; group 4 (11 rats) received the pellet plus amitrole in the drinking-water; group 5 (20 rats) received the pellet followed by administration of drinking-water providing a dose of 5 mg/day of *N*-butyl-*N*-nitrosourea (BNU) for 30 days starting at 50–55 days of age; and group 6 (19 rats) received the pellet followed by administration of BNU and, 7 days after BNU treatment, amitrole in the drinking-water. Groups 3–6 received the implants at the same time as they were castrated. Rats that lived beyond 230 days of age were considered to be effective animals; all survivors were killed at 14 months of age. Neoplastic nodules and hepatocellular carcinomas developed in 4/9 rats in group 3 and 15/17 in group 5, and pituitary tumours developed in 7/9 rats in group 3 and 12/17 in group 5. Addition of amitrole to these regimens (groups 4 and 6, respectively) had no effect on the incidence of pituitary tumours (8/11 and 10/14) but slightly (group 4; 2/11) and significantly (group 6; 3/14) reduced the incidences of neoplastic nodules and hepatocellular carcinomas. There were no pituitary or liver tumours in the untreated controls or in rats receiving amitrole alone (Sumi *et al.*, 1985).

4.   Other Data Relevant to an Evaluation of Carcinogenicity and its Mechanisms

4.1   Absorption, distribution, metabolism and excretion

4.1.1   *Humans*

Urinary excretion of unchanged amitrole at a concentration of 1 g/L was reported in a woman who ingested approximately 20 mg/kg bw of the herbicide (Geldmacher-von Mallinckrodt & Schmidt, 1970).

4.1.2   *Experimental systems*

Amitrole is rapidly and almost completely absorbed from the gut and lungs (Fang *et al.*, 1964; Burton *et al.*, 1974; Tjälve, 1975; Brown & Schanker, 1983). After intravenous or intragastric administration of radiolabelled amitrole to mice, the label accumulated in the bone marrow, spleen, thymus, liver and gut mucosa (Tjälve, 1975). After administration of an oral dose of radiolabelled compound to rats, the label disappeared from the heart, lung, spleen, testis and brain with a half-time of approximately 2.5 h. It was excreted mainly in the urine, with a small, variable amount found in the faeces

(Fang *et al.*, 1964). Six per cent of a 50-mg/kg bw oral dose was excreted in the urine of rats as 3-amino-5-mercapto-1,2,4-triazole and 3-amino-1,2,4-triazoyl-(5)-mercapturic acid (Grunow *et al.*, 1975).

When mice were given an intravenous dose of 3.4 mg/kg bw [^{14}C]amitrole, approximately 10% [estimated from data presented by the authors] of the radiolabel appeared to be irreversibly bound to liver tissue. The bound radiolabel was apparently located mainly centrilobularly, and the amount decreased very little over 24 h (Fujii *et al.*, 1984).

4.1.3   *Comparison of animals and humans*

No data were available to the Working Group.

4.2   **Toxic effects**

4.2.1   *Humans*

Intentional ingestion of a commercial mixture of amitrole and diuron at a dose equivalent to 20 mg/kg bw of amitrole was reported to have caused no symptoms of poisoning in a woman (Geldmacher-von Mallinckrodt & Schmidt, 1970).

English *et al.* (1986) reported on a 41-year-old weed control operator with a 6-month history of dermatitis involving his face, hands, back, thighs and feet. Patch testing with 1% amitrole revealed a strong positive vesicular reaction at 2 and 4 days, suggesting allergic contact dermatitis. Balkisson *et al.* (1992) reported on a 74-year-old, previously healthy man who sprayed an amitrole formulation (containing 19% amitrole, 17% ammonium thiocyanate) in a strong head-wind without any protective clothing for 2 h using 500 mL of the formulated material in 10 L of water. He developed a dry non-productive cough after 6–8 h. Diffuse, asymmetrical, severe alveolar damage in the lungs was detected, which was reversed by intravenous administration of high doses of corticosteroids.

The results of a study conducted on five men involved in spraying amitrole over 10 working days on utility right-of-ways in West Virginia (USA) were reported by WHO (1994; D.G. Baugher *et al.*, 1982). The amitrole was applied at a concentration of approximately 500 g of active ingredient per 100 L of water from hand-held hydraulic spray guns. Medical monitoring, particularly of the thyroid, was carried out both before and after spraying and included palpation of the thyroid gland and neck measurements 19 days before and 14 days after exposure, and thyroid function tests 19, 11 and 4 days before exposure and 0, 7 and 14 days after the last exposure. The thyroid function of all men was within the normal range, and no differences were found in any comparisons of thyroid function. It was estimated that the dermal exposure of each man over the 10-day period was approximately 340 mg/day. In a study reported by Miksche (1983), thyroid function was evaluated in five employees who had been engaged in the production and packaging of amitrole for between 3 and 16 years. Thyroid scintigrams and measurements of triiodothyronine (T3) and thyroxine (T4) revealed no evidence of thyroid dysfunction.

Legras *et al.* (1996) described a fatal case of poisoning with Radoxone TL (in which amitrole is the main active ingredient at 240 g/L, with ammonium thiocyanate at 215 g/L, which enhances the activity of amitrole). A 54-year-old man was hospitalized with unexplained coma, myoclonic contractions and vascular collapse. The concentrations of thiocyanate and amitrole in his blood were 750 mg/L and 138 mg/L, respectively, more than 12 h after ingestion of the preparation. Experimental studies and previously reported fatal cases suggest that thiocyanate is the predominant toxic substance in the herbicide mixture.

4.2.2   *Experimental systems*

Amitrole generally has little acute toxicity to experimental animals. The acute oral LD_{50} has been reported to be 14.7 g/kg bw in mice and 25 g/kg bw in rats (Kröller, 1966). An oral dose of 2 g/kg bw administered to sheep was fatal [details not given] (Hapke *et al.*, 1965). No pronounced toxicity was seen in mice, cats or dogs after intravenous injection of 1.6, 1.7 or 1.2 g/kg bw, respectively; mice tolerated an intraperitoneal injection of 4 g/kg bw amitrole (C.B. Shaffer, 1956; cited in Kröller, 1996). Acatalasaemic substrains of highly inbred C3H and C57BL mice were more resistant to the effects of amitrole, a known catalase inhibitor, on weight than mice with normal catalase activity (Feinstein *et al.*, 1978b). No sign of acute toxicity was seen in specific pathogen-free adult male or female rats given amitrole (99% pure) in aqueous solution by stomach tube at 4.0 g/kg bw or by dermal application at 2.5 g/kg bw (Gaines *et al.*, 1973). Intraperitoneal administration of 4.0 g/kg bw amitrole every 4 h for 24 h to male rats did not produce toxic effects (Kato, 1967).

Adult specific pathogen-free rats given diets containing 500 or 1000 mg/kg amitrole (99% pure) for 107–110 days gained 14–26% less body weight than did controls, but no reduction in weight gain was observed in rats fed diets containing 25 or 100 mg/kg amitrole for 240–247 days (Gaines *et al.*, 1973). The weight gain of specific pathogen-free rats, mice and golden hamsters was not affected by life-long administration of diets containing 10 mg/kg technical-grade amitrole (97% pure); however, a diet with 100 mg/kg amitrole resulted in a slight reduction in body weight in golden hamsters (Steinhoff *et al.*, 1983).

Amitrole markedly inhibited thyroid iodine uptake and the organic binding of iodine in rats (Alexander, 1959), and Strum and Karnovsky (1970) showed that amitrole reversibly inhibits thyroid peroxidase in this species. [Thyroperoxidase is the coupling enzyme that enhances the combination of thyroid hormone precursor molecules (e.g. mono- with diiodotyrosine, or diiodotyrosine with diiodotyrosine) into the biologically active forms of thyroid hormones (T3 and T4, respectively); see Figure 1 in General Remarks.] Male rats given drinking-water containing 0.04% (400 mg/L) amitrole developed goitre (i.e. thyroid gland enlargement due to follicular cell hypertrophy and hyperplasia) by 7 days (Strum & Karnovsky, 1971). In female rats given drinking-water containing 2.5 mg/mL amitrole, a small increase in the size of the thyroid was visible after 3 days, and the size of the gland had doubled by 10 days (Tsuda *et al.*, 1973). Continuous feeding of a diet containing 100 mg/kg amitrole resulted in the development of goitre in rats of each sex within 3 months, 25 mg/kg caused goitre in 4/10 females killed at 240 days, while rats receiving 10 mg/kg showed no goitrogenic effect within 24 months (Gaines *et al.*, 1973; Steinhoff *et al.*, 1983). Continuous feeding (up to 18 months) of a diet containing 100 mg/kg amitrole produced goitre in mice but not in golden hamsters; a dietary concentration of 10 mg/kg had no effect in either species (Steinhoff *et al.*, 1983).

In male rats (Blue Spruce Farms strain) fed diets containing 0, 0.25, 0.5, 2, 10 or 50 mg/kg amitrole for 11–13 weeks, several measures of thyroid function were affected: dose-related decreases in serum protein-bound iodine concentrations and thyroid ^{131}I uptake were observed in groups receiving > 2 mg/kg of diet 24 h after injection of the isotope; and morphological changes in the thyroid, consisting of follicular-cell hypertrophy and reduced luminal colloid, were observed at the two higher concentrations (Fregly, 1968).

Amitrole caused rapid inactivation of lactoperoxidase only in the presence of hydrogen peroxide. The kinetics is consistent with a suicide mechanism (Doerge & Niemczura, 1989). In view of the similarities between lactoperoxidase and thyroid peroxidase, the authors suggested a similar mechanism of inhibition of thyroid hormone synthesis by amitrole. In addition to its direct inhibitory effect on thyroperoxidase in thyroid follicular cells, amitrole has been reported to affect the peripheral metabolism and deiodination of T4, resulting in increased formation of reverse T3 (Cartier *et al.*, 1985). Amitrole did not inhibit 5′-deiodinase activity as did other goitrogens (e.g. propylthiouracil; see monograph in this volume) but rather stimulated the T4 5-deiodination pathway in peripheral tissues.

Studies on the time-course of the response of the thyroid to amitrole treatment in male Wistar rats given drinking-water containing 0.1% for 7 or 12 months showed a rapid rise in the concentration of thyroid-stimulating hormone (TSH) after a short lag phase of a few days (Wynford-Thomas *et al.*, 1983) that was paralleled by thyroid hypertrophy and hyperplasia. These effects peaked and plateaued after 3–4 months and thereafter remained relatively stable despite further exposure. Wynford-Thomas *et al.* (1982) reported striking decreases in T4 and T3 and marked increases in serum TSH concentrations resulting in increased thyroid weight due to increased follicular-cell numbers in male Wistar rats (aged 10–11 weeks at the start of the experiment) given amitrole at 0.1% in drinking-water (estimated equivalent dose, 500 mg/kg bw) daily for 3, 7, 14, 24, 46, 83, 116 or 153 days. Control groups (age-matched) were killed after 0, 25, 83 and 154 days. Mattioli *et al.* (1994) gave lower concentrations of amitrole in the drinking-water (1 g/L; estimated daily intake, 200 mg/kg bw) to male Sprague-Dawley albino rats (90–100 g) for 5, 8 or 12 days and found similar marked reductions in plasma T4 and T3 concentrations associated with a concurrent increase in both the mitotic index and frequency of S-phase cells, indicative of thyroid follicular-cell hyperplasia. A number of studies have shown that the goitrogenic action of amitrole is reversible on cessation of exposure (Jukes & Shaffer, 1960).

Enzymatically dispersed rat thyrocytes from the early plateau phase and involuting goitres were analysed for their capacity to form thyroid follicular units after transplantation into syngeneic recipients. The clonogenic fractions of goitres induced by either amitrole or $KClO_4$/Remington low-iodine diet were significantly smaller than in cells from control glands, and the clonogenic fraction of cells from the $KClO_4$-induced goitres was smaller than that of cells from amitrole-induced goitres, despite similar circulating TSH concentrations in the donor rats. The authors concluded that the capacity to proliferate clonally into follicular units is a specific trait that characterizes a unique subset of follicular cells and suggested that the hormonally responsive tumours that often develop in continuously stimulated rat thyroid glands arise from cells within this subset (Groch & Clifton, 1992).

In a study of the histopathological changes induced by amitrole in the liver, groups of male albino mice were given amitrole in the drinking-water at a concentration of 0.5, 1 or 2% for 30 days. Light microscopy revealed dose-related hypertrophy of hepatocytes, increased pyknotic nucleoli, increased vacuoles and lipid droplets in the cytoplasm. Electron microscopy revealed a dose-related proliferation of smooth endoplasmic reticulum (Reitze & Seitz, 1985).

4.3   Reproductive and prenatal effects

4.3.1   *Humans*

No data were available to the Working Group.

4.3.2   *Experimental systems*

When amitrole was last evaluated (IARC, 1986a), limited studies were reviewed in which Sherman rats were exposed to a dietary concentration of amitrole of 25, 100, 500 or 1000 mg/kg (equivalent to 2.5, 9.6, 43 or 87 mg/kg bw per day) for up to two generations. Pup weights were reduced at the two higher concentrations, atrophy of the thymus and spleen was observed, and the majority of pups died within 1 week of weaning. Reproduction was not affected at the two lower concentrations, but thyroid hyperplasia was observed at ≥ 100 mg/kg of diet (Gaines *et al.*, 1973).

4.4   Effects on enzyme induction or inhibition and gene expression

Amitrole inhibited catalase activity in the liver and iris–ciliary body in rats (Williams *et al.*, 1985) and in human cultured fibroblasts (Middelkoop *et al.*, 1991), and inhibited thyroperoxidase activity in rat thyroid follicular cells (Strum & Karnovsky, 1971).

4.5   Genetic and related effects

4.5.1   *Humans*

No data were available to the Working Group.

4.5.2   *Experimental systems* (see Table 3 for references)

Amitrole did not induce DNA damage or mutations in bacteria or mutations or chromosomal damage in cultured mammalian cells. It induced transformation in Syrian hamster embryo cells and chromosomal aberrations in plant root tips. Sporadic aneuploidy and recombinational effects were produced in yeast and fungi and in mammalian cells *in vitro*. No recessive lethal mutation, recombination or aneuploidy was seen in *Drosophila melanogaster*. Amitrole did not induce micronuclei in bone-marrow cells or unscheduled DNA synthesis in hepatocytes of mice treated *in vivo*.

Ki-*ras* mutation was detected in only 1/10 (10%) rat thyroid tumours induced by amitrole, while it was found in 8/15 (53%) radiation-induced tumours (Lemoine *et al.*, 1988).

4.6   Mechanistic considerations

An overall evaluation of the available data supports a mechanism of thyroid hormone imbalance in the development of follicular-cell neoplasia caused by amitrole in rats and mice because:

- Amitrole is considered not to be a genotoxic agent because of lack of activity in appropriate tests with bacteria, cultured mammalian cells and with rats and mice treated *in vivo*.
- Amitrole alters thyroid hormone homeostasis, decreases T4 and T3 and increases TSH concentrations in rats treated with doses that are within the range of those that produced tumours in the studies of carcinogenicity.
- The mechanism resulting in disturbed thyroid hormone synthesis is based on interference with the functioning of thyroid peroxidase.

On the basis of this information, which meets the criteria laid out in the IARC consensus report (Capen *et al.*, 1999), amitrole would be expected not to be carcinogenic to humans exposed to concentrations that do not lead to alterations in thyroid hormone homeostasis. Amitrole produces thyroid gland enlargement (goitre) in rats and mice as a result of follicular-cell hypertrophy and hyperplasia. The hyperplasia induced by amitrole in the thyroid gland is diffuse, in analogy with the morphological changes induced by TSH stimulation, rather than only multifocal, as would be induced by a genotoxic thyroid carcinogen (Hard, 1998). On the basis of the lack of genotoxicity, the liver tumours in mice and the benign pituitary tumours in rats were considered not to be produced by a genotoxic mechanism.

Table 3. Genetic and related effects of amitrole

Test system	Result[a]		Dose[b] (LED or HID)	Reference
	Without exogenous metabolic system	With exogenous metabolic system		
Prophage induction, SOS repair, DNA strand breaks, cross-links	NT	–	1000	Mamber et al. (1984)
Prophage induction, SOS repair, DNA strand breaks, cross-links	–	–	NR	Quillardet et al. (1985)
Prophage induction, SOS repair, DNA strand breaks, cross-links	–	–	1670	Nakamura et al. (1987)
Escherichia coli pol A, differential toxicity	–	–	250	Rosenkranz & Poirier (1979)
Escherichia coli rec, differential toxicity	–	NT	5000	Bamford et al. (1976)
Escherichia coli rec, differential toxicity	NT	–	4000	Mamber et al. (1983)
Bacteriophage, forward mutation	–	NT	25	Andersen et al. (1972)
Bacteriophage, reverse mutation	–	NT	200	Andersen et al. (1972)
Salmonella typhimurium TM677, forward mutation	NT	–	100	Skopek et al. (1981)
Salmonella typhimurium TA100, reverse mutation	NT	–	500 µg/plate	Hubbard et al. (1981)
Salmonella typhimurium TA100, reverse mutation	–	–	5000 µg/plate	MacDonald (1981)
Salmonella typhimurium TA100, TA1535, TA1537, TA98, reverse mutation	NT	–	5000 µg/plate	McCann et al. (1975)
Salmonella typhimurium TA100, TA1535, TA1536, TA1537, TA1538, TA98, reverse mutation	NT	–	250 µg/plate	Simmon (1979a)
Salmonella typhimurium TA100, TA1535, TA1537, TA1538, TA98, reverse mutation	–	–	333.3 µg/plate	Dunkel et al. (1984)
Salmonella typhimurium TA100, TA1535, TA1537, TA1538, TA98, reverse mutation	NT	–	4000 µg/plate	Mamber et al. (1984)
Salmonella typhimurium TA100, TA1535, TA1537, TA1538, TA98, reverse mutation	–	–	1000 µg/plate	Falck et al. (1985)

Table 3 (contd)

Test system	Result[a]		Dose[b] (LED or HID)	Reference
	Without exogenous metabolic system	With exogenous metabolic system		
Salmonella typhimurium TA100, TA1535, TA1537, TA1538, TA98, reverse mutation	−	−	10 000 µg/plate	Richold & Jones (1981)
Salmonella typhimurium TA100, TA1535, TA98, TA97, reverse mutation	−	−	3333 µg/plate	Zeiger *et al.* (1988)
Salmonella typhimurium TA1535, TA1537, TA1538, TA1536, reverse mutation	−	−	2000 µg/plate	Carere *et al.* (1978)
Salmonella typhimurium TA1535, TA1537, TA98, reverse mutation	−	−	500 µg/plate	Gatehouse (1981)
Salmonella typhimurium TA1535, TA1538, reverse mutation	−	−	250 µg/plate	Rosenkranz & Poirier (1979)
Salmonella typhimurium TA1537, TA98, reverse mutation	−	−	2000 µg/plate	MacDonald (1981)
Salmonella typhimurium TA98, reverse mutation	NT	−	10 000 µg/plate	Croker *et al.* (1992)
Salmonella typhimurium LT2 *trp*, reverse mutation	−	NT	4000 µg/plate	Bamford *et al.* (1976)
Escherichia coli, WP2 *uvrA*, reverse mutation	−	−	333.3 µg/plate	Dunkel *et al.* (1984)
Escherichia coli, WP2 *uvrA*, reverse mutation	−	−	1000 µg/plate	Falck *et al.* (1985)
Escherichia coli, WP2 *uvrA*, reverse mutation	−	−	500	Gatehouse (1981)
Saccharomyces wild type strain, differential toxicity	+	−	100	Sharp & Parry (1981a)
Saccharomyces cerevisiae, gene conversion	+	NT	300	Sharp & Parry (1981b)
Saccharomyces cerevisiae, gene conversion	NT	−	12 500	Zimmermann & Scheel (1981)
Saccharomyces cerevisiae, homozygosis	−	−	50 000	Simmon (1979b)
Saccharomyces cerevisiae, homozygosis	−	−	1000	Kassinova *et al.* (1981)
Saccharomyces cerevisiae, reverse mutation	−	−	1000	Mehta & von Borstel (1981)
Saccharomyces cerevisiae, aneuploidy	+	+	50	Parry & Sharp (1981)

Table 3 (contd)

Test system	Result[a] Without exogenous metabolic system	Result[a] With exogenous metabolic system	Dose[b] (LED or HID)	Reference
Saccharomyces coelicolor, forward mutation	(+)	NT	1000	Carere *et al.* (1978)
Aspergillus nidulans, forward mutation	–	NT	2000	Bignami *et al.* (1977)
Aspergillus nidulans, forward mutation	–	NT	10 000	Crebelli *et al.* (1986)
Aspergillus nidulans, crossing-over	(+)	NT	2000	Bignami *et al.* (1977)
Aspergillus nidulans, crossing-over	–	NT	10 000	Crebelli *et al.* (1977)
Aspergillus nidulans, aneuploidy	(+)	NT	400	Bignami *et al.* (1977)
Aspergillus nidulans, aneuploidy	–	NT	10 000	Crebelli *et al.* (1986)
Chromosomal aberrations, *Hordeum* spp.	+	NT	100	Wuu & Grant (1966)
Chromosomal aberrations, *Vicia faba*	+	NT	50	Wuu & Grant (1967)
Chromosomal aberrations, *Neatby's virescens* (wheat)	+	NT	1.25	Rédei & Sandhu (1988)
Drosophila melanogaster, mitotic recombination	–		1680	Vogel & Nivard (1993)
Drosophila melanogaster, wing spot test	?		840	Tripathy *et al.* (1990)
Drosophila melanogaster, white-ivory assay	?		1680	Consuegra *et al.* (1996)
Drosophila melanogaster, sex-linked recessive lethal mutations	–		10	Laamanen *et al.* (1976)
Drosophila melanogaster, sex-linked recessive lethal mutations	–		2000	Vogel *et al.* (1981)
Drosophila melanogaster, sex-linked recessive lethal mutations	–		20 000 feed[c]	Woodruff *et al.* (1985)
Drosophila melanogaster, aneuploidy and sex-linked recessive lethal mutations	–		10	Laamanen *et al.* (1976)
DNA fragmentation, rat hepatocytes *in vitro*	–	NT	1510	Mattioli *et al.* (1994)
Binding to RNA or protein *in vitro*	–	+	4	Krauss & Eling (1987)
Gene mutation, mouse lymphoma L5178Y cells, *Tk* locus *in vitro*	–	–	5000	McGregor *et al.* (1987)
Gene mutation, mouse lymphoma L5178Y cells, *Tk* locus *in vitro*	–	–	6000	Mitchell *et al.* (1988)

Table 3 (contd)

Test system	Result[a] Without exogenous metabolic system	Result[a] With exogenous metabolic system	Dose[b] (LED or HID)	Reference
Gene mutation, mouse lymphoma L5178Y cells, *Tk* locus *in vitro*	–	–	5000	Myhr & Caspary (1988)
Gene mutation, Syrian hamster embryo cells, *Hprt* and Na^+/K^+ ATPase *in vitro*	+	NT	0.3	Tsutsui *et al.* (1984)
Gene mutation, Syrian hamster embryo BP6T cells *in vitro*	–	NT	8400	Lesko *et al.* (1985)
Sister chromatid exchange, Chinese hamster lung V79 cells *in vitro*	–	+	1	Perry & Thomson (1981)
Chromosomal aberrations, Chinese hamster lung V79 cells *in vitro*	–	NT	1680	Ochi & Ohsawa (1985)
Chromosomal aberrations, Chinese hamster lung V79 cells *in vitro*	–	NT	2000	Sofuni & Ishidate (1988)
Cell transformation, Syrian hamster embryo cells, clonal assay	+	NT	1	Pienta *et al.* (1977)
Cell transformation, Syrian hamster embryo cells, clonal assay	+	NT	50	Inoue *et al.* (1981)
Cell transformation, Syrian hamster embryo cells, clonal assay	+	NT	0.3	Tsutsui *et al.* (1984)
Cell transformation, Syrian hamster embryo cells, clonal assay	(+)	NT	100	Mikalsen *et al.* (1990)
DNA fragmentation, human hepatocytes, human thyroid cells	–	NT	1510	Mattioli *et al.* (1994)
Gene mutation, diploid human fibroblasts HFW, *HPRT* gene mutation *in vitro*	–	NT	6720	Hwua & Yang (1998)
Chromosomal aberrations, human lymphocytes *in vitro*	–	NT	10 000	Meretoja *et al.* (1976)
Cell transformation, diploid human fibroblasts HFW, anchorage independence	–	NT	6720	Hwua & Yang (1998)
Host-mediated assay, mice and *Salmonella typhimurium* TA1950	–		245 po × 1	Braun *et al.* (1977)
Host-mediated assay, mice and *Salmonella typhimurium* TA1530	+		12 im × 1	Simmon *et al.* (1979)

Table 3 (contd)

Test system	Result[a]		Dose[b] (LED or HID)	Reference
	Without exogenous metabolic system	With exogenous metabolic system		
DNA fragmentation, thyroid and liver, rats *in vivo*	–		200 drinking-water, 12 days	Mattioli *et al.* (1994)
Unscheduled DNA synthesis, rat hepatocytes *in vivo*	–		1000 po × 1	Kornbrust *et al.* (1984)
Micronucleus formation, mice *in vivo*	–		135	Salamone *et al.* (1981)
Micronucleus formation, mice *in vivo*	–		500 ip × 2	Tsuchimoto & Matter (1981)

[a] +, positive; (+), weak positive; –, negative; ?, inconclusive; NT, not tested
[b] LED, lowest effective dose; HID, highest ineffective dose; in-vitro tests, µg/mL; in-vivo tests, mg/kg bw per day; NR, not reported; po, oral; im, intramuscular; ip, intraperitoneal
[c] Negative when given at 10 000 µg/mL to adults by injection

5. Summary of Data Reported and Evaluation

5.1　Exposure data

Amitrole is a herbicide, which has been used since the 1950s to control a wide range of weeds and grasses along roadsides, in vineyards and in orchards and in other applications, although contact with food crops is avoided. Amitrole is rapidly degraded in the environment, but occupational exposure may occur during its production and application.

5.2　Human carcinogenicity data

In a small cohort study of mortality among Swedish railroad workers who had sprayed herbicides, there was a statistically significant excess of cancers at all sites combined among men exposed to both amitrole and chlorophenoxy herbicides but not among those exposed mainly to amitrole.

5.3　Animal carcinogenicity data

Amitrole was tested in mice by oral administration, skin application and transplacental and perinatal exposure, in rats by oral and subcutaneous administration and in hamsters by oral administration. In mice, thyroid follicular-cell and hepatocellular tumours were produced after oral administration of amitrole. In rats, amitrole administered orally induced thyroid follicular-cell adenomas and carcinomas in males and females and a marginal increase in the incidence of pituitary adenomas in female rats at the highest dose. No carcinogenic effect was observed in hamsters.

In one experiment in rats, amitrole promoted thyroid follicular-cell tumours induced by N-nitrosobis(2-hydroxypropyl)amine.

5.4　Other relevant data

Amitrole is rapidly absorbed from the gastrointestinal tract and lung.

Amitrole caused thyroid gland enlargement (goitre) in rats and mice as a result of diffuse hypertrophy and hyperplasia of thyroid follicular cells. Administration of amitrole to rats under bioassay conditions that caused predominantly benign follicular-cell tumours resulted in alteration of thyroid hormone homeostasis, including increased secretion of thyroid-stimulating hormone. The underlying mechanism for the changes induced by amitrole is interference with the functioning of thyroid peroxidase.

No data were available on the genetic and related effects of amitrole in humans. Amitrole was not genotoxic in appropriate tests in bacteria and cultured mammalian cells or in rats and mice exposed *in vivo*. Amitrole induced chromosomal aberrations in plants, aneuploidy in some experiments in fungi and transformation of Syrian hamster embryo cells *in vitro*.

5.5 Evaluation

There is *inadequate evidence* in humans for the carcinogenicity of amitrole.

There is *sufficient evidence* in experimental animals for the carcinogenicity of amitrole.

Overall evaluation

Amitrole is *not classifiable as to its carcinogenicity to humans (Group 3)*.

In making its evaluation, the Working Group concluded that amitrole produces thyroid tumours in mice and rats by a non-genotoxic mechanism, which involves interference with the functioning of thyroid peroxidase, resulting in a reduction in circulating thyroid hormone concentrations and increased secretion of thyroid-stimulating hormone. Consequently, amitrole would not be expected to produce thyroid cancer in humans exposed to concentrations that do not alter thyroid hormone homeostasis.

An additional consideration of the Working Group, based on the lack of genotoxicity of amitrole, was that the liver tumours in mice and benign pituitary tumours in rats were also produced by a non-genotoxic mechanism.

Evidence from epidemiological studies and from toxicological studies in experimental animals provide compelling evidence that rodents are substantially more sensitive than humans to the development of thyroid tumours in response to thyroid hormone imbalance.

6. References

Alary, J., Bourbon, P., Escrieut, C. & Vandaele, J. (1984) Spectrophotometric determination of guanazole and aminotriazole in waters from an aminotriazole production plant. *Environ. Technol. Lett.*, **6**, 93–100

Alexander, N.M. (1959) Antithyroid action of 3-amino-12,4-triazole. *J. biol. Chem.*, **234**, 148–150

Allen, C.F.H. & Bell, A. (1946) 3-Amino-1,2,4-triazole (1,2,4-triazole, 3-amino). *Org. Synth.*, **26**, 11–12

American Conference of Governmental Industrial Hygienists (2000) *TLVs and other Occupational Exposure Values — 2000*, Cincinnati, OH [CD-ROM]

Andersen, K.J., Leighty, E.G. & Takahashi, M.T. (1972) Evaluation of herbicides for possible mutagenic properties. *J. agric. Food Chem.*, **20**, 649–656

Axelson, O. & Sundell, L. (1974) Herbicide exposure, mortality and tumor incidence. An epidemiological investigation on Swedish railroad workers. *Work Environ. Health*, **11**, 21–28

Axelson, O., Sundell, L., Andersson, K., Edling, C. & Hogstedt, C. (1980) Herbicide exposure and tumor mortality. An updated epidemiologic investigation on Swedish railroad workers. *Scand. J. Work Environ. Health*, **6**, 73–79

Balkisson, R., Murray, D. & Hoffstein, V. (1992) Alveolar damage due to inhalation of amitrole-containing herbicide. *Chest*, **101**, 1174–1176

Bamford, D., Sorsa, M., Gripenberg, U., Laamanen, I. & Meretoja, T. (1976) Mutagenicity and toxicity of amitrole. III. Microbial tests. *Mutat. Res.*, **40**, 197–202

Bignami, M., Aulicino, F., Velcich, A., Carere, A. & Morpurgo, G. (1977) Mutagenic and recombinogenic action of pesticides in *Aspergillus nidulans*. *Mutat. Res.*, **46**, 395–402

Braun, R., Schoneich, J. & Ziebarth, D. (1977) In vivo formation of *N*-nitroso compounds and detection of their mutagenic activity in the host-mediated assay. *Cancer Res.*, **37**, 4572–4579

Brown, R.A., Jr & Schanker, L.S. (1983) Absorption of aerosolized drugs from the rat lung. *Drug Metab. Disposition*, **11**, 355–360

Budavari, S., ed. (2000) *The Merck Index*, 12th Ed., Version 12:3, Whitehouse Station, NJ, Merck & Co. & Boca Raton, FL, Chapman & Hall/CRC [CD-ROM]

Burton, J.A., Gardiner, T.H. & Schanker, L.S. (1974) Absorption of herbicides from the rat lung. *Arch. environ. Health*, **29**, 31–33

Capen, C.C., Dybing, E., Rice, J.M. & Wilbourn, J.D., eds (1999) *Species Differences in Thyroid, Kidney and Urinary Bladder Carcinogenesis* (IARC Scientific Publications No. 147), Lyon, IARC*Press*

Carere, A., Ortali, V.A., Cardamone, G., Torracca, A.M. & Raschetti, R. (1978) Microbiological mutagenicity studies of pesticides *in vitro*. *Mutat. Res.*, **57**, 277–286

Carter, M.C. (1976) Amitrole. In: Kearney, P.C. & Kaufman, D.D., eds, *Herbicides: Chemistry, Degradation and Mode of Action*, New York, Marcel Dekker, pp. 377–398

Cartier, L.J., Williams, I.K., Holloszy, J. & Premachandra, B.N. (1985) Potentiation of thyroxine 5-deiodination by aminotriazole. *Biochim. biophys. Acta*, **843**, 68–72

CIS Information Services (2000) *Directory of World Chemical Producers (Version 2000.1)*, Dallas, TX [CD-ROM]

Consuegra, S., Ferreiro, J.A., Sierra, L.M. & Comendador, M.A. (1996) 'Non-genotoxic' carcinogens evaluated using the white-ivory assay of *Drosophila melanogaster*. *Mutat. Res.*, **359**, 95–102

Crebelli, R., Bellincampi, D., Conti, G., Conti, L., Morpurgo, G. & Carere, A. (1986) A comparative study on selected chemical carcinogens for chromosome malsegregation, mitotic crossing-over and forward mutation induction in *Aspergillus nidulans*. *Mutat. Res.*, **172**, 139–149

Croker, P., Bonin, A.M. & Stacey, N.H. (1992) Evaluation of amitrole mutagenicity in *Salmonella typhimurium* using prostaglandin synthase activation. *Mutat. Res.*, **283**, 7–11

Deutsche Forschungsgemeinschaft (2000) *List of MAK and BAT Values 2000* (Report No. 36), Weinheim, Wiley-VCH Verlag GmbH, p. 25

Doerge, D.R. & Niemczura, W.P. (1989) Suicide inactivation of lactoperoxidase by 3-amino-1,2,4-triazole. *Chem. Res. Toxicol.*, **2**,100–103

Dunkel, V.C., Zeiger, E., Brusick, D., McCoy, E., McGregor, D., Mortelmans, K., Rosenkranz, H.S. & Simmon, V.F. (1984) Reproducibility of microbial mutagenicity assays: I. Tests with *Salmonella typhimurium* and *Escherichia coli* using a standardized protocol. *Environ. Mutag.*, **6**, 1–254

English, J.S.C., Rycroft, R.J.G. & Calnan, C.D. (1986) Allergic contact dermatitis from aminotriazole. *Contact Derm.*, **14**, 255–256

Environmental Protection Agency (1984) *Amitrole: Pesticide Registration Standard and Guidance Document*, Washington DC, Office of Pesticides and Toxic Substances

Falck, K., Partanen, P., Sorsa, M., Suovaniemi, O. & Vainio, H. (1985) Mutascreen, an automated bacterial mutagenicity assay. *Mutat. Res.*, **150**, 119–125

Fang, S.C., George, M. &Yu, T.C. (1964) Metabolism of 3-amino-1,2,4-triazole-5-C^{14} by rats. *J. agric. Food Chem.*, **12**, 219–223

FAO/WHO (1999) *Pesticide Residues in Food — 1998* (FAO Plant Production and Protection Paper 152/1), Rome

Feinstein, R.N., Fry, R.J.M. & Staffeldt, E.F. (1978a) Carcinogenic and antitumor effects of aminotriazole on acatalasemic and normal catalase mice. *J. natl Cancer Inst.*, **60**, 1113–1116

Feinstein, R.N., Fry, R.J.M. & Staffeldt, E.F. (1978b) Comparative effects of aminotriazole on normal and acatalasemic mice. *J. environ. Pathol. Toxicol.*, **1**, 779–789

Fregly, M.J. (1968) Effect of aminotriazole on thyroid function in the rat. *Toxicol. appl. Pharmacol.*, **13**, 271–286

Fujii, T., Miyazaki, H. & Hashimoto, M. (1984) Autoradiographic and biochemical studies of drug distribution in the liver. III. [^{14}C]Aminotriazole. *Eur. J. Drug Metab. Pharmacokinet.*, **9**, 257–265

Gaines, T.B., Kimbrough, R.D. & Linder, R.E. (1973) The toxicity of amitrole in the rat. *Toxicol. appl. Pharmacol.*, **26**, 118–129

Gatehouse, D. (1981) Mutagenic activity of 42 coded compounds in the 'microtiter' fluctuation test. *Prog. Mutat. Res.*, **1**, 376–386

Geldmacher-von Mallinckrodt, M. & Schmidt, H.P. (1970) Toxicity and metabolism of aminotriazole in man. *Arch. Toxikol.*, **27**, 13–18

Groch, K.M. & Clifton, K.H. (1992) The plateau phase rat goiter contains a sub-population of TSH-responsive follicular cells capable of proliferation following transplantation. *Acta endocrinol.*, **126**, 85–96

Grunow, W., Altmann, H.-J. & Böhme, C. (1975) [Metabolism of 3-amino-1,2,4-triazole in rats.] *Arch. Toxicol.*, **34**, 314–324 (in German)

Hapke, H.-J., Rüssel, H. & Ueberschär, S. (1965) [Hazards in the use of aminotriazole.] *Dtsch. Tierärzt. Wochenschr.*, **72**, 204–206 (in German)

Hard, G.C. (1998) Recent developments in the investigation of thyroid regulation and thyroid carcinogenesis. *Environ. Health Perspectives*, **106**, 427–436

Hiasa, Y., Ohshima, M., Kitahori, Y., Yuasa, T., Fujita, T. & Iwata, C. (1982) Promoting effects of 3-amino-1,2,4-triazole on the development of thyroid tumors in rats treated with N-bis(2-hydroxypropyl)nitrosamine. *Carcinogenesis*, **3**, 381–384

Hodge, H.C., Maynard, E.A., Downs, W.L., Ashton, J.K. & Salerno, L.L. (1966) Tests on mice for evaluating carcinogenicity. *Toxicol. appl. Pharmacol.*, **9**, 583–596

Hoshino, M. (1960) Effect of 3-amino-1,2,4-triazole on the experimental production of liver cancer. *Nature*, **186**, 174–175

Hubbard, S.A., Green, M.H.L., Bridges, B.A., Wain, A.J. & Bridges, J.W. (1981) Fluctuation test with S9 and hepatocyte activation. *Prog. Mutat. Res.*, **1**, 361–370

Hwua, Y.-S. & Yang, J.-L. (1998) Effect of 3-aminotriazole on anchorage independence and mutagenicity in cadmium- and lead-treated diploid human fibroblasts. *Carcinogenesis*, **19**, 881–888

IARC (1974) *IARC Monographs on the Evaluation of the Carcinogenic Risk of Chemicals to Humans*, Vol. 7, *Some Anti-thyroid and Related Substances, Nitrofurans and Industrial Chemicals*, Lyon, IARC*Press*, pp. 31–43

IARC (1986a) *IARC Monographs on the Evaluation of the Carcinogenic Risk of Chemicals to Man*, Volume 41, *Some Halogenated Hydrocarbons and Pesticide Exposures*, Lyon, IARC*Press*, pp. 293–317

IARC (1986b) *IARC Monographs on the Evaluation of the Carcinogenic Risk of Chemicals to Man*, Volume 41, *Some Halogenated Hydrocarbons and Pesticide Exposures*, Lyon, IARC*Press*, pp. 357–406

IARC (1987) *IARC Monographs on the Evaluation of Carcinogenic Risks to Humans*, Suppl. 7, *Overall Evaluations of Carcinogenicity: An Updating of* IARC Monographs *Volumes 1 to 42*, Lyon, IARC*Press*, pp. 92–93

Innes, J.R.M., Ulland, B.M., Valerio, M.G., Petrucelli, L., Fishbein, L., Hart, E.R., Pallotta, A.J., Bates, R.R., Falk, H.L., Gart, J.J., Klein, M., Mitchell, I. & Peters, J. (1969) Bioassay of pesticides and industrial chemicals for tumorigenicity in mice: A preliminary note. *J. natl Cancer Inst.*, **42**, 1101–1114

Inoue, K., Katoh, Y. & Takayama, S. (1981) In vitro transformation of hamster embryo cells by 3-(N-salicyloyl)amino-1,2,4-triazole. *Toxicol. Lett.*, **7**, 211–215

Jukes, T.H. & Shaffer, C.B. (1960) Antithyroid effects of aminotriazole. *Science*, **132**, 296–297

Kassinova, G.V., Kovaltsova, S.V., Marfin, S.V. & Zakharov, I.A. (1981) Activity of 40 coded compounds in differential inhibition and mitotic crossing-over assays in yeast. *Prog. Mutat. Res.*, **1**, 434–455

Kato, R. (1967) Effect of administration of 3-aminotriazole on the activity of microsomal drug-metabolizing enzyme systems of rat liver. *Jpn. J. Pharmacol.*, **17**, 56–63

Kornbrust, D.J., Barfknecht, T.R., Ingram, P. & Shelburne, J.D. (1984) Effect of di(2-ethyl-hexyl)phthalate on DNA repair and lipid peroxidation in rat hepatocytes and on metabolic cooperation in Chinese hamster V-79 cells. *J. Toxicol. environ. Health*, **13**, 99–116

Krauss, R.S. & Eling, T.E. (1987) Macromolecular binding of the thyroid carcinogen 3-amino-1,2,4-triazole (amitrole) catalysed by prostaglandin H synthase, lactoperoxidase and thyroid peroxidase. *Carcinogenesis*, **8**, 659–664

Kröller, E. (1966) [Use and properties of 3-amino-1,2,4-triazole in relation to its residues in foodstuffs.] *Residue Rev.*, **12**, 162–192 (in German)

Laamanen, I., Sorsa, M., Bamford, D., Gripenberg, U. & Meretoja, T. (1976) Mutagenicity and toxicity of amitrole. I. Drosophila tests. *Mutat. Res.*, **40**, 185–190

Legras, A., Skrobala, D., Furet, Y., Kintz, P., Forveille, E., Dequin, P.F. & Perrotin, D. (1996) Herbicide: Fatal ammonium thiocyanate and aminotriazole poisoning. *Clin. Toxicol.*, **34**, 441–446

Lemoine, N.R., Mayall, E.S., Williams, D., Thurston, V. & Wynford-Thomas, D. (1988) Agent-specific ras oncogene activation in rat thyroid tumours. *Oncogene*, **3**, 541–544

Lesko, S.A., Trpis, L. & Yang, S.U. (1985) Induction of 6-thioguanine-resistant mutants by hyperoxia and gamma-irradiation: Effect of compromising cellular antioxidant systems. *Mutat. Res.*, **149**, 119–126

Lide, D.R. & Milne, G.W.A. (1996) *Properties of Organic Compounds*, Version 5.0, Boca Raton, FL, CRC Press [CD-ROM]

MacDonald, D.J. (1981) Salmonella/microsome tests on 42 coded chemicals. *Prog. Mutat. Res.*, **1**, 285–297

Mamber, S.W., Bryson, V. & Katz, S.E. (1983) The *Escherichia coli* WP2/WP100 rec assay for detection of potential chemical carcinogens. *Mutat. Res.*, **119**, 135–144

Mamber, S.W., Bryson, V. & Katz, S.E. (1984) Evaluation of the *Escherichia coli* K12 inductest for detection of potential chemical carcinogens. *Mutat. Res.*, **130**, 141–151

Mattioli, F., Robbiano, L., Fazzuoli, L. & Baracchini, P. (1994) Studies on the mechanism of the carcinogenic activity of amitrole. *Fundam. appl. Toxicol.*, **23**, 101–106

McCann, J., Choi, E., Yamasaki, E. & Ames, B. N. (1975) Detection of carcinogens as mutagens in the *Salmonella*/microsome test: Assay of 300 chemicals. *Proc. natl Acad. Sci. USA*, **72**, 5135–5139

McGregor, D.B., Martin, R., Cattanach, P., Edwards, I., McBride, D. & Caspary, W.J. (1987) Responses of the L5178Y tk+/tk− mouse lymphoma cell forward mutation assay to coded chemicals. I: Results for nine compounds. *Environ. Mutag.*, **9**, 143–160

Mehta, R.D. & von Borstel, R.C. (1981) Mutagenic activity of 42 encoded compounds in the haploid yeast reversion assay, strain XV185-14C. *Prog. Mutat. Res.*, **1**, 414–423

Meretoja, T., Gripenberg, U., Bamford, D., Laamanen, I. & Sorsa, M. (1976) Mutagenicity and toxicity of amitrole. II. Human lymphocyte culture tests. *Mutat. Res.*, **40**, 191–196

Middelkoop, A., Strijland, A. & Tager, J.M. (1991) Does aminotriazole inhibit import of catalase into peroxisomes by retarding unfolding? *FEBS Lett.*, **279**, 79–82

Mikalsen, S.-O., Kaalhus, O., Reith, A. & Sanner, T. (1990) Role of catalase and oxidative stress in hepatic peroxisome proliferator-induced morphological transformation of Syrian hamster embryo cells. *Int. J. Cancer*, **46**, 950–957

Mitchell, A.D., Rudd, C.J. & Caspary, W.J. (1988) Evaluation of the L5178Y mouse lymphoma cell mutagenesis assay: Intralaboratory results for sixty-three coded chemicals tested at SRI International. *Environ. mol. Mutag.*, **12** (Suppl. 13), 37–101

Mori, S., Takeuchi, Y., Toyama, M., Makino, S., Ohhara, T., Tochino, Y & Hayashi, Y. (1985) Amitrole: Strain differences in morphological response of the liver following subchronic administration to mice. *Toxicol. Lett.*, **29**, 145–152

Myhr, B.C. & Caspary, W.J. (1988) Evaluation of the L5178Y mouse lymphoma cell mutagenesis assay: Intralaboratory results for sixty-three coded chemicals tested at Litton Bionetics, Inc. *Environ. mol. Mutag.*, **12** (Suppl. 13), 103–194

Nakamura, S., Oda, Y., Shimada, T., Oki, I. & Sugimoto, K. (1987) SOS-inducing activity of chemical carcinogens and mutagens in *Salmonella typhimurium* TA1535/pSK1002: Examination with 151 chemicals. *Mutat. Res.*, **192**, 239–246

Napalkov, N.P. (1962) [Blastomogenic action of 3-amino-1,2,4-triazole.] *Gig. Tr. prof. Zabol.*, **6**, 48–51 (in Russian)

National Cancer Institute (1968) *Evaluation of Carcinogenic, Teratogenic, and Mutagenic Activities of Selected Pesticides and Industrial Chemicals. Volume I: Carcinogenic Study (PB-223 159)*, Springfield, VA, National Technical Information Service

National Institute for Occupational Safety and Health (2000) *National Occupational Exposure Survey 1981–83*, Cincinnati, OH, Department of Health and Human Services, Public Health Service

Occupational Safety and Health Administration (1998) *Sampling and Analytical Methods: Method PV2006 — Amitrole*, Washington DC, US Department of Labour

Ochi, T. & Ohsawa, M. (1985) Participation of active oxygen species in the induction of chromosomal aberrations by cadmium chloride in cultured Chinese hamster cells. *Mutat. Res.*, **143**, 137–142

Parry, J.M. & Sharp, D.C. (1981) Induction of mitotic aneuploidy in the yeast strain D6 by 42 coded compounds. *Prog. Mutat. Res.*, **1**, 468–480

Perry, P.E. & Thomson, E.J. (1981) Evaluation of the sister chromatid exchange method in mammalian cells as a screening system for carcinogens. *Prog. Mutat. Res.*, **1**, 560–569

Pienta, R.J., Poiley, J.A., & Lebherz, W.B., III (1977) Morphological transformation of early passage golden Syrian hamster embryo cells derived from cryopreserved primary cultures as a reliable in vitro bioassay for identifying diverse carcinogens. *Int. J. Cancer*, **19**, 642–655

Quillardet, P., De Bellecombe, C. & Hofnung, M. (1985) The SOS chromotest, a colorimetric bacterial assay for genotoxins: Validation study with 83 compounds. *Mutat. Res.*, **147**, 79–95

Rédei, G.P. & Sandhu, S.S. (1988) Aneuploidy detection with a short-term hexaploid wheat assay. *Mutat. Res.*, **201**, 337–348

Reitze, H.K. & Seitz, K.A. (1985) Light and electron microscopical changes in the liver of mice following treatment with aminotriazole. *Exp. Pathol.*, **27**, 17–31

Richold, M. & Jones, E. (1981) Mutagenic activity of 42 coded compounds in the Salmonella/microsome assay. *Prog. Mutat. Res.*, **1**, 314–322

Rosenkranz, H.S. & Poirier, L.A. (1979) Evaluation of the mutagenicity and DNA-modifying activity of carcinogens and noncarcinogens in microbial systems. *J. natl Cancer Inst.*, **62**, 873–892

Sadtler Research Laboratories (1980) *Sadtler Standard Spectra, 1980 Cumulative Molecular Formula Index*, Philadelphia, PA, p. 8

Salamone, M.F., Heddle, J.A. & Katz, M. (1981) Mutagenic activity of 41 compounds in the in vivo micronucleus assay. *Prog. Mutat. Res.*, **1**, 686–697

Savela, A., Vuorela, R. & Kauppinen, T. (1999) *ASA 1997* (Katsauksia 140), Helsinki, Finnish Institute of Occupational Health, p. 29 (in Finnish)

Sharp, D.C. & Parry, J.M. (1981a) Use of repair-deficient strains of yeast to assay the activity of 40 coded compounds. *Prog. Mutat. Res.*, **1**, 502–516

Sharp, D.C. & Parry, J.M. (1981b) Induction of mitotic gene conversion by 41 coded compounds using the yeast culture JD1. *Prog. Mutat. Res.*, **1**, 491–501

Simmon, V.F. (1979a) In vitro mutagenicity assays of chemical carcinogens and related compounds with *Salmonella typhimurium. J. natl Cancer Inst.*, **62**, 893–899

Simmon, V.F. (1979b) In vitro assays for recombinogenic activity of chemical carcinogens and related compounds with *Saccharomyces cerevisiae* D3. *J. natl Cancer Inst.*, **62**, 901–909

Simmon, V.F., Rosenkranz, H.S., Zeiger, E. & Poirier, L.A. (1979) Mutagenic activity of chemical carcinogens and related compounds in the intraperitoneal host-mediated assay. *J. natl Cancer Inst.*, **62**, 911–918

Sittig, M., ed. (1980) *Pesticide Manufacturing and Toxic Materials Control Encyclopedia*, Park Ridge, NJ, Noyes Data Corp., pp. 54–55

Skopek, T.R., Andon, B.M., Kaden, D.A. & Thilly, W. G. (1981) Mutagenic activity of 42 coded compounds using 8-azaguanine resistance as a genetic marker in Salmonella typhimurium. *Prog. Mutat. Res.*, **1**, 371–375

Sofuni, T. & Ishidate, M. (1988) Induction of chromosomal aberrations in active oxygen-generating systems. I. Effects of paraquat in Chinese hamster cells in culture. *Mutat. Res.*, **197**, 127–132

Steinhoff, D., Weber, H., Mohr, U. & Boehme, K. (1983) Evaluation of amitrole (aminotriazole) for potential carcinogenicity in orally dosed rats, mice, and golden hamsters. *Toxicol. appl. Pharmacol.*, **69**, 161–169

Strum, J.M. & Karnovsky, M.J. (1970) Cytochemical localization of endogenous peroxidase in thyroid follicular cells. *J. Cell Biol.*, **44**, 655–666

Strum, J.M. & Karnovsky, M.J. (1971) Aminotriazole goiter. Fine structure and localization of thyroid peroxidase activity. *Lab. Invest.*, **24**, 1–12

Sumi, C., Yokoro, K. & Matsushima, R. (1985) Inhibition by 3-amino-1*H*-1,2,4-triazole of hepatic tumorigenesis induced by diethylstilbestrol alone or combined with *N*-nitroso-butylurea in WF rats. *J. natl Cancer Inst.*, **74**, 1329–1334

Tjälve, H. (1975) The distribution of labelled aminotriazole in mice. *Toxicology*, **3**, 49–67

Tomlin, C.D.S., ed. (1999) *The e-Pesticide Manual*, 11th Ed., Version 1.1, Farnham, British Crop Protection Council [CD-ROM]

Tripathy, N.K., Würgler, F.E. & Frei, H. (1990) Genetic toxicity of six carcinogens and six non-carcinogens in the Drosophila wing spot test. *Mutat. Res.*, **242**, 169–180

Tsuchimoto, T. & Matter, B.E. (1981) Activity of coded compounds in the micronucleus test. *Prog. Mutat. Res.*, **1**, 705–711

Tsuda, H., Takahashi, M., Fukushima, S., Endo, Y. & Hikosaka, Y. (1973) Fine structure and localization of peroxidase activity in aminotriazole goiter. *Nagoya med. J.*, **18**, 183–190

Tsuda, H., Hananouchi, M., Tatematsu, M., Hirose, M., Hirao, K., Takahashi, M. & Ito, N. (1976) Tumorigenic effect of 3-amino-1*H*-1,2,4-triazole on rat thyroid. *J. natl Cancer Inst.*, **57**, 861–864

Tsuda, H., Takahashi, M., Murasaki, G., Ogiso, T. & Tatematsu, M. (1978) Effect of 3-amino-1*H*-1,2,4-triazole or low iodine diet on rat thyroid carcinogenesis induced by ethylenethiourea. *Nagoya med. J.*, **23**, 83–92

Tsutsui, T., Maizumi, H. & Barrett, J. C. (1984) Amitrole-induced cell transformation and gene mutations in Syrian hamster embryo cells in culture. *Mutat. Res.*, **140**, 205–207

Vesselinovitch, S.D. (1983) Perinatal hepatocarcinogenesis. *Biol. Res. Pregnancy Perinatol.*, **4**, 22–25

Vogel, E.W. & Nivard, M.J.M. (1993) Performance of 181 chemicals in a Drosophila assay predominantly monitoring interchromosomal mitotic recombination. *Mutagenesis*, **8**, 57–81

Vogel, E., Blijleven, W.G.H., Kortselius, M.J.H. & Zijlstra, J.A. (1981) Mutagenic activity of 17 coded compounds in the sex-linked recessive lethal test in *Drosophila melanogaster*. *Prog. Mutat. Res.*, **1**, 660–665

WHO (1994) *Amitrole* (Environmental Health Criteria No. 158), Geneva, International Programme on Chemical Safety

WHO (1999) *Inventory of IPCS and Other WHO Pesticide Evaluations and Summary of Toxicological Evaluations Performed by the Joint Meeting on Pesticide Residues [JMPR] through 1999*, 3rd Ed., Geneva, International Programme on Chemical Safety

Williams, R.N., Delamere, N.A. & Paterson, C.A. (1985) Inactivation of catalase with 3-amino-1,2,4-triazole: An indirect irreversible mechanism. *Biochem. Pharmacol.*, **34**, 3386–3389

Woodruff, R.C., Mason, J.M., Valencia, R. & Zimmering, S. (1985) Chemical mutagenesis testing in Drosophila. V. Results of 53 coded compounds tested for the National Toxicology Program. *Environ. Mutag.*, **7**, 677–702

Wuu, K.D. & Grant, W.F. (1966) Morphological and somatic chromosomal aberrations induced by pesticides in barley (*Hordeum vulgare*). *Can. J. genet. Cytol.*, **8**, 481–501

Wuu, K.D. & Grant, W.F. (1967) Chromosomal aberrations induced in somatic cells of *Vicia faba* by pesticides. *Nucleus*, **10**, 37–46

Wynford-Thomas, D., Stringer, B.M.J. & Williams, E.D. (1982) Desensitization of rat thyroid to the growth-stimulating action of TSH during prolonged goitrogen administration. *Acta endocrinol.*, **101**, 562–569

Wynford-Thomas, D., Stringer, B.M., Gomez Morales, M. & Williams, E.D. (1983) Vascular changes in early TSH-induced thyroid tumours in the rat. *Br. J. Cancer*, **47**, 861–865

Zeiger, E., Anderson, B., Haworth, S., Lawlor, T. & Mortelmans, K. (1988) Salmonella mutagenicity tests: IV. Results from the testing of 300 chemicals. *Environ. mol. Mutag.*, **11** (Suppl. 12), 1–157

Zimmermann, F.K. & Scheel, I. (1981) Induction of mitotic gene conversion in strain D7 of *Saccharomyces cerevisiae* by 42 coded chemicals. *Prog. Mutat. Res.*, **1**, 481–490

CHLORDANE AND HEPTACHLOR

Chlordane and heptachlor were considered together because of their close structural similarity and because technical-grade products each contain about 10–20% of the other compound.

These substances were considered by previous working groups, in 1978 (IARC, 1979), 1987 (IARC, 1987) and 1990 (IARC, 1991). Since that time, new data have become available, and these have been incorporated into the monograph and taken into consideration in the present evaluation.

1. Exposure Data

1.1 Chemical and physical data

1.1.1 *Synonyms, structural and molecular data*

Chemical Abstract Services Registry numbers, names and synonyms of chlordane and heptachlor and its epoxide are given in Table 1.

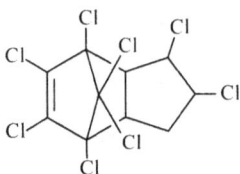

$C_{10}H_6Cl_8$ Chlordane   Relative molecular mass: 409.8

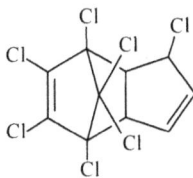

$C_{10}H_5Cl_7$ Heptachlor   Relative molecular mass: 373.5

Table 1. Chemical Abstract Services Registry numbers, names and synonyms of chlordane, heptachlor and its epoxide

Name	CAS Reg. Nos[a]	Chem. Abstr. names[b] and synonyms
Chlordane	57-74-9 (39400-80-1); 53637-13-1)	ENT 9932; **1,2,4,5,6,7,8,8-octachloro-2,3,3a,4,7,7a-hexahydro-4,7-methano-1*H*-indene;** 1,2,4,5,6,7,8,8-octachloro-2,3,3a,4,7,7a-hexahydro-4,7-methano-indene (IUPAC); octachloro-4,7-methanotetrahydro-indane; 1,2,4,5,6,7,8,8-octachloro-3a,4,7,7a-tetra-hydro-4,7-methanoindan; OMS 1437
Technical-grade chlordane	12789-03-6	
cis-Chlordane	5103-71-9 (152322-29-7; 22212-52-8; 26703-86-6; 28140-46-7)	α-Chlordan; α-chlordane; *cis*-chlordan; **(1α,2α,3aα,4β,7β,7aα)-1,2,4,5,6,7,8,8-octachloro-2,3,3a,4,7,7a-hexahydro-4,7-methano-1*H*-indene;** 1α,2α,4β,5,6,7β,8,8-octachloro-3aα,4,7,7aα-tetrahydro-4,7-methanoindan
trans-Chlordane[c]	5103-74-2 (152322-27-5; 17436-70-3; 28181-89-7)	β-Chlordan; β-chlordane; γ-chlordane; *trans*-chlordan; **(1α,2β,3aα,4β,7β,7aα)-1,2,4,5,6,7,8,8-octachloro-2,3,3a,4,7,7a-hexahydro-4,7-methano-1*H*-indene;** 1β,2α,4α,5,6,7α,8,8-octachloro-3aβ,4,7,7aβ-tetrahydro-4,7-methanoindan
'γ-Chlordane'[c]	5566-34-7[c]	γ-Chlordan; **2,2,4,5,6,7,8,8-octachloro-2,3,3a,4,7,7a-hexahydro-4,7-methano-1*H*-indene;** 2,2,4,5,6,7,8,8-octachloro-3a,4,7,7a-tetrahydro-4,7-methanoindan stereoisomer
Heptachlor	76-44-8 (23720-59-4; 37229-06-4)	3-Chlorochlordene; E 3314; ENT 15 152; **1,4,5,6,7,8,8-heptachloro-3a,4,7,7a-tetrahydro-4,7-methano-1*H*-indene;** 1,4,5,6,7,8,8-heptachloro-3a,4,7,7a-tetrahydro-4,7-methanoindene (IUPAC); OMS 193
Heptachlor epoxide	1024-57-3 (4067-30-5; 24699-42-1; 24717-72-4; 28044-82-8; 66429-35-4; 66240-71-9)	ENT 25584; epoxyheptachlor; 1,4,5,6,7,8,8-hepta-chloro-2,3-epoxy-3a,4,7,7a-tetrahydro-4,7-methanoindan; **(1aα,1bβ,2α,5α,5aβ,6β,6aα)-2,3,4,5,6,7,7-heptachloro-1a,1b,5,5a,6,6a-hexa-hydro-2,5-methano-2*H*-indeno(1,2-b)-oxirene;** heptachlor *cis*-oxide

[a] Deleted CAS Registry number(s) in parentheses

[b] In bold

[c] In most of the published literature, authors have used the term 'γ-chlordane' as a synonym for *trans*-chlordane, although the Chemical Abstracts Service has indexed such references with the 5566-34-7 CAS Registry Number. See also section 1.1.3.

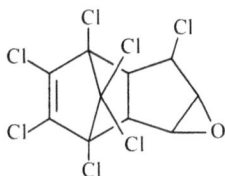

$C_{10}H_5Cl_7O$ Heptachlor epoxide   Relative molecular mass: 389.4

1.1.2   *Chemical and physical properties*

Chlordane

(a) *Description*: Light-yellow to amber-coloured, viscous liquid (technical product) (WHO, 1988a)

(b) *Boiling-point*: 175 °C at 1 mm Hg [0.13 kPa] (pure material) (Royal Society of Chemistry, 1989; Tomlin, 1999)

(c) *Melting-point*: 106–107 °C (*cis*-isomer); 104–105 °C (*trans*-isomer) (WHO, 1988a)

(d) *Spectroscopy data*: Infrared (prism [534]; grating [41094P]) spectroscopy data have been reported (Sadtler Research Laboratories, 1980).

(e) *Solubility*: Practically insoluble in water (1.0×10^{-4} g/L at 25 °C) but soluble in most organic solvents (e.g., acetone, cyclohexanone, ethanol, isopropanol, kerosene, trichloroethylene) (Worthing & Walker, 1987; Tomlin, 1999)

(f) *Stability*: Decomposed by alkalis, with loss of chlorine; ultraviolet irradiation induces a change in the skeletal structure and of the chlorine content; corrosive to iron, zinc and various protective coatings (Royal Society of Chemistry, 1989; Tomlin, 1999)

Heptachlor

(a) *Description*: White crystalline solid (Worthing & Walker, 1987; WHO, 1988b; Tomlin, 1999)

(b) *Boiling-point*: 135–145 °C at 1–1.5 mm Hg [0.13–0.20 kPa] (Tomlin, 1999)

(c) *Melting-point*: 95–96 °C (pure compound) (Worthing & Walker, 1987; Tomlin, 1999)

(d) *Spectroscopy data*: Infrared (prism/grating [74915]) and nuclear magnetic resonance (proton [47772]) spectral data have been reported (Sadtler Research Laboratories, 1990).

(e) *Solubility*: Practically insoluble in water (5.6×10^{-8} g/L at 25–29 °C); fairly soluble in organic solvents: acetone, benzene, ethanol and xylene (WHO, 1988b)

(f) *Stability*: Stable in daylight, air, moisture and moderate heat (160 °C); corrosive to metals; susceptible to epoxidation; slowly loses hydrogen chloride in alkaline media (WHO, 1988b; Royal Society of Chemistry, 1989; Tomlin, 1999)

Heptachlor epoxide

(a) *Description*: Solid (Agency for Toxic Substances and Disease Registry, 1989a)

(b) *Melting-point*: 160–161.5 °C (Environmental Protection Agency, 1987a)

(c) *Spectroscopy data*: Infrared (prism/grating [74932]) and nuclear magnetic resonance (proton [47783]) spectral data have been reported (Sadtler Research Laboratories, 1990).

(d) *Solubility*: Practically insoluble in water (3.5×10^{-4} g/L at 25 °C) (Environmental Protection Agency, 1987a)

1.1.3   *Trade names, technical products and impurities*

Examples of trade names for chlordane are Aspon, Belt, CD 68, Chlordan, Chlorindan, Chlor-Kil, Chlorotox, Corodane, Cortilan-neu, Dowchlor, Gold Crest C-100, HCS 3260, Intox, Kilex, Kypchlor, M-140, Niran, Octachlor, Oktaterr, Ortho-Klor, Penticklor, Prentox, Starchlor, Sydane, Synklor, Tat Chlor 4, Termex, Topichlor, Toxichlor, Unexan-Koeder and Velsicol 1068.

Examples of trade names for heptachlor are Aahepta, Agroceres, Arbinex 30TN, Basaklor, Biarbinex, Cupincida, Drinox, Fennotox, GPKh, Heptachlorane, Heptaf, Heptagran, Heptagranox, Heptamak, Heptamul, Heptasol, Heptox, Rhodiachlor, Soleptax and Velsicol 104. The trade names for heptachlor epoxide include GPKh epoxide, HCE, Hepox, Heptepoxide and Velsicol 53-CS-17.

The term 'chlordane' commonly refers to a complex mixture of chlordane isomers, other chlorinated hydrocarbons and by-products (WHO, 1988a). Technical-grade chlordane contains more than 140 components, consisting mainly of C_{10} alicyclic chlorinated hydrocarbons, the most abundant being *cis*- and *trans*-chlordane (Royal Society of Chemistry, 1989; Dearth & Hites, 1991; Tomlin, 1999). The nomenclature of *cis*- and *trans*-chlordane used in the literature has been confused. The *cis*-isomer, often referred to as 'α-chlordane', is described above under [5103-71-9]; the *trans*-isomer [5103-74-2], also usually known as 'γ-chlordane', is occasionally referred to as 'β-chlordane' (the term 'γ-chlordane' has also been assigned by the Chemical Abstracts Service to the 2,2,4,5,6,7,8,8-octachloroisomer [5566-34-7]). However, as the α/*cis* and γ/*trans* relationships have been reversed in some cases, particularly in the older literature, the α,β and γ nomenclature should be avoided (Buchert *et al.*, 1989). One description of the approximate composition of technical chlordane is as follows: *trans*-chlordane, 24%; *cis*-chlordane, 19%; chlordene isomers, 21.5%; heptachlor, 10%; nonachlor, 7% (Rostad, 1997); octachlorocyclopentene, 1%; hexachlorocyclopentadiene, 1%; other, 16.5% (Brooks, 1974). Several reviews give details of the composition of technical-grade chlordane (Cochrane & Greenhalgh, 1976; Sovocool *et al.*, 1977; Miyazaki *et al.*, 1985; Buchert *et al.*, 1989).

Chlordane has been available in various formulations, including 5–30% granules, oil solutions containing 2–300 g/L chlordane and emulsifiable concentrates containing

400–900 g/L (Royal Society of Chemistry, 1986; Worthing & Walker, 1987; WHO,1988a).

Technical-grade heptachlor contains about 72% heptachlor and 28% related compounds (20–22% *trans*-chlordane and 4–8% nonachlor). Formulations have included emulsifiable concentrates, wettable powders, dusts and granules containing various concentrations of active material (National Cancer Institute, 1977a; Izmerov, 1982; Worthing & Walker, 1987; WHO, 1988b; Tomlin, 1999). Two Finnish products which were used as components of plywood glues contained 17–25% heptachlor and 6–9% chlordanes. One of these products also contained 40% tetrachlorophenol and 1.5% tributyltin oxide (Mussalo-Rauhamaa *et al.*, 1991).

1.1.4   *Analysis*

Determination of chlordane residues is difficult because of the complex nature of the components and the fact that each component degrades independently. The resulting residues may bear little relation to the proportions in the technical product. Extraction from crops, other plant products, dairy products, plants and oils has been achieved with an 80–100% efficiency with the use of acetonitrile for extraction, petroleum ether for partitioning and clean-up on a Florisil column. Gel-permeation chromatography can also be used for clean-up, particularly of human adipose tissue. The method of choice for the qualitative and quantitative estimation of chlordane isomers and heptachlor is gas chromatography with electron-capture detection. Gas chromatographic analyses can be confirmed by gas chromatography–mass spectrometry, a method that can also provide good determination of some of the components, such as heptachlor epoxide. Analysis for total organically bound chlorine remains the preferred method for determination of technical-grade chlordane and heptachlor and of the active ingredient in formulations (WHO, 1988a,b).

Selected methods for the analysis of chlordane, heptachlor and heptachlor epoxide in various matrices are summarized in Table 2. Several reviews are available on the analysis of chlordane, heptachlor and heptachlor epoxide in technical products, formulations and as residues in various matrices. The methods include titrimetric, colorimetric, spectrophotometric, infrared spectroscopic and gas chromatographic methods (Bowery, 1964; Raw, 1970; Izmerov, 1982; WHO, 1984a,b; Williams, 1984a,b; Anon., 1985; Worthing & Walker, 1987; Agency for Toxic Substances and Disease Registry, 1989a,b; Royal Society of Chemistry, 1989; Fendick *et al.*, 1990; Tomlin, 1999).

1.2   Production

The chemistry and uses of chlordane and heptachlor and the problems associated with their technical-grade products have been reviewed (Brooks, 1974).

Table 2. Methods for the analysis of chlordane, heptachlor and heptachlor epoxide

Sample matrix	Sample preparation	Assay procedure	Limit of detection[a]	Reference
Air	Collect vapours on polyurethane foam (low or high volume); extract with 5–10% diethyl ether in hexane	GC/ECD	NR	Environmental Protection Agency (1999a,b) [Methods TO-04A, TO-10A]
	Collect vapours on Chromosorb 102; desorb with toluene	GC/ECD	0.1 µg/sample	Eller (1994) [Method 5510]
Water	Extract with hexane; inject extract	GC/ECD	0.14 (0.006, 0.012 µg/L)[b], 0.003, 0.004 µg/L	Environmental Protection Agency (1995a) [Method 505]
	Extract with dichloromethane; isolate extract; dry; concentrate with methyl *tert*-butyl ether (capillary column)	GC/ECD	0.0015[b], 0.01, 0.015 µg/L	Environmental Protection Agency (1995b) [Method 508.1]; AOAC International (2000) [Method 990.06]
	Extract by passing sample through liquid–solid extractor; elute with dichloromethane; concentrate by evaporation (capillary column)	GC/MS	Varies[c]	Environmental Protection Agency (1995c) [Method 525.2]
	Extract with methyl *tert*-butyl ether or pentane	GC/ECD	NA, 0.002–0.08, 0.002–0.2 µg/L	Environmental Protection Agency (1995d) [Method 551.1]
Municipal & industrial wastewater	Extract with dichloromethane; dry; concentrate; optional clean-up (acetonitrile partition or Florisil)	GC/ECD	NR, 0.004, 0.003 µg/L	Environmental Protection Agency (1993a) [Method 617]
	(1) If solids < 1%, extract with dichloromethane; (2) for nonsludges with solids 1–30%, dilute to 1% and extract with dichloromethane; if solids > 30%, sonicate with dichloromethane:acetone; (3) for sludges with solids < 30%, treat as in (2) above; if solids > 30%, sonicate with acetonitrile then dichloromethane; back extract with sodium sulfate; concentrate; clean-up	GC/ECD or GC/MCD or GC/ELCD	NR (8, 9 ng/L)[b], 5, 12 ng/L	US Environmental Protection Agency (1993b) [Method 1656]

Table 2 (contd)

Sample matrix	Sample preparation	Assay procedure	Limit of detection[a]	Reference
Municipal & industrial wastewater (contd)	Adjust to pH 11; extract with dichloromethane; dry; concentrate	GC/MS	NR, 1.9, 2.2 µg/L	APHA/AWWA/WEF (1999a) [Method 6410B]
	Extract with diethyl ether:hexane or dichloromethane:hexane; concentrate; clean-up with column adsorption chromatography	GC/ECD	NR	APHA/AWWA/WEF (1999b) [Method 6630B]
	Extract with dichloromethane; dry; exchange to hexane; clean-up with magnesia–silica gel; concentrate	GC/ECD	0.014, 0.003 0.083 µg/L	APHA/AWWA/WEF (1999c) [Method 6630C]
Liquid & solid waste	Extract with dichloromethane; dry; exchange to hexane; clean-up on Florisil	GC/ECD	0.014, 0.003, 0.083 µg/L	Environmental Protection Agency (1999c) [Method 608]
	Extract with dichloromethane; dry; concentrate (packed column)	GC/MS	NR, 1.9, 2.2 µg/L	Environmental Protection Agency (1999d) [Method 625]
	Extract with dichloromethane (liquid); hexane:acetone (1:1) or dichloromethane:acetone (1:1) (solid); clean-up	GC/ECD	groundwater: 1.5/1.8[b], 1.3, 1.5 µg/L; wastewater: 0.58[b], 0.56, 0.34 µg/L	Environmental Protection Agency (1996a) [Method 8081A]
	Mix with anhydrous sodium sulfate; extract with Soxhlet or sonication process; clean-up with Florisil or gel-permeation (capillary column)	GC/MS	NR	Environmental Protection Agency (1996b) [Method 8270C]
Soil	Extract with methanol; add aliquot and enzyme conjugate reagent to immobilized antibody; compare colour produced to reference reaction	Immuno-assay	20 µg/kg	Environmental Protection Agency (1996c) [Method 4041]

Table 2 (contd)

Sample matrix	Sample preparation	Assay procedure	Limit of detection[a]	Reference
Formulations (chlordane)	Dissolve in toluene or benzene, then toluene; extract with 0.1N silver nitrate solution	TCM	NR	AOAC International (2000) [Method 962.05]
	Dissolve in methanol:benzene or extract with pentane; add Davidow reagent[d], boil; cool; dilute with methanol; read absorbance at 550 nm	Colorimetry	NR	AOAC International (2000) [Method 965.14]
	Extract with acetone; filter or centrifuge	TLC	NR	AOAC International (2000) [Method 972.05]
	Dissolve and dilute with carbon disulfide; read absorbance at 13.3–14.1 µm for α-chlordane; at 7.19–7.75 µm for γ-chlordane	IRS	NR	AOAC International (2000) [Methods 973.15, 973.16]
Formulations (heptachlor)	Dissolve in acetic acid; add silver nitrate or extract with pentane; dissolve	ACM	NR	AOAC International (2000) [Method 962.07]
	Dissolve in carbon disulfide or extract with pentane; dissolve	GC/FID	NR	AOAC International (2000) [Methods 968.04, 973.17]
Selected vegetables	Extract with pentane; clean-up on Florex column; evaporate to dryness; react with Polen-Silverman reagent[e]; read absorbance at 560 nm for heptachlor and at 410 nm for heptachlor oxide	Colorimetry	NR, 0.02, 0.02–0.04 mg/kg	Food and Drug Administration (1989)
Nonfatty foods	Extract with acetone; partition or remove water; clean-up on Florisil; elute with dichloromethane	GC/ECD or GC/ELCD	NR	Food and Drug Administration (1999) [Method 302]
	Extract with acetonitrile or water/acetonitrile; partition into petroleum ether; clean-up on Florisil	GC/ECD or GC/ELCD	NR	Food and Drug Administration (1999) [Method 303]

Table 2 (contd)

Sample matrix	Sample preparation	Assay procedure	Limit of detection[a]	Reference
Fatty foods	Extract fat; partition into acetonitrile:petroleum ether; clean-up on Florisil	GC/ECD or GC/ELCD	NR	Food and Drug Administration (1999) [Method 304]
	Extract with acetonitrile; extract fat; dilute with water; extract residue into petroleum ether; clean-up on Florisil; elute with petroleum:ethyl ethers	GC/ECD-TD	NR	AOAC International (2000) [Method 970.52]
Fish tissue	Extract with petroleum ether; clean-up on Florisil	GC/ECD	NR	AOAC International (2000) [Method 983.21]

APHA/AWWA/WEF, American Public health Association/American Water Works Association/Water Environment Federation; ACM, active chlorine method; ECD, electron capture detection; ELCD, electrolytic conductivity detection; FID, flame ionization detection; GC, gas chromatography; IRS, infrared spectroscopy; MCD, microcoulometry detection; MS, mass spectrometry; TCM, total chlorine method; TD, thermionic detection; TLC, thin-layer chromatography

[a] The limits of detection are presented for chlordane, heptachlor and heptachlor epoxide, respectively; NA, not applicable; NR, not reported

[b] Detection limit(s) for *cis-/trans*-chlordane

[c] Limits of detection vary with extraction technique (cartridge or disc) and mass spectrometer (quadrupole or ion trap) from 0.061 to 0.17 μg/L for *cis*-chlordane; from 0.050 to 0.16 μg/L for *trans*-chlordane; from 0.059 to 0.15 μg/L for heptachlor; and from 0.048 to 0.13 μg/L for heptachlor epoxide

[d] Diethanolamine–potassium hydroxide solution

[e] Prepared by dissolving potassium hydroxide in distilled water, cooling to room temperature, adding butyl Cellosolve and monoethanolamine and diluting to 1 L with butyl Cellosolve. This solution, after standing for several days, is decanted from any sediment and diluted with an equal volume of benzene.

Chlordane was first produced commercially in the USA in 1947. In 1974, production in the USA amounted to 9500 tonnes (WHO, 1988a); the Environmental Protection Agency estimated that approximately 1600–1800 tonnes of chlordane were used in 1986. From 1 July 1983, the only use of chlordane approved in the USA was in the control of underground termites. This use was prohibited in April 1988. The amounts of chlordane both produced and used have decreased considerably (Environmental Protection Agency, 1987b; Agency for Toxic Substances and Disease Registry, 1989b, 1994).

Heptachlor was isolated from technical-grade chlordane in 1946. Production of heptachlor in the USA was 2700 tonnes in 1971, 900 tonnes in 1974, 590 tonnes in 1978, 180 tonnes in 1980 and 45 tonnes in 1982. Sales of heptachlor in the USA were voluntarily stopped by the sole local producer in August 1987, and, since April 1988, heptachlor can no longer be used for the underground control of termites in the USA (WHO, 1988b; Agency for Toxic Substances and Disease Registry, 1989a, 1993).

Chlordene, the starting material for the synthesis of both chlordane and heptachlor, is prepared by Diels-Alder condensation of hexachlorocyclopentadiene with cyclopentadiene (Agency for Toxic Substances and Disease Registry, 1989b). Chlordane is prepared by the Lewis acid-catalysed addition of chlorine to chlordene (WHO, 1984a), whereas heptachlor is prepared by free-radical chlorination of chlordene (Sittig, 1980).

Heptachlor epoxide can be prepared from heptachlor in a one-step oxidation. It is a metabolite as well as an environmental oxidation product of heptachlor (Anon., 1985).

Information available in 2000 indicated that chlordane is manufactured by two companies in India and one company in Argentina. The same source indicated that heptachlor is manufactured by one company each in India and Japan (CIS Information Services, 2000).

1.3   Use

Chlordane has been used as an insecticide since the 1950s. It is a versatile, broad-spectrum, contact insecticide and has been used mainly for non-agricultural purposes (primarily for the protection of structures, but also on lawns and turf, ornamental trees and drainage ditches). It has also been used on maize, potatoes and livestock (WHO, 1984a). The use pattern for chlordane in the USA in the mid-1970s was as follows: 35% by pest control operators, mostly on termites; 28% on agricultural crops, including maize and citrus; 30% for home lawn and garden use; and 7% on turf and ornamental plants (Agency for Toxic Substances and Disease Registry,1989b). Since the mid-1970s, the use of chlordane has been increasingly restricted in many countries (WHO, 1988a). By 1980, less than 4500 t of chlordane were being used yearly in the USA, mostly for termite control (Esworthy, 1985). By 1986, use had been reduced to 1800 t (Environmental Protection Agency, 1987b).

Heptachlor was first introduced as a contact insecticide in the USA in 1952 for foliar, soil and structural applications. It has also been used in the control of malaria. It is a non-systemic internal and contact insecticide (WHO, 1988b). The use pattern for heptachlor in the USA in the mid-1970s was as follows: 58% on maize, 27% by pest control operators, 13% as seed treatment and 2% for miscellaneous uses, including fire ant control, use on pineapples and possibly on citrus (Environmental Protection Agency, 1976). In 1970, the use of heptachlor throughout the world was as follows: Africa, 5%; Asia, 15%; Canada and the USA, 5%; Europe, 60%; and South America, 15% (WHO, 1988b). For example, in the Republic of Korea, average use of heptachlor was about 33 t/year over the period 1962–79 (Lee, 1982). The use of heptachlor has been increasingly restricted in many countries (WHO, 1988b). By 1986, less than 340 t of heptachlor were used in the USA, mainly for termite control (Environmental Protection Agency, 1987a).

1.4   Occurrence

1.4.1   *Occupational exposure*

According to the 1981–83 National Occupational Exposure Survey (National Institute for Occupational Safety and Health, 2000), about 3800 pesticide control workers in the USA were potentially exposed to chlordane, and about 1000 workers, including electrical power installers and pesticide control workers, were potentially exposed to heptachlor. According to the Finnish Register of Employees Exposed to Carcinogens, 18 laboratory workers were exposed to chlordane in Finland in 1997 (Savela *et al.*, 1999). Formerly, about 200 Finnish plywood workers were exposed to heptachlor, which was used in special glues in the production of plywood to be exported to tropical countries (Mussalo-Rauhamaa *et al.*, 1991).

Pesticide applicators were exposed on average to a concentration of 17 $\mu g/m^3$ (range, 0.6–116 $\mu g/m^3$) chlordane and 33 $\mu g/m^3$ (2.0–176 $\mu g/m^3$) heptachlor during the control of subterranean termites in the USA. Dermal exposure, monitored by collection on sterile gauze pads, was estimated to be higher (2.5 $\mu g/kg$ bw per h [194 $\mu g/h$] for chlordane, 1.8 $\mu g/kg$ bw per h [140 $\mu g/h$] for heptachlor) than that by inhalation (0.04 $\mu g/kg$ bw per h [3 $\mu g/h$] for chlordane, 0.08 $\mu g/kg$ bw per h [6 $\mu g/h$] for heptachlor), for a mean body weight of 77.5 kg (Kamble *et al.*, 1992). The concentrations of chlordane compounds (*trans*-nonachlor and oxychlordane) in the serum of Japanese pesticide spraymen who had been spraying chlordane formulations for < 3 and > 5 years were on average 2.4 ng/g and 5.1 ng/g, respectively (Takamiya, 1987). The concentration of heptachlor in the air of Finnish plywood mills was < 10–140 $\mu g/m^3$ during assembling, 1–50 $\mu g/m^3$ during hot pressing, 2–10 $\mu g/m^3$ during patching of veneers and 620 $\mu g/m^3$ (short-term exposure) during glue preparation (Kauppinen, 1986). The serum of these workers contained concentrations of heptachlor from below the level of detection to 0.3 ng/g heptachlor epoxide at up to 19.2 ng/g and chlordanes (oxychlordane, *trans*-nonachlor, *cis*-chlordane, *trans*-chlordane) at up to 1.3 ng/g (Mussalo-Rauhamaa *et al.*, 1991).

1.4.2   *Environmental occurrence*

Chlordane and heptachlor are persistent pesticides, the use of which has diminished substantially over the last two decades. These compounds have very low volatility and are essentially insoluble in water. Their biodegradation in soil is very slow, with half-times measured in decades. These chemicals are therefore persistent in the environment and can be expected to accumulate in sediment long after application has ceased.

The environmental occurrence of chlordane and heptachlor was reviewed previously (IARC, 1991). During the period when these compounds were being used as pesticides, a number of studies were carried out to determine the concentrations of chlordane, heptachlor and related compounds in foods. Most foods were found to contain low or undetectable concentrations of these chemicals, with the exception of meat, poultry and dairy products, in which significant concentrations were found.

The estimated dietary intake of heptachlor epoxide in the 1960s and 1970s in the USA was about 0.3–2 μg/day (Duggan & Corneliussen, 1972; Peirano, 1980; WHO, 1984b). Estimates of the intake of heptachlor epoxide in a Basque population in Spain in 1990–91 showed an average of < 0.1 μg/day (Urieta *et al.*, 1996). The estimated intake of total chlordane (chlordane, chlordene, *trans*-nonachlor, oxychlordane) in various age groups in the USA in 1982–84 ranged from 2 ng/kg bw per day for 14–16-year-old girls to 6.5 ng/kg bw per day for 2-year-old children (Gunderson, 1988).

Several studies published since the last evaluation (IARC, 1991), illustrating continuing detection of chlordane and heptachlor in the environment, are summarized below.

The concentrations of chlordane (measured as the sum of *cis*- and *trans*-chlordane) in coastal Nicaragua lagoons in 1995 ranged from 0.013 to 6.29 ng/g dry weight (*trans*-nonachlor, 0.005–2.0 ng/g dry weight), and the concentrations of heptachlor were < 0.004–65.4 ng/g dry weight (Carvalho *et al.*, 1999). A study of the transport of persistent organochlorine pesticides in suspended sediment along the Mississippi River from St Louis to New Orleans, USA, in 1988–90 showed concentrations of chlordane (reported as the sum of *cis*- and *trans*-chlordane) ranging from < 7 to 263 ng/g of organic carbon; similar amounts of nonachlor (*cis* + *trans*) were found. The annual transport of chlordane in suspended sediment from the Mississippi River to the Gulf of Mexico was estimated to be approximately 110 kg (nonachlor, 100 kg) (Rostad, 1997).

Chlordane and heptachlor present in sediments continue to enter the food chain by uptake by organisms in direct contact with the sediment. The National Contamination Biomonitoring Program in the USA determined the concentrations of various organo-chlorine pesticides in samples of freshwater fish taken from 107 sites in the USA in 1976–86. The annual geometric mean concentration ranged from 19 (1986) to 39 ng/g (1976–79) for the sum of *cis*- and *trans*-chlordane; from 48 (1986) to 82 ng/g (1978–79) for the sum of *cis*- and *trans*-chlordane, oxychlordane and *cis*- and *trans*-nonachlor; and from 5 (1984) to 10 ng/g (1978–79) for heptachlor epoxide. The annual maximum concentrations ranged from 490 (1986) to 3070 ng/g (1978–79) for the sum of *cis*- and *trans*-chlordane; from 980 (1986) to 6690 ng/g (1978–79) for the sum of *cis*- and *trans*-chlordane, oxychlordane and *cis*- and *trans*-nonachlor; and from 100 (1986) to 1170 ng/g (1978–79) for heptachlor epoxide (Schmitt *et al.*, 1999). The concentration of chlordane in a single 6.6-kg trout taken from Lake Tahoe, USA in 1993–94 was 17.7 ng/g wet weight, measured as the sum of *cis*- and *trans*-chlordane and 78 ng/g measured as *cis*- and *trans*-chlordane plus oxychlordane plus *trans*-nona-chlor (Datta *et al.*, 1999). The mean concentrations of the sum of *cis*- and *trans*-chlor-dane, oxychlordane and *cis*- and *trans*-nonachlor in yellowtail and winter flounder (flat fish) from off the coast of Newfoundland, Canada, at several locations in 1993 ranged from 0.35 to 6.25 ng/g wet weight (Ray *et al.*, 1998).

The concentrations of chlordane in beluga whale blubber from Alaska's north coast in 1992 ranged from 320 to 990 ng/g of fat in three females and were 2470 and 3880 ng/g of fat in two males. A single fetal specimen contained 690 ng/g of fat, comparable to the concentration in maternal fat of 620 ng/g (Wade *et al.*, 1997). A comprehensive review of the available data showed that the arithmetic mean concentrations of chlordane in traditional foods in northern and Arctic Canada, e.g. marine mammal meat, fish, birds and terrestrial animals, ranged from 2 to 34 ng/g wet weight (1160 ng/g wet weight for marine mammal blubber) (Chan, 1998).

Consumption of foods containing chlordane and heptachlor may result in measurable concentrations of these compounds in human tissues. A compilation of data from the 1960s and 1970s indicated that the mean concentration of heptachlor epoxide in adipose tissue from the general population ranged from 10 to 460 ng/g of fat (IARC, 1991). In a study in 1985–88 of 183 healthy German children, the mean concentration of heptachlor was 6 ng/g of fat (maximum, 87 ng/g of fat) and the mean concentration of heptachlor epoxide was 4 ng/g of fat (maximum, 86 ng/g of fat) (Teufel *et al.*, 1990). In Canadian newborns in 1993–95, the concentrations of *cis*- and *trans*-chlordane in cord blood from non-Inuit infants ranged from 0.01 to 0.07 µg/L, with 0.01–0.3 µg/L for *cis*-nonachlor, 0.01-0.17 µg/L for *trans*-nonachlor and 0.01-0.05 µg/L for oxychlordane, while the concentrations in cord blood from Inuit populations were 0.01–0.20 µg/L for *cis*-chlordane, 0.01–0.03 µg/L for *trans*-chlordane, 0.01–0.18 µg/L for *cis*-nonachlor, 0.01-1.13 µg/L for *trans*-nonachlor and 0.01-0.67 µg/L for oxychlordane. The concentrations in omental fat from Greenland Inuits at autopsy in 1993 were 11.6 ng/g of fat for *cis*- and *trans*-chlordane, 3.1 ng/g for *cis*-nonachlor, 1463 ng/g for *trans*-nonachlor and 862 ng/g for oxychlordane (Van Oostdam *et al.*, 1999).

The most significant source of exposure of infants to chlordane, heptachlor and their metabolites appears to be breast milk, in which the concentrations can be much higher than those in dairy milk. In a large international survey carried out in the 1970s, the mean concentrations of heptachlor and heptachlor epoxide in human breast milk ranged from 2 to 720 ng/g of fat; 2560 ng of heptachlor per gram of fat was found in a rural area in Spain (WHO, 1984b). The median concentration of heptachlor epoxide in breast milk of women in the USA reported in 1991 was 10 ng/g of fat, with a 90th percentile value of 100 ng/g of fat (Rogan *et al.*, 1991).

The concentrations of *cis*- and *trans*-chlordane in breast milk were higher in Inuit mothers from northern Quebec (3.7 ng/g of fat) than in southern Canadian residents (0.37 ng/g of fat) in 1989–92 (Van Oostdam *et al.*, 1999). The mean concentration of chlordane, measured as the sum of *cis*- and *trans*-chlordane, in 12 samples of breast milk from Arctic Canada in 1996 was 1.27 ng/g of fat, the values being 59 ng/g for oxychlordane, 4.29 ng/g for *cis*-nonachlor and 78 ng/g for *trans*-nonachlor (Newsome & Ryan, 1999).

1.5   Regulations and guidelines

The use of chlordane in agriculture has been banned or product registrations have been cancelled or withdrawn in many countries, beginning as early as 1968 and continuing through the 1970s and 1980s, because of concerns about risks to human health and the environment (WHO, 1988a; FAO/UNEP, 1996). For example, in the Joint FAO/UNEP Programme for the Operation of Prior Informed Consent for Banned or Severely Restricted Chemicals in International Trade (PIC Programme), more than 35 countries reported that the use of chlordane had been discontinued or severely restricted (e.g., to structural subterranean termite control) (FAO/UNEP, 1996).

Because of similar concerns and beginning as early as 1958, the agricultural use of heptachlor has been banned or product registrations cancelled or withdrawn in many countries (WHO, 1988b; Mussalo-Rauhamaa et al., 1991; FAO/UNEP, 1996). More than 29 countries reported to the PIC Programme that the use of heptachlor had been discontinued or severely restricted.

In those countries where use is restricted but may continue, the applications are restricted to seed treatment, structural termite control or wood treatment. In tropical and subtropical countries that have retained use for seed treatment or preplanting agricultural use, chlordane/heptachlor is restricted to crops that form the edible portions above ground and, in particular, to crops with long growing seasons that undergo processing before conception (FAO/UNEP, 1996).

Chlordane and heptachlor are among the 12 persistent organic pollutants being considered for international action to reduce or eliminate their releases under a global convention. As of December 2000, the participating governments had agreed to phase out use of chlordane and heptachlor and four other chlorinated pesticides, aldrin, endrin, hexachlorobenzene and toxaphene (Hogue, 2000).

In 1970, the FAO/WHO Joint Meeting on Pesticide Residues (JMPR) evaluated chlordane and established tolerances for residues in food of 0.02–0.5 mg/kg for the sum of cis- and trans-isomers of chlordane and oxychlordane (FAO/WHO, 1971). In 1986, an acceptable daily intake (ADI) in food of 0–0.0005 mg/kg bw was established (FAO/WHO, 1987). In 1994, the ADI was changed to a provisional tolerable daily intake (PTDI) value at the same level, 0.0005 mg/kg bw (WHO, 1999).

In 1966, JMPR also established an ADI in food of 0–0.0005 mg/kg bw for heptachlor/heptachlor epoxide; this value was reduced to 0–0.0001 mg/kg bw in 1991. In 1994, the ADI was changed to a PTDI value of 0.0001 mg/kg bw (WHO, 1999).

Extraneous residue limits (previously designed 'maximum residue levels' have been established by the Codex Alimentarius Commission for the sum of cis- and trans-chlordane or, in the case of animal products, the sum of cis- and trans-chlordane and 'oxychlordane' (fat-soluble residue) in or on the following commodities (in mg/kg): 0.05 for cottonseed oil (crude), linseed oil (crude), meat (fat), poultry meat (fat) and soya bean oil (crude); 0.02 for almonds, eggs, fruit, hazelnuts, maize, oats, pecan, rice (polished), rye, sorghum, soya bean oil (refined), cottonseed oil (edible), vegetables, walnuts and wheat; and 0.002 for milk (fat soluble) (FAO/UNEP, 1996).

Extraneous residue limits were established by the Codex Alimentarius Commission (1997) for the sum of heptachlor and heptachlor epoxide (fat-soluble residue) in or on the following commodities (in mg/kg): 0.5 for soya bean oil (crude); 0.2 for carrots, meat (fat) and poultry meat (fat); 0.05 for eggs and vegetables (except carrots, soya beans, sugar beets and tomatoes); 0.02 for cereal grains, cottonseed, tomatoes, soya beans (immature seeds) and soya bean oil (refined); 0.01 for citrus fruit and pineapples; and 0.006 for milk (fat soluble) (FAO/UNEP, 1996).

WHO (1993) recommended guideline values of 0.2 µg/L for chlordane (all isomers) and 0.03 µg/L for heptachlor and heptachlor epoxide in drinking-water. The Environmental Protection Agency (2000) in the USA has set maximum contaminant levels for chlordane, heptachlor and heptachlor epoxide in drinking-water of 0.002, 0.0004 and 0.0002 mg/L, respectively, and a goal of zero for all three chemicals. In Mexico, the maximum permissible concentrations of chlordane in ambient water are 0.002 mg/L for coastal and estuarine waters and 0.003 mg/L for water treated for drinking; those of heptachlor in ambient water are 0.2 µg/L for coastal waters, 0.002 mg/L for estuarine waters and 0.018 mg/L for water treated for drinking (WHO, 1988a,b). The Environmental Protection Agency in the USA has established a national ambient water quality criterion for heptachlor of 0.28 µg/L (Agency for Toxic Substances and Disease Registry, 1989a).

National and regional pesticide residue limits for chlordane, heptachlor and heptachlor epoxide in foods were compiled by the Food and Drug Administration (1990), Health and Welfare Canada (1990) and IARC (1991). Tables 3 and 4 present occupational exposure limits and guidelines for chlordane and heptachlor in several countries.

2.   Studies of Cancer in Humans

2.1   Cohort studies

Deaths among workers at two plants in the USA, one producing chlordane and the other producing heptachlor, were analysed in a series of studies with slightly different inclusion criteria (Wang & MacMahon, 1979a; Ditraglia et al., 1981; Shindell & Ulrich, 1986; Infante & Freeman, 1987; Shindell, 1987; Brown, 1992). Pesticide production started in 1946 in the first plant and in 1951 in the other. Exposures to other chemicals, including chlorine and dicyclopentadiene (in the chlordane plant) and to endrin, chlorine, chlorendic anhydride, hexachlorocyclopentadiene and vinyl chloride (in the heptachlor plant), were also reported. As the bases of these studies overlap substantially, they do not provide independent information on the carcinogenicity of chlordane/heptachlor. Only the results of the most recent analysis with the longest follow-up are summarized below. In some (Wang & MacMahon, 1979a; Ditraglia et al., 1981) but not all of the previous reports, a non-significant excess of lung cancer, of 20–30%, was reported.

Table 3. Occupational exposure limits and guidelines for chlordane

Country	Year	Concentration (mg/m³)	Interpretation
Australia	1993	0.5 (Ca, sk)	TWA
		2	STEL
Austria	1993	0.5 (sk)	TWA
Belgium	1993	0.5 (sk)	TWA
		2	STEL
Denmark	1993	0.5 (Ca, sk)	TWA
Egypt	1993	0.5 (sk)	TWA
Finland	1993	(Ca)	TWA
France	1993	0.5 (sk)	TWA
Germany	2000	0.5 (IF, 3B, sk)	TWA
India	1993	0.5 (sk)	TWA
		2	STEL
Ireland	1997	0.5 (sk)	TWA
		2	STEL
Netherlands	1999	0.5 (sk)	TWA
Philippines	1993	0.5 (sk)	TWA
Russian Federation	1993	0.01 (sk)	STEL
Switzerland	1993	0.5 (sk)	TWA
Thailand	1993	0.5	TWA
Turkey	1993	0.5 (sk)	TWA
USA			
ACGIH (TLV)	2000	0.5 (A3, sk)	TWA
NIOSH (REL)	2000	0.5 (Ca, sk)	TWA
OSHA (PEL)	2000	0.5 (sk)	TWA

From American Conference of Governmental Industrial Hygienists (ACGIH) (2000); Deutsche Forschungsgemeinschaft (2000)

sk, danger of cutaneous absorption; TWA, time-weighted average; Ca, carcinogen; STEL, short-term exposure limit; IF, inhalable fraction of aerosol; 3B, substances for which in-vitro or animal studies have yielded evidence of carcinogenic effects that is not sufficient for classification of the substance in one of the other categories; further studies are required before a final decision can be made; a maximum acceptable concentration (MAC) value can be established provided no genotoxic effects have been detected; TLV, threshold limit value; A3, confirmed animal carcinogen with unknown relevance to humans; NIOSH, National Institute for Occupational Safety and Health; OSHA, Occupational Safety and Health Administration; REL, recommended exposure limit; PEL, permissible exposure limit

The most recent investigation included white men employed in the two plants for at least 6 months before 1965, with follow-up to the end of 1987 (Brown, 1992). Most workers in non-production jobs were excluded from this analysis. There were 405 workers in the chlordane manufacturing plant, one (0.25%) of whom was lost to follow-up; in the heptachlor/endrin production plant, there were 305 men, with one

Table 4. Occupational exposure limits and guidelines for heptachlor

Country	Year	Concentration (mg/m^3)	Interpretation
Australia	1993	0.5 (sk)	TWA
Belgium	1993	0.5 (sk)	TWA
Denmark	1993	0.5 (sk)	TWA
Finland	1993	0.5 (sk)	TWA
		1.5	STEL
Germany	2000	0.5 (IF, 3B, sk)	TWA
Ireland	1997	0.5 (sk)	TWA
		2	STEL
Netherlands	1999	0.5 (sk)	TWA
Philippines	1993	0.5 (sk)	TWA
Russian Federation	1993	0.01	STEL
Switzerland	1993	0.5 (sk)	TWA
Turkey	1993	1 (sk)	TWA
USA			
ACGIH (TLV)	2000	0.05 (A3, sk)[a]	TWA
NIOSH (REL)	2000	0.5 (Ca, sk)	TWA
OSHA (PEL)	2000	0.5 (sk)	TWA

From American Conference of Governmental Industrial Hygienists (ACGIH) (2000); Deutsche Forschungsgemeinschaft (2000)

sk, danger of cutaneous absorption; TWA, time-weighted average; Ca, carcinogen; STEL, short-term exposure limit; IF, inhalable fraction of aerosol; 3B, substances for which in-vitro or animal studies have yielded evidence of carcinogenic effects that is not sufficient for classification of the substance in one of the other categories; further studies are required before a final decision can be made; a maximum acceptable concentration (MAC) value can be established provided no genotoxic effects have been detected; TLV, threshold limit value; A3, confirmed animal carcinogen with unknown relevance to humans; NIOSH, National Institute for Occupational Safety and Health; OSHA, Occupational Safety and Health Administration; REL, recommended exposure limit; PEL, permissible exposure limit

[a] Heptachlor and heptachlor epoxide

(0.33%) lost to follow-up. The expected numbers of deaths were calculated from the mortality rates of white males in the USA. The results for cancers at all sites and for specific sites at which at least two cases were observed are shown in Table 5, including the results for the haematopoietic system.

Cancer risks were also evaluated among cohorts of pesticide applicators engaged in termite control, in which chlordane has until recently been the most widely used chemical. As pesticide applicators are exposed to several different pesticides, it is difficult to disentangle the effects of chlordane from those of the others.

A study by Wang and MacMahon (1979b) of deaths in a cohort of over 16 000 urban pesticide applicators was extended (MacMahon et al., 1988) to give a maximal period of follow-up of 18 years (from 1967 to 1984). For the 8% of deaths for which a certificate was not located, the numbers of deaths attributable to cancer at specific sites were estimated on the basis of the proportion among observed causes of death. A significant excess of lung cancer based on 108 estimated deaths (standardized mortality ratio [SMR], 1.4; 90% confidence interval [CI], 1.1–1.6) was observed, with nonsignificant excesses for cancers of the skin (1.3; 0.65–2.2) and urinary bladder (1.2; 0.50–2.5). No excess was observed for cancers of the digestive organs and peritoneum, with 45 esti-

Table 5. Studies on cohorts of workers exposed to chlordane/heptachlor in the USA

Reference	Cancer	No. of cases	SMR	95% CI	Comments
Brown (1992)	*Chlordane manufacturers*				Workers were also exposed to several other chemicals
	All sites	35	0.87	0.61–1.2	
	Stomach	4	2.1	0.57–5.4	
	Pancreas	2	0.93	0.11–3.4	
	Respiratory system	19	1.3	0.80–2.1	
	Lymphatic/ haematopoietic	4	1.1	0.30–2.8	
	Heptachlor/endrin manufacturers				
	All sites	18	1.0	0.60–1.6	
	Stomach	2	2.8	0.34–10	
	Respiratory system	6	0.88	0.32–1.9	
	Bladder	3	7.1	1.5–21	
	Lymphatic/ haematopoietic	1	0.58	0.01–3.2	
MacMahon et al. (1988)	*Entire cohort of applicators*				Pesticide applicators; chlordane and heptachlor were among the components used. 90% CI
	Lung	108	1.4	1.1–1.6	
	Skin	9	1.3	0.65–2.2	
	Bladder	5	1.2	0.50–2.5	
	Lymphatic/ haematopoietic	25	0.97	0.67–1.4	
	Termite control operators only				
	Lung	30	0.97	0.7–1.3	Chlordane and heptachlor were the main components used. 90% CI
	Skin	3	1.2	[0.4–2.9]	
	Bladder	2	1.3	[0.3–3.9]	
	Buccal cavity and pharynx	5	1.4	0.5–3.3	
	Stomach	5	1.1	0.4–2.5	
	Colon	11	1.1	0.6–2.0	
	Liver	2	1.1	0.1–4.0	
	Pancreas	6	1.0	0.4–2.2	
	Larynx	4	2.4	0.7–6.2	

Table 5 (contd)

Reference	Cancer	No. of cases	SMR	95% CI	Comments
Blair *et al.*	Lung	54	1.4	(1.0–1.8)	Pesticide applicators;
(1983);	Skin	2	0.9	0.1–3.1	chlordane and heptachlor
Pesatori	Prostate	5	0.8	0.2–1.8	were among the
et al.	Testis	2	2.9	0.3–11	components used.
(1994)	Bladder	3	1.0	0.2–3.0	
(Florida)	Kidney	2	0.7	0.1–2.5	
	Brain	8	2.2	0.9–4.4	
	Lymphatic/ haematopoietic	9	0.8	0.4–1.5	
	Leukaemia	4	1.2	0.4–2.7	
	Nested case–				Exposure to chlordane
	control study of	9	1.2	0.4–3.8	Dead controls
	lung cancer		0.5	0.2–1.3	Living controls

mated deaths (0.84; 0.64–1.1), nor of the lymphohaematopoietic system, with 25 estimated deaths (0.97; 0.67–1.4). When the analyses were restricted to termite control operators, who have a higher probability of exposure to chlordane and heptachlor, no excess of lung cancer deaths (30) was observed, with 31 estimated deaths (0.97; 0.7–1.3), while the SMRs for skin (1.2) and bladder (1.3) cancer were comparable with those of the whole cohort. The risk for lung cancer did not rise with increasing duration of employment. No thyroid cancers were reported.

In an investigation of 3827 white male pesticide applicators in Florida, USA, licensed during 1965–66 (Blair *et al.*, 1983), whose follow-up was subsequently extended until 1 January 1982, an overall excess of lung cancer (SMR,1.4 [95% CI,1.0–1.8]) was found (Pesatori *et al.*, 1994). Small numbers of deaths also occurred from leukaemia (1.2; 0.4–2.7), oral cancer (1.4; 0.5–3.3) and cancers of the larynx (2.4; 0.7–6.2), testis (2.9; 0.3–11) and brain (2.2; 0.9–4.4), but the nonsignificant excesses of skin and urinary bladder cancer observed in the first report were no longer present. For other lymphatic/haematopoietic cancers, the SMRs were below 1.0. In a nested case–control study conducted for lung cancer, surrogate responders were identified for 65 (83%) of the 78 lung cancer cases (some of which occurred after the closing date of the cohort). Five controls were randomly matched by age to each case: three living at the time of death of the case and two who died in the same year. For dead controls, next-of-kin were interviewed, and for living controls information up to the time of death of the case was used. Interviews were obtained for 122 (80%) of the 152 selected deceased controls and 172 (75%) of the 229 living controls. When information on specific pesticides reported by the surrogate responders was considered, the age- and smoking-adjusted odds ratio for lung cancer associated with use of chlordane was 1.2 (95% CI, 0.4–3.8) in comparison with deceased controls and 0.5 (0.2–1.3) in comparison with living controls.

2.2   Case–control studies

As chlordane and heptachlor accumulate in fat tissue in increasing amounts with age, those studies in which the confounding effect of age was not strictly controlled for are difficult to interpret.

The case–control studies that were considered valid are summarized in Table 6.

2.2.1   *Lymphohaematopoietic system*

A case–control study was conducted in western Washington State, USA, on 128 men with soft-tissue sarcoma and 576 men with non-Hodgkin lymphoma aged 20–79 years at diagnosis during 1981–84 and identified between 1983 and 1985 through a population-based tumour registry (Woods *et al.*, 1987). Of the 150 eligible patients with soft-tissue sarcoma who were alive at the time of interview, 97 (65%) were included in the study; of the 56 eligible deceased cases, 31 (55%) were included. The corresponding figures for non-Hodgkin lymphoma were 402 (76%) of 527 eligible living patients and 174 (79%) of 219 eligible deceased cases. Living controls were selected by random-digit dialling (for ages 20–64) or from the Health Care Financing Administration (ages 65–79), while deceased controls were identified from death certificates showing a cause other than cancer for residents of the same area. Men whose cause of death was suicide or homicide were not eligible. Included in the analysis were 475 (76%) of the 622 living controls identified as eligible and 219 (76%) of the 288 deceased controls. The age-adjusted odds ratio for men reporting exposure to chlordane was 1.6 for non-Hodgkin lymphoma (95% CI, 0.7–3.8) and 0.96 for soft-tissue sarcoma (95% CI, 0.2–4.8). Adjustment for exposure to other selected chemicals by regression analysis did not change the risk estimates substantially. In an additional report from the same study in which the analysis was restricted to farmers (Woods & Polissar, 1989), the odds ratio for non-Hodgkin lymphoma in relation to exposure to chlordane was again 1.6 (0.5–5.1). [The Working Group noted that the number of proxy interviews with living subjects was not reported.]

In a case–control study of non-Hodgkin lymphoma in the USA, cases were iden-tified through the Iowa State Health Registry and a special surveillance of Minnesota hospital and pathology laboratory records (Cantor *et al.*, 1992). Men were eligible as cases if they had been aged 30 years or more at the time of diagnosis, their lymphoma had been diagnosed between March 1981 and October 1983 in Iowa and between October 1980 and September 1982 in Minnesota, and they were resident in the state, excluding, for Minnesota, the cities of Minneapolis, St Paul, Duluth and Rochester. The diagnoses were reviewed by a panel of four experienced regional pathologists. Of the 780 identified patients, 694 (89%) were interviewed, and 622 were confirmed in the

Table 6. Case–control studies of exposure to chlordane/heptachlor

Reference and location	No of cases : controls (types of controls)	Exposure assessment	Exposure categories	Odds ratio (95% CI) or p value	Comments
Non-Hodgkin lymphoma					

Woods et al. (1987); Woods & Polissar (1989) Washington State, USA	576 : 694 (population) (men)	Self-reported exposure to chlordane	No
			Yes
			Among farmers:
			  No
			  Yes
				1
				1.6 (0.7–3.8)
				
				1
				1.6 (0.5–5.1)
					1.6% of study population exposed to chlordane

Cantor et al. (1992) Iowa and Minnesota, USA	622 : 1245 (population) (men)	Self-reported exposure to chlordane	Non-farmers Ever handled on animals Handled on animals prior to 1965 Ever handled on crops Handled on crops prior to 1965 Ever handled on animals without protective equipment Ever handled on crops without protective equipment	1 1.7 (1.0–2.9) 2.2 (1.2–4.2) 1.7 (0.9–3.2) 1.6 (0.7–3.6) 2.2 (1.2–4.2) 2.1 (1.1–4.3)	Proxy interviews for deceased cases and controls
Hardell et al. (1996, 1997) Sweden	27 : 17 (surgical patients) (men and women)	Self-reported exposure to heptachlor Chlordane metabolites in abdominal wall adipose tissue < 119 ng/g lipid > 119 ng/g lipid	Ever handled on animals Sum of chlordane metabolites	1.3 (0.7–2.2) 1 3.3 (0.7–16)	Adjusted

Table 6 (contd)

Reference and location	No of cases : controls (types of controls)	Exposure assessment	Exposure categories	Odds ratio (95% CI) or p value	Comments
Hoar-Zahm et al. (1988) Nebraska, USA	385 : 1432 (population) (men and women)	Self-reported exposure to chlordane	No	1	Abstract
			Yes	2.1	
Leukaemia					
Brown et al. (1990) Iowa and Minnesota, USA	578 : 1245 (population) (men)	Self-reported exposure to chlordane and heptachlor	Non-farmers	1	Proxy interviews for deceased cases and controls
			Chlordane		
			Ever handled on crops	0.7 (0.3–1.6)	
			Ever handled on animals	1.3 (0.7–2.3)	
			Handled on animals at least 20 years previously	1.5 (0.7–3.1)	
			Days/year of use on crops		
			1–4	0.3 (0.0–2.5)	
			5–9	1.5 (0.1–18)	
			≥ 10	0.3 (0.0–2.5)	
			Days/year of use on animals		
			1–4	1.1 (0.4–2.8)	
			5–9	0	
			≥ 10	3.2 (0.9–11)	
			Heptachlor		
			Ever handled on crops	0.9 (0.5–1.7)	
			Days/year of use on crops		
			1–4	1.2 (0.4–3.3)	
			5–9	1.0 (0.3–3.2)	
			≥ 10	0.2 (0.0–1.8)	

Table 6 (contd)

Reference and location	No of cases : controls (types of controls)	Exposure assessment	Exposure categories	Odds ratio (95% CI) or p value	Comments
Hairy-cell leukaemia					
Nordström et al. (2000) Sweden	54 : 54 (population)	Chlordane metabolites in blood samples (ng/g of lipid)	≤ 44 > 44	1 1.4 (0.5–4.1)	Blood samples obtained from patients a median of 7.1 years after diagnosis
		Epstein-Barr virus early antigen immunoglobulin G titre (EBV)	EBV < 40, chlordane ≤ 44 EBV > 40, chlordane ≥ 44	1 16 (2.8-111)	
Multiple myeloma					
Brown et al. (1993) Iowa, USA	173 : 650 (population)	Self-reported exposure to chlordane	Non-farmers Ever used on animals	1 1.6 (0.7–3.6)	
Soft-tissue sarcoma					
Woods et al. (1987) Washington State, USA	128 : 694 (population) (men)	Self-reported exposure to chlordane	No Yes	1 0.96 (0.2–4.8)	
Breast cancer					
Falck et al. (1992) Connecticut, USA	20 (carcinoma) : 20 (benign breast disease)	Heptachlor epoxide, oxychlordane and trans-nonachlor in breast fat (wet weight) (ng/g)	Carcinoma [116 ± 50] Benign disease [97 ± 49] Carcinoma [87 ± 37] Benign disease [96 ± 80]	$p = 0.22$ $p = 0.65$	Mean heptachlor epoxide and oxychlordane Mean trans-nonachlor

Table 6 (contd)

Reference and location	No of cases : controls (types of controls)	Exposure assessment	Exposure categories	Odds ratio (95% CI) or p value	Comments
Dewailly et al. (1994) Canada	20 : 17 (benign breast disease)	Oxychlordane and trans-nonachlor in breast fat (ng/g)	Controls [31 ± 12] Cases ER-negative [27 ± 7] Cases ER-positive [39 ± 14] Controls [42 ± 18] Cases ER-negative [35 ± 8] Cases ER-positive [50 ± 11]	$p = 0.59$ $p = 0.12$ $p = 0.37$ $p = 0.07$	Mean oxychlordane Mean trans-nonachlor
Høyer et al. (1998) Denmark	240 : 477 (population)	Several chlordane metabolites in serum		No association found [data not shown]	Samples collected prospectively
Dorgan et al. (1999) Missouri, USA	105 : 208 (population)	Several chlordane metabolites in serum	% above detection limit *Oxychlordane* Controls 13.0% Cases 16.2% trans-*Nonachlor* Controls 42.8% Cases 49.5% *Heptachlor* Controls 19.2% Cases 20.0%	$p = 0.55$ $p = 0.22$ $p = 0.90$	Samples collected prospectively

Table 6 (contd)

Reference and location	No of cases : controls (types of controls)	Exposure assessment	Exposure categories	Odds ratio (95% CI) or *p* value	Comments
Aronson *et al.* (2000) Canada	217 : 213 (benign breast disease)	Several chlordane metabolites in breast fat (ng/g)	*cis-Nonachlor* ≤ 4.3 4.4–6.5 6.6–10 ≥ 11	1 0.81 (0.47–1.4) 0.48 (0.27–0.86) 0.80 (0.41–1.5)	Results were similar for pre- and post-menopausal women
			trans-Nonachlor ≤ 31 32–43 44–64 ≥ 65	1 0.93 (0.54–1.6) 0.69 (0.39–1.2) 0.78 (0.40–1.5)	
			Oxychlordane ≤ 24 25–32 33–46 ≥ 47	1 0.68 (0.40–1.2) 0.61 (0.35–1.1) 0.59 (0.31–1.2)	
Demers *et al.* (2000) Canada	315 : 219 (hospital), 307 (population)	Several chlordane metabolites in serum (ng/g)	*Oxychlordane* Hospital controls < 8.4 8.4–< 10.6 10.6–< 12.6 12.6–< 16.3 ≥ 16.3	1 1.1 (0.58–2.1) 0.96 (0.49–1.9) 0.81 (0.41–1.6) 0.55 (0.27–1.1)	No effect on tumour size and lymph-node involvment
			Population controls < 8.4 8.4–< 10.6 10.6–< 12.6 12.6–< 16.3 ≥ 16.3	1 1.1 (0.65–1.8) 1.0 (0.59–1.7) 1.3 (0.74–2.2) 1.5 (0.83–2.6)	

Table 6 (contd)

Reference and location	No of cases : controls (types of controls)	Exposure assessment	Exposure categories	Odds ratio (95% CI) or p value	Comments
Demers et al. (2000) (contd)			trans-*Nonachlor*		
			Hospital controls		
			< 10.6	1	
			10.6–< 13.5	1.3 (0.64–2.4)	
			13.5–< 16.9	1.5 (0.77–2.8)	
			16.9–< 20.7	0.59 (0.29–1.2)	
			≥ 20.7	0.74 (0.38–1.5)	
			Population controls		
			< 10.6	1	
			10.6–< 13.5	0.82 (0.49–1.4)	
			13.5–< 16.9	1.5 (0.91–2.6)	
			16.9–< 20.7	0.69 (0.39–1.2)	
			≥ 20.7	1.2 (0.68–2.1)	
Zheng et al. (2000) Connecticut, USA	304 : 186 (benign breast disease)	trans-Nonachlor and oxychlordane in breast fat (ng/g)	*Oxychlordane*		
			< 26.0	1	
			26.0–33.6	0.7 (0.4–1.2)	
			33.7–47.5	0.7 (0.4–1.2)	
			≥ 47.6	0.7 (0.4–1.3)	
			trans-*Nonachlor*		
			< 36.4	1	
			36.4–53.1	1.2 (0.7–2.1)	
			53.2–71.0	0.7 (0.4–1.3)	
			≥ 71.1	1.1 (0.6–1.9)	

Table 6 (contd)

Reference and location	No of cases : controls (types of controls)	Exposure assessment	Exposure categories	Odds ratio (95% CI) or p value	Comments
Endometrial cancer					
Weiderpass et al. (2000) Sweden	154 : 205 (population)	Oxychlordane and trans-nonachlor in serum (quartiles)	*Oxychlordane* 1 (low) 2 3 4 (high) *p* for trend, 0.33 trans-*Nonachlor* 1 (low) 2 3 4 (high) *p* for trend, 0.56	1 1.1 (0.6–2.2) 1.0 (0.5–2.0) 1.4 (0.7–2.8) 1 1.2 (0.6–2.3) 1.3 (0.7–2.7) 1.2 (0.6–2.5)	
Pancreatic cancer					
Hoppin et al. (2000) California, USA	108 : 82 (population)	trans-Nonachlor in serum (ng/g)	0 (below detection limit) 0.1–75 > 75	1 0.9 (0.5–1.9) 1.7 (0.8–3.5)	

Table 6 (contd)

Reference and location	No of cases : controls (types of controls)	Exposure assessment	Exposure categories	Odds ratio (95% CI) or p value	Comments
Childhood brain cancer					
Davis *et al.* (1993) Missouri, USA	45 : 85 (friends of cases), 108 (cancer controls)	Reported by parents	*Termite treatment of home within 1 year before residence*		
			Yes versus no, friend controls	2.6 (0.9–7.5)	
			Yes versus no, cancer controls	2.3 (0.8–6.4)	
			Termiticide used between 7 months of age and diagnosis		
			Yes versus no, friend controls	1.4 (0.5–3.9)	
			Yes versus no, cancer controls	1.4 (0.5–3.8)	
			Any termite treatment		
			Yes versus no, friend controls	2.9 (1.3–7.1)	
			Yes versus no, cancer controls	3.0 (1.3–7.4)	
			Chlordane used for termite treatment		
			Yes versus no, friend controls	1.5 (0.5–4.9)	
			Yes versus no, cancer controls	1.5 (0.5–5.1)	

ER, estrogen receptor

review to have a non-Hodgkin lymphoma. The 1245 controls were frequency matched to cases by age, residence and vital status. Living subjects aged less than 65 years were selected by random-digit dialling or from Medicare rosters for those aged over 65, and deceased men were selected from death certificate files. The response rates for the various groups of controls were 77–79%. Proxy interviews were conducted for deceased or incompetent men (184 cases and 425 controls). A detailed history of farming and pesticide use was obtained by an interviewer from all subjects who had worked on a farm for at least 6 months since the age of 18 by means of a questionnaire to the participating subjects or proxy responders. Odds ratios were estimated by unconditional multiple logistic regression, allowing for the matching variables plus other potential risk factors; the reference category was those who had never worked or lived on a farm as adults (266 cases, 547 controls). Thirty-one patients and 38 controls had ever handled chlordane as an animal insecticide (odds ratio, 1.7; 95% CI, 1.0–2.9), and 21 patients and 26 controls had used it as crop insecticide (1.7; 0.9–3.2); 25 patients and 43 controls had ever handled heptachlor as an animal insecticide (1.3; 0.7–2.2). When the analysis was limited to those who had handled chlordane before 1965, the odds ratios became 2.2 (1.2–4.2) for use on animals and 1.6 (0.7–3.6) for use on crops; the results for heptachlor were similar to those for any handling. The corresponding figures for those who had handled chlordane without protective equipment were 2.2 (1.2–4.2) for use on animals and 2.1 (1.1–4.3) for use on crops. The odds ratios were similar in the two study areas for use on animals; but for use on crops, the odds ratios were 1.3 (0.5–3.3) for Iowa and 3.1 (0.7–15) for Minnesota [The Working Group noted that part of the excess risk may have been due to the fact that people who were not farmers were used as the reference category.]

In a study in Sweden, 27 consecutive patients in whom non-Hodgkin lymphoma (17 men and 10 women) was diagnosed between 1994 and 1995 and living in the Uppsala–Örebro region were compared with 17 surgical controls (nine men and eight women) without a history of malignancy (Hardell et al., 1996). None of the patients or controls reported use of or occupational exposure to chlordane. Six chlordane metabolites were identified in adipose tissue obtained from the abdominal wall of the patients, while two others were not detected. The mean sum of the metabolites was 180 ng/g of lipid for the cases (range, 48–680 ng/g) and 93 ng/g of lipid (37–160 ng/g) for the control group ($p = 0.002$). For 17 cases and five controls, the sum of the metabolites was above the median for the whole study population (119 ng/g lipid), giving a crude odds ratio of 4.1 (95% CI, 1.1–15). These estimates were not adjusted for age. As reported in a letter published subsequently (Hardell et al., 1997), the odds ratio adjusted for age and sex by multiple logistic regression was 3.3 (0.7–16). The authors reported that the age distribution of cases and controls was similar.

A population-based case–control study of non-Hodgkin lymphoma conducted in eastern Nebraska, USA, on 385 histologically confirmed non-Hodgkin lymphoma cases (201 men and 184 women) and 1432 controls (725 men and 707 women) was presented in an abstract (Hoar Zahm et al., 1988). The odds ratio associated with chlordane use was 2.1, but no further information on the association was given. A sub-sequent publication on the relation between non-Hodgkin lymphoma in men and expo-sure to 2,4-D gives more details of the study design, with no mention however of chlordane (Hoar Zahm *et al.*, 1990).

In a study of leukaemia in men parallel to that of non-Hodgkin lymphoma conducted in Iowa and Minnesota, described above (Cantor *et al.*, 1992), 578 cases of leukaemia (340 living and 238 deceased) and 1245 controls (820 living and 425 deceased) were included (Brown *et al.*, 1990). The odds ratios for farmers were 0.7 (95% CI, 0.3–1.6) for those who reported use of chlordane on crops and 0.9 (0.5–1.7) for those who had used heptachlor on crops. Those who reported use of chlordane on animals had an odds ratio of 1.3 (0.7–2.3), while that for those who had handled it at least 20 years before diagnosis was 1.5 (0.7–3.1). Among farmers using chlordane on animals, the risks rose inconsistently with frequency of use, from an odds ratio of 1.1 (0.4–2.8) for fewer than 5 days per year, to no exposed case and five exposed controls for use on 5–9 days per year and to an odds ratio of 3.2 (0.9–11) for use $\geq$ 10 days per year. The risk estimates were not adjusted for other agricultural exposures. There was no evidence of increasing risk with increasing frequency of use of chlordane or heptachlor on crops.

In a study conducted in Sweden, 121 cases of hairy-cell leukaemia, a rare lympho-haematopoietic malignancy, that were diagnosed between 1987 and 1992 were identified from the Swedish Cancer Registry, and 484 controls were drawn from the national population registry and matched to the cases on age, sex and county (Nordström *et al.*, 2000). Of these, 111 patients (91%) and 400 controls (83%) answered the mailed questionnaire. Blood samples were taken a median of 7.1 years after diagnosis from 71 cases and from 186 controls; owing to refusal and other technical problems, chlordane and other pesticides were measured in only 54 (76%) cases and 54 (29%) controls. The odds ratio for having a blood concentration of chlordane above the median of controls (44 ng/g) was 1.4 (95% CI, 0.5–4.1), estimated from logistic regression with adjustment for several confounding factors. Antibodies to Epstein-Barr virus early antigen immuno-globulin G_1 in blood were also measured, and the effect of the interaction with chlordane on the risk for hairy-cell leukaemia was evaluated. The odds ratios were 4.3 (1.1–19) for patients with antibody titres above the median of 40, 1.3 (0.4–5.2) for those with chlordane concentrations above the median (of 44 ng/g) and 16 (2.8–111) for those with both measures above the median. [The Working Group noted that the blood samples were taken after heavy treatment with immunosuppressive drugs.]

In a study on multiple myeloma conducted in men in Iowa in parallel to the studies of non-Hodgkin lymphoma and leukaemia among men in Iowa and Minnesota, described above (Brown *et al.*, 1990; Cantor *et al.*, 1992), 173 patients (101 alive, 72 deceased) and 650 controls (452 alive, 198 deceased) were included in the analysis (Brown *et al.*, 1993). Logistic regression was used to obtain adjusted odds ratios for (self-reported) mixing, handling or application of specific pesticides, relative to the rates of men who were not farmers. Nine cases and 29 controls had used chlordane as animal insecticides, and the estimated odds ratio was 1.6 (95% CI, 0.7–3.6). [The Working

Group noted that part of the excess may have been due to the fact that men who were not farmers were used as the reference category.]

2.2.2   *Breast and female genital tract*

Fat tissue samples from mastectomy or biopsy specimens were obtained from 50 white women with a palpable breast mass or mammographic abnormalities at Hartford Hospital, Connecticut, USA, between May and September 1987 (Falck *et al.*, 1992). Histological examination revealed that 23 women had a mammary carcinoma, while the remaining 27 had benign disease. Twenty samples were selected from women in each group (mean age of cases, 63, range 36–86 years; mean age of controls, 59, range, 45–76 years) for analysis of several pesticides, including three metabolites of chlordane (heptachlor epoxide, oxychlordane and *trans*-nonachlor). The mean value (wet weight basis ± standard deviation) of the sum of heptachlor epoxide and oxy-chlordane was 116 ± 50 ng/g for women with breast carcinoma and 97 ± 49 ng/g for those with benign disease (*t* test, $p = 0.22$). For *trans*-nonachlor, the corresponding figures were 87 ± 37 ng/g and 96 ± 80 ng/g ($p = 0.65$).

Between November 1991 and May 1992, adipose tissue was collected from 41 women aged 40–69 who had undergone a biopsy in a hospital in Québec City (Canada), and the organochlorine content was determined (Dewailly *et al.*, 1994). Twenty women had breast cancer (mean age, 54.1 years), and 17 had adenomas or lipomas (mean age, 51.2 years); four women with other diseases were excluded. The mean oxychlordane concentration was 31 ± 12 ng/g in breast adipose tissue from the 17 subjects with benign disease, 27 ± 7 ng/g (Student *t* test, $p = 0.59$) in the nine estrogen receptor-negative cases and 39 ± 14 ng/g ($p = 0.12$) in the nine estrogen receptor-positive cases. For *trans*-nonachlor, the mean concentrations in the three groups were 42 ± 18, 35 ± 8 ($p = 0.37$) and 50 ± 11 ng/g ($p = 0.07$), respectively. Estrogen receptor status was not determined for two cases. [The Working Group noted that estrogen receptor-negative cancers of the breast are more frequent among younger women.]

In 1976, baseline information and blood samples were obtained from 7712 women enrolled in the Copenhagen City Heart Study, who were randomly selected through the Civil Registration System (Høyer *et al.*, 1998). According to the Danish Cancer Registry, 268 of the women developed breast cancer between 1976 and 1993. For each case, two women free of breast cancer and matched for age, date of examination and vital status at the time of diagnosis were randomly selected as controls. Blood samples were available in 1995 for 240 cases and 477 controls. Heptachlor, heptachlor epoxide, α- and γ-chlordane, oxychlordane and *trans*-nonachlor were among the compounds measured. Conditional logistic regression was used to estimate odds ratios for categories of pesticide concentrations. The authors did not report the concentrations of chlordane metabolites but indicated that no association was found.

A total of 7224 women donated blood to the Columbia, Missouri, breast cancer serum bank (USA) between 1977 and 1987 (over 90% in 1980 or earlier) (Dorgan *et al.*,

1999). Although active postal follow-up continued until 1989, 70% of the cohort was last contacted in 1982–83. A histologically confirmed breast cancer was diagnosed in 105 of the 6426 women for whom at least 4 mL of serum remained in the bank and who had had no history of cancer at the time of blood collection. Two controls were selected for each case, who were alive and free of cancer and matched to the cases by age, date of blood sample collection and history of benign breast disease at enrolment. Since the serum samples of two controls could not be analysed, 208 controls were included in the analysis. Among the compounds measured by gas chromatography were heptachlor, heptachlor epoxide, cis- and trans-chlordane, oxychlordane and trans-nonachlor. None of the samples contained cis- or trans-chlordane or heptachlor epoxide at concentrations above the limit of detection. The concentrations of oxychlordane were above the limit of detection for 16.2% of cases and 13.0 % of controls (p = 0.55). The corresponding figures were 20.0% and 19.2 % (p = 0.90) for heptachlor and 49.5% and 42.8% (p = 0.22) for trans-nonachlor.

Of 824 women who were under the age of 80, were scheduled for biopsy in two hospitals in Toronto and Kingston (Canada) between July 1995 and June 1997, had no history of cancer, had not participated in tamoxifen trials, had not had a breast implant and were not too ill to participate, 735 (89%) agreed to participate in a case–control study and 663 (81%) completed a questionnaire by telephone or mail (Aronson et al., 2000). Organochlorine compounds were determined in benign tissue taken during biopsy from 217 women with in-situ or invasive breast cancer and in 213 women matched for age and study site whose biopsy samples showed no malignancy but most of whom had a diagnosis of some form of benign breast disease. Over 30% of the women had undetectable levels of α- and γ-chlordane. For other compounds, the women were divided into four categories according to the tissue concentration. For cis-nonachlor, the odds ratios estimated by logistic regression and adjusted for several potential confounders were 0.81 (95% CI, 0.47–1.4), 0.48 (0.27–0.86) and 0.80 (0.41–1.5) for women in the second (4.4–6.5 µg/kg tissue), third (6.6–10 µg/kg) and fourth (≥ 11 µg/kg) categories, respectively, as compared with the first (≤ 4.3 µg/kg). The corresponding odds ratios were 0.93 (0.54–1.6), 0.69 (0.39–1.2) and 0.78 (0.40–1.5) for trans-nonachlor (with concentration ranges of 32–43 µg/kg, 44–64 µg/kg and ≥ 65 µg/kg in the second, third and fourth categories, respectively, in comparison with ≤ 31 µg/kg in the first category) and 0.68 (0.40–1.2), 0.61 (0.35–1.1) and 0.59 (0.31–1.2) for oxychlordane (with concentration ranges of 25–32 µg/kg, 33–46 µg/kg and ≥ 47 µg/kg in the second, third and fourth categories, respectively, in comparison with ≤ 24 µg/kg in the first category). When analyses were conducted separately for pre- and postmenopausal women, the results were similar in the two groups.

A study conducted in Québec, Canada, between 1994 and 1997 included 315 women aged 30–70 years and residing in the Québec City area with histologically confirmed breast cancer, 219 controls recruited in four hospitals of the study area and free of gynaecological diseases and 307 controls selected from the general population (Demers et al., 2000). The participation rates were 91% for cases, 89% for hospital controls and

47% for population controls. Blood samples were obtained before therapy, and *cis*- and *trans*-chlordane, *cis*-nonachlor, *trans*-nonachlor and oxychlordane were measured. As *cis*- and *trans*-chlordane and *cis*-nonachlor were detected in less than 70% of the blood samples, they were excluded from further analysis. In comparison with the first quintile of oxychlordane serum concentration, the adjusted odds ratios for women with concentrations in subsequent quintiles were 1.1 (0.58–2.1), 0.96 (0.49–1.9), 0.81 (0.41–1.6) and 0.55 (0.27–1.1) in relation to hospital controls and 1.1 (0.65–1.8), 1.0 (0.59–1.7), 1.3 (0.74–2.2) and 1.5 (0.83–2.6) in relation to population controls. For *trans*-nonachlor, the corresponding figures were 1.3 (0.64–2.4), 1.5 (0.77–2.8), 0.59 (0.29–1.2) and 0.74 (0.38–1.5) in relation to hospital controls and 0.82 (0.49–1.4), 1.5 (0.91–2.6), 0.69 (0.39–1.2) and 1.2 (0.68–2.1) in relation to population controls. The concentrations of oxychlordane and *trans*-nonachlor in blood were associated with the extent of disease.

Between 1994 and 1997, women aged 40–79 without a previous diagnosis of cancer, who had undergone breast-related surgery at the Yale-New Haven Hospital, New Haven, Connecticut, USA, and whose breast specimen was suitable for chemical analysis were asked to participate in a case–control study (Zheng *et al.*, 2000). Of the 490 women enrolled, 304 had histologically confirmed breast cancer and 186 had histologically confirmed benign breast disease (excluding atypical hyperplasia). The participation rate was 79% for cases and 74% for controls. The age- and lipid-adjusted geometric mean adipose tissue concentrations of oxychlordane and *trans*-nonachlor were similar for cases and controls. In comparison with the lowest quartile of concentration, the odds ratios adjusted for several covariates were 0.7 (0.4–1.2), 0.7 (0.4–1.2) and 0.7 (0.4–1.3) for those with subsequent quartiles of oxychlordane and 1.2 (0.7–2.1), 0.7 (0.4–1.3) and 1.1 (0.6–1.9) for *trans*-nonachlor.

A case–control study of endometrial cancer was conducted between 1996 and 1997 in 12 Swedish counties, which included 288 (73%) of the 396 cases of histologically confirmed endometrial cancer identified through a network of personnel at the departments of gynaecology and gynaecological oncology in the study area (Weiderpass *et al.*, 2000). An additional 134 women were excluded since they had used hormone replacement therapy, thus leaving 154 cases. Of the 742 women selected as controls from population registers and frequency matched to cases by 5-year age group, 205 were included in the study; the others were excluded because they had undergone hysterectomy, had used hormone replacement therapy or refused to participate. Serum samples were taken from all participants and analysed for organochlorine compounds. The odds ratios were obtained by logistic regression and adjusted for age and body mass index. In comparison with women in the first quartile of serum concentrations of chlordane metabolites, the odds ratios were 1.1 (0.6–2.2), 1.0 (0.5–2.0) and 1.4 (0.7–2.8) for subsequent quartiles of oxychlordane (*p* for trend = 0.33) and 1.2 (0.6–2.3), 1.3 (0.7–2.7) and 1.2 (0.6–2.5) for *trans*-nonachlor (*p* for trend = 0.56).

2.2.3   *Other cancers*

A study was conducted between 1996 and 1998 on cases of exocrine pancreatic cancer diagnosed among persons aged 21–85 in hospitals of the San Francisco Bay Area (USA) (Hoppin *et al.*, 2000). Only 113 of 611 potential cases were included in the study (108 cases included in the analysis), the most common cause of exclusion being death of the patient (55%). Age- and sex-matched controls were selected by random-digit dialling (age, < 65) or from the Health Care Financing Administration lists (age ≥ 65). Eighty-two of the selected controls agreed to provide a blood sample, giving a participation rate of 78% for people < 65 and 65% for those ≥ 65. Cases had significantly higher median concentrations of *trans*-nonachlor than controls. The adjusted odds ratios relative to individuals with concentrations below the detection limit were 0.9 (0.5–1.9) for a blood concentration between 0.1 and 75 ng/g and 1.7 (0.8–3.5) for a blood concentration > 75 ng/g of lipid.

The relationship between pesticide use in the home and childhood brain cancer was examined in a case–control study of 45 white children with brain cancer diagnosed between 1985 and 1989, resident in Missouri (USA) and identified through the Missouri Cancer Registry (Davis *et al.*, 1993). The participation rate was 73%, and histological confirmation was made for 89%. Two groups of controls were selected: the first consisted of friends of the children with brain cancer or of children with acute lymphocytic leukaemia (85 children; participation rate, 94%), and the second consisted of 108 children with cancer (mostly of the lymphohaematopoietic system; 71 children; participation rate, 78%). The adjusted odds ratio associated with living in a home that had been treated for termites within 1 year before residence or during residence from pregnancy to diagnosis was 2.9 (95% CI, 1.3–7.1) when friends were used as controls and 3.0 (1.3–7.4) with cancer controls. Of the 21 patients who reported any termite control treatment, only seven reported specific use of chlordane, giving an odds ratio of 1.5 (0.5–4.9) for friend controls and 1.5 (0.5–5.1) for cancer controls.

3.   Studies of Cancer in Experimental Animals

3.1   Oral administration

Mouse: A study on chlordane conducted by the International Research and Development Corporation in 1973 but not published by that organization was later reported by Epstein (1976). Groups of 100 male and 100 female CD-1 mice, 6 weeks of age, were fed a diet containing 0 (control), 5, 25 or 50 mg/kg technical-grade chlordane [purity unspecified] for 18 months. When 10 animals from each group that were killed for interim study at 6 months were excluded, the mortality rate at 18 months was 27–49%, with the exception of males and females receiving 50 mg/kg of diet, in which the rates were 86 and 76%, respectively. In addition, a relatively large number of animals were lost because of autolysis. A review of the histopathology of liver samples from this study by a panel of the National Academy of Sciences (1977) indicated a significant increase in the incidence of hepatocellular carcinomas in males at the intermediate dietary concentration and in females at the two higher concentrations (Table 7). [The Working Group noted that the original report and data were not available.]

Groups of 50 male and 50 female B6C3F$_1$ hybrid mice, 5 weeks of age, were fed a diet containing analytical-grade chlordane (71.7% *cis*-chlordane, 23.1% *trans*-chlordane, 0.3% heptachlor, 0.6% nonachlor, 1.1% hexachlorocyclopentadiene, 0.25% chlordene isomers and other chlorinated compounds) for 80 weeks. Males received an initial concentration of 20 or 40 mg/kg of diet and females received 40 or 80 mg/kg of diet; the time-weighted average dietary concentrations were 30 and 56 mg/kg for males and 30 and 64 mg/kg for females. There were 20 male and 20 female matched controls. The survivors were killed at 90–91 weeks. The survival rates in all groups was relatively high, being > 60% of treated males, > 80% of treated females and > 90% of male and female controls (National Cancer Institute, 1977b). A review of the histo-pathology of liver samples from this study by the panel of the National Academy of Sciences (1977) indicated a significant increase in the incidence of hepatocellular carcinomas by linear trend analysis in males and females and a significant increase in the combined incidence of hepatocellular carcinomas and 'nodular changes' in males and females at the higher concentration (Table 8).

Groups of 210 male B6C3F$_1$ and 160 male B6D2F$_1$ mice, 9 weeks of age, were fed diets containing 55 mg/kg technical-grade chlordane. A 'stop group' of 75 B6C3F$_1$ mice was returned to normal diet when they were 70 weeks (491 days) of age. Groups of 100 male B6C3F$_1$ and 50 male B6D2F$_1$ mice were used as untreated controls. When the treated mice were about 8 months of age, the concentration in the diet was increased to 60 mg/kg. From 408 days of age, groups of 5–33 mice were killed for pathological examination. In B6C3F$_1$ mice, the prevalence of hepatocellular adenomas in conti-nuously treated animals exceeded 99% by 530 days, and the prevalence of hepato-cellular carcinomas was 89% at terminal killing at 568 days. In B6D2F$_1$ mice, the pre-valence of hepatocellular adenomas reached 91% and that of hepatocellular carcinomas 86% at the terminal killing, although there was a lag of more than 100 days for tumour development in this strain. The prevalence of hepatocellular tumours in controls was less than 22% in B6C3F$_1$ males and 9% in B6D2F$_1$ males throughout the study. In the 'stop group', the prevalence of adenomas decreased from 100% to 93% between 548 and 568 days and that of carcinomas from 80% to 54% between 526 and 568 days (Malarkey *et al.*, 1995).

A study on heptachlor and its epoxide by the Food and Drug Administration in the USA carried out in 1965 but not published by that organization, was later summarized by Epstein (1976). Three groups of 100 male and 100 female C3H mice [age unspecified] were fed diets containing 0 (control) or 10 mg/kg heptachlor or 10 mg/kg heptachlor epoxide [purity unspecified] for 24 months. A review of the histopathology of liver samples from this study by the panel of the National Academy of Sciences

Table 7. Tumour incidence in CD-1 mice treated with chlordane

Concentration (mg/kg of diet)	Males		Females	
	Hepatocellular carcinomas	Hepatocellular carcinomas and nodules	Hepatocellular carcinomas	Hepatocellular carcinomas and nodules
0 (controls)	1/33	4/33	0/44	1/44
5	1/55	11/55	0/61	0/61
25	11/51 ($p = 0.015$)	30/51 ($p < 0.001$)	11/51 ($p < 0.001$)	23/51 ($p < 0.001$)
50	7/44	25/44 ($p < 0.001$)	6/40 ($p < 0.001$)	22/40 ($p < 0.001$)

From National Academy of Sciences (1977)

Table 8. Tumour incidence in B6C3F$_1$ mice treated with analytical-grade chlordane or technical-grade heptachlor

Treatment	Males		Females	
	Hepatocellular carcinomas	Hepatocellular carcinomas and nodules	Hepatocellular carcinomas	Hepatocellular carcinomas and nodules
Controls	2/20	5/20	1/19	1/19
Chlordane (low dose)	5/45	16/45	0/46	2/46
Chlordane (high dose)	12/46 ($p = 0.031$)[a]	30/46 ($p = 0.003$)	7/47 ($p = 0.018$)[a]	20/47 ($p = 0.002$)
Controls	2/19	5/19	0/10	1/10
Heptachlor (low dose)	3/45	14/45	0/44	3/44
Heptachlor (high dose)	2/45	24/45 ($p = 0.042$)	2/42	21/42 ($p = 0.022$)

From National Academy of Sciences (1977)
[a] Armitage's test for linear trend

(1977) indicated a significant increase in the incidence of hepatocellular carcinomas in females but not in males given heptachlor and in both males and females given heptachlor epoxide (Table 9). [The Working Group noted that the original report and data were not available.]

Table 9. Tumour incidence in C3H mice treated with heptachlor or heptachlor epoxide

Treatment	Males		Females	
	Hepatocellular carcinomas	Hepatocellular carcinomas and nodules	Hepatocellular carcinomas	Hepatocellular carcinomas and nodules
Control	29/77	48/77	5/53	11/53
Heptachlor (10 mg/kg of diet)	35/85	72/85 ($p = 0.001$)	18/80 ($p = 0.04$)	61/80 ($p < 0.001$)
Heptachlor epoxide (10 mg/kg of diet)	42/78 ($p = 0.031$)	71/78 ($p < 0.001$)	34/83 ($p < 0.001$)	75/83 ($p < 0.001$)

From National Academy of Sciences (1977)

A study on heptachlor and its epoxide conducted by the International Research and Development Corporation in 1973 but not published by that organization, was later reported by Epstein (1976). Groups of 100 male and 100 female CD-1 mice, 7 weeks of age, were fed diets containing a mixture of 75% heptachlor epoxide and 25% heptachlor [purity unspecified] at a concentration of 0 (control), 1, 5 or 10 mg/kg for 18 months. After exclusion of 10 animals from each group that were killed for interim study at 6 months, the mortality rate at 18 months was 34–49%, with the exception of males and females receiving the 10 mg/kg concentration, for which the rate was approximately 70%. In addition, comparatively large numbers of animals from all groups were lost because of autolysis. A review of the histopathology of liver samples from this study by the panel of the National Academy of Sciences (1977) indicated a significant increase in the combined incidence of hepatocellular carcinomas and nodules in the groups at the high concentration (Table 10). [The Working Group noted that the original report and data were not available.]

Groups of 50 male and 50 female B6C3F$_1$ hybrid mice, 5 weeks of age, were fed a diet containing technical-grade heptachlor (72 ± 3% heptachlor, 18% *trans*-chlordane, 2% *cis*-chlordane, 2% nonachlor, 1% chlordene, 0.2% hexachlorobutadiene and 10–15 other compounds) for 80 weeks. Males received an initial dietary concentration of 10 or 20 mg/kg and time-weighted average concentrations of 6 and 14 mg/kg; females received an initial concentration of 20 or 40 mg/kg of diet and time-weighted average concentrations of 9 and 18 mg/kg of diet. These concentrations were reduced during the

Table 10. Tumour incidence in CD-1 mice treated with a mixture of heptachlor and heptachlor epoxide (25%:75%)

Concentration (mg/kg of diet)	Males		Females	
	Hepatocellular carcinomas	Hepatocellular carcinomas and nodules	Hepatocellular carcinomas	Hepatocellular carcinomas and nodules
0 (controls)	1/59	2/59	1/74	1/74
1	1/58	1/58	0/71	0/71
5	2/66	4/66	1/65	3/65
10	1/73	27/73 ($p < 0.001$)	4/52	16/52 ($p < 0.001$)

From National Academy of Sciences (1977)

experiment because of adverse toxic effects. Matched controls consisted of 20 males and 20 females. The survivors were killed at 90–91 weeks. The survival rates in all groups were relatively high, with > 70% of treated and control males and 60% of treated and control females still alive at 90 weeks. The survival of treated female mice showed a significant decreasing trend in comparison with controls (National Cancer Institute, 1977a). A review of the histopathology of liver samples from this study by the panel of the National Academy of Sciences (1977) indicated a significant increase in the combined incidence of hepatocellular carcinomas and 'nodular changes' ($p < 0.05$) in males and females receiving the higher concentration (Table 8).

Rat: Groups of 50 male and 50 female Osborne-Mendel rats, 5 weeks of age, were fed diets containing analytical-grade chlordane (71.7% *cis*-chlordane, 23.1% *trans*-chlordane, 0.3% heptachlor, 0.6% nonachlor, 1.1% hexachlorocyclopentadiene, 0.25% chlordene isomers and other chlorinated compounds) for 80 weeks at an initial concentration of 400 or 800 mg/kg for males and 200 or 400 mg/kg of diet for females. These concentrations were reduced during the experiment because of adverse toxic effects, and the time-weighted average dietary concentrations were 204 and 407 mg/kg for males and 121 and 242 mg/kg for females. There were 10 male and 10 female matched controls and 60 male and 60 female pooled controls from similar bioassays of other compounds. The survivors were killed at 109 weeks, at which time approximately 50% of treated and control males, 60% of treated females and 90% of control females were still alive. Treated females showed a marginal increase in the incidence of thyroid follicular-cell neoplasms: 6/32 at the higher dietary concentration (four adenomas, two carcinomas; $p < 0.05$), 4/43 at the lower concentration and 3/58 in pooled controls ($p = 0.03$, trend test). There was also a marginal increase in the incidence of malignant fibrous histiocytomas [site unspecified] in treated males: 7/44 at the higher concentration ($p < 0.05$), 1/44 at the lower concentration and 2/58 in pooled controls (National Cancer Institute, 1977b).

Groups of 80 male and 80 female Fischer 344 rats, 5 weeks of age, were fed diets containing 0 (control), 1, 5 or 25 mg/kg technical-grade chlordane (containing unspecified amounts of *cis*- and *trans*-chlordane, isomers of chlordene, heptachlor and nonachlor) for 130 weeks. Eight males and nine females in each group were killed for evaluation at 26 and 52 weeks. The survival rate in all groups was > 65% at 104 weeks. Combined evaluations by the original pathologist and a panel of seven other pathologists indicated incidences of hepatocellular adenomas in males of 2/64 in controls, 4/64 at the low concentration, 2/64 at 5 mg/kg of diet and 7/64 at 25 mg/kg ($p = 0.018$ trend test) (Khasawinah & Grutsch, 1989a).

Epstein (1976) reported on a study conducted by the Kettering Laboratories in 1959, but not published by that organization. Groups of 25 female CFN rats, 7 weeks of age, were fed diets containing heptachlor epoxide [purity unspecified] (added by spraying alcoholic solutions on chow pellets) at a concentration of 0.5, 2.5, 5.0, 7.5 or 10 mg/kg for 108 weeks. The survival rate at that time was > 45% in both treated and control groups. A review of the histopathology of liver samples from this study by the panel of the National Academy of Sciences (1977) found no increase in the incidence of liver tumours in treated animals. [The Working Group noted that the original report and data were not available and also noted the small number of animals and the uncertain concentrations in the feed.]

Groups of 50 male and 50 female Osborne-Mendel rats, 5 weeks of age, were fed diets containing technical-grade heptachlor (71.7% *cis*-chlordane, 23.1% *trans*-chlordane, 0.3% heptachlor, 0.6% nonachlor, 1.1% hexachlorocyclopentadiene, 0.25% chlordene isomers and other chlorinated compounds) for 80 weeks. Males received an initial dietary concentration of 80 or 160 mg/kg and a time-weighted average concentration of 39 or 78 mg/kg of diet; females received an initial concentration of 40 or 80 mg/kg of diet and a time-weighted average concentration of 26 or 51 mg/kg of diet. Matched controls consisted of 10 males and 10 females; and pooled controls consisted of 60 males and 60 females. At 111 weeks, 55–75% of all treated and control groups were still alive. Thyroid follicular-cell neoplasms (10 adenomas, five carcinomas) occurred in 14/38 females at the higher concentration ($p < 0.01$), 3/43 females at the lower concentration and 3/58 controls. Follicular-cell neoplasms were found in 9/38 (seven adenomas, four carcinomas) males at the lower concentration ($p < 0.05$), 3/38 males at the higher concentration and 4/51 controls. The incidence of follicular-cell hyperplasia was not significantly increased in treated animals (National Cancer Institute, 1977a).

3.2 Administration with known carcinogens

Mouse: Groups of male B6C3F$_1$ mice, 8 weeks of age, were given drinking-water containing 0 (control) or 20 mg/L *N*-nitrosodiethylamine for 14 weeks. After 4 weeks with no treatment, mice received diets containing 0 (control), 25 or 50 mg/kg technical chlordane or 5 or 10 mg/kg technical heptachlor for 25 weeks. All surviving animals were killed at 43 weeks; five mice from each group were killed after 8 and 16 weeks of administration of chlordane or heptachlor. Both agents significantly increased the incidence of hepatocellular adenomas and carcinomas combined over that with *N*-nitrosodiethylamine alone (Table 11) (Williams & Numoto, 1984).

To study the tumour-promoting activity of chlordane on mouse skin, groups of male and female CD-1 mice, 7–8 weeks of age, were treated dermally with 0.2 μmol of 7,12-dimethylbenz[*a*]anthracene, followed 1 week later by 0 (control) or 2 μmol (820 μg) of chlordane in 200 μL acetone three times per week for 20 weeks. No increase in the incidence of skin tumours was reported (Moser *et al.*, 1993). [The Working Group noted that numerical data were not presented.]

Table 11. Preneoplastic and neoplastic liver lesions in B6C3F$_1$ mice treated with chlordane or heptachlor after initiation with *N*-nitrosodiethylamine (NDEA)

Exposure	Foci, G6Pase-deficient		Liver-cell neoplasms		
	No./cm^2	Area (mm^2/cm^2)	Incidence	No. of adenomas	No. of carcinomas
Control	0.04 ± 0.11	21 ± 0	3/28	2	1
NDEA	1.27 ± 1.07	10.2 ± 12.5	8/20	11	2
NDEA + 25 mg/kg diet chlordane	3.01 ± 1.28	15.5 ± 15.9	17/21[a]	27	16
NDEA + 50 mg/kg diet chlordane	3.83 ± 2.07	30.1 ± 22.1	18/22[a]	42	10
NDEA + 5 mg/kg diet heptachlor	1.81 ± 1.14	27.3 ± 40.7	16/21[b]	24	9
NDEA + 10 mg/kg diet heptachlor	2.29 ± 1.70	31.0 ± 38.7	20/26[b]	34	9

From Williams & Numoto (1984); G6Pase, glucose-6-phosphatase
[a] Significantly different from group given NDEA alone at $p < 0.01$
[b] Significantly different from group given NDEA alone at $p < 0.05$

4. Other Data Relevant to an Evaluation of Carcinogenicity and its Mechanisms

The toxicology of chlordane and heptachlor has been reviewed (FAO/WHO, 1964, 1965, 1967, 1968, 1971, 1978, 1983; WHO, 1984a,b; FAO/WHO, 1987; Public Health Service, 1989a,b).

4.1   Absorption, distribution, metabolism and excretion

4.1.1   *Humans*

Technical-grade chlordane contains nonachlor, heptachlor as well as *cis-* and *trans-*chlordane, and is metabolized into epoxides (Cassidy *et al.*, 1994), and these are compounds to which humans are exposed from the continued use and environmental presence of chlordane. Thus, information on nonachlor and heptachlor epoxide is included here. Heptachlor epoxide was the first of the materials derived from technical-grade chlordane to be analysed routinely in human adipose tissue. Residues result from its use in agriculture and in households. Studies on the storage of heptachlor epoxide and oxychlordane in the adipose tissue of the general population in various countries are summarized in section 1. *trans*-Nonachlor has also been identified in the adipose tissue of people representative of the general population of the USA (Sovocool & Lewis, 1975). Components of technical-grade chlordane — chlordane, heptachlor and *trans*-nonachlor — have been identified in human blood after a variety of exposures, indicating that all are absorbed (Saito *et al.*, 1986). As these compounds are lipophilic, they stored mainly in the adipose tissue. *trans*- and *cis*-Chlordane are metabolized to oxychlordane, and heptachlor is metabolized to heptachlor epoxide. Elimination takes place via both urine (Curley & Garrettson, 1969) and faeces (Garrettson *et al.*, 1985). Breast milk is a supplementary excretory route in lactating women (WHO, 1984a,b). Components of technical-grade chlordane and their metabolites are excreted in human milk in quantities that vary with agricultural and household use, dietary habits, individual phenotype and time of milk sampling. Chlordane and its metabolites are accumulated over time (Hirasawa & Takizawa, 1989) and have been found in the blood of pest control operators and in indoor air of houses treated with chlordane (Saito *et al.*, 1986; Menconi *et al.*, 1988). The use of chlordane for termite control is reported to result in detectable levels of chlordane in breast milk of women living in treated houses (Taguchi & Yakushiji, 1988).

The mean blood concentrations of total chlordane (*trans*-nonachlor, oxychlordane and heptachlor epoxide) of pest control operators were correlated with the conditions under which they sprayed technical-grade chlordane, including the total amount of chlordane sprayed ($r = 0.68$) and the number of days on which they had sprayed within the past year ($r = 0.78$), particularly, within the past 3 months ($r = 0.81$) (Saito *et al.*, 1986). Analysis of blood for chlordane metabolites showed their presence in the descending order *trans*-nonachlor, oxychlordane, heptachlorepoxide and *cis*-nonachlor. Serum concentrations of triglycerides and the activities of creatine phosphokinase and lactate dehydrogenase (LDH) were also found to be higher in pest-control operators (Ogata & Izushi, 1991).

The presence of heptachlor epoxide in the adipose tissue of stillborn infants (Wassermann *et al.*, 1974) and in the cord blood of newborns (D'Ercole *et al.*, 1976) demonstrates placental transfer of heptachlor and/or heptachlor epoxide.

Human liver preparations had little capacity to convert *trans*-nonachlor (a minor component of technical-grade chlordane) to *trans*-chlordane in comparison with rat liver prepared similarly (Tashiro & Matsumura, 1978). In liver microsomes, heptachlor epoxide constituted 85.8% of the metabolized heptachlor in those from rats but only 20.4% in those from human liver. Other metabolites identified in the human liver microsome system were 1-hydroxy-2,3-epoxychlordene (5%), 1-hydroxychlordene (4.8%) and 1,2-dihydroxydihydrochlordene (0.1%); 68.6% was unmetabolized heptachlor (Tashiro & Matsumura, 1978).

4.1.2   *Experimental systems*

    (*a*)   *Chlordane*

The metabolism of chlordane (WHO 1984a; Nomeir & Hajjar, 1987) and of hepta-chlor (WHO, 1984b; Fendick *et al.*, 1990) in experimental animals has been reviewed.

    (i)   *Absorption and distribution*

Chlordane is readily absorbed from the gastrointestinal tract of rats and mice (Barnett & Dorough, 1974; Tashiro & Matsumura, 1977; Ewing *et al.*, 1985), from the skin of rats (Ambrose *et al.*, 1953) and from the respiratory system of rats (Nye & Dorough, 1976).

Chlordane absorbed after oral administration to rats was rapidly distributed, with the highest concentrations in fat and lower concentrations in other organs, in the order liver, kidney, brain and muscle. Treatment with *trans*-chlordane resulted in slightly higher tissue concentrations than with *cis*-chlordane. The patterns of distribution were similar after single and repeated oral dosing (Barnett & Dorough, 1974).

    (ii)   *Metabolism and elimination*

The major route of metabolism of chlordane in treated animals is via oxychlordane. Heptachlor is a minor metabolite of both optical isomers of chlordane. *cis*- and *trans*-Chlordane give rise qualitatively to the same metabolites (Tashiro & Matsumura, 1977). Four metabolic pathways for the metabolism of chlordane have been proposed (Nomeir & Hajjar, 1987, Figure 1):
- hydroxylation to form 3-hydroxychlordane, followed by dehydration to form the postulated precursor of oxychlordane, 1,2-dichlorochlordene;
- dehydrochlorination to form heptachlor, with subsequent formation of hepta-chlor epoxide and various hydroxylation products;
- dechlorination to monochlorodihydrochlordene;
- replacement of chlorine atoms by hydroxyl groups, with formation of mono-, di- and trihydroxy metabolites which are excreted or conjugated with glucu-ronic acid.

Rats and mice eliminated 80–≥ 90% of a single oral dose of [^{14}C]chlordane within 7 days (Barnett & Dorough, 1974; Tashiro & Matsumura, 1977; Ewing *et al.*, 1985). Most of the radiolabel was eliminated in faeces. C57BL/6JX mice showed two distinct excretory patterns: the vast majority were high excretors, their elimination rate during the first day after dosing being 20 times faster than that of the low excretors (Ewing *et al.*, 1985).

Mice were given repeated doses of technical-grade chlordane (containing 5.88% *trans*- and 1.45% *cis*-nonachlor) in olive oil by gavage at 0.48 mg/mouse every other day for 29 days. No increase in the body burden of *trans*- or *cis*-chlordane was noted; rather, the levels decreased continuously, indicating that chlordane induced its own metabolism. The concentrations of *trans*- and *cis*-nonachlor and of oxychlordane, however, increased throughout the study period (Hirasawa & Takizawa, 1989).

Figure 1. Metabolic pathways of chlordane

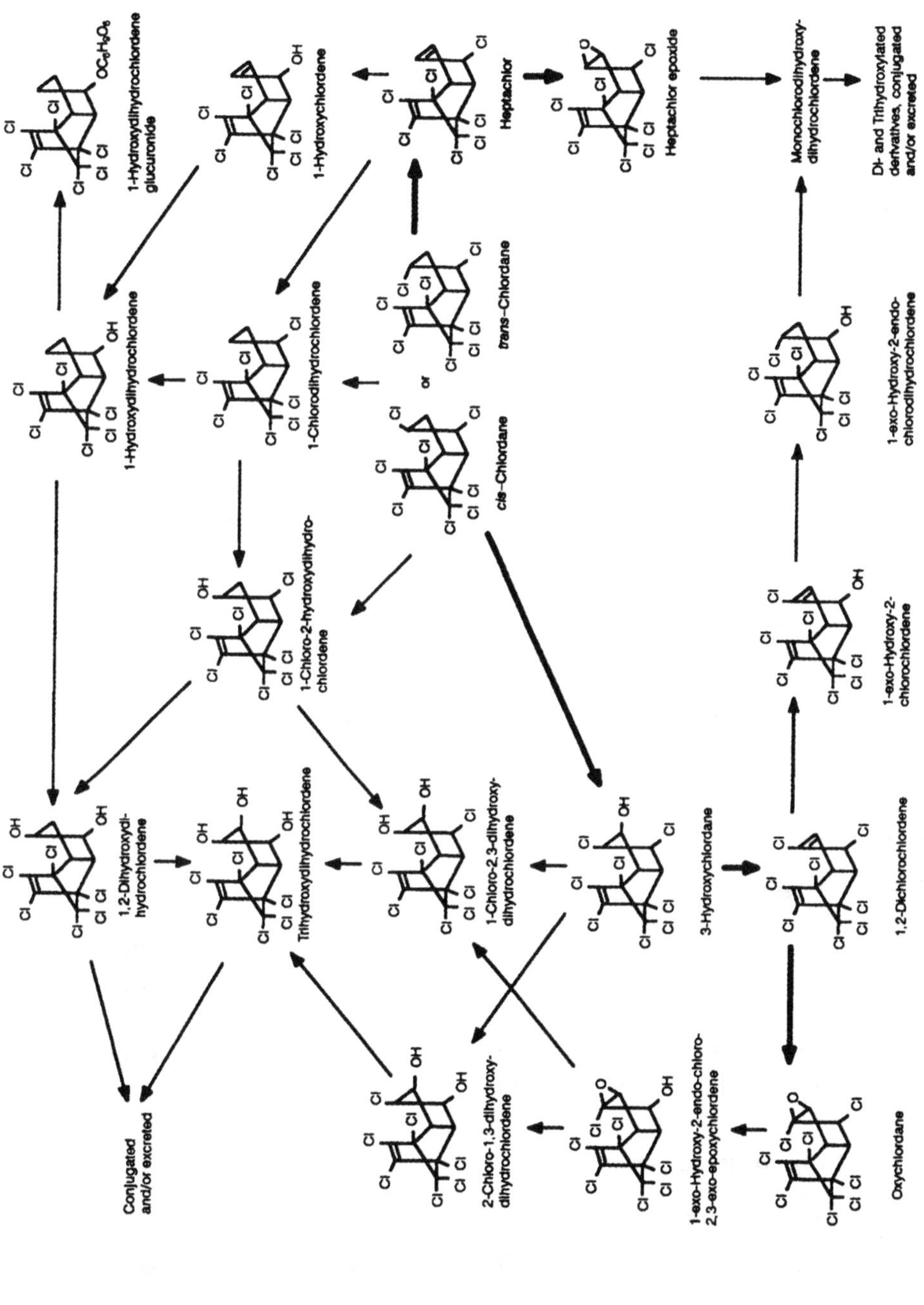

From Nomeir and Hajjar (1987)

(b)   *Heptachlor*

(i)   *Absorption and distribution*

Heptachlor is readily absorbed after intake by most routes and is readily metabolized to heptachlor epoxide by mammals (Public Health Service, 1989a; Fendick *et al.*, 1990). Heptachlor epoxide is stored mainly in fat but also in liver, kidney and muscle in rats and dogs. In rats fed 30 mg/kg of diet heptachlor for 12 weeks, the maximal concentrations of heptachlor epoxide were found in fat within 2–4 weeks; 12 weeks after cessation of exposure, heptachlor epoxide had completely disappeared from the adipose tissue (Radomski & Davidow, 1953). Heptachlor is also stored in fat as heptachlor epoxide in steers (Bovard *et al.*, 1971) and laying hens (Kan & Tuinstra, 1976). Heptachlor epoxide and a hydrophilic metabolite, 1-*exo*-hydroxy-2,3-epoxychlordene, were excreted in the faeces and urine of rat and rabbits treated with heptachlor (Klein *et al.*, 1968). Another metabolite, a dehydrogenated derivative of 1-hydroxy-2,3-epoxychlordene, was isolated from rat faeces (Matsumura & Nelson, 1971).

(ii)   *Metabolism*

Phenobarbital pretreatment significantly enhanced the metabolism of heptachlor in rats, causing a 6–11-fold increase in the formation of heptachlor epoxide in liver (Miranda *et al.*, 1973).

4.1.3   *Comparison of human and animal data*

In humans, *trans*- and *cis*-chlordane are metabolized to oxychlordane; heptachlor is metabolized to its epoxide. In experimental animals, the metabolism has been studied more extensively but is similar.

4.2   Toxic effects

4.2.1   *Humans*

Case reports and epidemiological studies of poisoning with technical-grade chlordane and heptachlor after occupational exposures and due to exposure of the general population are summarized in Table 12.

Sublethal exposure to chlordane has not been found to cause delayed neurotoxic effects (Grutsch & Khasawinah, 1991).

4.2.2   *Experimental systems*

(a)   *Chlordane*

The toxic effects of chlordane have been reviewed (WHO, 1984a).

The oral LD_{50} of chlordane in peanut oil was 335 (299–375) mg/kg bw for male and 430 (391–473) mg/kg bw for female Sherman rats (Gaines, 1960). The oral LD_{50} values

Table 12. Case reports, health surveys and epidemiological studies of cases of poisoning with technical-grade chlordane and technical-grade heptachlor

Population	Clinical features	Reference
22 workers manufacturing and formulating chlordane, aldrin, dieldrin	No evidence of adverse health effects	Princi & Spurbeck (1951)
24 workers employed for 2 months to 5 years in a plant manufacturing chlordane	No evidence of adverse health effects	Alvarez & Hyman (1953)
A female worker spilled a mixture of pesticides including chlordane on her clothing	Confusion, generalized convulsions, death; congestion of brain, lung and stomach mucosa	Derbes *et al.* (1955)
Suicide of a 32-year-old woman who ingested a 5% chlordane talc formulation; estimated ingested dose of chlordane, 6 g (104 mg/kg bw)	Vomiting, dry cough, agitation and restlessness, haemorrhagic gastritis, bronchopneumonia, muscle twitching, convulsions, death after 9.5 days	Derbes *et al.* (1955)
15 workers exposed for 1–15 years to chlordane during manufacture	No evidence of adverse health effects	Fishbein *et al.* (1964)
A 20-month-old boy drank an unknown quantity of a 74% technical-grade chlordane formulation	Vomiting and seizures 45 min after ingestion; serum alkaline phosphatase activity and thymal turbidity slightly elevated after 3 months	Curley & Garrettson (1969)
A 4-year-old girl ingested an unknown amount of 45% chlordane	Convulsions, increased excitability, loss or coordination, dyspnoea, tachycardia	Aldrich & Holmes (1969)
A segment of municipal water system in Chattanooga, TN (USA), 1976, was contaminated with chlordane, initially up to 1200 mg/L. Of 105 residents in affected houses, 71 reported contact with contaminated water	13/71 (18%) described mild symptoms (gastro-intestinal and/or neurological) compatible with chlordane exposure	Harrington *et al.* (1978)

Table 12 (contd)

Population	Clinical features	Reference
Case reports of blood dyscrasias associated with exposure to chlordane or heptachlor alone or in combination with other agents	25 previously reported and six new cases included 22 of aplastic anaemia, three of acute leukaemia, two of leukopenia and one each of hypoplastic anaemia, haemolytic anaemia, megaloblastic anaemia and thrombocytopenia	Infante *et al.* (1978)
Workers employed for more than 3 months in the manufacture of chlordane and heptachlor, 1946–76 [study population overlaps with that of Shindell & Ulrich (1986)]	17 deaths from cerebrovascular disease observed versus 9.3 expected	Wang & MacMahon (1979a)
Cohort of 16 126 men employed as pesticide applicators for ≥ 3 months in 1967, 1968 and 1976, including group of 6734 termite control operators	All deaths, 311 (SMR, 84); cerebrovascular disease among termite control operators (SMR, 39)	Wang & MacMahon (1979b)
A 62-year-old man accidentally ingested ~ 300 mL of 75% chlordane.	Unresponsive to verbal commands, generalized tonic seizures, profuse diarrhoea, transient increase in liver enzymes; recovery by 2 months	Olanoff *et al.* (1983)
A 59-year-old man with a history of Alzheimer disease inadvertently drank from a bottle containing a chlordane formulation	Rapid occurrence of convulsions, death despite cardiopulmonary resuscitation and treatment	Kutz *et al.* (1983)
A 30-year-old woman exposed to chlordane through excessive household use	Numbness around mouth and nose and in arm used for spraying; nausea, vomiting, persistent fatigue and anorexia, menometrorrhagia	Garrettson *et al.* (1985)
Workers employed in the manufacture of chlordane for ≥ 3 months, in 1946–85 [study population overlaps with that of Wang & MacMahon (1979a)]	20 deaths from cerebrovascular disease observed versus 11.7 expected	Shindell & Ulrich (1986)

Table 12 (contd)

Population	Clinical features	Reference
45 members of dairy-farm families who consumed milk and milk products contaminated with heptachlor metabolites	No heptachlor-related metabolic effects observed in routine liver function tests or specific assays for hepatic enzyme induction	Stehr-Green *et al.* (1986)
25 case reports of blood dyscrasias associated with exposure to chlordane and heptachlor; of 16 cases for which exposure data available, 75% involved home and garden applications and 25% professional applications	Aplastic anaemia, thrombocytopenic purpura, leukaemia, pernicious anaemia, megaloblastic anaemia	Epstein & Ozonoff (1987)
261 residents of 85 households treated with chlordane for termite control	Headache in 22% of cases; sore throat and respiratory infections in 16%; fatigue, 14%; sleeping difficulties, blurred vision and fainting also frequent	Menconi *et al.* (1988)

SMR, standardized mortality ratio

for *cis*- and *trans*-chlordane were reported to be similar (392 and 327 mg/kg bw, respectively). The oral LD_{50} of the major metabolite, oxychlordane, in rats was reported to be 19.1 mg/kg bw; the values for several other metabolites were > 4600 mg/kg bw. The signs associated with acute chlordane poisoning include ataxia, convulsions, respiratory failure and cyanosis, followed by death (WHO, 1984a).

An oral dose of chlordane of 50 mg/kg bw per day for 15 days resulted in convulsions and death in rats, whereas a dose of 25 mg/kg bw per day had no such effect (Ambrose *et al.*, 1953).

Cumulative autonomic, neuromuscular and sensorimotor neurotoxic effects were reported in female Fischer 344 rats at doses of up to 156 mg/kg bw of chlordane (Moser *et al.*, 1995). The neurotoxic effects of heptachlor occurred at much lower doses, but did not include neuromuscular or sensorimotor effects.

Mice treated with chlordane at doses of 0.1–8 mg/kg bw for 14 days showed a dose-related increase in cell-mediated immunity, as evaluated *in vitro*. Expression of delayed hypersensitivity and the antibody response to sheep red blood cells *in vivo* were unaltered (Johnson *et al.*, 1986).

(i)   *Studies related to liver toxicity*

During the first week of long-term studies (see section 3), chlordane caused tremor in female rats fed the high dietary concentration of 25 mg/kg. Later in the study, decreased body-weight gain and increased liver weights were observed in these animals (National Cancer Institute, 1977b; Khasawinah & Grutsch, 1989a). In mice, the liver was the target organ for non-neoplastic toxicity; the serum activities of aspartate and alanine aminotransferases were elevated in animals of each sex, and the liver weight was increased in males at 12.5 mg/kg of diet. Increased liver-cell volume was seen in males and females at 5 or 12.5 mg/kg of diet, and hepatocyte degeneration and necrosis were seen only in treated males (Khasawinah & Grutsch, 1989b).

Rats were given 100 mg/kg bw per day chlordane by stomach tube or 50 mg/kg bw per day chlordane by intraperitoneal injection once a day for 4 days. The total cholesterol and serum triglycerides concentrations and the activities of creatinine phosphokinase and LDH were increased by chlordane treatment. The isoenzyme patterns suggested that the increase in enzyme activities was related to skeletal muscle. Furthermore, significant increases in liver weight, liver water content and total lipid, triglyceride and phospholipid concentrations were recorded. Chlordane induced lipid peroxidation in the liver, with a dose–response relationship. Although no appreciable effect on mitochondrial function and latent ATPase activity was observed, 2,4-dinitrophenol-stimulated ATPase activity was inhibited. Histological examination of the liver confirmed fatty infiltration (Ogata & Izushi, 1991).

Administration of a single dose of chlordane at 120 mg/kg bw by gavage to female Sprague-Dawley rats resulted in significant increases in hepatic lipid peroxidation, measured as thiobarbituric acid-reactive substances (Hassoun *et al.*, 1993).

Chlordane was administered orally at two 0.25 LD_{50} doses to female Sprague-Dawley rats at 0 h and 21 h, and the animals were killed at 24 h. A threefold increase in hepatic lipid peroxidation was observed, while an increase in lipid peroxidation (measured as thiobarbituric acid-reactive substances) of 2.1-fold was observed in brain homogenates. After incubation of hepatic and brain tissues with 1 nmol/mL of chlordane *in vitro*, maximum increases in chemiluminescence, a measure of the generation of reactive oxygen species, occurred within 4–7 min of incubation and persisted for over 10 min. Increases of 2.7-fold were observed in chemiluminescence after incubation of the liver homogenates with chlordane, while an increase of 1.8-fold was observed in the brain homogenates. An increase of 2.3-fold was observed in the chemiluminescence responses in the liver homogenates from animals treated with chlordane, while an increase of twofold was observed in the brain homogenates. In an experiment in which cultured neuroactive PC-12 cells were incubated with chlordane, the release of LDH into the medium was used as an indicator of cell damage and cytotoxicity. Maximal release of LDH from cultured PC-12 cells was observed at a concentration of 100 nmol/L of the pesticide. An increase of 2.5-fold was observed in LDH leakage after incubation of the PC-12 cells with chlordane (Bagchi *et al.*, 1995).

(ii)   *Studies related to thyroid function and liver toxicity*

The effect of chlordane on the concentration of radiolabel from [^{125}I]thyroxine in plasma was studied in male CD rats given an intraperitoneal injection of 25 or 75 mg/kg bw per day chlordane for 5 days and 24 h later an injection of [^{125}I]thyroxine–[^{131}I]albumin; the animals were bled 35 min later. The concentration of radiolabel in plasma was statistically significantly decreased ($p < 0.001$), and increased uptake in the liver was found. The results at the two doses did not differ significantly. Similar effects were found when phenobarbital (see monograph in this volume) was administered at a dose of 100 mg/kg bw (Bernstein *et al.*, 1968).

Wistar rats and cynomolgus monkeys (*Macaca fascicularis*) were exposed to chlordane by inhalation at a concentration close to 0.1, 1 or 10 mg/m^3 for 8 h/day on 5 days per week for 90 days. In rats, the liver was the main target organ, and the liver weights were significantly increased in animals of each sex exposed to 10 mg/m^3. Histopathological changes, such as centrilobular hepatocyte enlargement, were observed in males and females at 1 and 10 mg/m^3. In male rats, increased height of the follicular thyroid epithelium was observed in 11/35 animals at 10 mg/m^3. A dose-related increase in cytochrome P450 and microsomal protein content was evident in animals of each sex. Essentially all of the observed changes were reversed within 90 days after cessation of exposure. No significant finding was made in male or female cynomolgus monkeys; however, cytochrome P450 and microsomal protein were not measured (Khasawinah *et al.*, 1989).

The time course over 6 months of liver and thyroid cell proliferation was studied in C57BL/10J mice fed 50 mg/kg of diet chlordane and killed on day 4, 5, 8, 15, 29, 99 or 190 after the start of dosing. Groups were withdrawn from treatment during days

29–99 and days 190–247. Replicating cells were labelled with bromodeoxyuridine delivered by an osmotic minipump for 3 days before necropsy. The peak labelling index was seen in the thyroid on day 5 ($5.99 \pm 2.90\%$ versus $1.00 \pm 20\%$ in controls) and in the liver on day 8 ($9.0 \pm 1.6\%$ versus $0.5 \pm 0.4\%$ in controls). Both organs showed an elevated labelling index during the first month of dosing, but while that in thyroid follicular cells was not statistically significantly increased at 190 days, that in liver cells was significantly elevated at all times, except in the withdrawal groups (Barrass *et al.*, 1993).

Chlordane at 200 μmol/L stimulated protein kinase C activity in preparations from mouse brains, liver and epidermis *in vitro*. The stimulation was calcium- and phospholipid-dependent and could be inhibited by quercetin, a known inhibitor of protein kinase C activity (Moser & Smart, 1989).

(b)   Heptachlor

The toxic effects of heptachlor have been reviewed (WHO, 1984b; Fendick *et al.*, 1990).

The acute oral LD_{50} of heptachlor in peanut oil was 100 (74–135) mg/kg bw for male and 162 (140–188) mg/kg bw for female Sherman rats (Gaines, 1960). The signs associated with acute heptachlor poisoning include hyperexcitability, tremors, convulsions and paralysis. Liver damage may occur as a late manifestation (WHO, 1984b). Administration of a single dose of 23 mg/kg bw heptachlor by gavage to female Fischer 344 rats resulted in necrotic lymphocytes in the spleen and thymus (Berman *et al.*, 1995).

Heptachlor epoxide is more acutely toxic than the parent compound, e.g. the oral LD_{50} of the epoxide in rats was 62 mg/kg bw (Sperling & Ewinike, 1969), and the intravenous LD_{100} values for heptachlor and heptachlor epoxide in mice were 40 and 10 mg/kg bw, respectively (WHO, 1984b).

Oral doses of pure heptachlor at 50 and 100 mg/kg bw per day were lethal to rats after 10 days. In animals given 5 mg/kg bw, hyperreflexia, dyspnoea and convulsions occurred, and pathological changes were observed in the liver, kidney and spleen (Pelikan *et al.*, 1968).

Dogs given 5 mg/kg bw heptachlor per day orally died within 21 days (Lehman, 1952).

Mink (*Mustela vison*) were fed diets that contained heptachlor at a concentration of 0, 12.5, 25, 50 or 100 mg/kg (as the technical-grade formulation) for 28 days, followed by a 7-day observation period. Concentrations ≥ 25 mg/kg resulted in a significant decrease in feed consumption, while concentrations ≥ 50 mg/kg caused a significant reduction in body weight. Deaths (37.5%) occurred only in the group at 100 mg/kg. Animals at the highest concentration also had reduced relative weights of the spleen and kidney and an increased relative weight of the adrenal glands when necropsied at the time of death or at termination of the study (Aulerich *et al.*, 1990).

Groups of mice were given heptachlor by intraperitoneal injection (50 mg/kg bw per day for 3 days), by gavage (10 mg/kg bw twice a week for 92 days) or in the diet (30 mg/kg of diet for 180 days). All groups showed increased activity of serum alanine aminotransferase; only the group that received heptachlor in the diet showed decreased serum cholinesterase activity. Serum creatine phosphokinase activity was increased significantly in the groups that received heptachlor by intraperitoneal injection or in the diet. Significant differences in serum lipid concentrations from those of controls were seen in all treated groups, as heptachlor has a known effect on lipid metabolism. Except in the group that received heptachlor orally, lipid peroxidation in the liver, expressed as malondialdehyde concentration, was also increased significantly (Izushi & Ogata, 1990).

Addition of heptachlor at a final concentration of 50 μmol/L to rat liver mitochondria, with succinate as the substrate, decreased the respiratory control index by markedly inhibiting state 3 respiration and slightly inhibiting state 4 respiration. Heptachlor at 100 μmol/L, with succinate as the substrate, suppressed states 3 and 4 respiration almost completely. In contrast, heptachlor at a final concentration of 50–100 μmol/L with β-hydroxybutylate as the substrate slightly decreased the respiratory control index, and use of ascorbate plus N,N,N',N'-tetramethylphenylene diamine as the substrate decreased the index hardly at all. Heptachlor at a concentration of 50 μmol/L in the presence of succinate also decreased the ADP:oxygen ratio of mitochondria. The mode of inhibition of succinate oxidation by heptachlor was apparently non-competitive, as seen in a Lineweaver-Burk plot (Meguro et al., 1990).

Cell death was observed when ML-1 cells were treated with heptachlor at concentrations > 80 μmol/L. At lower concentrations, heptachlor induced cell adherence and formation of extended cytoplasmic pseudopodia. At 80 μmol/L, there was cell differentiation to monocyte or macrophage types (Chuang & Chuang, 1991).

The effects of exposure to organochlorine pesticides on the chemotactic functions of rhesus monkey (Macaca mulatta) neutrophils and monocytes was investigated with a 48-well chemotaxis chamber. The chemokines interleukin-8 and RANTES (the natural ligand for the CC chemokine receptor 5) were used as the chemoattractants to induce chemotaxis. When the neutrophils and monocytes were treated with heptachlor, chlordane or toxaphene for 1 h at 37 °C, inhibition of chemotaxis was seen in all samples at concentrations as low as 10^{-14} to 10^{-5} mol/L. Toxaphene was the least effective of the three compounds in preventing monocytes from migrating towards RANTES (Miyagi et al., 1998).

Administration of approximately 2 mg/kg bw heptachlor to male albino rats [strain not specified] by gavage daily for 21 days did not alter serum thyroxine, triiodothyronine or thyroid-stimulating hormone concentrations (Akhtar et al., 1996). [The Working Group noted the low dose of heptachlor used in this experiment.]

4.3   Reproductive and developmental effects

4.3.1   *Humans*

An ecological study was carried out to compare the incidence rates of 37 congenital malformations in Hawaii with those in the USA as a whole (Le Marchand *et al.*, 1986), after contamination of milk on Oahu Island with heptachlor between the autumn of 1980 and December 1982, which was traced to contaminated foliage of pineapple plants used as cattle feed. Data on birth defects were obtained from the Birth Defects Monitoring Program, which covers 62–76% of all births in Hawaii. Temporal and geographical comparisons were made (Table 13). Increased incidence rates were reported on Oahu for cardiovascular malformations and hip dislocation: in 1978–80, the incidence of vascular malformations was 63.2/10 000 births on Oahu Island and 24.9 on the other Hawaian islands; in 1981–83, these rates were 76.2 and 24.4, respectively. For hip dislocation, the only increase occurred in 1981–83: the rates were 42.2/10 000 on Oahu and 22.4 on the other islands. All the increased rates on Oahu were statistically significant ($p < 0.01$). The authors noted that the increase in the incidence of cardiovascular malformations and hip dislocation began in 1978–80, which included only the first few months of contamination. [The Working Group noted that the incidence rates for hip dislocation were unstable.]

Table 13. Incidence rates per 10 000 births of cardiovascular malformations and hip dislocation on Oahu Island and on the other Hawaiian islands, 1970–83

Defect	Oahu				Other islands			
	1970–74	1975–77	1978–80	1981–83	1970–74	1975–77	1978–80	1981–83
Cardiovascular malformations	38.3	33.6	63.2	76.2	21.3	23.4	24.9	24.4
Hip dislocation	12.6	8.8	29.3	42.2	9.9	30.8	31.1	22.4

From Le Marchand *et al.* (1986)

4.3.2   *Experimental systems*

(*a*)   *Chlordane*

Chlordane has a range of effects on the reproductive system, including effects on circulating concentrations of hormones and gonadotropins and reductions in uterine and seminal vesicle weights (reviewed by Cassidy *et al.*, 1994). A thorough study of the developmental toxicity of chlordane was conducted by Cassidy *et al.* (1994), in which Sprague-Dawley rats were given technical-grade chlordane in peanut butter at a concentration resulting in a dose of 100, 500 or 5000 µg/kg bw per day. The dams were dosed from gestation day 4 to postnatal day 21 (i.e., through lactation). The pups were then exposed from 22 to 80 days of age. The lowest dose was designed to generate serum concentrations of heptachlor epoxide and oxychlordane similar to those found at the 99th percentile of exposure in the population of the USA. The end-points investigated included testosterone concentration in pups; general toxicity; neurobehavioural effects, in tests for learning (water maze), sex-specific reproductive behaviour, open-field activity and response to auditory startle; and a neurochemical parameter (γ-amino butyric acid-stimulated synaptosomal chloride uptake) in the whole brain. Exposure of the dams resulted in measurable concentrations of heptachlor and other metabolites in the offspring and in the dams' milk. Pre- and postnatal chlordane treatment lowered the concentrations of testosterone to 40% of the control level in female, but not in male, offspring in a dose-dependent fashion. These exposures also affected male mating behaviour, reducing the latency to intromission and increasing the total number of intromissions. In females, exposure to chlordane improved performance in the water maze, reducing the time for completing trials and reducing error rates; in males, no effects on maze behaviour was observed. Open-field behaviour was not changed. In tests of acoustic startle, there was some increase in maximum response but not in latency. There was a significant decrease in γ-amino butyric acid-mediated chloride uptake by synaptosomes from male rats exposed to the highest dose of chlordane; it should be noted that chlordane decreases chloride uptake *in vitro*, as has been reported for other cyclodiene pesticides (Gant *et al.*, 1987).

(b) Heptachlor

A study of developmental toxicity was conducted to test interactions of chemical mixtures, including heptachlor, trichloroethylene and diethylhexylphthalate (Narotsky & Kavlock, 1995; Narotsky *et al.*, 1995). Fischer 344 rats were given 0, 5.1, 6.8, 9.0 or 12 mg/kg bw per day heptachlor (99% pure) by gavage on gestational days 6–15. At the two higher doses, heptachlor decreased maternal weight gain and increased postnatal loss. Heptachlor interacted with diethylhexylphthalate in terms of increasing maternal death and decreasing pup weights on postnatal days 1 and 6. No terata were observed in heptachlor-exposed offspring (Amita-Rani & Krishnakumari, 1995). Other studies indicated that chlordane can affect testicular tissues in mice (Balash *et al.*, 1987; Al-Omar *et al.*, 2000) and gonadal production of progesterone and estradiol measured *ex vivo* after exposure of rats to 5–30 mg/kg bw heptachlor by subcutaneous injection every other day for 18 days (Oduma *et al.*, 1995). Oduma *et al.* (1995) also reported that exposure of female Sprague-Dawley rats to 5 or 20 mg/kg bw heptachlor (99% pure) by subcutaneous injection every other day for 18 days affected cyclicity, maternal body-weight gain, gestational length and litter size. [The Working Group noted that the data on cyclicity were not analysed statistically, but visual inspection indicated some disruptions at the higher dose.] Gestational length was increased in three of the 10 dams at the highest dose, and their litter size was reduced. No effects on pup survival were observed. Amita-Rani and Krishnakumari (1995) also reported that exposure of either female rats to a total dose of 25 or 50 mg/kg bw heptachlor (technical-grade) over 14 days by gavage or males to a total dose of 45.25 or 90.5 mg/kg bw over 90 days increased the number of resorptions.

In a study of the effects of heptachlor on reproductive function in mink (*Mustela vison*), the animals were given diets containing heptachlor (purity, 72%) at 6.25, 12.5 or 25 mg/kg from 6 weeks before mating for a total of 181 days. The highest concentration, stated to be equivalent to 3.1 mg/kg bw per day, was lethal to all animals, causing seizures and ataxia before death, which followed cessation of feeding. At a dietary concentration of 6.25 mg/kg, no effects were observed on gestational length or litter size, or on sperm motility or morphology in male mink. However, postnatal growth and pup survival were significantly reduced at 12.5 mg/kg of diet (Crum *et al.*, 1993).

The offspring of pregnant BALB/c mice given an oral dose of 0.16, 2, 4 or 8 mg/kg bw per day technical-grade chlordane in peanut butter for 19 days had enhanced overall resistance to influenza virus after infection at 38 days of life (Menna *et al.*, 1985). Other studies on the effects of prenatal exposure to chlordane on immune function followed the work of Spyker-Cranmer *et al.* (1982), who reported that exposure of mice *in utero* to analytical-grade chlordane at 0.16 or 8 mg/kg bw per day throughout gestation depressed cell-mediated immunity in adulthood.

The more recent studies showed that prenatal exposure of BALB/c mice to 4 or 8 mg/kg bw per day chlordane impaired contact hypersensitivity and delayed-type hypersensitivity reactions (see Blaylock *et al.*, 1995). Effects have also been reported on macrophage function, myeloid stem and progenitor cells and colony-forming unit (CFU) responses in adulthood. Theus *et al.* (1992) reported that BALB/c mice exposed *in utero* by feeding dams 8 mg/kg bw per day chlordane in peanut butter throughout gestation had significantly decreased functioning of inflammatory macrophages. Blyler *et al.* (1994) exposed BALB/c mice orally to 8 mg/kg bw per day chlordane (analytical-grade) on days 1–18 of gestation. At 6 weeks of postnatal life, bone-marrow cells were harvested and assayed for CFU. Sex-specific effects were observed, with significant increases in bone-marrow cellularity in males and females but a depression of CFU number only in females. Similar effects of the same treatment were reported on fetal liver-colony formation (Barnett *et al.*, 1998). Exposure of pregnant BALB/c mice to a diet containing chlordane at a concentration resulting in a dose of 8 mg/kg bw per day during the first 18 days of gestation had no effect on circulating T lymphocyte responses in either male or female offspring, but a small increase in natural killer cell activity was seen at 100 days of age (Blaylock *et al.*, 1990).

Male Sprague-Dawley rats were injected subcutaneously with 0, 5, 10, 15, 20 or 25 mg/kg bw heptachlor every other day for 2 weeks. At all doses, significantly suppressed plasma testosterone concentration ($p < 0.05$) and significantly increased plasma luteinizing hormone ($p < 0.01$) and cortisol ($p < 0.02$) concentrations were seen in treated rats as compared with corn oil-treated controls. Luteinizing hormone and testosterone concentrations were strongly correlated ($r = 0.69$; $p < 0.05$). The testes of rats treated with 25 mg/kg bw heptachlor showed some pathological changes (Wango *et al.*, 1997).

4.4   Effects on enzyme induction or inhibition and gene expression

4.4.1   *Humans*

No data were available to the Working Group.

4.4.2   *Experimental systems*

(*a*)   *Studies of liver*

Chlordane induced hepatic drug-metabolizing enzymes in experimental animals (WHO, 1984a; Fendick *et al.*, 1990) and enhanced estrone metabolism in rats and mice (Welch *et al.*, 1971). Studies of liver cytosol and microsomes from male Holtzman rats showed induction of hexobarbital and aminopyrine by chlordane; the stimulation was maximal 8 days after a single intraperitoneal injection of 10 mg/kg bw (Hart *et al.*, 1963). Chlordane has been classified as an inducer of cytochrome P450 (CYP) isozymes of the phenobarbital type (Okey, 1990).

Heptachlor blocks the cell cycle by preventing progression into S phase; this is associated with deactivation in cyclin-dependent kinase cdk2 and dephosphorylation of cdc2 (Chuang *et al.*, 1999).

Administration of a diet containing 2 mg/kg heptachlor for 2 weeks induced aniline hydroxylase and aminopyrine demethylase in rats (Den Tonkelaar & Van Esch, 1974). Heptachlor inhibited oxidative phosphorylation in rat liver mitochondria (Nelson, 1975) and (at 200 μmol/L) stimulated protein kinase C activity in preparations from mouse brain (Moser & Smart, 1989).

No H- or K-*ras* mutations were detected in chlordane-induced hepatocellular tumours in B6C3F$_1$ mice (15 adenomas and 15 carcinomas) or B6D2F$_1$ mice (10 adenomas and 10 carcinomas) obtained from a bioassay in which mice were exposed to 55 mg/kg of diet chlordane for up to 505 days. All acidophilic adenomas and carcinomas induced by chlordane showed increased expression of *bcl*-X$_L$ (Malarkey *et al.*, 1995; Christensen *et al.*, 1999).

Female B6C3F$_1$ mice were initiated with *N*-nitrosodiethylamine (5 mg/kg bw; intraperitoneally) and were then given hepatocarcinogenic concentrations of various chemicals, including chlordane (25 mg/kg of diet), for 4 or 8 months. In the chlordane-treated animals, none of the 39 basophilic hepatic foci that were evaluated showed immunoreactivity to tumour growth factor α (TGFα), but all 63 acidophilic foci were immunoreactive. There was no significant difference in the mean hepatic labelling index, as measured by incorporation of 5-bromo-2'-deoxyuridine, between foci immunoreactive and non-immunoreactive to TGFα. The incidence of immuno-reactivity to TGFα was greater in hepatocellular tumours that were predominantly of the basophilic phenotype. A similar pattern was seen for immunoreactivity to epidermal growth factor receptor, which was lacking in basophilic foci (0/16, 0%) and basophilic hepatocellular adenomas (0/6, 0%) and present in acidophilic foci (7/30, 23%) and acidophilic adenomas (2/9, 22%), suggesting an autocrine mechanism for the development of mouse liver tumours. The increased incidence of TGFα immunoreactivity in basophilic liver tumours suggests that TGFα is a marker of tumour progression in mouse liver. Furthermore, modulations of TGFα were dependent on phenotype rather than treatment, indicating inherent differences in the expression of TGFα in basophilic and acidophilic hepatic lesions (Moser *et al.*, 1997).

(b)   Studies of other systems

Expression of *ras* proto-oncogene mRNA in human myeloblastic leukaemia (ML-1) cells was analysed as a function of cDNA amplification by the polymerase chain reaction (PCR). In a pair of oligonucleotides that flank exon-2 from opposite strands (5′ and 3′) of H-*ras* cDNA for PCR amplification, ML-1 cells were found to express a 112-base pair segment of the *ras* transcript. A rapid decline in the expression of this transcript was seen in cells treated with heptachlor (80 μmol/L for up to 12 h), but addition of serum inhibited the effect of heptachlor and restored the expression of *ras* proto-oncogene mRNA. Expression of the same *ras* segment was not affected by treatment of ML-1 with the tumour promoter 12-*O*-tetradecanoylphorbol-13-acetate (Chuang & Chuang, 1991).

In peripheral blood mononuclear cells isolated form rhesus monkeys, heptachlor and chlordane affected mitogenic stimulation. At 80 μmol/L, both inhibited mitogen-induced proliferation and interleukin-2 release from the monocytes (Chuang *et al.*, 1992).

Addition of 50 μmol/L heptachlor to cultured human CEM×174 lymphocytic cells reduced the cellular levels of mitogen-activated protein kinase (MAPK) cascade proteins, including ERK1 (a 44-kDa MAPK), ERK2 (a 42-kDa MAPK), an 85-kDa and a 54-kDa MAPK, MEK1 (a 45-kDa ERK) and MEKK (a 78-kDa MEK). However, heptachlor treatment caused a marked increase in the expression of activated ERK1 and ERK2 (Thr- and Tyr-dually phosphorylated) in the cells (Chuang & Chuang, 1998).

In LLC-PK1 pig kidney cells transiently cotransfected with (CYP3A23)₂-tk-CAT and mouse pregnenolone X receptor, chlordane (20 μmol/L, 24 h) induced the CYP3A23 DR-3 element, and this activation required the pregnenolone X receptor (Schuetz *et al.*, 1998).

In transfection experiments, chlordane (10 μmol/L, 48 h) was found to antagonize estrogen-related receptor α-1 (ERRα-1) expression of the reporter chloramphenicol acetyltransferase activity in SK-BR-3 breast cancer cells. ERRα-1 is a member of the orphan nuclear receptor family, as its ligand has not been identified. Chlordane can suppress aromatase activity and aromatase expression by antagonizing ERRα-1 (Yang & Chen, 1999).

Experiments with CEM×174 cells, a hybrid of human T and B cells, were performed to investigate the effects of the tumour promoter heptachlor and its congeners chlordane and toxaphene on retinoblastoma (*Rb*) gene expression. Heptachlor, chlordane and toxaphene, at concentrations of 10–50 μmol/L, reduced Rb protein expression in a concentration-dependent manner. In the case of heptachlor, the reduction could be seen as early as 12 h and was time-dependent. Analysis of Rb mRNA revealed no detectable difference over the same concentration range. In a similar experiment, *p53* protein expression was decreased, with no change in that of mRNA (Rought *et al.*, 1998, 1999).

4.5 Genetic and related effects

4.5.1 *Humans*

No data were available to the Working Group.

4.5.2 *Experimental systems* (see Tables 14 and 15 for references)

Chlordane induced neither DNA damage nor point mutations in bacteria. It caused SOS repair and prophage induction in *Escherichia coli* and gene conversion in *Saccharomyces cerevisiae*. In cultured mammalian cells, it did not induce unscheduled DNA synthesis but did induce gene mutations at the *Tk* and Na^+/K^+ ATPase loci. It inhibited gap-junctional intercellular communication in cultured mammalian cells. In single studies with cultured human cells, evidence was obtained for the induction of unscheduled DNA synthesis and sister chromatid exchange, but not for the induction of gene mutations. Sister chromatid exchange was induced in intestinal cells of *Umbra limi* (mud minnow) *in vivo*. Chlordane caused micronucleus formation and chromosomal aberrations in the bone marrow of mice treated *in vivo*, and nuclear aberrations (micronucleated and apoptotic cells) in hair follicle cells of these mice. No evidence was found of adduct formation with chlordane in liver DNA of mice treated *in vivo*. No dominant lethal mutation was found in mice.

Heptachlor did not induce DNA damage or point mutations in bacteria, gene conversion in *Saccharomyces cerevisiae* or sex-linked recessive lethal mutations in *Drosophila melanogaster*. It did not induce unscheduled DNA synthesis in cultured rodent cells in the absence of metabolic activation, but did so in human fibroblasts with metabolic activation. It induced gene mutations at the *Tk* but not at the *Hprt* locus in rodent cells. Heptachlor inhibited gap-junctional intercellular communication in cultured rodent and human cells. It did not induce gene mutation in *lacI* transgenic mice or dominant lethal mutations in mice *in vivo*[1].

---

[1] The Working Group was aware of unpublished studies of sister chromatid exchange (positive) and chromosomal aberrations (negative) in Chinese hamster ovary cells *in vitro*.

Table 14. Genetic and related effects of chlordane

Test system	Result[a] Without exogenous metabolic system	Result[a] With exogenous metabolic system	Dose[b] (LED or HID)	Reference
ColE1 plasmid DNA strand breaks (from *Escherichia coli* K12 ColE1)	–	NT	100	Griffin & Hill (1978)
Escherichia coli WP2$_s$ (λ) prophage induction	+	+	20 000	Houk & DeMarini (1987)
SOS repair (*SulA*) induction in *Escherichia coli* PQ37	+	NT	NR	Venkat *et al.* (1995)
Bacillus subtilis rec strains, differential toxicity	–	–	50	Matsui *et al.* (1989)
Salmonella typhimurium, TA1538, TA1978, differential toxicity	–	NT	2000 µg/disk	Rashid & Mumma (1986)
Escherichia coli WP2, K12, differential toxicity	–	NT	2000 µg/disk	Rashid & Mumma (1986)
Salmonella typhimurium TA100, TA1535, TA1537, TA1538, TA98, reverse mutation	NT	–	5000 µg/plate	Simmon *et al.* (1977)
Salmonella typhimurium TA100, TA1535, TA1537, TA1538, TA98, G46, C3076, D3052, reverse mutation	–	–	NR	Probst *et al.* (1981)
Salmonella typhimurium TA100, TA1535, TA1537, TA1538, TA98, reverse mutation	–	–	NR	Gentile *et al.* (1982)
Salmonella typhimurium TA100, TA1535, TA1537, TA98, reverse mutation	–	–	1000 µg/plate	Mortelmans *et al.* (1986)
Escherichia coli WP2, WP2 *uvrA*, reverse mutation	–	–	NR	Probst *et al.* (1981)
Saccharomyces cerevisiae D4, gene conversion	–	+	6.6	Gentile *et al.* (1982)
Unscheduled DNA synthesis, Fischer 344 rat, CD-1 mouse and Syrian hamster primary hepatocytes *in vitro*	–	NT	4.1	Maslansky & Williams (1981)
DNA single-strand breaks, PC-12 adrenal phaeochromocytoma cells *in vitro*	+	NT	0.041	Bagchi *et al.* (1995)
Unscheduled DNA synthesis, Fischer 344 rat primary hepatocytes *in vitro*	–	NT	41	Probst *et al.* (1981)
Unscheduled DNA synthesis, Fischer 344 rat primary hepatocytes *in vitro*	–	NT	4.1	Williams *et al.* (1989)

Table 14 (contd)

Test system	Result[a]		Dose[b] (LED or HID)	Reference
	Without exogenous metabolic system	With exogenous metabolic system		
Gene mutation, Chinese hamster lung V79 cells, *Hprt* locus *in vitro*	–	NT	1.6	Tsushimoto et al. (1983)
Gene mutation, Chinese hamster lung V79 cells, ouabain resistance *in vitro*	+	NT	4.1	Ahmed et al. (1977a)
Gene mutation, Chinese hamster lung V79 cells, diphtheria toxin resistance *in vitro*	–	NT	1.6	Tsushimoto et al. (1983)
Gene mutation, mouse lymphoma L5178Y cells, *Tk* locus *in vitro*	+	NT	25	McGregor et al. (1988)
Gene mutation, rat liver epithelial ARL cells *in vitro*, *Hprt* locus	–	NT	41	Telang et al. (1982)
Micronucleus formation, beluga whale skin fibroblasts *in vitro*	+	–	5	Gauthier et al. (1999)
Cell transformation, Syrian hamster embryo cells, focus assay	+	NT	8[c]	Bessi et al. (1995)
Covalent binding to DNA (^{32}P-postlabelling), Syrian hamster embryo cells	–	NT	10	Bessi et al. (1995)
Unscheduled DNA synthesis, human VA-4 fibroblasts *in vitro*	+	–	0.4	Ahmed et al. (1977b)
Gene mutation, human fibroblasts *in vitro*[d]	–	–	41	Tong et al. (1981)
Sister chromatid exchange, human LAZ-007 lymphocytes *in vitro*	+	+	0.41	Sobti et al. (1983)
Inhibition of intercellular communication, rat liver epithelial ARL cells *in vitro*	+	NT	2.1	Telang et al. (1982)
Inhibition of intercellular communication, V79 cells *in vitro*	(+)	NT	0.41	Tsushimoto et al. (1983)
Inhibition of intercellular communication, male B6C3F$_1$ mouse primary hepatocytes *in vitro*	+	NT	20.5	Ruch et al. (1990)
Inhibition of intercellular communication, male Fischer 344 rat primary hepatocytes *in vitro*	+	NT	20.5	Ruch et al. (1990)
Inhibition of intercellular communication, Syrian hamster embryo and V79 cells *in vitro*	+	NT	5	Bessi et al. (1995)

Table 14 (contd)

Test system	Result[a] Without exogenous metabolic system	Result[a] With exogenous metabolic system	Dose[b] (LED or HID)	Reference
DNA single-strand breaks, Sprague-Dawley rat liver cells in vivo (12-h treatment)	+		120 po × 1	Hassoun et al. (1993)
DNA single-strand breaks, Sprague-Dawley rat liver cells in vivo	+		60 po × 2	Bagchi et al. (1995)
Sister chromatid exchange, Umbra limi intestinal cells in vivo	+		0.00002	Vigfusson et al. (1983)
Micronucleus formation, male CD-1 Swiss mouse bone-marrow cells in vivo	(+)		205 µmol/kg, dermal × 1	Schop et al. (1990)
Chromosomal aberrations, male Swiss mouse bone-marrow cells in vivo	+		10 po × 1	Sarkar et al. (1993)
Nuclear aberrations, male CD-1 Swiss mouse hair follicle cells in vivo	+		51 µmol/kg, dermal × 1	Schop et al. (1990)
Dominant lethal mutation, male ICR/Ha Swiss mice	–		240 ip × 1	Epstein et al. (1972)
Dominant lethal mutation, male ICR/Ha Swiss mice	–		50 po × 5	Epstein et al. (1972)
Dominant lethal mutation, male CD-1 mice	–		100 ip × 1	Arnold et al. (1977)
Dominant lethal mutation, male CD-1 mice	–		100 po × 1	Arnold et al. (1977)
Covalent binding to DNA (^{32}P-postlabelling), male and female B6C3F$_1$ mouse liver in vivo	–		50 po × 1 or 200 mg/kg of diet, 14 days	Whysner et al. (1998)

[a] +, positive; (+), weak positive; –, negative; NT, not tested

[b] LED, lowest effective dose; HID, highest ineffective dose; in-vitro tests, µg/mL; in-vivo tests, mg/kg bw per day; NR, not reported; po, oral; ip, intraperitoneal

[c] Three applications were given.

[d] Mediated by rat primary hepatocytes

Table 15. Genetic and related effects of heptachlor and heptachlor epoxide

Test system	Result[a]		Dose[b] (LED/HID)	Reference
	Without exogenous metabolic system	With exogenous metabolic system		
Heptachlor				
ColE1 plasmid DNA strand breaks (from *Escherichia coli* K12 ColE1)	–	NT	100	Griffin & Hill (1978)
Escherichia coli WP2, K12, differential toxicity	–	NT	2000 µg/disk	Rashid & Mumma (1986)
Salmonella typhimurium TA1538, TA1978, differential toxicity	–	NT	2000 µg/disk	Rashid & Mumma (1986)
Bacillus subtilis rec strains, differential toxicity	–	–	356	Matsui et al. (1989)
Salmonella typhimurium TA100, TA1535, TA1537, TA1538, TA98, reverse mutation	NT	–	5000 µg/plate	Simmon et al. (1977)
Salmonella typhimurium TA100, TA1535, TA1537, TA1538, TA98, G46, C3076, D3052, reverse mutation	–	–	NR	Probst et al. (1981)
Salmonella typhimurium TA100, TA1535, TA98, reverse mutation	–	(+)[c]	10 µg/plate	Gentile et al. (1982)
Salmonella typhimurium TA100, TA1535, TA1537, TA1538, TA98, reverse mutation	–	–	5000 µg/plate	Moriya et al. (1983)
Salmonella typhimurium TA100, TA1535, TA1537, TA98, reverse mutation	–	–	333 µg/plate	Zeiger et al. (1987)
Salmonella typhimurium TA100, TA102, TA98, TA97, reverse mutation	–	–	1000 µg/plate	Mersch-Sundermann et al. (1988)
Escherichia coli WP2, WP2 *uvr*A, reverse mutation	–	–	NR	Probst et al. (1981)
Escherichia coli WP2, reverse mutation	–	–	5000 µg/plate	Moriya et al. (1983)
Saccharomyces cerevisiae D4, gene conversion	–	–	NR	Gentile et al. (1982)
Drosophila melanogaster, sex-linked recessive lethal mutations	–		1 ng, injection	Benes & Šrám (1969)
Unscheduled DNA synthesis, rat, mouse and Syrian hamster primary hepatocytes *in vitro*	–	NT	3.7	Maslansky & Williams (1981)

Table 15 (contd)

Test system	Result[a] Without exogenous metabolic system	With exogenous metabolic system	Dose[b] (LED/HID)	Reference
Unscheduled DNA synthesis, Fischer 344 rat primary hepatocytes in vitro	–	NT	3.7	Probst et al. (1981)
Unscheduled DNA synthesis, rat primary hepatocytes in vitro	–	NT	3.7	Williams et al. (1989)
Gene mutation, mouse lymphoma L5178Y cells, Tk locus in vitro	+	NT	25	McGregor et al. (1988)
Gene mutation, rat liver epithelial ARL cells in vitro, Hprt locus	–	NT	37	Telang et al. (1982)
Unscheduled DNA synthesis, human VA-4 fibroblasts in vitro	–	+	37	Ahmed et al. (1977b)
Inhibition of intercellular communication, rat liver epithelial ARL cells in vitro	+	NT	0.37	Telang et al. (1982)
Inhibition of intercellular communication, Chinese hamster V79 cells in vitro	+	NT	10	Kurata et al. (1982)
Inhibition of intercellular communication, male Fischer 344 rat primary hepatocytes in vitro	+	NT	18.7	Ruch et al. (1990)
Inhibition of intercellular communication, male B6C3F$_1$ mouse primary hepatocytes in vitro	+	NT	18.7	Ruch et al. (1990)
Inhibition of intercellular communication, human breast epithelial cells in vitro	+	NT	10	Nomata et al. (1996)
Gene mutation, lacI transgenic mouse liver assay in vivo	–		20 mg/kg of diet, 120 days	Gunz et al. (1993)
Dominant lethal mutation, male ICR/Ha Swiss mice	–		24 ip × 1; 10 po × 5	Epstein et al. (1972)
Heptachlor epoxide				
Aspergillus nidulans, forward mutation	–	NT	10 450	Crebelli et al. (1986)
Aspergillus nidulans, mitotic crossing-over	–	NT	10 000	Crebelli et al. (1986)
Aspergillus nidulans, aneuploidy	–	NT	10 000	Crebelli et al. (1986)

472 IARC MONOGRAPHS VOLUME 79

Table 15 (contd)

Test system	Result[a]		Dose[b] (LED/HID)	Reference
	Without exogenous metabolic system	With exogenous metabolic system		
Salmonella typhimurium TA1535, TA1536, TA1537, TA1538, reverse mutation	–	–	1000 µg/plate	Marshall *et al.* (1976)
Unscheduled DNA synthesis, human VA-4 fibroblasts *in vitro*	–	+	3.9	Ahmed *et al.* (1977b)
Inhibition of intercellular communication (dye transfer), rat liver WB F344 cells *in vitro*	+[d]	NT	10	Matesic *et al.* (1994)
Inhibition of intercellular communication, human breast epithelial cells *in vitro*	+[d]	NT	1	Nomata *et al.* (1996)

[a] +, positive; (+), weak positive; –, negative; NT, not tested
[b] LED, lowest effective dose; HID, highest ineffective dose; in-vitro tests, µg/mL; in-vivo tests, mg/kg bw per day; NR, not reported; ip, intraperitoneal; po, oral
[c] Technical grade
[d] Loss of intercellular communication was characterized by a substantial, sustained loss of connexin 43 immunostaining within 15–60 min of treatment; at least in human cells, there was no reduction of connexin 43 mRNA.

Heptachlor epoxide did not induce forward mutation, mitotic crossing-over or aneuploidy in *Aspergillus* or reverse mutation in *Salmonella typhimurium*. It did induce unscheduled DNA synthesis in human fibroblasts *in vitro* with metabolic activation, and inhibited gap-junctional intercellular communication in rat liver and human breast epithelial cells *in vitro*, without metabolic activation.

4.6   Mechanistic considerations

Both chlordane and heptachlor have shown some potential to inhibit gap-junctional intercellular communication and to induce genetic toxicity in cultured mammalian cells. Chlordane has been reported to induce DNA damage in rat liver, but the induction of DNA repair has not been observed. While the evidence is not strong, it remains possible that such events, should they also occur *in vivo,* could play a role in the carcinogenesis induced by these compounds.

Chlordane induces hepatic microsomal metabolism and increased CYP content in rats. It also produces increased cell proliferation in the thyroid gland of mice. Chlordane administered by intraperitoneal injection has been found to lower thyroxine concentrations in rats. However, no information was available on the concentrations of thyroxine, triiodothyronine or thyroid-stimulating hormone in long-term bioassays in rodents. Therefore, while hepatic metabolism of thyroxine resulting in increased thyroid-stimulating hormone is possibly involved in the induction of thyroid tumours in rats, the other mechanisms cannot be excluded because the information is incomplete.

Chlordane is toxic to the liver in rats and mice. In mice, increased hepatocellular proliferation has been found at doses that produce hepatocellular cancer in mice. In rats, liver toxicity has been shown to be accompanied by enhanced lipid peroxidation and generation of reactive oxygen species. Chlordane has been shown to promote liver tumours in mice.

5.   Summary of Data Reported and Evaluation

5.1   Exposure data

Chlordane and heptachlor are structurally related organochlorine insecticides; the technical-grade product of each contains about 10–20% of the other compound. They have been used since the 1950s for termite control, on agricultural crops, on lawns, on livestock and for other purposes. Their use has currently been banned or severely restricted in many countries. In these countries, human exposure is still possible owing to their persistence in the environment and their consequent occurrence in meat, fish and other fat-containing foodstuffs, but the mean daily intake has probably decreased.

5.2   Human carcinogenicity data

Several cohort studies, with different inclusion criteria and lengths of follow-up, have been conducted to investigate the mortality of workers at two plants in the USA, one producing chlordane and the other heptachlor and endrin. The workers were also exposed to other chemicals. Although no excess was seen in the rate of mortality from all cancers, some, but not all, of the studies showed a slight excess of lung cancer. A similar small excess of mortality from lung cancer was observed in two cohorts of pesticide applicators in the USA; however, when the analyses were limited to the workers more likely to be exposed to chlordane, the mortality rate for lung cancer was lower than in the overall cohort.

A number of case–control studies were conducted to investigate the risks for cancers of the lymphohaematopoietic system, breast and a few other sites in relation to exposure to chlordane. These studies differed widely in size and methods and in exposure assessment, which was either reported by the subjects themselves (or proxy respondents) or estimated from measures of the concentrations of chlordane metabolites in samples of fat tissue or blood. The populations studied also varied widely, some studies including higher proportions of farmers, who are occupationally exposed to pesticides, while the subjects in others (including most studies of women) had no occupational exposure to chlordane. In most studies, exposure to many other organochlorine or other types of pesticides was also assessed. Four case–control studies of non-Hodgkin lymphoma showed a consistent but modest increase in the risk associated with exposure to chlordane, although it was almost impossible to separate the effect of chlordane from those related to farming *per se* or to exposure to other pesticides. One case–control study each of hairy-cell leukaemia, leukaemia not otherwise specified, soft-tissue sarcoma and multiple myeloma yielded no notable results with respect to chlordane. No association with chlordane concentrations in blood or fat tissue was found in six of seven case–control studies of breast cancer conducted in Denmark and North America, in two of which blood samples were collected prospectively, or in one study on endometrial cancer conducted in Sweden. No clear pattern emerged in a study of pancreatic cancer in the USA, while a small study of brain cancer in children showed elevated risks associated with termite control treatment, also in comparison with children with cancer of the lymphohaematopoietic system.

5.3   Animal carcinogenicity data

Chlordane, technical-grade chlordane, heptachlor, technical-grade heptachlor, heptachlor epoxide and a mixture of heptachlor and heptachlor epoxide have been tested for carcinogenicity by oral administration in several strains of mice and rats. In the studies in mice, increased incidences of hepatocellular neoplasms (including carcinomas) were seen in both males and females. Increased incidences of thyroid follicular-cell adenomas and carcinomas were seen in one study each with chlordane and technical-grade heptachlor in rats. In a third study in rats, technical-grade chlordane marginally increased the incidence of liver adenomas in male rats. In initiation–promotion studies in mice, administration of chlordane or heptachlor after N-nitroso-diethylamine resulted in increased incidences of hepatocellular tumours.

5.4   Other relevant data

Chlordane is primarily metabolized to oxychlordane and to a minor extent may also be dehydrochlorinated to heptachlor. Heptachlor, which is also a component of technical-grade chlordane, is biotransformed to its epoxide. Subsequent dechlorination reactions lead to hydroxylated compounds, which are excreted primarily as glucu-ronides. Minor metabolites include heptachlor and heptachlor epoxide.

Accidental or intentional exposure to chlordane has resulted in signs of neurotoxicity and, in some cases, death. In experimental animals, the toxic effects of chlordane on the liver include lipid peroxidation and cell proliferation secondary to cytotoxicity. In the thyroid, chlordane has been shown to decrease thyroxine concentrations in rats. Both chlordane and heptachlor induce hepatic and gonadal microsomal oxidative enzymes and also steroid hormone metabolism.

Chlordane and heptachlor are toxic to reproduction and development in mice, rats and mink. Pre- and postnatal exposures to chlordane affected the development of the immune system in rodents. Impaired cell-mediated immunity after prenatal exposure to chlordane has been observed in female BALB/c mice.

No data were available on the genetic and related effects of chlordane or heptachlor in humans. Both compounds inhibited gap-junctional intercellular communication and induced gene mutations in rodent cells. Likewise, both compounds induced unscheduled DNA synthesis in human fibroblasts but not in rodent hepatocytes. Chlordane induced DNA damage in liver cells of rats treated *in vivo*, but heptachlor did not induce mutations in hepatocytes of *lacI* transgenic mice treated *in vivo*. Neither chlordane nor heptachlor caused dominant lethal mutation in mice. Neither chlordane nor heptachlor was mutagenic to bacteria, and only chlordane damaged bacterial or plasmid DNA.

5.5   Evaluation

There is *inadequate evidence* in humans for the carcinogenicity of chlordane and heptachlor.

There is *sufficient evidence* in experimental animals for the carcinogenicity of chlordane and of heptachlor.

Overall evaluation

Chlordane and heptachlor are *possibly carcinogenic to humans (Group 2B)*.

6. References

Agency for Toxic Substances and Disease Registry (1989a) *Toxicological Profile for Heptachlor/Heptachlor Epoxide* (Report No. ATSDR/TP-88/16; NTIS PB89-194492), Washington DC, Public Health Service, Department of Health and Human Services

Agency for Toxic Substances and Disease Registry (1989b) *Toxicological Profile for Chlordane* (Report No. ATSDR/TP-89/06; NTIS PB90-168709), Washington DC, Public Health Service, Department of Health and Human Services

Agency for Toxic Substances and Disease Registry (1993) *Toxicological Profile for Heptachlor/Heptachlor Epoxide (Update)* (Report No. ATSDR/TP-92/11; NTIS PB93-182467), Atlanta, GA, Public Health Service, Department of Health and Human Services

Agency for Toxic Substances and Disease Registry (1994) *Toxicological Profile for Chlordane (Update)* (Report No. ATSDR/TP-93/03; NTIS PB95-100111), Atlanta, GA, Public Health Service, Department of Health and Human Services

Ahmed, F.E., Lewis, N. J. & Hart, R.W. (1977a) Pesticide induced ouabain resistant mutants in Chinese hamster V79 cells. *Chem.-biol. Interactions*, **19**, 369–374

Ahmed, F.E., Hart, R.W. & Lewis, N. J. (1977b) Pesticide induced DNA damage and its repair in cultured human cells. *Mutat. Res.*, **42**, 161–173

Akhtar, N., Kayani, S.A., Ahmad, M.M. & Shahab, M. (1996) Insecticide-induced changes in secretory activity of the thyroid gland in rats. *J. appl. Toxicol.*, **16**, 397–400

Aldrich, F.D. & Holmes, J.H. (1969) Acute chlordane intoxication in a child. Case report with toxicological data. *Arch. environ. Health*, **19**, 129–132

Al-Omar, M.A., Abbas, A.K. & Al-Obaidy, S.A. (2000) Combined effect of exposure to lead and chlordane on the testicular tissues of Swiss mice. *Toxicol. Lett.*, **115**, 1–8

Alvarez, W.C. & Hyman, S. (1953) Absence of toxic manifestations in workers exposed to chlordane. *Arch. ind. Hyg. occup. Med.*, **19**, 480–483

Ambrose, A.M., Christensen, H.E., Robbins, D.J. & Rather, L.J. (1953) Toxicological and pharmacological studies on chlordane. *Arch. ind. Hyg. occup. Med.*, **8**, 197–210

American Conference of Governmental Industrial Hygienists (2000) *TLVs and other Occupational Exposure Values — 2000 CD-ROM*, Cincinnati, OH, ACGIH®

Amita-Rani, B.E. & Krishnakumari, M.K. (1995) Prenatal toxicity of heptachlor in albino rats. *Pharmacol. Toxicol.*, **76**, 112–114

Anon. (1985) Epoxy heptachlor. *Dangerous Prop. ind. Mater. Rep.*, **5**, 63–74

American Public Health Association/American Water Works Association/Water Environment Federation (1999a) Method 6410B. Liquid–liquid extraction gas chromatographic/mass spectrometric method. In: *Standard Methods for the Examination of Water and Wastewater*, 20th Ed., Atlanta, GA

American Public Health Association/American Water Works Association/Water Environment Federation (1999b) Method 6630B. Liquid–liquid extraction gas chromatographic method I. In: *Standard Methods for the Examination of Water and Wastewater*, 20th Ed., Atlanta, GA

American Public Health Association/American Water Works Association/Water Environment Federation (1999c) Method 6630C. Liquid–liquid extraction gas chromatographic method II. In: *Standard Methods for the Examination of Water and Wastewater*, 20th Ed., Atlanta, GA

AOAC International (2000) *Official Methods of Analysis of AOAC International*, 17th Ed., Gaithersburg, MD [CD-ROM] [Methods 962.05, 962.07, 965.14, 968.04, 970.52, 972.05, 973.15, 973.16, 973.17, 983.21, 990.06]

Arnold, D.W., Kennedy, G.L., Jr, Keplinger, M.L., Calandra, J.C. & Calo, C.J. (1977) Dominant lethal studies with technical chlordane, HCS-3260 and heptachlor: heptachlor epoxide. *J. Toxicol. environ. Health*, **2**, 547–555

Aronson, K.J., Miller, A.B., Woolcott, C.G., Sterns, E.E., McCready, D.R. & Lickley, L.A. (2000) Breast adipose tissue concentrations of polychlorinated biphenyls and other organochlorines and breast cancer risk. *Cancer Epidemiol. Biomarkers Prev.*, **9**, 55–63

Aulerich, R.J., Bursian, S.J. & Napolitano, A.C. (1990) Subacute toxicity of dietary heptachlor to mink (*Mustela vison*). *Arch. environ. Contam. Toxicol.*, **19**, 913–916

Bagchi, D., Bagchi, M., Hassoun, E.A. & Stohs, S.J. (1995) In vitro and in vivo generation of reactive oxygen species, DNA damage and lactate dehydrogenase leakage by selected pesticides. *Toxicology*, **104**, 129–140

Balash, K.J., Al-Omar, M.A. & Abdul-Latif, B.M. (1987) Effect of chlordane on testicular tissues of Swiss mice. *Bull. environ. Contam. Toxicol.*, **39**, 434–442

Barnett, J.R. & Dorough, H.W. (1974) Metabolism of chlordane in rats. *J. agric. Food Chem.*, **22**, 612–619

Barnett, J.B., Blaylock, B.L., Gandy, J., Menna, J.H., Denton, R. & Soderberg, L.S. (1998) Alteration of fetal liver colony formation by prenatal chlordane exposure. *Fundam. appl. Toxicol.*, **15**, 820–822

Barrass, N., Steward, M., Warburton, S., Aitchison, J., Jackson, D., Wadsworth, P., Marsden, A. & Orton, T. (1993) Cell proliferation in the liver and thyroid of C57B1/10J mice after dietary administration of chlordane. *Environ. Health Perspectives*, **101**, 219–224

Benes, V. & Šrám, R. (1969) Mutagenic activity of some pesticides in *Drosophila melanogaster*. *Ind. Med.*, **38**, 442–444

Berman, E., Schlicht, M., Moser, V.C. & MacPhail, R.C. (1995) A multidisciplinary approach to toxicological screening: I. Systemic toxicity. *J. Toxicol. environ. Health*, **45**, 127–143

Bernstein, G., Artz, S.A., Hasen, J. & Oppenheimer, J.H. (1968) Hepatic accumulation of ^{125}I-thyroxine in the rat: Augmentation by phenobarbital and chlordane. *Endocrinology*, **82**, 406–409

Bessi, H., Rast, C., Rether, B., Nguyen-Ba, B.G. & Vasseur, P. (1995) Synergistic effects of chlordane and TPA in multistage morphological transformation of SHE cells. *Carcinogenesis*, **16**, 237–244

Blair, A., Grauman, D.J., Lubin, J.H. & Fraumeni, J.F., Jr (1983) Lung cancer and other causes of death among licensed pesticide applicators. *J. natl Cancer Inst.*, **71**, 31–37

Blaylock, B.L., Soderberg, L.S.F., Gandy, J., Menna, J.H., Denton, R. & Barnett, J.B. (1990) Cytotoxic T-lymphocyte and NK responses in mice treated prenatally with chlordane. *Toxicol. Lett.*, **51**, 41–49

Blaylock, B.L., Newsom, K.K., Holladay, S.D., Shipp, B.K., Bartow, T.A. & Mehendale, H.M. (1995) Topical exposure to chlordane reduces the contact hypersensitivity resonse to oxazolone in BALB/c mice. *Toxicol. Lett.*, **81**, 205–211

Blyler, G., Landreth, K.S. & Barnett, J.B. (1994) Gender-specific effects of prenatal chlordane exposure on myeloid cell development. *Fundam. appl. Toxicol.*, **23**, 188–193

Bovard, K.P., Fontenot, J.P. & Priode, B.M. (1971) Accumulation and dissipation of heptachlor residues in fattening steers. *J. anim. Sci.*, **33**, 127–132

Bowery, T.G. (1964) Heptachlor. In: Zweig, G., ed., *Analytical Methods for Pesticides, Plant Growth Regulators, and Food Additives*, Vol. II, *Insecticides*, New York, Academic Press, pp. 245–256

Brooks, G.T. (1974) *Chlorinated Insecticides*, Vol. 1, *Technology and Application*, Cleveland, OH, CRC Press, pp. 85–158

Brown, D.P. (1992) Mortality of workers employed at organochlorine pesticide manufacturing plants — An update. *Scand. J. Work Environ. Health*, **18**, 155–161

Brown, L.M., Blair, A., Gibson, R., Everett, G.D., Cantor, K.P., Schuman, L.M., Burmeister, L.F., Van-Lier, S.F. & Dick, F. (1990) Pesticide exposures and other agricultural risk factors for leukemia among men in Iowa and Minnesota. *Cancer Res.*, **50**, 6585–6591

Brown, L.M., Burmeister, L.F., Everett, G.D. & Blair, A. (1993) Pesticide exposures and multiple myeloma in Iowa men. *Cancer Causes Control*, **4**, 153–156

Buchert, H., Class, T. & Ballschmiter, K. (1989) High resolution gas chromatography of technical chlordane with electron capture- and mass selective detection. *Fresenius Z. anal. Chem.*, **333**, 211–217

Cantor, K.P., Blair, A., Everett, G., Gibson, R., Burmeister, L.F., Brown, L.M., Schuman, L. & Dick, F.R. (1992) Pesticides and other agricultural risk factors for non-Hodgkin's lymphoma among men in Iowa and Minnesota. *Cancer Res.*, **52**, 2447–2455

Carvalho, F.P., Montenegro-Guillen, S., Villeneuve, J.-P., Cattini, C., Bartocci, J., Lacayo, M. & Cruz, A. (1999) Chlorinated hydrocarbons in coastal lagoons on the Pacific Coast of Nicaragua. *Arch. environ. Contam. Toxicol.*, **36**, 131–139

Cassidy, R.A., Vorhees, C.V., Minnema, D.J. & Hastings, L. (1994) The effects of chlordane exposure during pre- and postnatal periods at environmentally relevant levels on sex steroid-mediated behaviors and functions in the rat. *Toxicol. appl. Pharmacol.*, **126**, 326–337

Chan, H.M. (1998) A database for environmental contaminants in traditional foods in northern and Arctic Canada: Development and applications. *Food Add. Contam.*, **15**, 127–134

Christensen, J.G., Romach, E.H., Healy, L.N., Gonzales, A.J., Anderson, S.P., Malarkey, D.E., Corton, J.C., Fox, T.R., Cattley, R.C. & Goldsworthy, T.L. (1999) Altered bcl-2 family expression during non-genotoxic hepatocarcinogenesis in mice. *Carcinogenesis*, **20**, 1583–1590

Chuang, L.F. & Chuang, R.Y. (1991) The effect of the insecticide heptachlor on ras proto-oncogene expression in human myeloblastic leukemia (ML-1) cells. *Toxicology*, **70**, 283–292

Chuang, L.F. & Chuang, R.Y. (1998) Heptachlor and the mitogen-activated protein kinase module in human lymphocytes. *Toxicology*, **128**, 17–23

Chuang, L.F., Liu, Y., Killam, K., Jr & Chuang, R.Y. (1992) Modulation by the insecticides heptachlor and chlordane of the cell-mediated immune proliferative responses of rhesus monkeys. *In Vivo*, **6**, 29–32

Chuang, L.F., Rought, S.E. & Chuang, R.Y. (1999) Differential regulation of the major cyclin-dependent kinases, cdk2 and cdc2, during cell cycle progression in human lymphocytes exposed to heptachlor. *In Vivo*, **13**, 455–461

CIS Information Services (2000) *Directory of World Chemical Producers (Version 2000.1)*, Dallas, TX [CD-ROM]

Cochrane, W.P. & Greenhalgh, R. (1976) Chemical composition of technical chlordane. *J. Assoc off. anal. Chem.*, **59**, 696–702

Codex Alimentarius Commission (1997) *Codex Maximum Limits for Pesticide Residues*, Rome, FAO

Crebelli, R., Bellincampi, D., Conti, G., Conti, L., Morpurgo, G. & Carere, A. (1986) A comparative study on selected chemical carcinogens for chromosome malsegregation, mitotic crossing-over and forward mutation induction in *Aspergillus nidulans*. *Mutat. Res.*, **172**, 139–149

Crum, J.A., Bursian, S.J., Auberich, R.J., Polin & D. & Braselton, W.E. (1993) The reproductive effects of dietary heptachlor in mink (*Mustela vison*). *Arch. environ. contam. Toxicol.*, **24**, 156–164

Curley, A. & Garrettson, L.K. (1969) Acute chlordane poisoning. Clinical and chemical studies. *Arch. environ. Health*, **18**, 211–215

Datta, S., Ohyama, K., Dunlap, D.Y. & Matsumura, F. (1999) Evidence for organochlorine contamination in tissues of salmonids in Lake Tahoe. *Ecotoxicol. environ. Saf.*, **42**, 94–101

Davis, J.R., Brownson, R.C., Garcia, R., Bentz, B.J. & Turner, A. (1993) Family pesticide use and chilhood brain cancer. *Arch. environ. Contam. Toxicol.*, **24**, 87–92

Dearth, M.A. & Hites, R.A. (1991) Complete analysis of technical chlordane using negative ionization mass spectrometry. *Environ. Sci. Technol.*, **25**, 245–254

Demers, A., Ayotte, P., Brisson, J., Dodin, S., Robert, J. & Dewailly, E. (2000) Risk and aggressiveness of breast cancer in relation to plasma organochlorine concentrations. *Cancer Epidemiol. Biomarkers Prev.*, **9**, 161–166

Den Tonkelaar, E.M. & Van Esch, G.J. (1974) No-effect levels of organochlorine pesticides based on induction of microsomal liver enzymes in short-term toxicity experiments. *Toxicology*, **2**, 371–380

Derbes, V.J., Dent, J.H., Forrest, W.W. & Johnson, M.F. (1955) Fatal chlordane poisoning. *J. Am. med. Assoc.*, **158**, 1367–1369

D'Ercole, A.J., Arthur, R.D., Cain, J.D. & Barrentine, B.F. (1976) Insecticide exposure of mothers and newborns in a rural agricultural area. *Pediatrics*, **57**, 869–874

Deutsche Forschungsgemeinschaft (2000) *List of MAK and BAT Values 2000* (Report No. 36), Weinheim, Wiley-VCH Verlag GmbH, pp. 36, 63

Dewailly, E., Dodin, S., Verreault, R., Ayotte, P., Sauve, L., Morin, J. & Brisson, J. (1994) High organochlorine body burden in women with estrogen receptor-positive breast cancer. *J. natl Cancer Inst.*, **86**, 232–234

Ditraglia, D., Brown, D.P., Namekata, T. & Iverson, N. (1981) Mortality study of workers employed at organochlorine pesticide manufacturing plants. *Scand. J. Work Environ. Health*, **7** (Suppl. 4), 140–146

Dorgan, J.F., Brock, J.W., Rothman, N., Needham, L.L., Miller, R., Stephenson, H.E, Jr, Schussler, N. & Taylor, P.R. (1999) Serum organochlorine pesticides and PCBs and breast cancer risk: Results from a prospective analysis (USA). *Cancer Causes Control*, **10**, 1–11

Duggan, R.E. & Corneliussen, P.E. (1972) Dietary intake of pesticide chemicals in the United States (III), June 1968–April 1970. *Pestic. Monit. J.*, **5**, 331–341

Eller, P.M., ed. (1994) Method 5510. In: *NIOSH Manual of Analytical Methods (DHHS (NIOSH) Publ. No. 94-113)*, 4th Ed., Cincinnati, OH, National Institute for Occupational Safety and Health

Environmental Protection Agency (1976) Velsicol Chemical Co., consolidated heptachlor/chlordane hearing. *Fed. Regist.*, **41**, 7552–7572

Environmental Protection Agency (1987a) *Heptachlor and Heptachlor Epoxide*, Washington DC, Office of Drinking Water

Environmental Protection Agency (1987b) *Chlordane, Heptachlor, Aldrin and Dieldrin* (Technical Report Document), Washington DC, Office of Pesticides and Toxic Substances

Environmental Protection Agency (1993a) Method 617. The determination of organohalide pesticides and PCBs in municipal and industrial wastewater. In: *Methods for the Determination of Nonconventional Pesticides in Municipal and Industrial Wastewater* (EPA Report No. EPA-821/R-93-010-A), Washington DC

Environmental Protection Agency (1993b) Method 1656. The determination of organo-halide pesticides in municipal and industrial wastewater. In: *Methods for the Determination of Nonconventional Pesticides in Municipal and Industrial Wastewater* (EPA Report No. EPA-821/R-93-010-A), Washington DC

Environmental Protection Agency (1995a) Method 505. Analysis of organohalide pesticides and commercial polychlorinated biphenyl (PCB) products in water by microextraction and gas chromatography [Rev. 2.1]. In: *Methods for the Determination of Organic Compounds in Drinking Water*, Supplement III (EPA Report No. EPA-600/R-95-131; US NTIS PB-216616), Cincinnati, OH, Environmental Monitoring Systems Laboratory

Environmental Protection Agency (1995b) Method 508.1. Determination of chlorinated pesticides, herbicides, and organohalides by liquid–solid extraction and electron capture gas chromatography [Rev. 2.0].]. In: *Methods for the Determination of Organic Compounds in Drinking Water*, Supplement III (EPA Report No. EPA-600/R-95-131; US NTIS PB-216616), Cincinnati, OH, Environmental Monitoring Systems Laboratory

Environmental Protection Agency (1995c) Method 525.2. Determination of organic compounds in drinking water by liquid–solid extraction and capillary column gas chromatography/mass spectrometry [Rev. 2.0]. In: *Methods for the Determination of Organic Compounds in Drinking Water*, Supplement III (EPA Report No. EPA-600/R-95/131; US NTIS PB-216616), Cincinnati, OH, Environmental Monitoring Systems Laboratory

Environmental Protection Agency (1995d) Method 551.1. Determination of chlorination by-products, chlorinated solvents, and halogenated pesticides/herbicides in drinking water by liquid–liquid extraction and gas chromatography with electron-capture detection [Rev. 1.0]. In: *Methods for the Determination of Organic Compounds in Drinking Water*, Supplement III (EPA Report No. EPA-600/R-95/131; US NTIS PB-216616), Cincinnati, OH, Environmental Monitoring Systems Laboratory

Environmental Protection Agency (1996a) Method 8081A. Organochlorine pesticides by gas chromatography [Rev. 1]. In: *Test Methods for Evaluating Solid Waste — Physical/Chemical Methods* (EPA Report No. SW-846), Washington DC, Office of Solid Waste

Environmental Protection Agency (1996b) Method 8270C. Semivolatile organic compounds by gas chromatography/mass spectrometry (GC/MS) [Rev. 3]. In: *Test Methods for Evaluating Solid Waste — Physical/Chemical Methods* (EPA Report No. SW-846), Washington DC, Office of Solid Waste

Environmental Protection Agency (1996c) Method 4041. Soil screening for chlordane by immunoassay [Rev. 0]. In: *Test Methods for Evaluating Solid Waste — Physical/Chemical Methods* (EPA Report No. SW-846), Washington DC, Office of Solid Waste

Environmental Protection Agency (1999a) Method TO-04A. Determination of pesticides and polychlorinated biphenyls in ambient air using high volume polyurethane foam (PUF) sampling followed by gas chromatographic/multi-detector detection (GC/MD). In: *Compendium of Methods for the Determination of Toxic Compounds in Ambient Air*, 2nd Ed. (EPA Report No. EPA-625/R-96-010b), Cincinnati, OH, Center for Environmental Research Information

Environmental Protection Agency (1999b) Method TO-10A. Determination of pesticides and polychlorinated biphenyls in ambient air using low volume polyurethane foam (PUF) sampling followed by gas chromatographic/multi-detector detection (GC/MD). In: *Compendium of Methods for the Determination of Toxic Compounds in Ambient Air*, 2nd Ed. (EPA Report No. EPA-625/R-96-010b), Cincinnati, OH, Center for Environmental Research Information

Environmental Protection Agency (1999c) Methods for organic chemical analysis of municipal and industrial wastewater. Method 608 — Organochlorine pesticides and PCBs. *US Code Fed. Regul., Title 40*, Part 136, App. A, pp. 114–134

Environmental Protection Agency (1999d) Methods for organic chemical analysis of municipal and industrial wastewater. Method 625 — Base/neutrals and acids. *US Code Fed. Regul., Title 40*, Part 136, App. A, pp. 202–228

Environmental Protection Agency (2000) *Drinking Water Standards and Health Advisories* (EPA Report No. EPA-882/B-00-001), Washington DC, Office of Water

Epstein, S.S. (1976) Carcinogenicity of heptachlor and chlordane. *Sci. total Environ.*, **6**, 103–154

Epstein, S.S. & Ozonoff, D. (1987) Leukemias and blood dyscrasias following exposure to chlordane and heptachlor. *Teratog. Carcinog. Mutag.*, **7**, 527–540

Epstein, S.S., Arnold, E., Andrea, J., Bass, W. & Bishop, Y. (1972) Detection of chemical mutagens by the dominant lethal assay in the mouse. *Toxicol. appl. Pharmacol.*, **23**, 288–325

Esworthy, R.F. (1985) *Preliminary Quantitative Usage Analysis of Chlordane*, Washington DC, US Environmental Protection Agency, Office of Pesticide Programs

Ewing, A.D., Kadry, A.M. & Dorough, H.W. (1985) Comparative disposition and elimination of chlordane in rats and mice. *Toxicol. Lett.*, **26**, 233–239

Falck, F., Jr, Ricci, A., Jr, Wolff, M.S., Godbold, J. & Deckers, P. (1992) Pesticides and poly-chlorinated biphenyl residues in human breast lipids and their relation to breast cancer. *Arch. environ. Health*, **47**, 143–146

FAO/UNEP (1996) *Prior Informed Consent Decision Guidance Documents: Chlordane/Chlordimeform/EDB/Heptachlor/Mercury Compounds*, Geneva, Rotterdam Convention on the Prior Informed Consent Procedure for Certain Hazardous Chemicals and Pesticides in International Trade (http://www.fao.org/ag/agp/agpp/pesticid/pic/dgdhome.htm)

FAO/WHO (1964) *Evaluation of the Toxicity of Pesticide Residues in Food. Report of a Joint Meeting of the FAO Committee on Pesticides in Agriculture and the WHO Expert Committee on Pesticide Residues* (FAO Meeting Report No. PL/1963/13; WHO/Food Add /23), Rome

FAO/WHO (1965) *Evaluation of the Toxicity of Pesticide Residues in Food. Report of a Joint Meeting of the FAO Committee on Pesticides in Agriculture and the WHO Expert Committee on Pesticide Residues* (FAO Meeting Report No. PL: CP/15; WHO/Food Add./67.32), Rome

FAO/WHO (1967) *Evaluation of the Toxicity of Pesticide Residues in Food. Report of a Joint Meeting of the FAO Committee on Pesticides in Agriculture and the WHO Expert Committee on Pesticide Residues* (FAO Meeting Report No. PL:CP/15; WHO/Food Add./67.32), Rome

FAO/WHO (1968) *Evaluation of the Toxicity of Pesticide Residues in Food. Report of a Joint Meeting of the FAO Committee on Pesticides in Agriculture and the WHO Expert Committee on Pesticide Residues* (FAO Meeting Report No. PL: 1967/M/11/1; WHO/Food Add./68.30), Rome

FAO/WHO (1971) *Evaluation of the Toxicity of Pesticide Residues in Food. Report of a Joint Meeting of the FAO Committee on Pesticides in Agriculture and The WHO Expert Committee on Pesticide Residues* (AGP:1970/M/12/1; WHO/Food Add. 71.42), Rome

FAO/WHO (1978) *Pesticide Residues in Food: 1977 Evaluations* (FAO Plant Production and Protection Paper 10 Supp.), Rome

FAO/WHO (1983) *Pesticide Residues in Food — 1982 Evaluations. Data and Recommendations of the Joint Meeting of the FAO Panel of Experts on Pesticide Residues in Food and the Environment and the WHO Expert Group on Pesticide Residues* (FAO Plant Production and Protection Paper 49), Rome

FAO/WHO (1987) *Pesticide Residues in Food — 1986. Report of the Joint Meeting of the FAO Panel of Experts on Pesticide Residues in Food and the Environment and a WHO Expert Group on Pesticide Residues* (FAO Plant Production and Protection Paper 77), Rome

Fendick, E.A., Mather-Mihaich, E., Houck, K.A., St Clair, M.B., Faust, J.B., Rockwell, C.H. & Owens, M. (1990) Ecological toxicology and human health effects of heptachlor. *Rev. environ. Contam. Toxicol.*, **111**, 61–142

Fishbein, W.I., White, J.V. & Isaacs, H.J. (1964) Survey of workers exposed to chlordane. *Ind. Med. Surg.*, **33**, 726–727

Food and Drug Administration (1989) *Pesticide Analytical Manual*, Vol. II, *Methods Which Detect Multiple Residues*, Washington DC, Department of Health and Human Services

Food and Drug Administration (1990) Action levels for residues of certain pesticides in food and feed. *Fed. Reg.*, **55**, 14359–14363

Food and Drug Administration (1999) Methods 302, 303 and 304. In: Makovi, C.M. & McMahon, B.M., eds., *Pesticide Analytical Manual, Vol. I: Multiresidue Methods*, 3rd Rev. Ed., Washington DC, Management Methods Branch

Gaines, T.B. (1960) The acute toxicity of pesticides to rats. *Toxicol. appl. Pharmacol.*, **2**, 88–89

Gant, D.B., Eldefrawi, M.E. & Eldefrawi, A.T. (1987) Cyclodiene insecticides inhibit GABA receptor-regulated chloride transport. *Toxicol. appl. Pharmacol.*, **88**, 313–321

Garrettson, L.K., Guzelian, P.S. & Blanke, R.V. (1985) Subacute chlordane poisoning. *Clin. Toxicol.*, **22**, 565–571

Gauthier, J.M., Dubeau, H. & Rassart, E. (1999) Induction of micronuclei in vitro by organochlorine compounds in beluga whale skin fibroblasts. *Mutat. Res.*, **439**, 87–95

Gentile, J.M., Gentile, G.J., Bultman, J., Sechriest, R., Wagner, E.D. & Plewa, M.J. (1982) An evaluation of the genotoxic properties of insecticides following plant and animal activation. *Mutat. Res.*, **101**, 19–29

Griffin, D.E., III & Hill, W.E. (1978) In vitro breakage of plasmid DNA by mutagens and pesticides. *Mutat. Res.*, **52**, 161–169

Grutsch, J.F. & Khasawinah, A. (1991) Signs and mechanisms of chlordane intoxication. *Biomed. environ. Sci.*, **4**, 317–326

Gunderson, E.L. (1988) Chemical contaminants monitoring. FDA total diet study, April 1982–April 1984, dietary intakes of pesticides, selected elements, and other chemicals. *J. Assoc. off. anal. Chem.*, **71**, 1200–1209

Gunz, D., Shephard, S.E. & Lutz, W.K. (1993) Can nongenotoxic carcinogens be detected with the lacI transgenic mouse mutation assay? *Environ. mol. Mutag.*, **21**, 209–211

Hardell, L., Liljegren, G., Lindström, G., van Bavel, B., Broman, K., Fredrikson, M., Hagberg, M., Nordström, M. & Johansson, B. (1996) Increased concentrations of chlordane in adipose tissue from non-Hodgkin's lymphoma patients compared with controls without a malignant disease. *Int. J. Oncol.*, **9**, 1139–1142

Hardell, L., Liljegren, G., Lindström, G., van Bavel, B., Fredrikson, M. & Hagberg, H. (1997) Polychlorinated biphenyls, chlordanes, and the etiology of non-Hodgkin's lymphoma (Letter to the Editor). *Epidemiology*, **6**, 689

Harrington, J.M., Baker, E.L., Jr, Folland, D.S., Saucier, J.W. & Sandifer, S.H. (1978) Chlordane contamination of a municipal water system. *Environ. Res.*, **15**, 155–159

Hart, L.G., Shultice, R.W. & Fouts, J.R. (1963) Stimulatory effects of chlordane on hepatic microsomal drug metabolism in the rat. *Toxicol. appl. Pharmacol.*, **5**, 371–386

Hassoun, E., Bagchi, M., Bagchi, D. & Stohs, S.J. (1993) Comparative studies on lipid peroxidation and DNA-single strand breaks induced by lindane, DDT, chlordane and endrin in rats. *Comp. Biochem. Physiol.*, **104C**, 427–431

Health and Welfare Canada (1990) *National Pesticide Residue Limits in Foods*, Ottawa, Bureau of Chemical Safety, Food Directorate, Health Protection Branch

Hirasawa, F. & Takizawa, Y. (1989) Accumulation and declination of chlordane congeners in mice. *Toxicol. Lett.*, **47**, 109–117

Hoar Zahm, S., Weisenburger, D.D., Babbitt, P.A., Saal, R.C., Cantor, K.P. & Blair, A. (1988) A case–control study of non Hodgkin's lymphoma and agricultural factors in eastern Nebraska (Abstract). *Am. J. Epidemiol.*, **128**, 901

Hoar Zahm, S., Weisenburger, D.D., Babbitt, P.A., Saal, R.C., Vaught, J.B., Cantor, K.P. & Blair, A. (1990) A case–control study of non-Hodgkin's lymphoma and the herbicide 2,4-dichlorophenoxyacetic acid (2,4-D) in eastern Nebraska. *Epidemiology*, **1**, 349–356

Hogue, C. (2000) Dioxins to be major issue at treaty negotiations. *Chem. Eng. News*, **20 March**, 35

Hoppin, J.A., Tolbert, P.E., Holly, E.A., Brook, J.W., Korrick, S.A., Altshul, L.M., Zhang, R.H., Bracci, P.M., Burse, V.W. & Needham, L.L. (2000) Pancreatic cancer and serum organochlorine levels. *Cancer Epidemiol. Biomarkers Prev.*, **9**, 199–205

Houk, V.S. & DeMarini, D.M. (1987) Induction of prophage lambda by chlorinated pesticides. *Mutat. Res.*, **182**, 193–201

Høyer, A.P., Grandjean, P., Jorgensen, T., Brock, J.W. & Hartvig, H.B. (1998) Organochlorine exposure and risk of breast cancer. *Lancet*, **352**, 1816–1820

IARC (1979) *IARC Monographs on the Evaluation of the Carcinogenic Risk of Chemicals to Humans*, Vol. 20, *Some Halogenated Hydrocarbons*, Lyon, IARCPress, pp. 45–65, 129–154

IARC (1987) *IARC Monographs on the Evaluation of Carcinogenic Risks to Humans*, Suppl. 7, *Overall Evaluations of Carcinogenicity: An Updating of* IARC Monographs *Volumes 1 to 42*, Lyon, IARCPress, pp. 146–148

IARC (1991) *IARC Monographs on the Evaluation of Carcinogenic Risks to Humans*, Vol. 53, *Occupational Exposures in Insecticide Application, and Some Pesticides*, Lyon, IARC*Press*, pp. 115–175

Infante, P.F. & Freeman, C. (1987) Cancer mortality among workers exposed to chlordane (Letter to the Editor). *J. occup. Med.*, **29**, 908–909

Infante, P.F., Epstein, S.S. & Newton, W.A., Jr (1978) Blood dyscrasias and childhood tumors and exposure to chlordane and heptachlor. *Scand. J. Work Environ. Health*, **4**, 137–150

Izmerov, N.F., ed. (1982) *International Register of Potentially Toxic Chemicals. Scientific Reviews of Soviet Literature on Toxicity and Hazards of Chemicals: Heptachlor* (Issue 3), Moscow, Centre of International Projects, United Nations Environment Programme

Izushi, F. & Ogata, M. (1990) Hepatic and muscle injuries in mice treated with heptachlor. *Toxicol. Lett.*, **54**, 47–54

Johnson, K.W., Holsapple, M.P. & Munson, A.E. (1986) An immunotoxicological evaluation of gamma-chlordane. *Fundam. appl. Toxicol.*, **6**, 317–326

Kamble, S.T., Ogg, C.L., Gold, R.E. & Vance, A.D. (1992) Exposure of applicators and residents to chlordane and heptachlor when used for subterranean termite control. *Arch. environ. Contam. Toxicol.*, **22**, 253–259

Kan, C.A. & Tuinstra, L.G.M.T. (1976) Accumulation and excretion of certain organochlorine insecticides in broiler breeder hens. *J. agric. Food Chem.*, **24**, 775–778

Kauppinen, T. (1986) Occupational exposure to chemical agents in the plywood industry. *Ann. occup. Hyg.*, **30**, 19–29

Khasawinah, A.M. & Grutsch, J.F. (1989a) Chlordane: Thirty-month tumorigenicity and chronic toxicity test in rats. *Regul. Toxicol. Pharmacol.*, **10**, 95–109

Khasawinah, A.M. & Grutsch, J.F. (1989b) Chlordane: 24-month tumorigenicity and chronic toxicity test in mice. *Regul. Toxicol. Pharmacol.*, **10**, 244–254

Khasawinah, A.M., Hardy, C.J. & Clark, G.C. (1989) Comparative inhalation toxicity of technical chlordane in rats and monkeys. *J. Toxicol. environ. Health*, **28**, 327–347

Klein, W., Korte, F., Weisgerber, I., Kaul, R., Mueller, W. & Djirsarai, A. (1968) [The metabolism of endrin, heptachlor and telodrin.] *Qual. Plant Mater. Veg.*, **15**, 225–238 (in German)

Kurata, M., Hirose, K. & Umeda, M. (1982) Inhibition of metabolic cooperation in Chinese hamster cells by organochlorine pesticides. *Jpn. J. Cancer Res. (Gann)*, **73**, 217–221

Kutz, F.W., Strassman, S.C., Sperling, J.F., Cook, B.T., Sunshine, I. & Tessari, J. (1983) A fatal chlordane poisoning. *J. Toxicol. clin. Toxicol.*, **20**, 167–174

Lee, S.-R. (1982) [Overall assessment of organochlorine insecticide residues in Korean foods.] *Korean J. Food Sci. Technol.*, **14**, 82–93 (in Korean)

Lehman, A.J. (1952) Chemicals in foods: A report to the Association of Food and Drug Officials on current developments. Part II. Pesticides. Section III: Subacute and chronic toxicity. *Q. Bull. Assoc. Food Drug Off. US*, **16**, 47–53

Le Marchand, L., Kolonel, L.N., Siegel, B.Z. & Dendle, W.H., III (1986) Trends in birth defects for a Hawaiian population exposed to heptachlor and for the United States. *Arch. environ. Health*, **41**, 145–148

MacMahon, B., Monson, R.R., Wang, H.H. & Zheng, T. (1988) A second follow-up of mortality in a cohort of pesticide applicators. *J. occup. Med.*, **30**, 429–432

Malarkey, D.E., Devereux, T.R., Dinse, G.E., Mann, P.C. & Maronpot, R.R. (1995) Hepato-carcinogenicity of chlordane in B6C3F1 and B6D2F1 male mice: Evidence for regression in B6C3F1 mice and carcinogenesis independent of *ras* proto-oncogene activation. *Carcinogenesis*, **16**, 2617–2625

Marshall, T.C., Dorough, H.W. & Swim, H.E. (1976) Screening of pesticides for mutagenic potential using *Salmonella typhimurium* mutants. *J. agric. Food Chem.*, **24**, 560–563

Maslansky, C.J. & Williams, G.M. (1981) Evidence for an epigenetic mode of action in organo-chlorine pesticide hepatocarcinogenicity: A lack of genotoxicity in rat, mouse and hamster hepatocytes. *J. Toxicol. environ. Health*, **8**, 121–130

Matesic, D.F., Rupp, H.L., Bonney, W.J., Ruch, R.J. & Trosko, J.E. (1994) Changes in gap-junction permeability, phosphorylation, and number mediated by phorbol ester and non-phorbol-ester tumor promoters in rat liver epithelial cells. *Mol. Carcinog.*, **10**, 226–236

Matsui, S., Yamamoto, R. & Yamada, H. (1989) The *Bacillus subtilis*/microsome rec-assay for the detection of DNA damaging substances which may occur in chlorinated and ozonated waters. *Water Sci. Technol.*, **21**, 875–887

Matsumura, F. & Nelson, J.O. (1971) Identification of the major metabolic product of hepta-chlor epoxide in rat feces. *Bull. environ. Contam. Toxicol.*, **5**, 489–492

McGregor, D.B., Brown, A., Cattanach, R., Edwards, I., McBride, D., Riach, C. & Caspary, W.J. (1988) Responses of the L5178Y tk$^+$/tk$^-$ mouse lymphoma cell forward mutation assay: III. 72 coded chemicals. *Environ. mol. Mutag.*, **12**, 85–154

Meguro, T., Izushi, F. & Ogata, M. (1990) Effect of heptachlor on hepatic mitochondrial oxi-dative phosphorylation in rat. *Ind. Health*, **28**, 151–157

Menconi, S., Clark, J.M., Langenberg, P. & Hryhorczuk, D. (1988) A preliminary study of potential human health effects in private residences following chlordane applications for termite control. *Arch. environ. Health*, **43**, 349–352

Menna, J.H., Barnett, J.B. & Soderberg, L.S.F. (1985) Influenza type A virus infection of mice exposed in utero to chlordane: Survival and antibody studies. *Toxicol. Lett.*, **24**, 45–52

Mersch-Sundermann, V., Dickgiesser, N., Hablizel, U. & Gruber, B. (1988) [Examination of the mutagenicity of organic microcontaminants on the environment. I. The mutagenicity of selected herbicides and insecticides in the *Salmonella* microsome test (Ames test) in relation to the pathogenetic potency of contaminated ground- and drinking-water.] *Zbl. Bakt. Mikrobiol. Hyg B.*, **186**, 247–260 (in German)

Miranda, C.L., Webb, R.E. & Ritchey, S.J. (1973) Effect of dietary protein quality, phenobarbital and SKF 525-A on heptachlor metabolism in the rat. *Pestic. Biochem. Physiol.*, **3**, 456–461

Miyagi, T., Lam, K.M., Chuang, L.F. & Chuang, R.Y. (1998) Suppression of chemokine-induced chemotaxis of monkey neutrophils and monocytes by chlorinated hydrocarbon insecticides. *In Vivo*, **12**, 441–446

Miyazaki, T., Yamagishi, T. & Matsumoto, M. (1985) Isolation and structure elucidation of some components in technical grade chlordane. *Arch. environ. Contam. Toxicol.*, **14**, 475–483

Moriya, M., Ohta, T., Watanabe, K., Miyazawa, T., Kato, K. & Shirasu, Y. (1983) Further muta-genicity studies on pesticides in bacterial reversion assay systems. *Mutat. Res.*, **116**, 185–216

Mortelmans, K., Haworth, S., Lawlor, T., Speck, W., Tainer, B. & Zeiger, E. (1986) Salmonella mutagenicity tests: II. Results from the testing of 270 chemicals. *Environ. Mutag.*, **8** (Suppl. 7), 1–119

Moser, G.J. & Smart, R.C. (1989) Hepatic tumor-promoting chlorinated hydrocarbons stimulate protein kinase C activity. *Carcinogenesis*, **10**, 851–856

Moser, G.J., Robinette, C.L. & Smart, R.C. (1993) Characterization of skin tumor promotion by mirex: Structure–activity relationships, sexual dimorphism and presence of Ha-*ras* mutation. *Carcinogenesis*, **14**, 1155–1160

Moser, V.C., Cheek, B.M. & MacPhail, R.C. (1995) A multidisciplinary approach to toxicological screening: III. Neurobehavioral toxicity. *J. Toxicol. environ. Health*, **45**, 173–210

Moser, G.J., Wolf, D.C. & Goldsworthy, T.L. (1997) Quantitative relationship between transforming growth factor-alpha and hepatic focal phenotype and progression in female mouse liver. *Toxicol. Pathol.*, **25**, 275–283

Mussalo-Rauhamaa, H., Pyysalo, H. & Antervo, K. (1991) Heptachlor, heptachlor epoxide, and other chlordane compounds in Finnish plywood workers. *Arch. environ. Health*, **46**, 340–346

Narotsky, M.G. & Kavlock, R.J. (1995) A multidisciplinary approach to toxicological screening: II. Developmental toxicity. *J. Toxicol. environ. Health*, **45**, 145–171

Narotsky, M.G., Weller, E.A., Chinchilli, V.M. & Kavlock, R.J. (1995) Nonadditive developmental toxicity in mixtures in trichloroethylene, di(2-ethylhexyl) phthalate, and heptachlor in a 5 × 5 × 5 design. *Fundam. appl. Toxicol.*, **27**, 203–216

National Academy of Sciences (1977) *An Evaluation of the Carcinogenicity of Chlordane and Heptachlor*, Washington DC

National Cancer Institute (1977a) *Bioassay of Heptachlor for Possible Carcinogenicity* (Technical Report Series No. 9; DHEW Publ. No. (NIH) 77-809), Washington DC, Department of Health, Education, and Welfare

National Cancer Institute (1977b) *Bioassay of Chlordane for Possible Carcinogenicity* (Technical Report Series No. 8; DHEW Publ. No. (NIH) 77-808), Washington DC, Department of Health, Education, and Welfare

National Institute for Occupational Safety and Health (2000) *National Occupational Exposure Survey 1981–83*, Cincinnati, OH, Department of Health and Human Services, Public Health Service

Nelson, B.D. (1975) The action of cyclodiene pesticides on oxidative phosphorylation in rat liver mitochondria. *Biochem. Pharmacol.*, **24**, 1–19

Newsome, W.H. & Ryan, J.J. (1999) Toxaphene and other chlorinated compounds in human milk from northern and southern Canada: A comparison. *Chemosphere*, **39**, 519–526

Nomata, K., Kang, K.-S., Hayashi, T., Matesic, D., Lockwood, L., Chang, C.C. & Trosko, J.E. (1996) Inhibition of gap junctional intercellular communication in heptachlor- and heptachlor epoxide-treated normal human breast epithelial cells. *Cell Biol. Toxicol.*, **12**, 69–78

Nomeir, A.A. & Hajjar, N.P. (1987) Metabolism of chlordane in mammals. *Rev. environ. Contam. Toxicol.*, **100**, 1–22

Nordström, M., Hardell, L., Lindstrom, G., Wingfors, H., Hardell, K. & Linde, A. (2000) Concentrations of organochlorines related to titers to Epstein-Barr virus early antigen IgG as risk factors for hairy cell leukemia. *Environ. Health Perspectives*, **108**, 441–445

Nye, D.E. & Dorough, H.W. (1976) Fate of insecticides administered endotracheally to rats. *Bull. environ. Contam. Toxicol.*, **15**, 291–296

Oduma, J.A., Wango, E.O., Oduor-Okelo, D., Makawiti, D.W. & Odonog, H. (1995) In vivo and in vitro effects of degraded doses of the pesticide heptachlor on female sex steroid hormone production in rats. *Comp. Biochem. Physiol.*, **111C**, 191–196

Ogata, M. & Izushi, F. (1991) Effects of chlordane on parameters of liver and muscle toxicity in man and experimental animals. *Toxicol. Lett.*, **56**, 327–337

Okey, A.B. (1990) Enzyme induction in the cytochrome P-450 system. *Pharmacol. Ther.*, **45**, 241–298

Olanoff, L.S., Bristow, W.J., Colcolough, J., Jr & Reigart, J.R. (1983) Acute chlordane intoxication. *J. Toxicol clin. Toxicol.*, **20**, 291–306

Peirano, W.B. (1980) *Heptachlor — Maximum Acceptable Limit in Drinking Water*, Washington DC, Environmental Protection Agency

Pelikan, Z., Halacka, K., Polster, M. & Cerny, E. (1968) [Long-term intoxication of rats by small doses of heptachlor.] *Arch. belg. Méd. traum. Méd. Ig.*, **26**, 529–538 (in French)

Pesatori, A.C., Sontag, J.M., Lubin, J.H., Consonni, D. & Blair, A. (1994) Cohort mortality and nested case–control study of lung cancer among structural pest control workers in Florida (United States). *Cancer Causes Control*, **5**, 310–318

Princi, F. & Spurbeck, G.H. (1951) A study of workers exposed to the insecticides chlordane, aldrin, dieldrin. *Arch. ind. Hyg. occup. Med.*, **3**, 64–72

Probst, G.S., McMahon, R.E., Hill, L.E., Thompson, C.Z., Epp, J.K. & Neal, S.B. (1981) Chemically-induced unscheduled DNA synthesis in primary rat hepatocyte cultures: A comparison with bacterial mutagenicity using 218 compounds. *Environ. Mutag.*, **3**, 11–32

Public Health Service (1989a) *Agency for Toxic Substances and Disease Registry Toxicological Profile for Heptachlor/Heptachlor Epoxide* (Report No. ATSDR/TP-88/16; NTIS PB 89-194492), Washington DC

Public Health Service (1989b) *Agency for Toxic Substances and Disease Registry Toxicological Profile for Chlordane* (Report No. ATSDR/TP-89/06; NTIS PB90-168709), Washington DC

Radomski, J.L. & Davidow, B. (1953) The metabolite of heptachlor, its estimation, storage and toxicity. *J. Pharmacol. exp. Ther.*, **107**, 266–272

Rashid, K.A. & Mumma, R.O. (1986) Screening pesticides for their ability to damage bacterial DNA. *J. environ. Sci. Health*, **B21**, 319–334

Raw, G.R., ed. (1970) *CIPAC Handbook*, Vol. 1, Cambridge, Collaborative International Pesticides Analytical Council, pp. 420–427

Ray, S., Bailey, M., Paterson, G., Metcalfe, T. & Metcalfe, C. (1998) Comparative levels of organochlorine compounds in flounders from the northeast coast of Newfoundland and an offshore site. *Chemosphere*, **36**, 2201–2210

Rogan, W.J., Blanton, P.J., Portier, C.J. & Stallard, E. (1991) Should the presence of carcinogens in breast milk discourage breast feeding? *Regul. Toxicol. Pharmacol.*, **13**, 228–240

Rostad, C.E. (1997) Concentration and transport of chlordane and nonachlor associated with suspended sediment in the Mississippi River, May 1988 to June 1990. *Arch. environ. Contam. Toxicol.*, **33**, 369–377

Rought, S.E., Yau, P.M., Schnier, J.B., Chuang, L.F. & Chuang, R.Y. (1998) The effect of heptachlor, a chlorinated hydrocarbon insecticide, on p53 tumor suppressor in human lymphocytes. *Toxicol. Lett.*, **94**, 29–36

Rought, S.E., Yau, P.M., Chuang, L.F., Doi, R.H. & Chuang, R.Y. (1999) Effect of the chlorinated hydrocarbons heptachlor, chlordane, and toxaphene on retinoblastoma tumor suppressor in human lymphocytes. *Toxicol. Lett.*, **104**, 127–135

Royal Society of Chemistry (1986) *European Directory of Agrochemical Products*, Vol. 3, *Insecticides, Acaricides, Nematicides*, Cambridge, pp. 112, 331–332

Royal Society of Chemistry (1989) *The Agrochemicals Handbook* [Dialog Information Services (File 306)], Cambridge

Ruch, R.J., Fransson, R., Flodstrom, S., Warngard, L. & Klaunig, J.E. (1990) Inhibition of hepatocyte gap junctional intercellular communication by endosulfan, chlordane and heptachlor. *Carcinogenesis*, **11**, 1097–1101

Sadtler Research Laboratories (1980) *The Standard Spectra, 1980, Cumulative Molecular Formula Index*, Philadelphia, PA, p. 354

Sadtler Research Laboratories (1990) *The Sadtler Standard Spectra, 1981–1990, Supplementary Index*, Philadelphia, PA

Saito, I., Kawamura, N., Uno, K., Hisanaga, N., Takeuchi, Y., Ono, Y., Iwata, M., Gotoh, M., Okutani, H., Matsumoto, T., Fukaya, Y., Yoshitomi, S. & Ohno, Y. (1986) Relationship between chlordane and its metabolites in blood of pest control operators and spraying conditions. *Int. Arch. occup. environ. Health*, **58**, 91–97

Sarkar, D., Sharma, A. & Talukder, G. (1993) Differential protection of chlorophyllin against clastogenic effects of chromium and chlordane in mouse bone marrow in vivo. *Mutat. Res.*, **301**, 33–38

Savela, A., Vuorela, R. & Kauppinen, T. (1999) *ASA 1997* (Katsauksia 140), Helsinki, Finnish Institute of Occupational Health, p. 30 (in Finnish)

Schmitt, C.J., Zajicek, J.L., May, T.W. & Cowman, D.F. (1999) Organochlorine residues and elemental contaminants in US freshwater fish, 1976–1986: National contaminant biomonitoring program. *Rev. environ. Contam. Toxicol.*, **162**, 43–104

Schop, R.N., Hardy, M.H. & Goldberg, M.T. (1990) Comparison of the activity of topically applied pesticides and the herbicide 2,4-D in two short-term in vivo assays of genotoxicity in the mouse. *Fundam. appl. Toxicol.*, **15**, 666–675

Schuetz, E.G., Brimer, C. & Schuetz, J.D. (1998) Environmental xenobiotics and the anti-hormones cyproterone acetate and spironolactone use the nuclear hormone pregnenolone X receptor to activate the *CYP3A23* hormone response element. *Mol. Pharmacol.*, **54**, 1113–1117

Shindell, S. (1987) Cancer mortality among workers exposed to chlordane (Reply to a letter to the Editor). *J. occup. Med.*, **29**, 909–911

Shindell, S. & Ulrich, S. (1986) Mortality of workers employed in the manufacture of chlordane: An update. *J. occup. Med.*, **28**, 497–501

Simmon, V.F., Kauhanen, K. & Tardiff, R.G. (1977) Mutagenic activity of chemicals identified in drinking water. *Dev. Toxicol. environ. Sci.*, **2**, 249–258

Sittig, M., ed. (1980) *Pesticide Manufacturing and Toxic Materials Control Encyclopedia*, Park Ridge, NJ, Noyes Data Corp., pp. 445–448

Sobti, R.C., Krishan, A. & Davies, J. (1983) Cytokinetic and cytogenetic effect of agricultural chemicals on human lymphoid cells in vitro. II. Organochlorine pesticides. *Arch. Toxicol.*, **52**, 221–231

Sovocool, G.W. & Lewis, R.G. (1975) The identification of trace levels of organic pollutants in human tissues: Compounds related to chlordane/heptachlor exposure. *Trace Subst. environ. Health*, **9**, 265–280

Sovocool, G.W., Lewis, R.G., Harless, R.L., Wilson, N.K. & Zehr, R.D. (1977) Analysis of technical chlordane by gas chromatography/mass spectrometry. *Anal. Chem.*, **49**, 734–740

Sperling, F. & Ewinike, H. (1969) Changes in LD_{50} of parathion and heptachlor after turpentine pretreatment (Abstract No. 24). *Toxicol. appl. Pharmacol.*, **14**, 622

Spyker-Cranmer, J.M., Barnett, J.B., Avery, D.L. & Cranmer, M.F. (1982) Immunoteratology of chlordane: Cell-mediated and humoral immune responses in adult mice exposed in utero. *Toxicol. appl. Pharmacol.*, **62**, 402–408

Stehr-Green, P.A., Schilling, R.J., Burse, V.W., Steinberg, K.K., Royce, W., Wohlleb, J.C. & Donnell, H.D. (1986) Evaluation of persons exposed to dairy products contaminated with heptachlor (Letter to the Editor). *J. Am. med. Assoc.*, **256**, 3350–3351

Taguchi, S. & Yakushiji, T. (1988) Influence of termite treatment in the home on the chlordane concentration in human milk. *Arch. environ. Contam. Toxicol.*, **17**, 65–71

Takamiya, K. (1987) Residual levels of plasma oxychlordane and *trans*-nonachlor in pest control operators and some characteristics of these accumulations. *Bull. environ. Contam. Toxicol.*, **39**, 750–755

Tashiro, S. & Matsumura, F. (1977) Metabolic routes of *cis*- and *trans*-chlordane in rats. *J. agric. Food Chem.*, **25**, 872–880

Tashiro, S. & Matsumura, F. (1978) Metabolism of trans-nonachlor and related chlordane components in rat and man. *Arch. environ. Contam. Toxicol.*, **7**, 113–127

Telang, S., Tong, C. & Williams, G.M. (1982) Epigenetic membrane effects of a possible tumor promoting type on cultured liver cells by the non-genotoxic organochlorine pesticides chlordane and heptachlor. *Carcinogenesis*, **3**, 1175–1178

Teufel, M., Niessen, K.H., Sartoris, J., Brands, W., Lochbühler, H., Waag, K., Schweizer, P. & von Oelsnitz, G. (1990) Chlorinated hydrocarbons in fat tissue: Analyses of residues in healthy children, tumor patients, and malformed children. *Arch. environ. Contam. Toxicol.*, **19**, 646–652

Theus, S.A., Lau, K.A., Tabor, D.R., Soderberg, L.S. & Barnett, J.B. (1992) In vivo prenatal chlordane exposure induces development of endogenous inflammatory macrophages. *J. Leukocyte Biol.*, **51**, 366–372

Tomlin, C.D.S., ed. (1999) *The e-Pesticide Manual — A World Compendium*, 11th Ed., Version 1.1, Farnham, British Crop Protection Council

Tong, C., Fazio, M. & Williams, G.M. (1981) Rat hepatocyte-mediated mutagenesis of human cells by carcinogenic polycyclic aromatic hydrocarbons but not organochlorine pesticides. *Proc. Soc. exp. Biol. Med.*, **167**, 572–575

Tsushimoto, G., Chang, C.C., Trosko, J.E. & Matsumura, F. (1983) Cytotoxic, mutagenic, and cell–cell communication inhibitory properties of DDT, lindane and chlordane on Chinese hamster cells *in vitro. Arch. environ. Contam. Toxicol.*, **12**, 721–730

Urieta, I., Jalón, M. & Eguileor, I. (1996) Food surveillance in the Basque country (Spain). II. Estimation of the dietary intake of organochlorine pesticides, heavy metals, arsenic, aflatoxin M_1, iron and zinc through the total diet study, 1990/91. *Food Addit. Contam.*, **13**, 29–52

Van Oostdam, J., Gilman, A., Dewailly, E., Usher, P., Wheatley, B., Kuhnlein, H., Neve, S., Walker, J., Tracy, B., Feeley, M., Jerome, V. & Kwavnick, B. (1999) Human health implications of environmental contaminants in Arctic Canada: A review. *Sci. total Environ.*, **230**, 1–82

Venkat, J.A., Shami, S., Davis, K., Nayak, M., Plimmer, J.R., Pfeil, R. & Nair, P.P. (1995) Relative genotoxic activities of pesticides evaluated by a modified SOS microplate assay. *Environ. mol. Mutag.*, **25**, 67–76

Vigfusson, N.V, Vyse, E.R., Pernsteiner, C.A. & Dawson, R.J. (1983) In vivo induction of sister-chromatid exchange in *Umbra limi* by the insecticides endrin, chlordane, diazinon and guthion. *Mutat. Res.*, **118**, 61–68

Wade, T.L., Chambers, L., Gardinall, P.R., Sericano, J.L. & Jackson, T.J. (1997) Toxaphene, PCB, DDT, and chlordane analyses of beluga whale blubber. *Chemosphere*, **34**, 1351–1357

Wang, H.H. & MacMahon, B. (1979a) Mortality of workers employed in the manufacture of chlordane and heptachlor. *J. occup. Med.*, **21**, 745–748

Wang, H.H. & MacMahon, B. (1979b) Mortality of pesticide applicators. *J. occup. Med.*, **21**, 741–744

Wango, E.O., Onyango, D.W., Odongo, H., Okindo, E. & Mugweru, J. (1997) In vitro production of testosterone and plasma levels of luteinising hormone, testosterone and cortisol in male rats treated with heptachlor. *Comp. Biochem. Physiol.*, **118C**, 381–386

Wassermann, M., Tomatis, L., Wassermann, D., Day, N.E., Groner, Y., Lazarovici, S. & Rosenfeld, D. (1974) Epidemiology of organochlorine insecticides in the adipose tissue of Israelis. *Pestic. Monit. J.*, **8**, 1–7

Weiderpass, E., Adami, H.O., Baron, J.A., Wicklund-Glynn, A., Aune, M., Atuma, S. & Persson, I. (2000) Organochlorines and endometrial cancer risk. *Cancer Epidemiol. Biomarkers Prev.*, **9**, 487–493

Welch, R.M., Levin, W., Kuntzman, R., Jacobson, M. & Conney, A.H. (1971) Effect of halogenated hydrocarbon insecticides on the metabolism and uterotropic action of estrogens in rats and mice. *Toxicol appl. Pharmacol.*, **19**, 234–246

WHO (1984a) *Chlordane* (Environmental Health Criteria 34), Geneva

WHO (1984b) *Heptachlor* (Environmental Health Criteria 38), Geneva

WHO (1988a) *Chlordane Health and Safety Guide* (Health and Safety Guide No. 13), Geneva

WHO (1988b) *Heptachlor Health and Safety Guide* (Health and Safety Guide No. 14), Geneva

WHO (1993) *Guidelines for Drinking-water Quality*, 2nd Ed., Vol. 1, *Recommendations*, Geneva

WHO (1999) *Inventory of IPCS and Other WHO Pesticide Evaluations and Summary of Toxicological Evaluations Performed by the Joint Meeting on Pesticide Residues [JMPR] through 1999*, 3rd Ed., Geneva, International Programme on Chemical Safety

Whysner, J., Montandon, F., McClain, R.M., Downing, J., Verna, L.K., Steward, R.E. & Williams, G.M. (1998) Absence of DNA adduct formation by phenobarbital, polychlorinated biphenyls, and chlordane in mouse liver using the ^{32}P-postlabeling assay. *Toxicol. appl. Pharmacol.*, **148**, 14–23

Williams, S., ed. (1984a) *Official Methods of Analysis of the Association of Official Analytical Chemists*, 14th Ed., Washington DC, Association of Official Analytical Chemists, pp. 111–113

Williams, S., ed. (1984b) *Official Methods of Analysis of the Association of Official Analytical Chemists*, 14th Ed., Washington DC, Association of Official Analytical Chemists, pp. 533–543

Williams, G.M. & Numoto, S. (1984) Promotion of mouse liver neoplasms by the organo-chlorine pesticides chlordane and heptachlor in comparison to dichlorodiphenyltrichloro-ethane. *Carcinogenesis*, **5**, 1689–1696

Williams, G.M., Mori, H. & McQueen, C.A. (1989) Structure–activity relationships in the rat hepatocyte DNA-repair test for 300 chemicals. *Mutat. Res.*, **221**, 263–286

Woods, J.S. & Polissar, L. (1989) Non-Hodgkin's lymphoma among phenoxy herbicide-exposed farm workers in western Washington State. *Chemosphere*, **18**, 401–406

Woods, J.S., Polissar, L., Severson, R.K., Heuser, L.S. & Kulander, B.G. (1987) Soft tissue sarcoma and non-Hodgkin's lymphoma in relation to phenoxyherbicide and chlorinated phenol exposure in western Washington. *J. natl Cancer Inst.*, **78**, 899–910

Worthing, C.R. & Walker, S.B., eds (1987) *The Pesticide Manual — A World Compendium*, 8th Ed., Thornton Heath, British Crop Protection Council, pp. 145–146, 455–456

Yang, C. & Chen, S. (1999) Two organochlorine pesticides, toxaphene and chlordane, are anta-gonists for estrogen-related receptor alpha-1 orphan receptor. *Cancer Res.*, **59**, 4519–4524

Zeiger, E., Anderson, B., Haworth, S., Lawlor, T., Mortelmans, K. & Speck, W. (1987) *Salmo-nella* mutagenicity tests: III. Results from the testing of 255 chemicals. *Environ. Mutag.*, **9** (Suppl. 9), 1–110

Zheng, T., Holford, T.R., Tessari, J., Mayne, S.T., Hoar Zahm, S., Owens, P.H., Zhang, B., Ward, B., Carter, D., Zhang, Y., Zhang, W., Dubrow, R. & Boyle, P. (2000) Oxychlordane and trans-nonachlor in breast adipose tissue and risk of female breast cancer. *J. Epidemiol. Biostat.*, **5**, 153–160

HEXACHLOROBENZENE

This substance was considered by previous working groups, in 1978 (IARC, 1979) and 1986 (IARC, 1987). Since that time, new data have become available, and these have been incorporated into the monograph and taken into consideration in the present evaluation.

1. Exposure Data

1.1 Chemical and physical data

1.1.1 *Nomenclature*

Chem. Abstr. Serv. Reg. No.: 118-74-1
Chem. Abstr. Name: Hexachlorobenzene
IUPAC Systematic Name: Hexachlorobenzene
Synonyms: HCB; pentachlorophenyl chloride; perchlorobenzene

1.1.2 *Structural and molecular formulae and relative molecular mass*

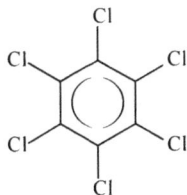

C_6Cl_6 Relative molecular mass: 284.78

1.1.3 *Chemical and physical properties of the pure substance*

(*a*) *Description*: White needles (Lide & Milne, 1996; WHO, 1997; Budavari, 2000)
(*b*) *Boiling-point*: 325 °C (Lide & Milne, 1996)
(*c*) *Melting-point*: 231.8 °C (Lide & Milne, 1996)

(*d*) *Spectroscopy data*: Infrared [prism (4545), grating (410)], ultraviolet and mass spectral data have been reported (Sadtler Research Laboratories, 1980; Lide & Milne, 1996).

(*e*) *Solubility*: Practically insoluble in water (5×10^{-6} g/L at 25 °C); very soluble in benzene; soluble in chloroform and diethyl ether; slightly soluble in ethanol (Lide & Milne, 1996; WHO, 1997)

(*f*) *Volatility*: Vapour pressure, 1.09×10^{-5} mm Hg [1.45 mPa] at 20 °C (Budavari, 2000)

(*g*) *Stability*: Flash-point, 242 °C (Budavari, 2000)

(*h*) *Octanol/water partition coefficient (P)*: log P, 5.5 (WHO, 1997)

1.1.4 *Technical products and impurities*

Technical-grade hexachlorobenzene was commercially available in the past as a wettable powder, liquid and dust. It was reported to contain about 98% hexachlorobenzene, 1.8% pentachlorobenzene and 0.2% 1,2,4,5-tetrachlorobenzene in the USA (IARC, 1979). Several other impurities have been detected, including hepta- and octa-chlorodibenzofurans, octachlorodibenzo-*para*-dioxin and decachlorobiphenyl (WHO, 1997).

Trade names for hexachlorobenzene include Amatin, Anticarie, Bunt-Cure, Bunt-No-More, Co-op Hexa Granox NM, HexaCB, Julin's Carbon Chloride, No Bunt, Sanocide, Smut-Go and Snieciotox.

1.1.5 *Analysis*

Methods for the analysis of hexachlorobenzene in various matrices are summarized in Table 1.

1.2 Production

Industrial synthesis of hexachlorobenzene involves the chlorination of benzene at 150–200 °C with a ferric chloride catalyst or distillation of residues from the production of tetrachloroethylene (WHO, 1997).

Few recent data on the quantities of hexachlorobenzene produced are available. Worldwide production of pure hexachlorobenzene was estimated to be 10 000 t/year for the years 1978–81. Hexachlorobenzene was produced or imported in the European Community at 8000 t/year in 1978, and a company in Spain reportedly produced an estimated 150 t/year. Approximately 1500 t/year of hexachlorobenzene were manufactured in Germany for the production of rubber chemicals, but this production was discontinued in 1993. Intentional production of hexachlorobenzene has declined as a result of restrictions on its use since the 1970s, but it may still be produced as an incidental by-product in some processes (see section 1.4) (WHO, 1997).

Table 1. Methods for analysis of hexachlorobenzene

Sample matrix	Sample preparation	Assay procedure	Limit of detection	Reference
Air	Trap on glass-fibre filter and XAD-2; extract with toluene	HRGC/ LRMS	0.18 pg/m^3	Hippelein *et al.* (1993)
	Adsorb on polyurethane foam; extract with diethyl ether in hexane	GC/ECD	< 0.1 μg/m^3	Lewis & MacLeod (1982)
	Adsorb on polyurethane foam; extract with hexane; fractionate by HPLC	GC/ECD	Low pg/m^3 range	Oehme & Stray (1982)
	Adsorb on polyurethane foam or Tenax-GC resin; reflux with dichloromethane; reflux with hexane; clean-up by alumina chromatography	GC/ECD	NR	Billings & Bidleman (1980)
	Adsorb on Amberlite XAD-2; desorb with carbon tetrachloride	GC/PID	0.815 mg/m^3	Langhorst & Nestrick (1979)
	Collect vapours on polyurethane foam; extract with 5–10% diethyl ether in hexane	GC/ECD	NR	Environmental Protection Agency (1999a,b) [Methods TO-04A, TO-10A]
	Collect on polyurethane foam; Soxhlet extraction; concentrate	GC/ECD or GC/ECD and GC/MS	5 ng/m^3	Hsu *et al.* (1988)
Water	Extract with hexane; inject extract	GC/ECD	0.002 μg/L	Environmental Protection Agency (1995a) [Method 505]
	Extract with dichloromethane; isolate extract; dry; concentrate with methyl *tert*-butyl ether (capillary column)	GC/ECD	0.001 μg/L	Environmental Protection Agency (1995b) [Method 508.1]
	Extract by passing sample through liquid–solid extractor; elute with dichloromethane; concentrate by evaporation (capillary column)	GC/MS	0.049–0.13 μg/L[a]	Environmental Protection Agency (1995c) [Method 525.2]

Table 1 (contd)

Sample matrix	Sample preparation	Assay procedure	Limit of detection	Reference
Water (contd)	Extract with methyl *tert*-butyl ether or pentane	GC/ECD	0.001 µg/L	Environmental Protection Agency (1995d) [Method 551.1]
	Strip from water with stream of air; adsorb on activated carbon filter; extract with carbon disulfide or dichloromethane	GC/MS or GC/FID	0.001 µg/L	APHA/AWWA/ WEF (1999a) [Method 6040B]
	Adjust pH; concentrate on XAD-4; clean-up on silica gel	GC/MS	0.1 µg/L	Garrison & Pellizzari (1987)
Ground-water	Solvent extraction; solvent exchange	GC/ECD	0.12 µg/L	Munch *et al.* (1990) [National Pesticide Survey Method 2]
River water	Centrifuge; digest with chromic acid; extract	GC/ECD	NR	Driscoll *et al.* (1991)
Soil, chemical waste samples	Extract with hexane	GC/ECD	10 mg/kg	DeLeon *et al.* (1980)
Municipal & industrial discharges	Extract with dichloromethane; dry; exchange to hexane; concentrate	GC/ECD	0.05 µg/L	Environmental Protection Agency (1999c) [Method 612]
	Extract with dichloromethane; dry; concentrate (packed column)	GC/MS	1.9 µg/L	Environmental Protection Agency (1999d) [Method 625]
	Adjust to pH 11; extract with dichloromethane; dry; concentrate	GC/MS	1.9 µg/L	APHA/AWWA/ WEF (1999b) [Method 6410B]
	Add isotope-labelled analogue; extract with dichloromethane; dry over sodium sulfate; concentrate	GC/MS	10 µg/L	Environmental Protection Agency (1999e) [Method 1625]
Liquid & solid waste	Extract with dichloromethane (liquid); hexane:acetone (1:1) or dichloromethane:acetone (1:1) (solid); clean-up	GC/ECD	NR	Environmental Protection Agency (1996a) [Method 8081A]

Table 1 (contd)

Sample matrix	Sample preparation	Assay procedure	Limit of detection	Reference
Soil, waste & water	Extract with dichloromethane (liquid); dichloromethane:acetone (1:1) (solid); clean-up	GC/ECD	5.6 ng/L (reagent water)	Environmental Protection Agency (1994a) [Method 8121]
Air sampling media, soil, solid waste & water	Liquid–liquid extraction or Soxhlet extraction or ultrasonic extraction or waste dilution or direct injection; clean-up with Florisil or gel-permeation (capillary column)	GC/MS	10 µg/L (aqueous); 660 µg/kg (soil/sediment) (EQL)	Environmental Protection Agency (1996b) [Method 8270C]
Soil, sludge & solid waste	Thermal extraction; concentrate; thermal desorption	TE/GC/MS	0.01–0.5 mg/kg	Environmental Protection Agency (1996c) [Method 8275A]
Sediment, soil, solid waste and waste-water	Liquid–liquid extraction (water); Soxhlet or ultrasonic extraction (sediment, soil or waste)	GC/FT-IR	20 µg/L	Environmental Protection Agency (1994b) [Method 8410]
Soil	Extract with light petroleum; liquid–liquid partition; clean-up with sulfuric acid	GC/ECD	NR	Waliszewski & Szymczynski (1985)
Sediment	Extract with dichloromethane; subject to acid fractionation; subject base or neutral fraction to silica gel chromatography	GC/MS	NR	Lopez-Avila et al. (1983)
	Microwave; extract; centrifuge; filter	GC/ECD	NR	Onuska & Terry (1993)
Fish tissue	Grind with sodium sulfate; extract with hexane:acetone; clean-up on Na_2SO_4:alumina: silica gel:Florisil column followed by a H_2SO_4 column on silica gel	GC/ECD	[~ 0.05 µg/kg]	Oliver & Nicol (1982)
	Extract with hexane:isopropanol; solvent and sulfuric acid partitioning	GC/ECD	NR	Lunde & Ofstad (1976)
	Macerate; Soxhlet extract; clean-up with sulfuric acid:silica gel	GC/ECD	5 µg/kg (lipid basis)	Rahman et al. (1993)

Table 1 (contd)

Sample matrix	Sample preparation	Assay procedure	Limit of detection	Reference
Fish tissue (contd)	Sulfuric acid digestion; silica gel column chromatography; methylation; alumina column chromatography	GC/ECD	10–15 µg/kg	Lamparski *et al.* (1980)
	Homogenize; Soxhlet extract; GPC fractionate; silica gel fractionate	GC/MS	12.5 µg/kg	ATSDR (1998)
Fish, aquatic biota	Homogenize with solvent; solvent exchange; clean-up on Florisil	GC/ECD	50 µg/kg wet weight	Miskiewicz & Gibbs (1994)
Aquatic organisms	Homogenize; Soxhlet extract; GPC fractionate; SPE fractionate; solvent exchange	GC/ECD	NR	Shan *et al.* (1994) [USGS method]
Oyster tissue	Extract with acetone:acetonitrile; partition into petroleum ether; clean-up with silica gel chromatography	GC/ECD	NR	Murray *et al.* (1980)
Adipose tissue (chicken)	Extract with hexane; subject to Florisil clean-up and one-fraction elution	GC/ECD	NR	Watts *et al.* (1980)
Adipose tissue	Extract; GPC clean-up; fractionate on Florisil	GC/MS	12 µg/kg	Stanley (1986)
	Soxhlet extraction; clean-up on Florisil	GC/ECD	1 µg/kg	Alawi & Ababneh (1991)
	Extract with solvent; remove bulk lipid; fractionate on Florisil	HRGC/MS	12 µg/kg	Stanley (1986)
	Extract with benzene:acetone; filter; fractionate on Florisil	GC/ECD	0.12 µg/kg	Mes (1992)
	SFE with alumina (to remove lipids); purify by column chromatography	GC/ECD	10 µg/kg	ATSDR (1998)
	Extract fat; dissolve in hexane; elute with hexane; concentrate	GC/ECD	NR	AOAC International (2000) [Method 980.22]

Table 1 (contd)

Sample matrix	Sample preparation	Assay procedure	Limit of detection	Reference
Fatty foods	SFE/SFC (on-line clean-up)	GC/ECD	4 µg/kg	Nam & King (1994)
	Extraction and pretreat; clean-up on Florisil	GC/ECD; TLC	10 µg/kg	ATSDR (1998) [DFG Method S9]
	Extract fat; partition into acetonitrile:petroleum ether; clean-up on Florisil	GC/ECD or GC/ELCD	NR	Food and Drug Administration (1999) [Method 304]
	Extract fat; clean-up on Florisil; elute with acetonitrile; separate with petroleum ether	GC/ECD	NR	AOAC International (2000) [Method 977.19]
Milk	Solvent extraction; solvent partition; solvent exchange; GPC clean-up; optional alumina clean-up	GC/ECD	0.5 µg/L	Trotter & Dickerson (1993)
Non-fatty foods	Extract with acetone; partition or remove water; clean-up on Florisil; elute with dichloromethane	GC/ECD or GC/ELCD	NR	Food and Drug Administration (1999) [Method 302]
	Extract with acetonitrile or water:acetonitrile; partition into petroleum ether; clean-up on Florisil	GC/ECD or GC/ELCD	NR	Food and Drug Administration (1999) [Method 303]
Vegetable oils, oil seeds	Sandwich-type extraction; fractionate	GC/ECD	0.1–2 µg/kg	Seidel & Linder (1993)
Fruit, vegetables	Chop and blend; blend with solvent; partition with water; dry	GC/ECD, GC/MS	2 µg/kg	Pylypiw (1993)
Crops and foods	Solvent extraction; GPC clean-up; optional silica gel clean-up	GC/ECD	NR	ATSDR(1998) [DFG Method S19]
Urine	Extract with carbon tetrachloride; clean-up on silica gel; concentrate	GC/PID	4.1 µg/L	Langhorst & Nestrick (1979)

Table 1 (contd)

Sample matrix	Sample preparation	Assay procedure	Limit of detection	Reference
Blood	Extract with carbon tetrachloride; clean-up on silica gel; concentrate	GC/PID	16 µg/L	Langhorst & Nestrick (1979)
	Extract with hexane:isopropanol	GC/ECD	NR	Lunde & Bjorseth (1977)
	Extract with hexane; concentrate	GC/ECD	0.016 µg/L	Bristol et al. (1982)
	Homogenize with benzene; filter; fractionate on Florisil	GC/ECD	0.01 µg/L	Mes (1992)
Serum	Extract denatured serum with solvent; fractionate on Florisil; acid treatment and clean-up on silica gel	GC/ECD	1 µg/L	Burse et al. (1990)
Breast milk	Separate fats; column clean-up	GC/ECD	0.4 µg/kg fat	Abraham et al. (1994)
	Extract with acetone:benzene; fractionate on Florisil	GC/ECD	0.033 µg/L	Mes et al. (1993)
Semen	Solvent extraction; clean-up on Florisil; concentrate	GC/ECD	0.3 µg/L	Stachel et al. (1989)
Formulations	Dissolve in toluene or methanol:toluene	GC/FID	NR	AOAC International (2000) [Method 999.04]

APHA/AWWA/WEF, American Public Health Association/American Water Works Association/Water Environment Federation; ATSDR, Agency for Toxic Substances and Disease Registry; USGS, United States Geological Survey; DFG, Deutsche Forschungsgemeinschaft; ECD, electron capture detection; ELCD, electrolytic conductivity detection; GC, gas chromatography; FID, flame ionization detection; FT-IR, Fourier transform infrared spectrometry; GPC, gel permeation chromatography; HPLC, high-performance liquid chromatography; HRGC, high-resolution gas chromatography; LRMS, low-resolution mass spectrometry; MS, mass spectrometry; NR, not reported; PID, photoionization detection; SFC, supercritical fluid chromatography; SFE, supercritical fluid extraction; TE, thermal extraction; TLC, thin-layer chromatography

[a] Limit of detection varies with extraction technique (cartridge or disc) and mass spectrometer (quadrupole or ion trap).

Information available in 2000 indicated that hexachlorobenzene was manu-factured by five companies in China and one company in Argentina (CIS Information Services, 2000).

1.3   Use

In the past, hexachlorobenzene had many uses in industry and agriculture. The major agricultural application was as a seed dressing for crops such as wheat, barley, oats and rye to prevent growth of fungi. The use of hexachlorobenzene in such appli-cations was discontinued in many countries in the 1970s owing to concerns about adverse effects on the environment and human health. Hexachlorobenzene may continue to be used for this purpose in some countries; for example, hexachlorobenzene was still used in 1986 as a fungicide, seed-dressing and scabicide in sheep in Tunisia (Government of Canada, 1993; WHO, 1997).

In industry, hexachlorobenzene has been used directly in the manufacture of pyro-technics, tracer bullets and as a fluxing agent in the manufacture of aluminium. It has also been used as a starting material in the production of pentachlorophenol, a porosity-control agent in the manufacture of graphite anodes, and as a peptizing agent in the production of nitroso and styrene rubber for tyres. It is likely that some or all of these applications have been discontinued (WHO, 1987, 1997).

1.4   Occurrence

Although hexachlorobenzene production has ceased in most countries, it may still be generated as an inadvertent by-product in the manufacture of chlorinated solvents, chlorinated aromatics and chlorinated pesticides. It was estimated in 1986 that approxi-mately 4130 t/year of hexachlorobenzene were generated as a waste product in the USA and that nearly 77% of this was produced from the manufacture of three chlorinated solvents: carbon tetrachloride, trichloroethylene and tetrachloroethylene. The remainder was produced by the chlorinated pesticide industry (WHO, 1997). According to the Environmental Protection Agency's Toxic Chemical Release Inventory, in 1997 about 18 t of hexachlorobenzene were reported as waste product (Environmental Protection Agency, 2000). In 1977, about 300 t of hexachlorobenzene were generated in Japan as a waste by-product in the production of tetrachloroethylene, almost all of which was incinerated. It was estimated that > 5000 t/year hexachlorobenzene were produced as a by-product during tetrachloroethylene production in the former Federal Republic of Germany in 1980. Estimates from the European Chlorinated Solvent Association indi-cated that up to 4000 t/year of hexachlorobenzene are produced in Europe as a by-product during certain tetrachloroethylene production processes, and that over 99% of this by-product is incinerated (WHO, 1997).

While hexachlorobenzene can also be a contaminant in commercial-grade chlorinated solvents, it was not detected (detection limit, 5 mg/L) in carbon tetrachloride or tetrachloroethylene in an investigation in Canada in the late 1980s or in production lots of tri- and tetrachloroethylene produced in Europe in 1996 (detection limit, 2 μg/L solvent) (WHO, 1997).

Some chlorinated pesticides contain hexachlorobenzene as an impurity in the final product, usually at a concentration of less than 1%, although higher concentrations have been reported when inappropriate procedures were used for the synthesis and purification stages (WHO, 1997).

1.4.1 *Occupational exposure*

According to the 1981–83 National Occupational Exposure Survey (National Institute for Occupational Safety and Health, 2000), about 1000 workers in the chemical industry were potentially exposed to hexachlorobenzene in the USA. According to the Finnish Register of Employees Exposed to Carcinogens, 15 laboratory workers were exposed in Finland in 1997 (Savela *et al.*, 1999).

Hexachlorobenzene has been detected in workplace air during the production of pentachlorophenol in the Russian Federation (Melnikova *et al.*, 1975). The blood of 11 workers in a factory where chlorinated solvents were made in the USA in 1974 contained 14–233 μg/L (Burns & Miller, 1975). In 1994, the average concentration of hexachlorobenzene in the serum of 57 workers in a Spanish organochlorine compound factory was 120 μg/L. Maintenance workers had a higher average concentration (247 μg/L, n = 12) than production (105 μg/L, n = 36), laboratory (49 μg/L, n = 6) or administrative (16 μg/L, n = 3) workers (Sala *et al.*, 1999a). The concentration of hexachlorobenzene was [36 μg/L] (1–160 μg/L) in the serum of 41 workers in a Brazilian organochlorine compound plant (da Silva Augusto *et al.*, 1997). The average plasma concentration in nine Swedish aluminium foundry workers who used hexachloroethane for degassing was 313 ng/g of lipid (controls, 67 ng/g of lipid) in 1992 (Seldén *et al.*, 1997).

1.4.2 *Environmental occurrence*

Hexachlorobenzene is a persistent pesticide the use of which has diminished substantially over the past two decades. This compound has low volatility and is practically insoluble in water. Its biodegradation in soil is very slow, with a half-time measured in decades. Hence, hexachlorobenzene persists in the environment and may be expected to accumulate in sediment long after application has ceased.

Recent reviews of environmental exposure to hexachlorobenzene by WHO (1997) and by the Agency for Toxic Substances and Disease Registry (1998) in the USA offer an overview of past environmental concentrations of this chemical. During the period when it was being used as a pesticide, a number of studies were carried out to determine its concentration in food. Most foods were found to contain low or undetectable concentrations, with the exception of meat and dairy products, in which significant concentrations were found.

The Total Diet Study, a marketbasket survey conducted in 1985–91 in the USA, demonstrated the presence of hexachlorobenzene in several foods which may be eaten by infants or children, at concentrations of 0.1–5.0 µg/kg (Yess *et al.*, 1993). The estimated mean dietary intake of this chemical from these studies in 1982–84 was 0.0011–0.002 µg/kg bw per day depending on age and sex. By 1991, it was estimated that the dietary intake had fallen to 0.0002–0.0004 µg/kg bw per day (Agency for Toxic Substances and Disease Registry, 1998).

The concentrations of hexachlorobenzene in air are generally low, although they were higher in the past. In 1976–79, air was measured for this chemical throughout the USA, and 49% of samples showed detectable concentrations, with a mean value of about 0.1 ng/m^3. In 1977, 12% of these values exceeded 1.5 ng/m^3. In a study in the Great Lakes region of the USA in 1981, the concentrations ranged from 0.09 to 0.28 ng/m^3. Measurements between July 1988 and September 1989 in Egbert, Ontario (Canada), showed a wide range of concentrations in air, from 0.04 pg/m^3 to 640 pg/m^3. The indoor concentrations in Jacksonville, FL, and Springfield, MA, in the USA in 1986–88 revealed ranges of 0.3–1.3 ng/m^3 and 0.1 ng/m^3, respectively, whereas the values were not detected to 0.2 ng/m^3 and not detected, respectively, in paired outdoor samples, suggesting indoor sources of this chemical in Jacksonville. Measurements near chlorinated solvent and pesticide manufacturing facilities in 1974 revealed much higher concentrations in air, ranging from 24 to 23 296 ng/m^3 (Agency for Toxic Substances and Disease Registry, 1998).

In 1986–91, the average concentrations of hexachlorobenzene in precipitation samples ranged from 0.108 to 0.174 ng/L in the Great Lakes region, while drinking-water supplies in the vicinity of Lake Ontario showed a somewhat broader mean range of 0.06–0.2 ng/L. The Great Lakes themselves had average ambient concentrations of 0.02–0.10 ng/L in 1982. The St Lawrence River had concentrations ranging from not detected to 0.09 ng/L in 1991. The Niagara River, which drains a more heavily industrialized area, showed more variable and generally higher concentrations, ranging from 0.02 to 17 ng/L, in 1982. Under polluted conditions, much higher concentrations can occur (Agency for Toxic Substances and Disease Registry, 1998).

The concentrations in sediments ranged from 0.2 to 97 µg/kg in Lake Ontario in 1982. Sediments at 1–2 cm depth had even higher concentrations, with an average of about 460 µg/kg. Previous studies suggest that the contamination was greater when hexachlorobenzene use was common. A study of agricultural sites in 37 states in the USA in 1972 indicated concentrations varying from 0.01 to 0.44 mg/kg, depending on the type of treatment the soil had experienced. Urban sites in the 1970s also had concentrations of 0.01–0.59 mg/kg. Uncontrolled hazardous waste sites established in the early 1970s are some of the most heavily contaminated areas. Concentrations as high as 20 mg/kg were found in soil at a scenic highway site near Baton Rouge, LA. Deep soil cores from the same site showed concentrations as high as 400 mg/kg (Agency for Toxic

Substances and Disease Registry, 1998). Carvalho *et al.* (1999) reported concentrations of hexachlorobenzene of 0.004–1.1 ng/g dry weight in sediment in coastal Nicaragua lagoons in 1995.

Hexachlorobenzene in sediments can enter the food chain by uptake by small organisms in direct contact with sediment. The measured concentrations in composited fish samples from the Great Lakes ranged from < 2.0 to 3470 µg/kg in 1980–81. More recent results show a decrease in concentrations in the Great Lakes, the concentrations in trout ranging from 0.22 to 9.0 µg/kg. In Galveston Bay, TX, fish, crab and oyster samples were found to contain 0.31–9.6 µg/kg wet weight in 1980–81. Hexachlorobenzene has also been found in wildlife, most notably in birds, with concentrations between 6 and 64 µg/kg in 1983–84. Hexachlorobenzene is preferentially sequestered in fat, and the typical concentration in duck muscle was only 0.4–0.9 µg/kg, whereas the concentration in fat was as high as 70 µg/kg of lipid in water fowl in 1993 (Agency for Toxic Substances and Disease Registry, 1998).

Ray *et al.* (1998) reported mean concentrations of hexachlorobenzene in yellow-tail flounder from off the coast of Newfoundland at several locations ranging from 0.09 to 0.61 µg/kg wet weight in 1993.

Van Oostdam *et al.* (1999) reported an estimated daily intake of hexachlorobenzene intake from breast milk by Inuit infants of 0.6 µg/kg bw per day. Newsome and Ryan (1999) reported a study of breast milk from various populations in northern and southern Canada in 1986, 1992 and 1996. The median and mean concentrations of hexachlorobenzene were 43.5 and 43 ng/g of lipid in northern Canada, which were substantially higher than those in southern Canada. The mean concentration in breast milk from Canadian women in a national study in 1992 was 14.5 ng/g of lipid (mean, 13 ng/g of lipid) (Newsome et al., 1995).

Hexachlorobenzene is found in human tissues, including blood, with mean values of 3 µg/L in Spain (To-Figueras *et al.*, 1995) and 0.7 µg/L in Germany (Gerhard *et al.*, 1998). The concentration in cord blood of newborns ranged from 0.01 to 1.4 µg/L for non-Inuit populations and from 0.02 to 1.2 µg/L for Inuit populations (Van Oostdam *et al.*, 1999).

1.5   Regulations and guidelines

Occupational exposure limits for hexachlorobenzene in several countries are presented in Table 2.

The Joint FAO/WHO Meeting on Pesticide Residues in 1974 established a conditional acceptable daily intake for hexachlorobenzene of 0–0.0006 mg/kg bw, which was withdrawn in 1978 (WHO, 1999). WHO (1993) recommended a guideline limit value of 1 µg/L for hexachlorobenzene in drinking-water.

Because of concerns about risks to human health and the environment, the use of hexachlorobenzene has been discontinued in many countries. For example, according to voluntary national reporting to the Joint FAO/UNEP Programme for the Operation of

Table 2. Occupational exposure limits and guidelines for hexachlorobenzene

Country	Year	Concentration (mg/m^3)	Interpretation
Czech Republic	1993	1	TWA
		2	STEL
France	1993	(Ca)	
Germany	1999	4^a	–
Netherlands	1999	0.03	TWA
Poland	1998	0.5 (sk)	TWA
Russian Federation	1993	0.9 (sk)	STEL
USA			
ACGIH (TLV)	2000	0.002 (A3, sk)	TWA

From American Conference of Governmental Industrial Hygienists (ACGIH) (2000); Deutsche Forschungsgemeinschaft (2000)
TWA, time-weighted average; STEL, short-term exposure limit; Ca, carcinogen; sk, danger of cutaneous absorption; A3, confirmed animal carcinogen with unknown relevance to humans; 4, substances with carcinogenic effects in which genotoxicity plays little or no role.
^{a} Biological Tolerance Value, 150 µg/L in plasma or serum

Prior Informed Consent for Banned or Severely Restricted Chemicals in International Trade, hexachlorobenzene is banned or product registrations have been withdrawn in the Member States of the European Union and the Members associated with the European Union in the European Economic Area, effective in 1979, and in at least six other countries: Australia (1987), Japan (1979), Morocco (1984), New Zealand (1972), Switzerland (1986) and the USA (1987) (FAO/UNEP, 1997).

Hexachlorobenzene is one of 12 persistent organic pollutants being considered for international action to reduce or eliminate their releases under a global convention. As of December 2000, the participating governments had agreed to phase out hexachlorobenzene and five other chlorinated pesticides (aldrin, chlordane, endrin, heptachlor and toxaphene) Hogue, 2000).

2.   Studies of Cancer in Humans

2.1   Descriptive studies

During periods of relative famine in the mid-1950s in south-eastern Turkey, seed grain treated with hexachlorobenzene (approximately 2 kg/t of seed) was diverted for bread production, resulting in numerous cases of severe intoxication and an epidemic of porphyria cutanea tarda. Of the estimated 3000–4000 people affected by the disease over the years 1955–59, 252 patients of an average age of 36 years were traced and offered a clinical and biochemical examination between 1977 and 1987, i.e. 20–30 years after exposure (Peters *et al.*, 1982; Gocmen *et al.*, 1989). No case of malignant hepatic or thyroid tumour was found. During the examinations, 56 samples of milk were obtained from lactating women (Peters *et al.*, 1982) which had an average hexachlorobenzene content of 510 ng/g (standard deviation, 750 ng/g), whereas milk from unexposed controls contained 70 ng/g (Gocmen *et al.*, 1989). [The Working Group noted that the study subjects were relatively young and that the clinical investigation for tumours of the liver and thyroid was restricted to the subgroup of patients who survived to the date of examination, which may have resulted in an underestimation of risk.]

In a descriptive study of mortality (1984–91) and cancer incidence (1980–89) among approximately 5000 inhabitants of a small town located in the vicinity of an organo-chlorine-contaminating electrochemical factory in Catalonia, Spain, Grimalt *et al.* (1994) observed small clusters among men of incident cases of thyroid cancer (standard incidence ratio [SIR], 6.7; 95% confidence interval [CI], 1.6–28; two cases), soft-tissue sarcoma (5.5; 1.7–18; three cases), brain tumour (2.7; 1.0–7.2; four cases) and cancer of unknown origin (2.4; 1.25–4.4; 10 cases), while the incidence of and mortality from all types of cancers combined were found to be compatible with those expected on the basis of population-based regional incidence and mortality rates. Among the women in the population, no significant associations for equivalent sites were seen. The average concentration of hexachlorobenzene in 40 air samples taken from the area was 35 ng/m^3, which was approximately 100 times higher than the average concentration measured in five samples taken in a control city (Barcelona). Similarly, the average concentration of hexachlorobenzene in sera from 13 local volunteers (26 µg/L; range 7.5–69 µg/L) was significantly higher ($p < 0.001$) than that found in samples from 13 subjects chosen in a hospital in the control city (4.8 µg/L; 1.5–15 µg/L).

In the same population, Sala *et al.* (1999b) conducted a cross-sectional study 4 years later of 1800 inhabitants, over 14 years of age, who were interviewed to obtain information on personal health, 16 selected chronic medical conditions and all diseases, cancer included, for which an association with hexachlorobenzene had previously been suspected. In addition, 608 of the 1800 study participants donated blood samples, which were analysed by gas chromotography for content of organo-chlorine compounds. The median concentration of hexachlorobenzene in all serum samples was 16.5 µg/L. In men, the concentrations were highest among those employed at the factory (geometric mean, 54.6–60.3 µg/L). A benign or malignant neoplasm was reported by 13% of the female participants and 4.5% of the male parti-cipants. The confirmed cancer prevalence was non-significantly higher among inhabitants employed at the electrochemical factory than among the other study parti-cipants (odds ratio, 1.9).

2.2   Case–control studies

Information on body uptake of hexachlorobenzene and other organochlorine compounds has been reported primarily in studies of breast cancer. Body uptake was
measured either by cumulated concentrations of hexachlorobenzene in breast adipose
tissue samples, or in serum samples, or both. The case–control studies of breast cancer
are grouped according to whether biological samples were collected during diagnosis
or treatment (contemporary samples) or whether they were collected from banked
serum samples (archival samples). The results of these studies and of studies of cancers
at other sites are summarized in Table 3. As hexachlorobenzene accumulates in fat
tissue in increasing amounts with age, those studies in which the confounding effect of
age was not strictly controlled for are difficult to interpret.

2.2.1   *Studies of breast cancer based on contemporary biological samples*

In a hospital-based case–control study from Helsinki, Finland, Mussalo-Rauhamaa
et al. (1990) collected 10–20 g of breast adipose tissue from 44 patients in whom breast
cancer had been diagnosed in 1985 or 1986. The tissue samples were analysed for the
content of neutral organochlorine compounds and polycyclic aromatic hydrocarbons by
gas chromatography, and the concentrations were compared with those seen in breast
tissue samples obtained during routine post-mortem examinations of 33 accidental fata-
lities. A total of 41 samples from cases (93%) and all 33 samples from controls showed
detectable concentrations of hexachlorobenzene, yielding a mean concentration in
positive samples of 140 ng/g (standard deviation, 80) and 110 (50) ng/g of fat, respectively, with an associated *p* value of 0.48. [The Working Group noted that the criteria
for selection of study subjects were not given in the report.]

In another small hospital-based case–control study, from Connecticut, USA, Falck
et al. (1992) measured and compared the concentrations of organochlorine compound
residues in 0.5-g samples of breast fat obtained during 1987 from 20 women with
breast cancer (cases) and 20 women with benign breast disease (controls), who were
all referred to the hospital for initial surgical evaluation. The patients' height, weight
and smoking histories were obtained from the medical records or from brief telephone
interviews. The mean ages were similar for the two groups (63 and 59 years for cases
and controls, respectively), but more controls had a history of current or past smoking
(15 of 20) than did cases (six of 20). The mean concentrations of hexachlorobenzene
were 23 ng/g of fat (wet weight) in tissues of women with breast cancer and 20 ng/g
in women with benign breast disease, with an associated *p* value in a test unadjusted
for other variables of 0.32. [The Working Group noted that the criteria for selection of
study subjects were not given in the report.]

In a further, small, hospital-based case–control study, from Québec, Canada,
Dewailly *et al.* (1994) studied the content of organochlorine compounds in samples of
0.2–1 g of breast adipose tissue from 20 women with breast adenocarcinoma (cases) and

Table 3. Case–control studies of hexachlorobenzene and risk for breast cancer

Reference and location	Subjects in the analysis	Biological sample	Exposure estimates	Mean concentration (ng/g)	Odds ratio (95% CI) or p value	Comments
Studies of breast cancer with contemporary samples						
Mussalo-Rauhamaa et al. (1990) Finland	44 patients 33 controls	Breast fat	Test-positive controls (n = 33) Test-positive cases (n = 41)	110 140	p = 0.48	Only test-positive cases included
Falck et al. (1992) Connecticut, USA	20 patients 20 controls	Breast fat (wet weight)	All control samples All case samples	20 23	p = 0.32	No adjustment for other variables
Dewailly et al. (1994) Québec, Canada	20 patients 17 controls	Breast fat	All control samples Estrogen receptor-negative Estrogen receptor-positive	33 31 42	p = 0.53 p = 0.29	
Güttes et al. (1998) Hesse, Germany	45 patients 20 controls	Breast fat	All control samples All case samples	261 309	p = 0.40	Adjustment for age
Liljegren et al. (1998) Sweden	43 patients 35 controls	Breast fat	Any > 40 ng/g – postmenopausal cases – estrogen receptor-positive – both		1.3 (0.3–4.5) 1.9 (0.4–7.2) 2.0 (0.6–7.5) 7.1 (1.1–45)	Adjustment for age and parity
Moysich et al. (1998) New York, USA	154 patients 192 controls	Serum	All women – first tertile (low) – second tertile – third tertile (high) Parous; never lactated – first tertile (low) – second tertile – third tertile (high)	0–0.34 0.35–0.44 0.45–1.35 0–0.34 0.35–0.44 0.45–1.35	1 0.6 (0.3–1.0) 0.8 (0.4–1.5) 1 1.3 (0.4–4.0) 1.8 (0.6–5.4)	Adjustment for other variables; all women postmenopausal

Table 3 (contd)

Reference and location	Subjects in the analysis	Biological sample	Exposure estimates	Mean concentration (ng/g)	Odds ratio (95% CI) or p value	Comments
Moysich et al. (1998) (contd)			Parous; ever lactated			
			– first tertile (low)	0–0.34	1	
			– second tertile	0.35–0.44	0.3 (0.1–0.7)	
			– third tertile (high)	0.45–1.35	0.5 (0.2–1.1)	
Zheng et al., (1999) Connecticut, USA	304 cases 186 controls	Breast fat	All women	< 12.5 (low)	1	Adjustment for other variables; control women had benign breast disease
				12.5–15.9	0.7 (0.4–1.3)	
				16.0–21.0	0.7 (0.4–1.2)	
				≥ 21.1 (high)	0.9 (0.5–1.6)	
			Premenopausal women	< 12.5 (low)	1	
				≥ 19.5 (high)	0.8 (0.3–2.0)	
			Postmenopausal women	< 13.2 (low)	1	
				≥ 23.8 (high)	0.8 (0.4–1.8)	
			Parous; never lactated	> 12.4 (low)	1	
				≥ 21.1 (high)	0.7 (0.3–1.7)	
			Parous; ever lactated	< 12.5 (low)	1	
				≥ 23.7 (high)	0.5 (0.2–1.4)	
Mendonça et al. (1999) Rio de Janeiro, Brazil	162 cases 331 controls	Serum	> 0.2 ng/mL Test-positive cases (n = 4) Test-positive controls (n = 7)		[1.2 (0.3–3.9)]	Unadjusted
Aronson et al. (2000) Ontario, Canada	217 cases 213 controls	Breast fat	All women	≤ 21	1	Adjustment for other variables; control women had benign breast disease
				22–31	1.0 (0.6–1.7)	
				32–51	0.8 (0.4–1.4)	
				≥ 52	1.2 (0.6–2.3)	
			Premenopausal women	≤ 21	1	
				≥ 32	1.0 (0.5–2.4)	
			Postmenopausal women	≤ 21	1	
				≥ 32	0.6 (0.3–1.5)	

Table 3 (contd)

Reference and location	Subjects in the analysis	Biological sample	Exposure estimates	Mean concen- tration (ng/g)	Odds ratio (95% CI) or p value	Comments
Study of breast cancer with archival samples						
Dorgan et al. (1999) Missouri, USA	105 cases 208 controls	Serum	All women	0–62 63–83 84–105 106–406	1 2.5 (1.2–5.3) 1.9 (0.9–4.3) 2.3 (1.0–5.0) p = 0.38 for trend	Matched on age, benign breast disease diagnosis, month and year of blood collection
			Time since blood collection: ≤ 2.7 years	0–93 94–153 154–406	1 1.6 (0.7–3.9) 2.6 (1.1–6.2)	
			> 2.7 years	0–93 94–153 154–406	1 1.9 (0.8–4.4) 0.6 (0.2–1.7)	
Endometrial cancer						
Weiderpass et al. (2000) Sweden	154 cases 205 controls	Serum	All control samples All case samples	66.2 70.3	p = 0.08	Adjustment for lipid content in serum
			All subjects – first quartile (cases/controls)	40.8/40.2 (median)	1	Multivariate, adjusted for age and body mass index
			– second quartile – third quartile – fourth quartile (cases/controls)	94.2/109.5 (median)	1.2 (0.6–2.2) 1.0 (0.5–1.9) 1.0 (0.5–1.9)	

Table 3 (contd)

Reference and location	Subjects in the analysis	Biological sample	Exposure estimates	Mean concentration (ng/g)	Odds ratio (95% CI) or p value	Comments
Pancreatic cancer						
Hoppin et al. (2000) San Francisco, USA	108 cases 82 controls	Serum	All control samples All case samples	22 28	$p = 0.22$	Adjustment for lipid content of serum
			All subjects	0 0.1–32 > 32	1 0.9 (0.4–1.9) 1.6 (0.8–3.4)	Multivariate adjustment for age, race and sex
Hairy-cell leukaemia						
Nordström et al. (2000) Sweden	54 cases 54 controls	Serum	All control samples All case samples	45.2 44.7	$p = 0.11$	Unadjusted
			Antibodies to EBV early antigen – low/low – high/high		1 11 (2.2–69)	Adjusted for age and body mass index

EBV, Epstein-Barr virus

17 women with breast adenomas or lipomas (controls). The study subjects were chosen from among 41 women who were referred to the medical centre for a biopsy because of a breast mass and who volunteered to participate in the study; four were excluded as they had lesions of borderline malignancy. The estrogen receptor status of the adenocarcinomas was determined, and fat organochlorine concentrations, including hexachlorobenzene, were measured by high-resolution gas chromatography. The mean ages of cases and controls were 54 and 51 years, respectively. The mean adipose tissue concentrations of hexachlorobenzene were 33 ng/g (standard deviation, 13) in the 17 control subjects, 42 ng/g (16) in nine estrogen receptor-positive subjects and 31 ng/g (11.5) in nine receptor-negative subjects. The associated p values in significance tests unadjusted for other variables were 0.29 and 0.53, respectively.

Güttes *et al.* (1998) used surgically removed breast tissue from 45 women with breast cancer (cases) and 20 women with various benign breast diseases (controls) to study the relationship between accumulated concentrations of organochlorine compounds in fat tissue and risk for breast cancer. Tissue samples of 0.5–2 g were obtained during 1993 and 1994 from two hospitals in the region of central Hesse, Germany. The mean ages of the breast cancer patients and control subjects were 61 and 50 years, respectively. Data on risk factors for breast cancer other than age were not available. The unadjusted mean concentrations of hexachlorobenzene were 343 ng/g of breast fat (range, 47–2224) in tissue samples from breast cancer patients and 206 ng/g (95–607) in samples from control subjects. However, the authors found that the concentrations of hexachlorobenzene and certain other organochlorine compounds showed a strong, positive correlation with the age of the woman at the time the sample was donated, and a regression analysis with adjustment for age differences between cases and controls gave mean concentrations of 309 and 261 ng/g, respectively, with an associated p value of 0.40.

Liljegren *et al.* (1998) studied 78 consecutive patients operated at one clinic in Sweden during 1993–95 for invasive breast cancer (43 cases) or a benign lesion in the breast (35 controls). A sample of approximately 10 g, free of tumour, was taken from the breast during the surgical procedure; fat was extracted, cleaned and analysed by high-resolution gas chromatography and mass spectrometry for hexachlorobenzene and other organochlorine compounds. Data on potential confounders, including parity, lactation, menopausal status, hormonal therapy, smoking habits and family history of breast cancer were assessed from a self-administered standardized questionnaire. Information on estrogen receptor status was obtained from the medical records of the breast cancer patients. The mean ages of breast cancer patients and control subjects were 58 and 54 years, respectively. The mean concentrations of hexachlorobenzene, unadjusted for age or other potential confounding factors, were 72.6 ng/g of fat (range, 12–490 ng/g) in the samples from cancer patients and 48.1 ng/g (17–400) in samples from control subjects. In a multivariate logistic regression analysis, age and parity were found to be the only potential confounders of importance. An odds ratio for breast cancer of 1.3 (95% CI, 0.3–4.5) was estimated for exposure to hexachlorobenzene after adjustment for age, parity, familial breast cancer history and smoking. Subanalyses with inclusion only of postmenopausal women (32 cases, 21 controls) or of estrogen receptor-positive cancers (32 cases, 35 controls) yielded adjusted risk estimates of 1.9 (0.4–7.2) and 2.0 (0.6–7.5). A further analysis that included only postmenopausal women with estrogen receptor-positive cancers (23 cases, 21 controls) yielded an odds ratio of 7.1 (1.1–45) in association with exposure to hexachlorobenzene. [The Working Group noted that there was no information on the cut-off points used in the multivariate analysis for hexachlorobenzene or other organochlorine compounds in the fat tissue samples.]

Moysich *et al.* (1998) conducted a population-based case–control study of postmenopausal breast cancer in Erie and Niagara counties in western New York, USA, during the period 1986–91. Of 777 white women with histologically confirmed, postmenopausal breast cancer who were eligible for study, 439 (57%) were interviewed; of 1076 postmenopausal community controls, identified from public administrative listings, 494 (45%) agreed to participate. Information on usual diet, reproductive and medical histories and other lifestyle characteristics were obtained at a structured personal interview. Of the women who provided interviews, 262 cases (60%) and 319 controls (65%) agreed to donate a blood sample. However, patients were included only if their blood had been drawn before chemotherapy or radiation and within 3 months of surgery, leaving a total of 154 postmenopausal women with breast cancer for study. Finally, 192 of the 319 controls for whom stored blood was available were frequency matched to cases by date of blood draw (± 3 months) and age (± 3 years). The content of hexachlorobenzene and other organochlorine compounds in the sera was quantified by high-resolution gas chromatography. The mean serum concentrations, adjusted in a multivariate analysis for age and serum lipids, were 0.41 ng/mL of serum (standard deviation, 0.19) in postmenopausal women with breast cancer and 0.42 ng/mL (0.19) in female community controls. Exposure categories were examined in tertiles, on the basis of the distribution of hexachlorobenzene concentrations in the controls, and associated odds ratios for breast cancer were calculated by unconditional logistic regression. With the lower exposure category as reference, the odds ratios for breast cancer in the middle and upper exposure categories, adjusted for age, reproductive factors and other potential confounders, were 0.6 (95% CI, 0.3–1.0) and 0.8 (0.4–1.5), respectively. In order to determine any modifying effect of lactation, women were also stratified by history of breastfeeding, excluding 48 nulliparous women. Within the subgroup of 191 women who had ever breastfed, the middle and upper exposure categories for hexachlorobenzene were associated with odds ratios of 0.3 (95% CI, 0.1–0.7) and 0.5 (0.2–1.1), respectively, while similar analyses within the subgroup of 107 women who had never breastfed showed odds ratios of 1.3 (0.4–4.0) and 1.8 (0.6–5.4), respectively.

From the files of a surgical pathology department of one medical centre in Connecticut, USA, where records of newly completed breast-related surgery were kept, Zheng *et al.* (1999) identified 385 consecutive breast cancer patients aged 40–79 years who were treated surgically during 1994–97 and from whose breast specimen at least 0.4 g of residual breast adipose tissue was available. Of these, 304 (79%) agreed to participate in the study (cases). The same files were used to identify 251 potential controls who had had breast-related surgery at the centre in whom benign breast disease was histologically diagnosed, besides fulfilling the same inclusion criteria (age, period and available fat sample) as those applied to cases. Of these, 186 (74%) agreed to participate in the study (controls). Information on major known or suspected risk factors for breast cancer was obtained at personal interviews, and the content of hexachlorobenzene in fat tissue samples was determined by gas chromotography. The cases (mean age, 56 years) were significantly older than controls (mean age, 53 years). The mean concentrations of hexachlorobenzene, adjusted in a multivariate analysis for age and sample lipid composition, were similar for breast cancer cases and benign breast disease controls overall (21 ng/g; standard deviation, 17.7 versus 19.1 ng/g; standard deviation, 15; $p = 0.21$) and by menopausal status. Cases and controls also did not differ significantly in the mean concentrations of hexachlorobenzene in adipose tissue when the cases were stratified by estrogen receptor or progesterone status. Quartiles of adipose tissue concentrations of hexachlorobenzene were formed on the basis of the frequency distribution in controls, and a linear logistic regression model was used to adjust for confounders when estimating the exposure–disease relationship. When the lower exposure quartile was used as the standard exposure category (< 12.5 ng/g), women in the second (12.5–15.9 ng/g), third (16.0–21.0 ng/g) and upper (≥ 21.1 ng/g) quartiles had adjusted odds ratios for breast cancer of 0.7 (95% CI, 0.4–1.3), 0.7 (0.4–1.2) and 0.9 (0.5–1.6), respectively. For 186 parous women who reported ever having breastfed, an odds ratio of 0.5 (0.2–1.4) was observed when the highest quartile was compared with the lowest; the equivalent risk estimate for parous women who reported never having breastfed was 0.7 (0.3–1.7).

In a case–control study in Rio de Janeiro, Brazil, Mendonça *et al.* (1999) studied 177 women with invasive breast cancer admitted to one hospital during 1995 and 1996 and 350 controls selected among female visitors to the same hospital. In addition to information obtained at a personal interview with a standardized questionnaire, 10-mL blood samples were taken. Of 162 blood samples available from cases and 331 available from controls, four (2.5%) and seven (2.1%), respectively, showed detectable hexachlorobenzene (> 0.2 ng/mL) [unadjusted odds ratio, 1.2; 95% CI, 0.3–3.9].

Aronson *et al.* (2000) conducted a hospital-based case–control study in two cities in Ontario, Canada, during 1995–97. Of 824 women eligible for study (under the age of 80, no previous diagnosis of cancer, no breast implants and not too ill) who were all scheduled for excision biopsy of a suspected breast cancer, 663 (80.5%) agreed to participate and completed a questionnaire by telephone interview or by mail. The majority of the questionnaires, providing information on known and suspected risk factors for breast cancer, were completed before the participants knew their diagnosis. After biopsy, the histological records of study subjects were reviewed: the cases were subjects in whom in-situ or invasive breast cancer was diagnosed and the controls were subjects with no malignancy (but often with some form of benign breast disease). Organochlorine compounds were determined in tissue from all case women for whom at least 0.2 g of benign tissue was available ($n = 217$) and in tissue from a subset of control women ($n = 213$) frequency matched by age in 5-year groups and study site. The cases were on average 4 years older than the controls. The geometric mean concentrations of hexachlorobenzene, unadjusted for age, were 32 ng/g (95% CI, 29.3–34.8) in fat samples from cases and 30.1 ng/g (27.8–32.5) in samples from controls. Exposure to organochlorine compounds was examined in four categories, with the cut-point for the upper category at the 85th percentile of the control concentration, and odds ratios were assessed in an unconditional logistic regression analysis. When the lower concentration of hexachlorobenzene (≤ 21 ng/g of fat) was used as the standard exposure category, women in the second (22–31 ng/g), third (32–51 ng/g) and upper (≥ 52 ng/g) exposure categories showed odds ratios adjusted for potential confounders of 0.97 (0.6–1.7), 0.75 (0.4–1.4) and 1.2 (0.6–2.3), respectively. Similar patterns were seen after stratification of study subjects by menopausal status at diagnosis.

2.2.2   *Study of breast cancer based on archival biological samples*

In a case–control study nested in a cohort from the Columbia, Missouri Breast Cancer Serum Bank, USA, Dorgan *et al.* (1999) examined the relationship between exposure to organochlorine pesticides and polychlorinated biphenyls and breast cancer. Of 7224 women initially free of cancer who donated blood to the bank on one or more occasions between 1977 and 1987, 6426 had at least 4 mL of serum remaining in the bank and were included in the study. During up to 9.5 years of follow-up, a histologically confirmed breast cancer was diagnosed in 105 women. For each breast cancer case, two controls were selected from among the eligible women, matched to the case on age, benign breast disease diagnosis during the previous 2 years and month and year of blood collection ($n = 208$). The concentration of hexachlorobenzene was measured by gas chromatography and was corrected for the total lipid content in the sample. Information on clinical status, age, height, weight, menstrual and reproductive histories, smoking, use of medication and family history of breast cancer was obtained by initial self-reporting or medical record review. The case women tended to be better educated than the controls and were more likely to be nulliparous and to have a first-degree relative with a history of breast cancer. Smoking was significantly inversely associated with breast cancer. The percentages of case and control women with concentrations of hexachlorobenzene at or above the limit of detection of the assay were 98.1 and 95.2, respectively ($p = 0.16$). For use in the risk analysis, the women were stratified into quartiles on the basis of the concentration of hexachlorobenzene per gram of serum lipids relative to the distribution in controls. The relative risk, adjusted for potential confounders, was estimated by conditional logistic regression. When the lower exposure quartile was used as the standard exposure category (0–62 ng/g of serum lipid), the second (63–83 ng/g), third (85–105 ng/g) and upper (106–406 ng/g) quartiles showed relative risks of 2.5 (95% CI, 1.2–5.3), 1.9 (0.9–4.3) and 2.3 (1.0–5.0), with a *p* value of 0.38 in a test for trend. The presence of hexachlorobenzene was significantly positively associated with the occurrence of breast cancer among women who received their diagnosis close to the time of blood collection (≤ 2.7 years), but not among women whose cancer was diagnosed later (> 2.7 years). In summary, the results of the study do not support the hypothesis that women who are exposed to organochloride pesticides are at increased risk for breast cancer.

2.2.3   *Studies of cancers at other sites*

Weiderpass *et al.* (2000) conducted a case–control study of women, 50–74 years of age in the populations of 12 coastal counties in Sweden, with incident histologically confirmed endometrial cancer diagnosed during 1996–97. The women, who were identified at departments of gynaecology and gynaecological oncology in the study area, were eligible if they were born in Sweden, had not had a hysterectomy and had never used hormone replacement therapy. Of 396 reported patients, 288 (73%) volunteered to donate blood samples and complete a questionnaire. Subsequently, 134 case women were excluded because they had used hormorne replacement therapy, leaving 154 in the study. Population controls, frequency-matched to the case by 5-year age groups were randomly selected from the population registers of the study area. Of 742 control women selected, 492 (66%) responded to the questionnaire and donated blood samples. After the exclusion of 287 women because of hysterectomy or use of hormone replacement therapy, 205 control women were included in the study. The self-administered questionnaire requested information on weight, height, reproductive history, diet, hormone use, smoking, physical activity and medical history. Serum samples from the study subjects were analysed for their content of hexachlorobenzene and other organochlorine compounds in the lipid fraction by high-resolution gas chromatography. The mean serum concentrations of hexachlorobenzene, unadjusted for any potential confounder, were 70.3 ng/g of lipid in women with endometrial cancer and 66.2 ng/g in female community controls ($p = 0.08$). Exposure categories were examined in quartiles on the basis of the distribution of hexachlorobenzene concentrations in the controls, and associated odds ratios for endometrial cancer were calculated by unconditional logistic regression. With the lower exposure category as reference, the odds ratio for endometrial cancer in the second, third and fourth quartiles was 1.2 (0.6–2.2), 1.0 (0.5–1.9) and 1.0 (0.5–1.9), respectively. The data do not support the hypothesis that the exposure to the organochlorides studied increased the risk for endometrial cancer.

In a case–control study in the San Francisco Bay Area, USA, conducted during 1996–98, Hoppin *et al.* (2000) studied 108 of 611 patients with incident pancreatic cancer, diagnosed when they were aged 32–85 years, and 82 of 253 control subjects. The controls were frequency-matched to the cases on age and sex by random digit dialling and random sampling of Health Care Financing Administration lists. A personal interview was conducted in which questions on occupational exposures, tobacco use, diet and medical history were posed, and a blood sample was drawn. The serum samples were analysed for their content of hexachlorobenzene and other organochlorine compounds in the lipid fraction by high-resolution gas chromatography. The mean concentration of hexachlorobenzene, adjusted for the lipid content of serum, was 28 ng/g of lipid in patients with pancreatic cancer and 22 ng/g in control subjects ($p = 0.22$). The exposure categories were examined in tertiles, and the associated odds ratios for pancreatic cancer were calculated by unconditional logistic regression. With the lower exposure category as reference, the odds ratio for pancreatic cancer in the middle and upper exposure categories, adjusted for potential confounders, were 0.9 (95% CI, 0.4–1.9) and 1.6 (0.8–3.4), respectively.

In a small, population-based case–control study in Sweden, Nordström et al. (2000) studied 54 of 121 male patients notified to the Swedish Cancer Registry with a diagnosis of hairy cell leukaemia in 1987–92 and 54 of 484 controls drawn from the national population registry and matched to the case on age, sex and county. A questionnaire mailed to study subjects requested information about previous occupations, exposure to potential risk factors for leukaemia and present height and weight. A blood sample was drawn and analysed for hexachlorobenzene and other organochlorine compounds in the serum lipid fraction by high-resolution gas chromatography. Samples were also analysed for titres of antibodies to Epstein-Barr virus early antigen immunoglobulin G. The mean concentration of hexachlorobenzene, unadjusted for the lipid content of serum, was 44.7 ng/g of lipid in patients with hairy cell leukaemia and 45.2 ng/g in control subjects ($p = 0.11$). When concentrations below 43.9 ng/g (the median concentration for controls) were used as the reference category, the odds ratio associated with higher concentrations, adjusted for age and body mass index, was 1.0 (95% CI, 0.4–2.7). A further subdivision of study subjects into those with a high titre of antibodies to Epstein-Barr virus early antigen and those with a low titre (again with the median value of controls as the cut-off) revealed a significantly increased odds ratio for hairy cell leukaemia of 11 (95% CI, 2.2–69) in the subgroup with high antibody titres and a high serum content of hexachlorobenzene. However, the estimate was based on few study subjects. [The Working Group noted that the blood samples were taken after intensive treatment with immunosuppressive drugs.]

3.   Studies of Cancer in Experimental Animals

3.1   Oral administration

Mouse: Groups of 30–50 male and 30–50 female Swiss mice, 6–7 weeks of age, were fed diets containing 0 (control), 50, 100 or 200 mg/kg hexachlorobenzene (> 99.5% pure) until they were 120 weeks old, at which time all survivors were killed. A fifth group was given 300 mg/kg hexachlorobenzene for only 15 weeks. At 90 weeks of age, the percentage survival rates in males and females in the five groups were 50 and 48; 30 and 40; 27 and 30; 4 and 0; and 13 and 57%, respectively. The incidence of lymphomas and lung tumours was not increased in treated animals. No liver-cell tumours were found in the controls or in the group receiving hexachlorobenzene at 50 mg/kg of diet. The incidences of liver-cell tumours in surviving male and female mice at the time the first liver-cell tumour was observed were 3/12, 7/29 and 1/3 in males and 3/12, 14/26 and 1/10 in females for the groups receiving 100, 200 and 300 mg/kg diet, respectively. The effective intakes of hexachlorobenzene that induced liver-cell tumours were 12–24 mg/kg bw per day (Cabral *et al.*, 1979; Cabral & Shubik, 1986).

Rat: Groups of 12 and 14 female Argus rats and four and six female MRC-Wistar rats, 5–7 weeks of age, were fed either control diet or a diet containing 100 mg/kg hexachlorobenzene (99.5% pure) for 90 weeks. The incidences of liver-cell tumours were 0/12 and 14/14 for the Argus control and treated groups, respectively, and 0/4 and 4/6 for the MRC-Wistar control and treated groups, respectively (Smith & Cabral, 1980).

Groups of 10–12 male and 10 female Fischer 334 rats, 6–7 weeks of age, were fed a diet containing 0 (control) or 200 mg/kg hexachlorobenzene for 90 weeks. Liver tumours were observed only in surviving treated female rats, the incidence in this group being 5/10 with neoplastic nodules and 5/10 with 'carcinomas' (Smith *et al.*, 1985).

Groups of 94 male and 94 female weanling Sprague-Dawley rats [age unspecified] were fed diets containing 0 (control), 75 or 150 mg/kg hexachlorobenzene (purity, > 99.5%) for up to 104 weeks. Small numbers of animals were killed at intervals for biochemical and pathological analyses. The tumour incidences at the end of the study are shown in Table 4. Increased incidences of tumours of the liver and kidney were reported. The types of liver tumours diagnosed included hepatocellular carcinomas, bile-duct adenomas and haemangiomas, while the kidney tumours were all adenomas (Ertürk *et al.*, 1986).

Table 4. Incidence of tumours in rats fed hexachlorobenzene

Tumour type	Concentration in the diet (mg/kg)					
	Control		75		150	
	Males	Females	Males	Females	Males	Females
Liver haemangioma	0/54	0/52	10/52	23/56	11/56	35/55
Hepatocellular carcinoma	0/54	0/52	3/52	36/56	4/56	48/55
Bile-duct adenoma	0/54	1/52	2/52	19/56	2/56	29/55
Renal-cell adenoma	7/54	1/52	41/52	7/56	42/56	15/55

From Ertürk *et al.* (1986)

Hamster: A total of 159 female and 157 male Syrian golden hamsters, 6 weeks of age, were given dietary concentrations of 0 (control), 50, 100 or 200 mg/kg hexachlorobenzene (> 99.5% pure) for life, equivalent to a dose of 0, 4, 8 or 16 mg/kg bw per day.

The incidences of hepatomas, liver haemangioendotheliomas and thyroid follicular-cell adenomas were increased by exposure to hexachlorobenzene. The incidences of hepatomas were 0/40, 14/30, 26/30 and 49/57 in males and 0/39, 14/30, 17/30 and 51/60 in females at 0, 50, 100 and 200 mg/kg of diet, respectively. A 'hepatoma' was first observed in a female hamster after 18 weeks of treatment. The incidences of liver haemangioendotheliomas in males and females receiving the highest concentration were 20/57 and 7/60, respectively, compared with 0/40 male and 0/39 female controls. Three of the haemangioendotheliomas metastasized [organ not specified]. A significant increase in the incidence of alveolar adenomas of the thyroid was found in treated animals, with rates of 0/40, 0/30, 1/30 and 8/57 ($p < 0.05$) in males and 0/39, 2/30, 1/30 and 3/60 in females at 0, 50, 100 and 200 mg/kg of diet, respectively (Cabral $et\ al.$, 1977; Cabral & Shubik, 1986).

3.2   Perinatal administration

$Rat:$ Groups of male and female Sprague-Dawley rats were fed diets containing 0 (control), 0.32, 1.6, 8 or 40 mg/kg hexachlorobenzene. After 90 days on test, the F_0 rats were mated on a one-to-one basis within each treatment group; the F_1 pups were weaned at 21 days of age, divided into groups of 50 males and 50 females and continued on their parents' diets for up to 130 weeks. The mortality curves for control and treated rats were similar in both generations. No statistically significant increase in the incidence of thyroid follicular-cell tumours was found in the F_1 generation, but there were marginally increased incidences of tumours at other sites. In males, parathyroid adenomas were found in 2/48, 4/48, 2/48, 1/49 and 12/49 ($p < 0.05$, Fisher's exact test) at 0, 0.32, 1.6, 8 and 40 mg/kg of diet, respectively, and in females, the incidences of 'neoplastic nodules' of the liver were 0/49, 0/49, 2/50, 2/49 and 10/49 ($p < 0.01$, Fisher's exact test). The incidence of adrenal pheochromocytomas was increased in a linear trend ($p < 0.05$, Cochran-Armitage test) in both sexes: males — 10/48, 12/48, 7/48, 13/48 and 17/40; females — 2/49, 4/49, 4/50, 5/49 and 17/49 ($p < 0.01$, Fisher's exact test) (Arnold $et\ al.$, 1985; Arnold & Krewski, 1988).

3.3   Administration with known carcinogens or modifying factors

$Mouse$: Groups of 35 male ICR mice, 7 weeks of age, were fed diets containing 10 or 50 mg/kg hexachlorobenzene (99.9%), 250 or 500 mg/kg of diet polychlorinated terphenyl or 50 mg/kg of diet hexachlorobenzene combined with 250 mg/kg of diet polychlorinated terphenyl for 24 weeks. All surviving animals were killed after 40 weeks. Hexachlorobenzene alone induced no liver tumours. Nodular hyperplasia of the liver occurred in 3/28 animals given 250 mg/kg of diet polychlorinated terphenyl. When polychlorinated terphenyl was given in combination with hexachlorobenzene, 23/28 rats developed nodular hyperplasia and 8/28 developed hepatocellular carcinomas (Shirai $et\ al.$, 1978).

Groups of male C57BL/10ScSn and DBA/2 mice, 7–10 weeks of age, received an injection of iron dextran (600 mg/kg bw Fe) and 7 days later were fed a diet containing 0 (control) or 100 mg/kg hexachlorobenzene for up to 18 months. None of 11 surviving C57BL/10ScSn mice treated with hexachlorobenzene alone developed liver hyperplastic nodules [authors' terminology] or hepatocellular carcinomas, whereas 10/10 and 9/10 of those given iron dextran plus hexachlorobenzene developed nodules and carcinomas. respectively. All surviving DBA/2 mice were killed at 10 months; no focal hyperplasia was seen with the combined treatment (Smith *et al.*, 1989).

Rat: Groups of male and female Fischer 344/N rats, 10 weeks of age, were given drinking-water containing *N*-nitrosodiethylamine (NDEA) at a concentration of 0 (control) or 0.015% for 3 weeks. After a 2-week recovery period, the animals were fed a diet containing 0 or 200 mg/kg hexachlorobenzene for 30 weeks. No tumours or hyperplastic nodules of the liver were found in animals treated with hexachlorobenzene alone. The average numbers of visible liver tumours > 3 mm and > 10 mm in size were 10.1 and 4.4 in males receiving NDEA plus hexachlorobenzene and 4.0 and 0.6 in rats treated with NDEA alone. In females, the respective numbers were 5.1 and 1.5 compared with 1.2 and 0.3 (Stewart *et al.*, 1989).

Groups of 15–16 male Fischer 344 rats, 6 weeks of age and weighing approximately 120 g, were given a single intraperitoneal injection of 200 mg/kg bw NDEA, followed 2 weeks later by a diet containing 0 (control), 0.6, 3, 15, 75 or 150 mg/kg hexachlorobenzene. Other groups of 10 males received the diets containing hexachlorobenzene only. The numbers and areas of foci positive for glutathione-*S*-transferase-placental form (GST-P) in the livers were increased in a concentration-related manner, and the increase was statistically significant ($p < 0.001$) at the three highest concentrations (Cabral *et al.*, 1996). Similar results were reported by Gustafson *et al.* (2000) for male Fischer 344 rats given oral doses of hexachlorobenzene (0.1 or 0.4 mmol/kg [29 or 114 mg/kg] bw) daily for 3 weeks after initiation with NDEA.

Groups of male and female Sprague-Dawley rats weighing 175–225 g were subjected to partial hepatectomy or sham operation and 24 h later were treated by oral gavage with 0.3 mmol/kg [31 mg/kg] bw NDEA or distilled water. Four days after NDEA administration, the rats were fed a diet containing 0 or 100 mg/kg hexachlorobenzene for 45 days. One week later, all surviving animals were killed, and liver sections stained for γ-glutamyltranspeptidase (γ-GT)-positive foci. Hexachlorobenzene significantly enhanced the number of foci per cm^2, both with and without partial hepatectomy. Females were more sensitive than males (Pereira *et al.*, 1982).

4. Other Data Relevant to an Evaluation of Carcinogenicity and its Mechanisms

4.1   Absorption, distribution, metabolism and excretion

4.1.1   *Humans*

Hepta- and octachlorodibenzodioxins and dibenzofurans have been found in technical-grade hexachlorobenzene (IARC, 1979), and there has been some dispute in the literature as to whether these dioxins play a role in the toxic effects associated with exposure to hexachlorobenzene (e.g., Jones & Chelsky, 1986).

Hexachlorobenzene is characterized by a very long half-time and high lipophilicity. The bioconcentration factor for hexachlorobenzene in humans is estimated to be 320, and estimates of the half-time in humans are between 4 and 8 years. Hexachlorobenzene crosses the placenta and is found in fetuses, cord blood, follicular fluid and breast milk. In an investigation of the concentrations of hexachlorobenzene in human placenta, maternal blood, milk and cord blood in 36 healthy pregnant women living in rural Japan, a significant linear correlation was found between the concentration of hexachlorobenzene in placenta and in cord blood and also between placenta and milk (Ando *et al.*, 1985).

Pentachlorothiophenol was initially detected and quantified in all urine samples from 40 persons in the general population with high body burdens of hexachlorobenzene (To-Figueras *et al.*, 1992). In a second study, serum and urine from 100 persons in a general population who had been heavily exposed to airborne hexachlorobenzene were analysed. Hexachlorobenzene was detected in all serum samples, at concentrations ranging between 1.1 and 953 ng/mL. Pentachlorophenol was detected in all urine samples, with values ranging between 0.58 and 13.9 µg excreted within 24 h, with a geometric mean of 2.05 µg. A sulfur derivative that, after hydrolysis, yielded pentachlorobenzenethiol was also identified and quantified in all the urine samples, with values ranging between 0.18 and 84.0 µg within 24 h and a geometric mean of 1.39 µg. The sulfur derivative assessed as pentachlorobenzenethiol appeared to be the main metabolite, its urinary concentrations surpassing those of pentachlorophenol in persons with an accumulated concentration of hexachlorobenzene in serum > 32 ng/mL. The concentrations of pentachlorobenzenethiol in urine collected over 24 h showed a strong association with the concentrations of hexachlorobenzene in serum; the association was stronger in men than in women. A weaker association was found between the concentrations of pentachlorophenol in urine and hexachlorobenzene in serum, which was statistically significant only for men. These results suggested that formation of the cysteine conjugate is a quantitatively important metabolic pathway in humans, especially in persons with high hexachlorobenzene body burdens. Moreover, pentachlorobenzenethiol is a urinary marker of the internal dose of hexachlorobenzene and of glutathione-mediated metabolism (To-Figueras *et al.*, 1997).

4.1.2   *Experimental systems*

(*a*)   *Absorption and distribution*

Hexachlorobenzene administered orally to rats was absorbed slowly from the gut, mainly via the lymphatic system, and was stored extensively in the fat after 48 h (Iatropoulos *et al.*, 1975). In rats fed hexachlorobenzene for 4 weeks, subsequent food deprivation appeared to enhance the toxic response (liver hypertrophy), implying decreased mobilization of hexachlorobenzene residues into fat and resulting in greater accumulation of hexachlorobenzene in plasma, liver, brain and adrenal glands (Villeneuve *et al.*, 1977).

In rhesus monkeys (*Macaca mullata*) given hexachlorobenzene at a dose of 8, 32, 64 or 128 mg/kg bw per day by gavage for 60 days, body fat and bone marrow had the highest concentrations, followed by adrenal glands, liver, kidney, brain, ovaries, muscle and serum. The serum concentrations did not appear to correspond to the dose (Knauf & Hobson, 1979). After administration of a single intravenous injection of hexachlorobenzene to male beagles, the chemical was initially found primarily in the lung (2 h) but after 8 h was found primarily in the fat. Excretion in these dogs occurred essentially through the bile and faeces, urinary excretion being of less importance (Sundlof *et al.*, 1982). Absorption of hexachlorobenzene applied dermally to male Fischer 344 rats increased from 1% to 9.7% between 6 and 72 h, and the blood concentrations increased linearly with time (Koizumi, 1991).

In adult female Sprague-Dawley rats dosed with 50 mg/kg bw hexachlorobenzene by gavage, the chemical was found to concentrate primarily in the fat and also in endocrine glands with large lipid components, such as the follicular fluid of the ovary and thyroid. The concentrations of residues of hexachlorobenzene in nine rats given 50 mg/kg bw per day were significantly ($p < 0.05$) greater in the periovarian fat than in the thyroid gland and were significantly ($p < 0.05$) greater in the thyroid gland than in the adrenal gland and ovary. The concentrations of residues of hexachlorobenzene in the ovary were greater than those in the thymus, liver or lung (Foster *et al.*, 1993).

Hexachlorobenzene was found in the milk of cows given the compound (Fries & Marrow, 1976) and in the organs of 18-day-old offspring of rat dams fed a diet containing hexachlorobenzene (Mendoza *et al.*, 1975).

Toxicokinetics demonstrated that hexachlorobenzene is transferred across the placenta and into breast milk in rodents (Courtney & Andrews, 1985; Courtney *et al.*, 1985; Nakashima *et al.*, 1997). Dose-dependent increases in fetal tissues were found when CD-1 mice or CD rats received a single dose of hexachlorobenzene by gavage on day 11 or 16 of gestation or treatment on days 6–11 or 6–16 at a dose of 10, 50 or 100 mg/kg bw per day (Courtney *et al.*, 1979). A similar 6-day study of pregnant hamsters and guinea-pigs showed that the hamster fetuses had fivefold greater concentrations of hexachlorobenzene than the guinea-pig fetuses (Courtney *et al.*, 1985). In a study in which lactating rhesus monkeys were given hexachlorobenzene by gavage for 60 days at a dose of 64 mg/kg bw per day, the infant serum concentrations were two- to fivefold higher than those in maternal serum, and their tissue concentrations were also generally higher than those of their mothers. The distribution in infants showed concentration in fat, bone marrow and adrenal glands (Bailey *et al.*, 1980). When pregnant Sprague-Dawley rats were given a diet containing hexachlorobenzene during gestation and lactation (35 nmol/100 g diet [100 μg/kg diet]), about 0.39% of the total intake during gestation was transferred to the fetuses. A large proportion of the hexachlorobenzene body burden was lost during lactation, and the concentration in the stomach contents of suckling pups was highest on day 2 after birth (Nakashima *et al.*, 1997).

(b)   Metabolism and excretion

Quantitative recovery of intraperitoneally and orally administered [^{14}C]hexachlorobenzene in rats was dose-dependent, but more label was recovered from faeces than from the urine. The major urinary metabolites were pentachlorophenol, tetrachlorohydroquinone and pentachlorothiophenol. The other urinary metabolites were tetrachlorobenzene, pentachlorobenzene, 2,4,5- and 2,4,6-trichlorophenols and 2,3,4,6- and 2,3,5-6-tetrachlorophenols; 2,3,4-trichlorophenol and other tetrachlorophenols were present in traces amounts. These metabolites were excreted as conjugates or in free form in the urine. Unchanged hexachlorobenzene was found in the faeces and in fat (Mehendale *et al.*, 1975; Engst *et al.*, 1976; Koss *et al.*, 1976; Renner & Schuster, 1977) (see Figure 1).

After 110 μg/day [^{14}C]hexachlorobenzene were given orally to *Macaca mulatta* monkeys for 11–15 months, 50% of the radiolabel found in the urine was associated with pentachlorophenol and 25% with pentachlorobenzene, the remaining being associated with unidentified metabolites and unchanged hexachlorobenzene. In the faeces, 99% of the radiolabel was attached to unchanged hexachlorobenzene. During the last 10 days of the experiment, males excreted 7.2% of the administered dose in the urine and 51.9% in the faeces and females excreted 4.6 and 42.2%, respectively (Rozman *et al.*, 1977).

Examination of 1 g of liver tissue from adult female Wistar rats given 178 μmol/kg bw [50.7 mg/kg bw] hexachlorobenzene after 9 weeks revealed the presence of 1 μmol hexachlorobenzene, 50 nmol pentachlorophenol, 5 nmol tetrachlorohydroquinone, 0.1 nmol pentachlorothiophenol and pentachlorothioanisole. The authors hypothesized that the sulfur in the latter two compounds was derived from glutathione (Koss *et al.*, 1978, 1979).

Male and female Fischer 344 rats were dosed every other day for 103 days with 50 μmol/kg bw [14.2 mg/kg bw] hexachlorobenzene by esophageal intubation. This dose produced hepatic porphyria, especially in females. Urine was collected periodically and analysed for pentachlorophenol, 2,3,5,6-tetrachlorobenzene-1,4-diol and pentachlorothiophenol. The combined urinary excretion of these metabolites was greater in females than males, especially during the first 10 weeks. Pentachlorothiophenol was present at particularly high concentrations in the urine of females. The male:female ratios for pentachlorophenol and pentachlorothiophenol in bile were identical to those

Figure 1. Urinary metabolites of hexachlorobenzene

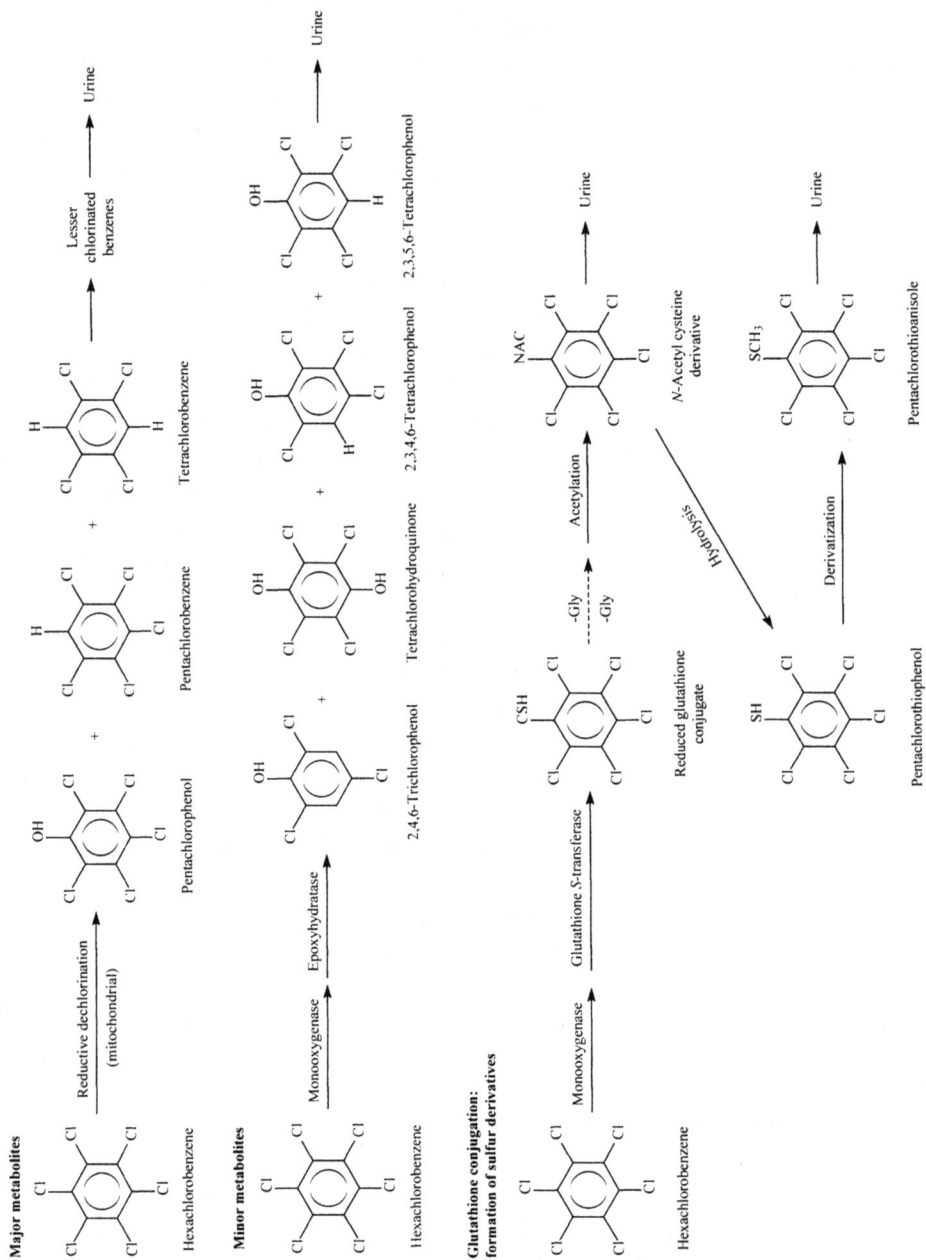

Modified from Agency for Toxic Substances and Disease Registry (1998)

for these compounds in faeces. Excretion of metabolites by both males and females was stimulated by pretreatment with diethylstilbestrol. No sex differences in metabolism were observed in immature rats (Rizzardini & Smith, 1982).

A study of the metabolism of hexachlorobenzene in isolated hepatocytes from male and female Fischer 344 adult rats showed that sex differences in metabolism did not explain the differences in porphyria development. The significant metabolites were pentachlorophenol, pentachlorothiophenol and tetrachloro-1,4-benzenedithiol. Likewise, covalent binding of [^{14}C]hexachlorobenzene to protein after incubation with hepatocytes could not account for the sex-dependent porphyrogenic activity (Stewart & Smith, 1987).

Sexually immature male and female Wistar rats given hexachlorobenzene showed initially no differences in the excretion of *N*-acetyl-*S*-(pentachlorophenyl)cysteine, but 5–8 days after weaning, the urinary concentrations of the sulfur derivative began to increase in females, until a 10-fold difference between the sexes was established. Studies *in vitro* and analysis of tissues after administration of pentachloronitrobenzene *in vivo* showed that conjugation with glutathione and hydrolysis of the conjugates to yield free pentachlorothiophenol did not differ between males and females. These findings tend to reinforce the view that an active renal secretory mechanism, probably induced by estrogens during sexual maturation, is responsible for the highly efficient excretion of sulfur derivatives of hexachlorobenzene and pentachloronitrobenzene by female rats (To-Figueras *et al.*, 1991).

The metabolism of [^{14}C]hexachlorobenzene was studied in microsomes derived from 12-week-old male Wistar rats. The metabolites formed were pentachlorophenol and tetrachlorohydroquinone. In addition, a considerable amount of covalent binding of radiolabel to protein was found: 11 pmol covalent binding per 4 mg microsomal protein in an incubation mixture containing 25 µmol/L hexachlorobenzene. In order to establish the potential role of reductive dechlorination in the covalent binding, the anaerobic metabolism of hexachlorobenzene was investigated. Incubation at low oxygen concentrations indicated a relationship between covalent binding and microsomal oxidation of hexachlorobenzene. The finding of conversion-dependent covalent binding indicated that less than 10% of the covalent binding occurs during conversion of hexachlorobenzene to pentachlorophenol, and the remainder is produced during conversion of pentachlorophenol to tetrachlorohydroquinone, which is in redox equilibrium with the corresponding semiquinone and quinone (chloranil). The covalent binding is inhibited by addition of ascorbic acid or glutathione. These results indicate the involvement of chloranil or the semiquinone radical in covalent binding during microsomal hexachlorobenzene metabolism (van Ommen *et al.*, 1986).

In rats given diets containing either hexachlorobenzene or its metabolite pentachlorobenzene for 13 weeks, both compounds were oxidized to pentachlorophenol and tetrachlorohydroquinone, which were the only two common metabolites excreted in urine. Additional urinary metabolites of hexachlorobenzene were *N*-acetyl-*S*-(pentachlorophenyl)cysteine, which appeared to be quantitatively the most important product, and mercaptotetrachlorothioanisole, which was excreted as a glucuronide. The biotransformation of hexachlorobenzene and pentachlorobenzene was modulated by selective inhibition of cytochrome P450 (CYP) 3A1/2 in rats by combined treatment with hexachlorobenzene or pentachlorobenzene and triacetyloleandomycin. Rats receiving this diet excreted much less pentachlorophenol and tetrachlorohydroquinone than rats fed hexachlorobenzene or pentachlorobenzene alone, indicating the involvement of CYP3A in the oxidation of both compounds (den Besten *et al.*, 1994).

Male and female Sprague-Dawley rats were given five consecutive doses of 1 g/kg bw hexachlorobenzene by gavage over 2 days. The cumulative dose produced porphyria in female but not male rats after a delay of 6 weeks. The animals were killed 0, 6, 12, 18 or 24 h after the last dose. The hepatic glutathione concentration showed a diurnal cycle in both male and female rats, which was more pronounced in males; the minimum concentration was observed 12 h after dosing. The glutathione concentration in hexachlorobenzene-treated male rats was significantly lower than that in controls at 6, 18 and 24 h, whereas no significant difference was observed in hexachlorobenzene-treated female rats. Biliary excretion of a metabolite originating from glutathione conjugation of hexachlorobenzene was higher in male than in female rats. These results suggested that hepatic glutathione conjugation of hexachlorobenzene is more important in male than in female rats, which may be related to the lower incidence of liver porphyria observed in hexachlorobenzene-treated male than female rats (D'Amour & Charbonneau, 1992).

4.2   Toxic effects

4.2.1   *Humans*

An epidemic of 4000 cases of porphyria cutanea tarda occurred in Turkey between 1955 and 1959 as a result of human consumption of grain that had been treated with hexachlorobenzene. The estimated intake of hexachlorobenzene was 50–200 mg/day over a relatively long period before the disease became apparent (Peters *et al.*, 1966; Mazzei & Mazzei, 1973; Peters, 1976; Peters *et al.*, 1978). The majority of the patients were children, mostly boys, aged 4–14 years (Cam & Nigogosyan, 1963). A mortality rate of 14% was reported within several years (Peters *et al.*, 1966, 1978). The exposure to hexachlorobenzene led to the development of bullae on sun-exposed areas, hyperpigmentation, hypertrichosis and porphyrinuria. The condition was known as 'kara yara' or 'black sore'. Children under the age of 4 rarely developed porphyria, but in breastfed infants a condition known as 'pink sore' was reported, with a mortality rate greater than 95% (Cam, 1960; Peters, 1976). Samples of breast milk from the mothers of these infants were shown to contain hexachlorobenzene (Peters *et al.*, 1966). Follow-up studies of 32 of the patients have shown that abnormal porphyrin metabolism and active symptomatology persisted 20 years after ingestion of hexachlorobenzene (Peters *et al.*, 1978; Cripps *et al.*, 1980).

In a later follow-up that included examination of 204 patients from this population, the following signs and symptoms were still present: weakness, paraesthesia, neuritis, myotonia, severe residual scarring from the initial bullae, hyperpigmentation and hirsutism. After exposure beginning in childhood, small stature, small hands and painless arthritis were present. Of particular note, enlarged thyroids were present in 25% of men and 60% of women in comparison with 5% of unexposed persons from this region of Turkey. Two persons died of liver failure; one was a 27-year-old man and the other a 54-year-old woman during treatment for tuberculosis (Cripps *et al.*, 1984; Peters *et al.*, 1986). In another follow-up of 252 persons with a history of porphyria after the Turkish incident 20–30 years earlier, similar findings were reported. Many of the patients had dermatological, neurological and orthopaedic symptoms and signs. The observed clinical findings include scarring of the face and hands (83.7%), hyperpigmentation (65%), hypertrichosis (44.8%), pinched facies (40.1%), painless arthritis (70.2%), small hands (66.6%), sensory shading (60.6%), myotonia (37.9%), cogwheeling (41.9%), enlarged thyroid (34.9%) and enlarged liver (4.8%). When urine and stool porphyrin concentrations were determined in all patients, 17 had an elevated concentration of at least one of the porphyrins. A total of 56 specimens of human milk obtained from mothers with porphyria were analysed for hexachlorobenzene. The average value was 0.51 mg/L in hexachlorobenzene-exposed patients and 0.07 mg/L in unexposed controls. The children of mothers with three decades of hexachlorobenzene-induced porphyria appeared to be normal. Three persons had undergone thyroidectomy, which revealed colloidal goitre. One additional person, a 47-year-old woman, had died of liver cirrhosis (Gocmen *et al.*, 1989).

A group of 52 men were exposed to hexachlorobenzene as a by-product in a chemical manufacturing plant in Brazil. The serum immunoglobulin (IgG, IgM and IgA) concentrations of these men were examined and compared with those of unexposed, age- and sex-matched individuals. At the time of testing, the exposed population had a mean concentration of hexachlorobenzene in blood of 38.4 μg/L, with a range of 1–160 μg/L. Increased IgG and IgM concentrations were found in the hexachlorobenzene-exposed workers ($p < 0.05$ and $p < 0.01$, respectively). The IgM concentrations were positively correlated with the length of exposure ($r = 0.367$) and the activities of aspartate aminotransferase ($r = 0.367$) and alanine aminotransferase ($r = 0.507$) (Queiroz *et al.*, 1998a). In 66 exposed workers from this plant, the lytic activity of neutrophils in the presence of antigens from *Candida albicans* and *C. pseudotropicalis* was found to be impaired (Queiroz *et al.*, 1998b).

The average concentration of hexachlorobenzene in the plasma of people living near a hexachlorobenzene manufacturing plant but not exposed occupationally was 3.6 μg/L; there was no evidence of porphyria, but the plasma coproporphyrin concentrations were abnormally high (Burns & Miller, 1975). Urine specimens from nine male aluminium foundry workers in smelters where aluminium was degased with hexachloroethane at six different companies, and from 18 controls, matched for sex, age, residence and socioeconomic status, were analysed for total porphyrins and porphyrin isomers.

Workers exposed to hexachlorobenzene and octachlorostyrene (thermal by-product of hexachloroethane) had a statistically significant increase in total urinary porphyrins over that in controls (mean ± standard deviation: 13.63 ± 11.13 μmol/mol creatinine and 6.24 ± 3.84 μmol/mol creatinine, respectively; $p = 0.02$) (Seldén *et al.*, 1999).

In a cross-sectional study of 1800 inhabitants of a small village in the south of Catalonia, Spain, which surrounds an electrochemical factory characterized by high concentrations of hexachlorobenzene in the air, biological samples were obtained during 1994 from 615 persons. Self-reported health outcomes were validated against clinical records and cancer registry data. The serum concentrations of hexachlorobenzene were very high in men who worked in the electrochemical factory (geometric mean, 54.6 μg/L in randomized participants) and were lower among subjects who had never worked in the electrochemical factory (women, 14.9 μg/L; men, 9.0 μg/L). Perceived health and the prevalence of self-reported common chronic conditions, porphyria cutanea tarda, thyroid disease, Parkinson disease, cancer and reproductive outcomes were within the ranges observed in other studies (Sala *et al.*, 1999b).

4.2.2 *Experimental systems*

The oral LD_{50} of hexachlorobenzene in rats varied from 3500 to 10 000 mg/kg bw (Booth & McDowell, 1975).

(a) *Effects on the thyroid*

Male Syrian hamsters were fed diets containing hexachlorobenzene at 100 mg/kg for 28 weeks, 200 mg/kg of diet for 18 or 28 weeks or 500 mg/kg of diet for 6 weeks. All the animals had an at least 2.5–3-fold increase in thyroid size, mainly due to enlargement of some follicles. Serum thyroxine (T4) concentrations were unchanged, whereas those of triiodothyronine (T3) were eventually depressed by more than 60%. The uptake of ^{131}I into the thyroid was induced approximately threefold in hamsters given 500 mg/kg of diet for 3 or 6 weeks. The effects of hexachlorobenzene in hamsters differed from those in rats, as exposure of rats to 500 mg/kg of diet for 6 weeks produced only a small increase in thyroid size (1.3-fold), only a slightly depression in serum concentrations of T3 but a 74% reduction in those of T4 (Smith *et al.*, 1986, 1987).

Administration of 1 g/kg bw hexachlorobenzene for 4 weeks to female Wistar rats resulted in a sixfold increase in T4 metabolic clearance and in the distribution space. Decreased serum T4 concentrations resulted from an increase in both deiodinative and faecal disposal. The metabolism of T3 was only slightly affected. The enhanced peripheral disposition of T4 appeared to lead to increased thyroid function, as measured by augmented thyroid-stimulating hormone (TSH) serum concentrations and ^{125}I uptake in the thyroid. Serum binding of T4 was not affected (Kleiman de Pisarev *et al.*, 1989).

When female Wistar rats were given 1 g/kg bw hexachlorobenzene by gavage daily for 1 or 8 weeks, porphyria and changes in thyroid function and thyroid hormone metabolism were seen. Serum T4 concentrations were depressed, and a 50% reduction in protein-bound iodine was found, whereas the concentration of T3 was not depressed significantly at either treatment time. Hexachlorobenzene altered T4 metabolism in rat liver slices, increasing dehalogenation. Administration of hexachlorobenzene for 1 week inhibited porphyrinogen decarboxylase activity for uroporphyrinogen disappearance by 25% and coproporphyrinogen formation by 51%. After 8 weeks of hexachlorobenzene administration, the rats showed characteristic porphyria (Kleiman de Pisarev *et al.*, 1990).

Groups of WAG-RIJ rats received oral doses of 0–3.5 mmol/kg bw [0–1 g/kg bw] hexachlorobenzene three times per week for 2 or 4 weeks (highest dose only). Measurements of thyroid hormone status after 2 weeks showed a dose-dependent decrease in total T4 concentration, decreased free T4 concentrations and little change in total T3 concentrations. The effects on thyroid hormone status were more pronounced after 4 weeks and included increased TSH concentrations. The major metabolite, pentachlorophenol, interacted competitively with thyroid hormone-binding proteins in serum to produce a rapid, dose-dependent decrease in total and free T4 concentrations, but not in total T3 concentration, in serum. The decrease in total serum T4 concentrations was attributed to competitive interactions of pentachlorophenol with hormone serum-binding proteins and increased metabolism induced by hexachlorobenzene, to an equal degree. At lower doses and with the shorter dosing, increased metabolism of T4 was the main cause of the decrease in total serum T4 concentration. Therefore, similar effects were produced simultaneously by the parent compound and its metabolite, through different, independent mechanisms (van Raaij *et al.*, 1993a).

In WAG/MBL rats exposed to 1 g/kg bw hexachlorobenzene orally three times a week for 4 weeks, the T4 concentration was lowered by 35.5% whereas that of T3 was unchanged. Analysis of bile by high-performance liquid chromatography revealed a more than threefold increase in T4 glucuronide and a concomitant reduction in unconjugated T4. T4 UDP-glucuronosyltransferase (UGT) activity in hepatic microsomes was increased more than 4.5-fold in animals exposed to hexachlorobenzene, and *para*-nitrophenol UGT showed a comparable increase. T3 UGT activity was increased 2.5-fold by hexachlorobenzene, but androsterone UGT activity was unchanged. These results suggest that T4 is a substrate for hexachlorobenzene-inducible *para*-nitrophenol UGT and T3 for androsterone UGT. In the absence of the latter, T3 is also glucuronidated to some extent by *para*-nitrophenol UGT. Type 1 iodothyronine deiodinase activity was decreased by hexachlorobenzene treatment (van Raaij *et al.*, 1993b).

In Wistar rats treated with 1 g/kg bw hexachlorobenzene by gavage daily for 1 or 4 weeks, depletion of T4 but no change in T3 concentrations were observed in serum. In the liver, mitochondrial L-glycerolphosphate dehydrogenase activity did not change significantly, but the cytosolic enzymes, malic enzyme, glucose-6-phosphate dehydrogenase and 6-phosphogluconate dehydrogenase, were induced by hexachlorobenzene, only in animals with an intact thyroid. The absence of cytosolic enzyme induction in thyroidectomized rats treated with hexachlorobenzene indicates that this compound is not intrinsically thyromimetic. The induction of the hepatic cytosolic enzymes in hexachlorobenzene-treated thyroidectomized rats was dependent on the presence of thyroid hormone, administered intraperitoneally at a daily dose of 100 μg/kg bw. The unchanged activity of the thyroid-regulated mitochondrial L-glycerolphosphate dehydrogenase, in contrast to the increased activities of the cytosolic enzymes, was not considered consistent with a shift in functional thyroid status after treatment with hexachlorobenzene (Kleiman de Pisarev *et al.*, 1995).

WAG/RIJ-MBL rats were given either hexachlorobenzene, pentachlorophenol or tetrachlorohydroquinone as a single equimolar intraperitoneal dose of 0.056 mmol/kg bw (i.e. 16, 15 or 14 mg/kg bw, respectively). Hexachlorobenzene did not alter serum T4 or T3 concentrations for up to 96 h after dosing, but pentachlorophenol and tetra-chlorohydroquinone both reduced the serum T4 concentrations, with a maximum effect between 6 and 24 h after exposure. Tetrachlorohydroquinone was more effective in repressing T3 than T4 blood concentrations. In another experiment, rats received pentachlorophenol or tetrachlorohydroquinone intraperitoneally at various doses. The reduction in T4 concentration by pentachlorophenol was inversely related to the serum concentration of this compound, on the basis of toxicokinetics and dose–response profiles. Furthermore, the concentration of pentachlorophenol in serum after adminis-tration of hexachlorobenzene appeared to be too low to have an effect. The results of this study indicate that not hexachlorobenzene itself, but rather its metabolites penta-chlorophenol and tetrachlorohydroquinone, are involved in the reduced serum thyroid hormone concentrations seen after administration of hexachlorobenzene to rats (van Raaij *et al.*, 1991a).

In a competition assay *in vitro*, pentachlorophenol was an effective competitor for the T4-binding sites of serum carriers, whereas hexachlorobenzene was ineffective. Ex-vivo experiments demonstrated occupation of T4-binding sites in sera from penta-chlorophenol-exposed animals but not in sera from hexachlorobenzene- or tetrachloro-hydroquinone-treated animals. Competing ability for T4-binding sites was still present in the sera of pentachlorophenol-exposed animals but was absent in hexachloro-benzene- and tetrachlorohydroquinone-exposed animals. The results suggest that thyroid hormone displacement by the major metabolite pentachlorophenol may play a role in hexachlorobenzene-induced hypothyroidism (van Raaij *et al.*, 1991b).

Serum T4 and the free T4 index were significantly ($p < 0.05$) suppressed in hexachlorobenzene-treated female Sprague-Dawley rats given 50 mg/kg bw per day by gavage when compared with a control group ($n = 8$). In contrast, no significant differences in the serum concentrations of estradiol or progesterone or in the percentage of T3 uptake were observed. In a second experiment, 16 adult female Sprague-Dawley rats were dosed as above and superovulated by subcutaneous admi-nistration of pregnant mare serum gonadotrophin (10 IU) and human chorionic gonadotrophin (20 IU). The circulating concentrations of progesterone were signifi-cantly ($p < 0.05$) higher than those in the control group ($n = 8$). The per cent uptake of T3 and the serum concentration of T4 were significantly ($p = 0.05$) suppressed when compared with controls, with no effect on the free T4 index. These results suggest that the effects of hexachlorobenzene on thyroid parameters may be modulated by hormonal changes in female rats (Foster *et al.*, 1993).

(b)   *Effects on the liver*

Hexachlorobenzene has a range of toxic effects on the liver. Those observed in rats after long-term feeding of a diet containing up to 1000 mg/kg bw technical-grade hexachlorobenzene (93–95% pure) included hepatocellular hypertrophy and necrosis, spleen enlargement and porphyria. The survival rates were 70% and 5% for males and females, respectively, at the highest concentration (Kimbrough & Linder, 1974).

Doses of hexachlorobenzene ranging from 0.05 to 50 mg/kg bw per day administered to pigs for 90 days induced porphyria. Animals given the highest dose died. Increased urinary excretion of coproporphyrin was observed in groups receiving 0.5 and 5 mg/kg bw per day after 8 weeks; in those receiving 5 mg/kg bw per day, induction of microsomal liver enzymes, accompanied by increased liver weight, was also observed (den Tonkelaar *et al.*, 1978).

Hexachlorobenzene fed in the diet at 0.1% to rats for 15 days caused marked hepatomegaly and increased microsomal CYP and protein contents. Flow-cytometric analysis revealed no changes in hepatocyte ploidy, and the changes noted were associated with increased hepatocyte size (Rizzardini *et al.*, 1990).

A great deal of research has been focused on the porphyrogenic effects of hexachlorobenzene. Rats can be made porphyrinogenic by long-term administration of 50–1000 mg/kg bw hexachlorobenzene (Koss *et al.*, 1978; Rios de Molína *et al.*, 1980; Krishnan *et al.*, 1991), and the resulting porphyria is associated with inhibition of uroporphyrinogen decarboxylase, similar to spontaneous porphyria cutanea tarda, which has been described in episodes of human poisoning (see above).

Porphyrins accumulate in the urine, liver, kidney and spleen, suggesting an effect on the activity of uroporphyrinogen decarboxylase (UROD) (Doss *et al.*, 1976; Kuiper-Goodman *et al.*, 1977; Goerz *et al.*, 1978). Dosing of female Wistar rats at 50 mg/kg bw per day resulted in increasing concentrations of porphyrins in the liver and urine and of δ-aminolaevulinic acid (ALA) and porphorbilinogen in the urine (Koss *et al.*, 1978).

The course of events associated with hexachlorobenzene-induced porphyria was investigated in female Wistar rats given 0.1 g/kg bw hexachlorobenzene every other day for 6 weeks and then kept for an additional 18 months without treatment. During the first phase, the hexachlorobenzene concentration in the liver was almost constant, and the activity of UROD gradually decreased. Then, the porphyrin concentration increased, and there was complete inhibition of UROD. Next, after cessation of hexachlorobenzene administration, the porphyrin concentration continued to increase, and UROD activity continued to be inhibited. Finally, the porphyrin concentration decreased and the activity of UROD returned (Koss *et al.*, 1983).

During exposure of rats to 200 mg/kg of diet hexachlorobenzene for 4–29 weeks, some females showed elevated γ-GT activity throughout the periportal regions of the liver, but all those examined at 29 weeks had a few γ-GT-positive foci. The livers of males were not affected at 29 weeks, but after 90 weeks of feeding, males also had elevated periportal γ-GT activity and a number of γ-GT-positive foci (Manson & Smith, 1984).

In rats fed 0.3% hexachlorobenzene in the diet for 8 weeks, urinary excretion of ALA, coproporphyrin and uroporphyrin increased to reach 2.4, 3.3 and 3.8 times the control values, respectively. In the liver, an increase was observed in ALA synthetase activity and decreases in ALA dehydratase and uroporphyrinogen decarboxylase activities (Kondo & Shimizu, 1986).

Cytosol from female Wistar rat livers was incubated with uroporphyrinogen III and 1-mmol/L concentrations of chlorinated phenols, thiophenols, thioanisoles and benzenes. UROD was inhibited by tetrachlorohydroquinone, pentachlorophenol, pentachlorothiophenol and 1,2,3,5- and 1,2,4,5-tetrachlorobenzene. Other compounds including hexachlorobenzene, which was tested for comparative reasons, did not impair UROD activity, but the concentration used was 0.1 mmol/L. In the presence of tetrachlorohydroquinone, uroporphyrinogen was decarboxylated to hepta- and hexa-carboxyporphyrinogen; in the presence of the four compounds with inhibitory effects, pentacarboxyporphyrinogen and coproporphyrinogen were formed in addition. Copro-porphyrinogen formation was inhibited completely by tetrachlorohydroquinone, while pentachlorophenol decreased its formation by about 50% and pentachlorothiophenol and 1,2,3,5- and 1,2,4,5-tetrachlorobenzene by < 10% (Billi de Catabbi et al., 1986).

In another study of the inhibitory effects of hexachlorobenzene and its metabolites on UROD, hydroxylated products including pentachlorophenol, 2,3,4,6-tetrachloro-phenol and 2,4,5- or 2,4,6-trichlorophenol were active, whereas hexachlorobenzene had no effect (Rios de Molína et al., 1980). In chick embryo liver cells in culture, the main metabolite did not induce porphyria but pentachlorothioanisole and tetrachlorothio-anisole did. Inhibition of hepatic drug metabolism by piperonyl butoxide prevented the accumulation of porphyrins, whereas pre-incubation of liver cell cultures with β-naptho-flavone markedly enhanced porphyrin accumulation. The antioxidants ascorbic acid and vitamin E also prevented hexachlorobenzene-induced porphyria, implying a role of a pro-oxidant. Inhibition of UROD was postulated to be the primary lesion induced by hexachlorobenzene, in view of the pattern of porphyrins found in the culture (Debets et al., 1980, 1981a).

Significantly higher concentrations of N-acetyl-S-(pentahalophenyl)cysteine were found in the urine of hexachlorobenzene-exposed rats than in that of hexafluoro-benzene-exposed rats; furthermore, hexafluorobenzene did not cause porphyria, whereas hexachlorobenzene resulted in significantly elevated concentrations of both urinary and liver porphyrins. These results indicate that the extent of metabolism of hexahalogenated benzenes into urinary metabolites resulting from glutathione conjugation is a better indication of their porphyrinogenic action than the extent of their metabolism to phenolic metabolites (Rietjens et al., 1995).

The porphyrinogenic effects of hexachlorobenzene are stronger in female than in male Fischer and Sprague-Dawley rats (Rizzardini & Smith, 1982; Smith et al., 1985; Krishnan et al., 1991), and this sex-dependent susceptibility is correlated with tumorigenicity. After 90 weeks of hexachlorobenzene treatment, 100% of the surviving female Fisher 344 rats had multiple liver tumours which were strongly γ-GT-positive and classified histologically as neoplastic nodules or hepatocellular carcinomas. In contrast, only 16% of males developed tumours, which were smaller and fewer per liver than those in females. The sex difference in tumour response could not be explained by differences in hepatic hexachlorobenzene concentrations (Smith et al., 1985). Female BDVI rats were given 3 mg/kg bw per day NDEA for 5 weeks by gavage beginning at 4 weeks of age. When the animals were 40 weeks old, 1 g/kg bw hexachlorobenzene was administered daily by gavage for 5 weeks to some animals, and the animals were killed between 46 and 56 weeks of age. The urinary concentration of porphyrins increased during the 5 weeks of treatment with hexachlorobenzene in both NDEA-exposed animals and controls. When the tumour tissue was compared with surrounding parenchyma and tissue from animals receiving hexachlorobenzene only, the concentrations of porphyrins in the tumours were not significantly different from those in controls, whereas there were large accumulations in hexachlorobenzene-exposed 'normal' liver. Also, the activity of ALA synthetase was increased in the latter but not the former (Wainstok de Calmanovici et al., 1991).

Iron is important in the development of porphyria after treatment with hexachlorobenzene. This was demonstrated in an experiment in which female Wistar rats were fed a diet deficient in iron or given a subcutaneous injection of 25 mg/kg bw iron dextran on the first day of the experiment. On day 8, the rats received an intraperitoneal injection of about 1 g/kg bw hexachlorobenzene; all rats were killed on day 60. The uroporphyrin content of the liver of animals treated with iron and hexachlorobenzene was 10 000-fold greater than that in controls and 20-fold greater than that in animals given hexachlorobenzene alone. No uroporphyrin could be detected in the iron-deficient groups, with or without hexachlorobenzene, and iron alone had little effect on the uroporphyrin concentration. Lipid peroxidation, as measured by malondialdehyde formation, was increased, especially in the group given iron plus hexachlorobenzene and to a lesser extent in the group given iron only. Animals given hexachlorobenzene plus iron showed evidence of protein–protein cross-linking, as measured by sodium dodecyl sulfate gel electrophoresis (Alleman et al., 1985).

In female AGUS and Fischer 344 rats given diets containing hexachlorobenzene for 65 weeks at 0.01 or 0.02% and pretreatment with an iron-loading subcutaneous injection of iron–dextran complex, hepatocellular necrosis and fibrin deposition in the areas of sinusoidal dilatation were more marked, and sinusoidal telangiectasis was accelerated. Control rats had none of these changes, except for an occasional macrophage with iron staining (Carthew & Smith, 1994).

Groups of 12 female Chbb THOM rats were given the iron chelator desferrioxamine by intramuscular injection of 100 mg/kg bw three times a week, hexachlorobenzene (1 g/kg bw per day) by gavage or desferrioxamine at the start of hexachlorobenzene treatment and throughout the experiment. All rats were killed after 12–14 weeks. Treatment with desferrioxamine delayed and diminished urinary excretion of precursors and porphyrins by reducing the liver iron concentration and reduced the accumulation of porphyrins in the liver induced by hexachlorobenzene by attenuating the activity of the enzymes porphyrinogen carboxylyase and ALA synthetase (Wainstock de Calmanovici et al., 1986).

Factors other than iron are also important. In a comparative study, female Wistar and Chbb THOM rats were given 1 g/kg bw per day hexachlorobenzene by gavage for 7 weeks. In Wistar rats, hepatic porphyrins were increased 140-fold and ALA synthetase activity fourfold, and UROD activity was inhibited by 70%. In Chbb THOM rats, these values were threefold, 1.7-fold and 22%, respectively. As the total iron content was similar in the two strains, the difference in susceptibility to porphyria was not wholly ascribable to differences in iron metabolism (Wainstok de Calmanovici et al., 1989).

The involvement of CYP3A in hexachlorobenzene-induced porphyria was established in biotransformation studies with microsomes derived from male Wistar rats treated with various inducers of CYP isoenzymes, and by selective inactivation of CYP3A by triacetyloleandomycin, resulting in strong inhibition of the microsomal conversion of hexachlorobenzene and pentachlorophenol. In-vivo inactivation of CYP3A was achieved by co-administration of hexachlorobenzene and triacetyloleandomycin. Female Wistar rats treated with these compounds in the diet (hexachlorobenzene, 0.03%; triacetyloleandomycin, 0.3%) for 10 weeks showed strongly diminished urinary excretion of the major oxidative metabolites (pentachlorophenol and tetrachlorohydroquinone), as compared with rats treated with hexachlorobenzene alone. Concomitant administration of triacetyloleandomycin resulted in complexation of 70% of the total amount of hepatic microsomal CYP. The group treated with hexachlorobenzene alone had a 600-fold increase in the amount of hepatic porphyrins, whereas concomitant administration of triacetyloleandomycin almost completely inhibited this effect. A strong correlation was found between the amounts of porphyrins and oxidative metabolites excreted, as a function of length of exposure (van Ommen et al., 1989).

Another study with triacetyloleandomycin confirmed the role of CYP3A in the development of porphyria. This study suggested that a putative reactive intermediate in the primary oxidative step plays a role in hexachlorobenzene-induced porphyria, since the degree of porphyria was highly correlated with the excretion of pentachlorophenol and much more weakly correlated with early excretion of tetrachlorohydroquinone (den Besten et al., 1993).

Modulating thyroid function also influences hexachlorobenzene-induced porphyria. The serum T4 concentrations in female Wistar rats were depressed after 8 days of administration of 1 g/kg bw per day hexachlorobenzene by gavage, whereas the concentrations of T3 were not altered. Administration of T4 at 100 μg/kg bw per day simultaneously with hexachlorobenzene resulted in hyperthyroxinaemia. A significant decrease in UROD activity was found after 8 days of treatment with hexachlorobenzene in T4-treated rats, but in rats with no T4 administration and in thyroidectomized rats this decrease in UROD activity was delayed to 21 and 30 days, respectively. Therefore, thyroid hormones seemed to enhance the induction of hexachlorobenzene-induced porphyria (Sopena de Kracoff *et al.*, 1994).

Hexachlorobenzene-induced porphyria was associated with lipid peroxidation in rats with iron loading. Female Sprague-Dawley rats were fed a diet containing hexachlorobenzene at 0.2% (w/w), carbonyl iron at 1.0% (w/w) or hexachlorobenzene plus iron for 8 weeks. The total hepatic porphyrin concentration was increased 100-fold in rats receiving hexachlorobenzene or hexachlorobenzene plus iron, and there was a significant increase in mitochondrial lipid peroxidation, as measured by the concentration of conjugated dienes, in these treated rats (Feldman & Bacon, 1989).

Female Wistar rats given 1 g/kg bw per day hexachlorobenzene for 1–8 weeks showed decreased UROD activity and the presence of an inhibitor of the enzyme during the first 2 weeks. This inhibitor was isolated from a supernatant obtained after centrifugation at 11 000 × g, which was filtered through Sephadex G-25, heated for 5 min at 100 °C and then centrifuged at 1000 × g for 10 min. The concentration of hepatic porphyrins began to increase during the second week of treatment, became statistically significant during the third week and continued to increase over subsequent weeks. During this period, measures of lipid peroxidation malondialdehyde and conjugated dienes also increased. The phospholipid content showed an initial increase, ascribed to a proliferation of membranes, and a later decrease, ascribed to toxic effects involving membrane destruction (Billi de Catabbi *et al.*, 1997).

After 30 days of treatment of male Wistar rats with 25 mg/kg bw per day hexachlorobenzene by gavage, increases in microsomal CYP content, thiobarbituric acid-reactive substances, adrenochrome production (a marker of superoxide production), NADPH cytochrome c reductase and NADPH oxidase were observed in the liver. In plasma, increases in malondialdehyde, ascorbic acid and urinary coproporphyrin concentrations were also found. The liver showed severe lesions with vacuolization and nuclear degeneration mainly in zone 3 hepatocytes. Plasma aspartate and alanine aminotransferase activities were also increased (Almeida *et al.*, 1997).

(c)   *Neurotoxic effects*

Adult mink (*Mustela vison*) and ferrets (*Mustela putorius furo*) were given diets containing hexachlorobenzene at a concentration of 1, 5 or 25 mg/kg for 47 weeks. The concentration of hypothalamic serotonin (5-HT) was significantly elevated at all doses in mink, and that of cerebellar 5-HT was significantly elevated at 1 mg/kg of diet in ferrets. Regional concentrations of brain biogenic amines were determined in the offspring of female mink given 1 or 5 mg/kg of diet hexachlorobenzene. The hypothalamic dopamine concentrations were significantly depressed in the kits at both concentrations. Animals receiving 125 or 625 mg/kg of diet hexachlorobenzene died before termination of the experiment, the female ferrets at 125 mg/kg of diet displaying abnormal aggressiveness and hyperexcitability just before death (Bleavins *et al.*, 1984).

(d) Nephrotoxicity

Groups of male and female Sprague-Dawley rats were given hexachlorobenzene in corn oil by gavage for 15 days (on days 1–5, 8–12 and 15) or 50 mg/kg bw hexachlorobenzene in 36 doses (on 5 days/week over 50 days). Urine was collected on days 1, 8 and 15 of the 15-day treatment and on day 50 of the 50-day treatment. In both males and females in the first study, hexachlorobenzene had induced glycosia by day 8. In males only, hexachlorobenzene induced proteinaemia in both studies. Histological examination of the kidneys of male rats revealed degenerative and regenerative cellular foci accompanied by increased accumulation of protein droplets in epithelial cells of the proximal tubules. Similar histological observations were made in male rats after 50 days of hexachlorobenzene treatment. No such histological alterations were observed in the kidneys of female rats. In male rats, the concentration of α_{2u}-globulin in kidney was increased 11-fold as compared with controls in the 15-day study; no results for this end-point were reported in the 50-day study. In addition, hexachlorobenzene was found to be bound reversibly to α_{2u}-globulin (Bouthillier *et al.*, 1991).

(e) Effects on the immune system

Male BALB/c mice fed a diet containing 167 mg/kg hexachlorobenzene for 6 weeks became immunosuppressed, as indicated by decreased serum globulin concentrations and a decreased response of spleen lymphocytes to sheep red blood cells (Loose *et al.*, 1977). Male Wistar rats receiving 0.5, 1 or 2 mg/kg bw per day hexachlorobenzene for 3 weeks showed increased numbers of neutrophils, monocytes and basophils and increased IgM concentrations. Hexachlorobenzene did not alter cell-mediated immunity but it altered humoral antibody responses (Vos *et al.*, 1979a). In the offspring of female rats given diets containing hexachlorobenzene at concentrations ≤ 150 mg/kg, suppression of cellular and humoral immunity was reported (Vos *et al.*, 1979b). In BALB/c mice fed a diet containing 167 mg/kg hexachlorobenzene, measures of humoral immune response were found to be decreased after 6 weeks, and increased susceptibility to *Plasmodium berghei* infection and endotoxin were found (Loose *et al.*, 1979). Some effects of hexachlorobenzene aerosols (3.5 and 35 mg/m³) on pulmonary bactericidal, macrophage phagocytic and alveolar macrophage enzyme activities were found in male Sprague-Dawley rats (Sherwood *et al.*, 1989).

Female Brown Norway, Lewis and Wistar rats were fed diets containing different doses of hexachlorobenzene (because of differences in toxicity in these strains) of 150–900 mg/kg for 4 weeks. Skin lesions were found, which were most severe in Norway and least severe in Wistar rats. The occurrence of pulmonary lesions was not strain-dependent, but immunomodulation varied somewhat by strain, Brown Norway rats showing the most splenomegaly; IgE or IgG concentrations were dose-dependent in this strain (Michielsen *et al.*, 1997). In a study of Brown Norway and genetically euthymic and athymic WAG/Rij rats with or without depletion of T cells caused by adult thymectomy, thymus-derived T cells were not required for the production of skin and lung lesions and splenic changes by hexachlorobenzene (Michielsen *et al.*, 1999).

In a study of male Wistar rats fed diets containing 0, 500 or 1000 mg/kg hexachlorobenzene for 3 weeks, the total IgM concentration was increased, as were the weights of the spleen and lymph nodes, but the IgG concentrations were unaffected (Schielen *et al.*, 1993). The immune effects in female Wistar rats in the studies of den Besten *et al.* (1993, 1994) (described in sections 4.1.2(b) and 4.2.2(b)) were probably due to the parent compound, hexachlorobenzene, or its non-oxidative metabolites and were not dependent on oxidative metabolism, in contrast to the production of porphyria. Therefore, the dose-dependently increased weights of lymph nodes and spleen and the increased serum concentrations of IgM, IgA and autoantibody-specific IgM were not secondary to porphyria (Schielen *et al.*, 1995).

A dose-dependent increase in interleukin-2 and interferon-α mRNA levels was found in cultured spleen cells derived from male Wistar rats fed diets containing 50, 150 or 450 mg/kg hexachlorobenzene for 6 weeks (Vandebriel *et al.*, 1998).

(*f*) *Effects on the parathyroid*

Human exposure to hexachlorobenzene has resulted in demineralization of bone and development of osteoporosis. Experiments were undertaken to investigate the effects of hexachlorobenzene on the homeostatic mechanism of calcium metabolism. Fischer 344 rats were given an intragastric dose of 0, 0.1, 1, 10 or 25 mg/kg bw hexachlorobenzene on 5 days/week for 5 weeks. Serum cholesterol, alanine aminotransferase activity, 1,25-dihydroxyvitamin D3 and parathyroid hormone concentrations were significantly higher than control values. The urinary calcium concentration decreased significantly with increasing dose of hexachlorobenzene, indicating conservation of calcium. In an experiment conducted for 5, 10 or 15 weeks, serum alkaline phosphatase activity was significantly decreased at the two higher doses after both 10 and 15 weeks of exposure. 1,25-Dihydroxyvitamin D3 was measured in the group exposed for 5 weeks and was found to be significantly elevated at the three higher doses. After 5 and 15 weeks of exposure to hexachlorobenzene, the concentration of parathyroid hormone was significantly elevated at the two higher doses at both times. Wet femur density was significantly increased at the two higher doses after 10 weeks of exposure and at the three higher doses after 15 weeks. Bone strength was also significantly increased at the three higher doses (Andrews *et al.*, 1988, 1989, 1990).

(g) *Other effects*

Decreases in circulating concentrations of corticosterone were found when hexachlorobenzene was administered by gavage at 1, 10 or 100 mg/kg bw per day for 30 days to ovariectomized Sprague-Dawley rats. The serum concentrations of progesterone and aldosterone were not altered (Foster *et al.*, 1995a).

Female Wistar and Chbb THOM rats were dosed with 1 g/kg bw hexachlorobenzene by gavage on 5 days/week for up to 4 weeks. The Wistar rats showed an increased porphyrin content in the Harderian gland and changes in phospholipid metabolism, whereas the other strain showed a decrease (Cochón et al., 1999).

4.3   Reproductive and developmental effects

4.3.1   Humans

Continuing occupational exposures (e.g., Grimalt et al., 1994) and the accidental exposure of Turkish populations in the 1950s (Peters et al., 1987) have provided extensive information on human health outcomes associated with exposure to hexachlorobenzene.

In the epidemic of poisoning that occurred in Turkey (see section 4.2.1), breastfed infants showed a condition known as 'pink-sore' and had a mortality rate > 95%. Samples of breast milk from the mothers of these infants were shown to contain hexachlorobenzene (Cam, 1960; Peters et al., 1966; Peters, 1976).

Positive associations were reported between hexachlorobenzene concentrations in breast milk (> 146 µg/kg of fat) and the risk for otitis media during the first year of life among Inuit infants in Canada (Dewailly et al., 2000). A case–control study of miscarriage in Germany reported a correlation between blood hexachlorobenzene concentration and small decreases in follicle-stimulating hormone concentration and decreases in immunological markers (CD8, CD4:CD8 ratio) in the women, but no apparent relationship between hexachlorobenzene concentration and the risk for miscarriage (Gerhard et al., 1998).

Jarrell et al. (1998) reviewed the reproductive outcomes associated with the Turkish episode and reported on the reproductive effects in women who were exposed as children in the 1950s. The serum concentrations of hexachlorobenzene were measured in persons with porphyria cutanea tarda and in two control groups 40 years after the original exposure. Little difference was found. The authors also found no relationship between current hexachlorobenzene and circulating hormone concentrations, but they did find a relationship between the rate of spontaneous abortion and the serum hexachlorobenzene concentration.

4.3.2   Experimental systems

Hexachlorobenzene has been reported to affect both reproduction and development. Prenatal exposure of CD-1 mice to 10 or 50 mg/kg bw hexachlorobenzene on days 6–17 of gestation caused significant postnatal mortality (Courtney et al., 1984). Exposure to hexachlorobenzene affected the female gonad histopathologically and endocrinologically. Hexachlorobenzene induced follicular degeneration and increased atresia in rodents and primates (Sims et al., 1991; Jarrell et al., 1993); it affected cyclicity in both rodents and primates (Foster et al., 1992a,b, 1995a,b), and it altered gonadal steroidogenesis (Foster *et al.*, 1992a,b, 1993, 1995a,b). The highest dose of hexachlorobenzene used (10 mg/kg bw per day orally for 90 days) specifically reduced the numbers of primordial follicles in cynomolgus monkeys (*Macaca fascicularis*) (Jarrell *et al.*, 1993). The effects of hexachlorobenzene on ovarian morphology and steroidogenesis can be induced at a dose as low as 0.1 mg/kg bw per day for 90 days in cynomolgus monkeys (Foster *et al.*, 1996). Alvarez *et al.* (2000) also reported altered cyclicity and reduced ovulation in response to daily exposure of male Wistar rats by gavage to 1 g/kg bw hexachlorobenzene for 30 days. Decreased uterine estrogen receptor concentrations were also observed in these rats, but no change was found in uterine weight. No data on the histological appearance of the uterus were presented. No studies were found on the effects of hexachlorobenzene on the male reproductive system.

Hexachlorobenzene also affects development. Exposure *in utero* and during lactation caused neonatal mortality in rats fed diets containing 60–140 mg/kg hexachlorobenzene (Kitchin *et al.*, 1982) and in monkeys given 64 mg/kg bw per day by gavage for 60 days (Bailey *et al.*, 1980). After more limited exposure *in utero*, hexachlorobenzene induced structural malformations, including cleft palate, enlarged kidneys and hydronephrosis, in CD-1 mice. The latter effects were observed in the pups of dams treated with 10 or 50 mg/kg bw per day on days 6–16 of gestation (Andrews & Courtney, 1986). These malformations were strikingly similar to the terata associated with exposure to dioxins *in utero*, as noted by these authors, which raises the issue of the possible presence of traces of dioxins in technical-grade hexachlorobenzene. A dose of 10 mg/kg bw hexachlorobenzene, even at 99% purity (Andrews & Courtney, 1986) could still result in exposure to dioxin of as much as 100 μg/kg bw, which is well within the range of doses of 2,3,7,8-tetrachlorodibenzo-*para*-dioxin (TCDD) that are teratogenic (see Dienhart *et al.*, 2000).

Prenatal exposure to hexachlorobenzene causes additional developmental effects. Barnett *et al.* (1987) reported that BALB/c mice exposed daily to 0.5 or 5 mg/kg bw hexachlorobenzene throughout gestation had alterations in immunological parameters. Both doses diminished delayed-type hypersensitivity responses in offspring tested at 40 days of age; the higher dose impaired mixed lymphocyte response to allogenic spleen cells; and, in adulthood, small changes in the relative proportion of T and B cells in the spleen were observed.

Two studies were conducted to determine the effects of exposure to hexachlorobenzene during development on neurobehavioural end-points. Female Sprague-Dawley rats were exposed before gestation to hexachlorobenzene by gavage at a dose of 2.5 or 25 mg/kg bw per day for 4 days. Two weeks later, they were mated with unexposed males. This treatment did not affect either maternal or pup body weight. In assessments of behaviour during the first 20 days after birth, hexachlorobenzene-exposed pups responded more quickly to negative geotaxis tests and in olfactory discrimination tests. They were also more active than controls up to postnatal day 60, and were less reactive to acoustic startle on postnatal day 23 but more reactive on postnatal day 90. The complexity of these effects makes it difficult to propose hypotheses about the mechanism of action, but the results demonstrate that hexachlorobenzene can affect neurobehavioural function in developing rats (Goldey & Taylor, 1992). Female albino Wistar WU rats were fed diets containing hexachlorobenzene at 4, 8 or 16 mg/kg before and during gestation and lactation. After weaning, the pups were given the same diet as their dams. No changes were found in open-field activity at postnatal day 21; however, in tests of operant learning begun at postnatal day 150, treated animals showed decreased response rates (Lilienthal et al., 1996).

4.4   Effects on enzyme induction or inhibition and gene expression

4.4.1   *Humans*

No data were available to the Working Group.

4.4.2   *Experimental systems*

The porphyrinogenic effects of hexachlorobenzene are associated with induction of several hepatic CYP enzymes, as shown in early studies (Grant et al., 1974; Mehendale et al., 1975; Stonard, 1975).

In groups of female AGUS or Wistar rats given 50 mg/kg bw hexachlorobenzene by gavage every other day for 8 weeks, large increases in ethoxyresorufin deethylase activity were found in both strains, although the activities were higher in AGUS rats; however, AGUS rats showed less induction of GST activity (Debets et al., 1981b). In adult female rats fed hexachlorobenzene at a concentration that induced porphyria, the activity of microsomal glucuronyltransferase was increased (Graef et al., 1982). Both crude and purified hexachlorobenzene were found to increase the activity of liver enzymes in male and female Sprague-Dawley rats 4 days after an intraperitoneal injection of 150 mg/kg bw. The enzyme activities induced included benzphetamine N-dealkylation, ethoxyresorufin deethylation and ethoxycoumarin O-dealkylation (Franklin et al., 1983).

The effect of a single dose of 200 mg/kg bw hexachlorobenzene was compared in male Syrian hamsters and male Fischer 344/N rats. Although the total CYP content of the liver was induced much more in hamsters (4.7-fold) than in rats (2.5-fold), there was little induction of either pentoxy- or ethoxyphenoxazone dealkylation in hamsters. In rats, the two enzyme activities were induced approximately 12- and fivefold, respectively (Smith et al., 1987).

Hexachlorobenzene and 2,3,4,4′,5-pentachlorobiphenyl induced a similar spectrum of CYP-dependent monooxygenase activities in rats, including 4-dimethylaminoantipyrine N-demethylase, aryl hydrocarbon (Ah) hydroxylase and ethoxyresorufin deethylase (Li et al., 1986).

Hexachlorobenzene induced both of the phenobarbital-inducible forms, cytochrome P450b and P450e [CYP2B1 and CYP2B2], and the 3-methylcholanthrene-inducible forms, cytochrome P450c and P450d [CYP1A1 and CYP1A2], in rat liver microsomes. The concentration of P450d [CYP1A2] was considerably greater than that of P450c [CYP1A1] in hexachlorobenzene-induced rat liver. Hexachlorobenzene increased the amounts of mRNAs for P450b, P450c and P450d [CYP2B1, CYP1A1 and CYP1A2] mRNA in rat liver polysomes, suggesting that it increases the synthesis of the corresponding proteins (Goldstein et al., 1986; Linko et al., 1986).

Feeding 0.1% hexachlorobenzene in the diet to female Sprague-Dawley rats for 55 days resulted in a fourfold increase in urinary porphyrin excretion and a significant decrease in serum T4 concentration (< 10 versus 38 µg/L in controls) and in T3 concentration (0.49 versus 0.64 µg/L in controls). The rats were then fed normal diet for an additional 42 days. During that time, one-third of the rats died, and the urinary porphyrin concentration increased to 100 times the control level. In the surviving animals killed at the end of the experiment, the liver microsomal enzymes ethoxyresorufin deethylase, pentoxyresorufin deethylase, aminopyrine N-demethylase and UGT were induced 10-fold, 12-fold, < 2-fold and 2-fold, respectively. It was further noted that, whereas the animals that died began wasting 5 days after cessation of intake of hexachlorobenzene, when relatively minor disturbances in porphyrins were found, the survivors developed major porphyrin disturbances without wasting; the deaths were therefore not correlated with porphyria (Rozman et al., 1986).

Microsomal cytochrome P450 was induced to a greater extent in male than in female Fischer rats, while cytochrome b_5 was induced only in males. Aminopyrine-N-demethylase activity doubled in animals of each sex after treatment, while that of Ah hydroxylase was 16 times the control value in females and 1.5 times the value in males. After hexachlorobenzene treatment, the phospholipid content of microsomal membranes in liver was increased, while the cholesterol content was unchanged. Analysis of the phospholipid pattern showed that hexachlorobenzene interfered with the biosynthesis of phospholipids containing choline. Hexachlorobenzene showed more pronounced features of a 'phenobarbital type' inducer in males than in females (Cantoni et al., 1987).

Hexachlorobenzene at a concentration of ≥ 1 µmol/L inhibited the specific binding of [³H]TCDD (0.3 nmol/L) to the Ah receptor in vitro, and the inhibition was competitive, with a K_i of approximately 2.1 µmol/L. In rats fed a diet containing 3000 mg/kg hexachlorobenzene for 4 h to 7 days, the specific binding of [³H]TCDD in hepatic cytosol was reduced by up to 40%, due principally to a decrease in the number of binding sites for [³H]TCDD rather than to competition from residual hexachlorobenzene. As shown by immunoblotting and radioimmunoassay, hexachlorobenzene induced CYP1A1 and CYP1A2, which are regulated by the Ah receptor, as well as the phenobarbital-inducible isozymes CYP2B1 and CYP2B2. Taken together, these results indicate that hexachlorobenzene is a weak agonist for the Ah receptor and suggest that some of its effects are mediated by its interaction with this gene-regulatory protein (Hahn et al., 1989).

A study in *Cyp1a2*(–/–) mice showed that the presence of CYP1A2 is essential for the production of the uroporphyria caused by hexachlorobenzene and iron (and by 3-methylcholanthrene). In this experiment, male wild-type C57BL/6J mice, which had been injected with 500 mg/kg bw iron dextran 3 days earlier, were compared with mice containing the *Ahr^b* allele and injected intraperitoneally with 100 mg/kg bw hexachlorobenzene. After 42 days, the mice were injected a second time with 75 mg/kg bw hexachlorobenzene and killed 20 days later. In wild-type mice, the hepatic uroporphyrin concentration ranged from 70 to 310 nmol/g of liver, whereas in null mice it was < 1 nmol/g of liver. Exposure of another group to iron dextran and hexachlorobenzene and to ALA in drinking-water for 58 days before sacrifice resulted in a uroporphyrin concentration of about 300 nmol/g of liver in all wild-type mice, but again < 1 nmol/g of liver in the null mice. Exposure of wild-type mice to iron dextran and ALA without hexachlorobenzene for 28–31 days resulted in uroporphyrin accumulation to a mean value of 50 nmol/g of liver; the null mice were found to have the same iron liver content as the wild-type. In another experiment, CYP1A2 and uroporphyrinogen oxidation were induced twofold in wild-type mice 6 days after injection of hexachlorobenzene, but no CYP1A2 was present in null mice. This study also showed that hexachlorobenzene did not increase hepatic microsomal uroporphyrinogen oxidation in *Cyp1a2*(-/-) mice (Sinclair *et al.*, 2000).

Hexachlorobenzene was studied in two congenic strains of C57BL/6J mice that differ only at the *AhR* locus. Female B6-Ah^b mice (Ah receptor, approximately 30–70 fmol/mg of cytosolic protein) and B6-Ah^d mice (Ah receptor, undetectable) were pretreated with iron at 500 mg/kg bw (given as iron dextran) and then fed a diet containing 0 or 200 mg/kg hexachlorobenzene for up to 17 weeks. Urinary excretion of porphyrins was increased after 7 weeks of hexachlorobenzene treatment in B6-Ah^b mice, and by 15 weeks was over 200 times greater than that of mice given only iron. In B6-Ah^d mice, porphyrin excretion did not begin to increase until after 13 weeks, and after 15 weeks was only six times greater than that of controls. Similar differences were seen in the hepatic porphyrin concentrations at 15 weeks: B6-Ah^b, 1110 ± 393; B6-Ah^d, 17.6 ± 14.5; controls, approximately 0.20 nmol/g. UROD activity was diminished by 70 and 20% in B6-Ah^b and B6-Ah^d mice, respectively, after 15 weeks of treatment with hexachlorobenzene. Hexachlorobenzene induced small amounts of a protein recognized by anti-CYP1A1 in B6-Ah^b mice, but not in B6-Ah^d mice. Relatively large amounts of a protein recognized by anti-CYP1A2 were induced in both strains, but to a somewhat greater extent in the B6-Ah^b mice. The results of this experiment indicate that the Ah locus influences the susceptibility of C57BL/6J mice to hexachlorobenzene-induced porphyria and are consistent with the suggestion that sustained induction of CYP1A2 and/or CYP1A1 is a causative factor in the development of this disease (Hahn *et al.*, 1988).

The combination of a single subcutaneous dose of iron (12.5 mg/mouse) and subsequent treatment with hexachlorobenzene at 0.02% in the diet caused progressive inhibition of hepatic UROD in male C57BL/10 mice, leading to accumulation of uroporphyrin within 4–6 weeks. The activity of the enzyme was only slightly inhibited in the absence of iron, and was not inhibited in the absence of hexachlorobenzene. Females were less sensitive than males. Comparisons of the C57BL/10, BALB/c, AKR and DBA/2 strains indicated that the susceptibility of the mice to the induction of porphyria did not completely correlate with their classification as Ah-responsive or Ah-non-responsive (Smith & Francis, 1983).

While there is a marked sex difference in hexachlorobenzene-induced porphyria (see above), the induction of oxidation of uroporphyrinogen I to uroporphyrin I by hepatic microsomes was not correlated with the sex difference in porphyria development. Ethoxyresorufin deethylase activity (associated with CYP1A1) and immuno-blotting with polyclonal antibodies to CYP1A1 and CYPA2 were significantly greater in hexachlorobenzene-exposed females. Immunocytochemical studies showed that, even after 30 weeks of exposure to hexachlorobenzene, CYP1A1 and CYP1A2 were still more highly induced in female liver, especially in the centrilobular region (Smith *et al.*, 1990).

After a single intraperitoneal administration of 200 mg/kg bw hexachlorobenzene to female rats, UROD activity was 61 and 69% of normal with and without iron loading, respectively, and the liver porphyrin concentrations were 96 and 25 mg/g, respectively. Hexachlorobenzene did not produce significant porphyric effects in male rats. Aroclor 1254 induced CYP1A to a greater extent in females than in males and to a greater extent than hexachlorobenzene, which showed a greater propensity to induce CYP2B. Overall, the correlation between decreased UROD activity and porphyrin accumulation was highest when fitted to an exponential curve, indicating the importance of extreme depression of UROD activity in evoking experimental porphyria by such chemicals (Franklin *et al.*, 1997).

Hexachlorobenzene was found to be a potent inducer of malic enzyme gene expression in the liver of female Wistar rats exposed to 1 g/kg bw by gavage for 9–15 days. No changes in T4 or T3 concentrations were found in rat liver, and the activities of other thyroid hormone-responsive enzymes were not found to be increased. In studies with H35 rat hepatoma cells exposed to 10 or 50 nmol/L hexachlorobenzene, the increase in malic enzyme mRNA was shown to occur through the thyroid response element (Loaiza-Perez *et al.*, 1999). In contrast, in brown adipose tissue of male Wistar rats given 1 g/kg bw hexachlorobenzene by gavage for 30 days, the activities of malic enzyme, glucose-6-phosphate dehydrogenase and L-glycerol-3-phosphate dehydrogenase were decreased in both euthyroid and thyriodectomized rats (Alvarez *et al.*, 1999).

Administration of hexachlorobenzene at 1 g/kg bw per day to female Wistar rats by gavage for up to 30 days resulted in time-dependent decreases in the activity of two membrane-bound enzymes, 5′-nucleotidase and Na+/K+ ATPase, and hexachlorobenzene was found to cause a significant rise in protein tyrosine kinase activity during the early stages of intoxication (day 2), followed by a significant decrease at 10 days and returning to control levels after 20 days of treatment. A stimulatory effect of hexachlorobenzene on endogenous microsomal protein phosphorylation *in vitro* was observed from day 2 of intoxication up to 30 days of treatment. Administration of 1 g/kg bw hexachlorobenzene to rats for 10 days caused a 50% reduction in epidermal growth factor receptor–ligand binding (Randi *et al.*, 1998).

In male Fischer 344 rats exposed by gavage to 0.4 mmol/kg bw per day hexachlorobenzene [114 mg/kg bw per day] or pentachlorobenzene for 6 weeks, a distinct pattern of non-focal expression of rGSTP1-1 was observed. The expression was localized to the centrilobular region, with the most intense staining nearest the central vein. A western blot analysis revealed five- and 15-fold induction of rGSTP1-1 with pentachlorobenzene and hexachlorobenzene on an equimolar basis, respectively. Evaluation of porphyrin fluorescence also revealed centrilobular accumulation, with average concentrations of porphyrin of 0.319, 0.580 and 0.206 μg/g tissue with pentachlorobenzene, hexachlorobenzene and in corn-oil controls, respectively. In view of the role of activator protein-1 in rGSTP1-1 expression and of CYP1A2 in the pathogenesis of porphyria cutanea tarda, immunohistochemical localization of *c-jun*, *c-fos* and *CYP1A2* was also performed. Increased expression and co-localization within the liver lobule were observed for *c-jun*, *c-fos*, *CYP1A2*, rGSTP1-1 and areas of porphyrin accumulation. These observations are consistent with the results of studies that have associated the induction of GST-P with *jun*- and *fos*-related gene products (Thomas *et al.*, 1998).

In a comparative study of chlorobenzenes given to male Fischer rats by gavage daily for 6 weeks, 1,2,4,5-tetrachlorobenzene, pentachlorobenzene and hexachlorobenzene, but not 1,4-dichlorobenzene, promoted GSTP1-1-positive preneoplastic foci formation in the liver after initiation with NDEA. The induction of CYP1A2 and CYP2B1/2 correlated with both the presence and degree of promotion of GSTP1-1 foci by the four chlorobenzenes. The authors concluded that induction of CYP1A2 or CYP2B1/2 by chlorobenzene isomers is associated with promotional ability (Gustafson *et al.*, 2000; see also section 3.3).

4.5   Genetic and related effects

The genetic toxicity of hexachlorobenzene has been reviewed (Brusick, 1986).

4.5.1   *Humans*

Measurement of micronucleus frequency in peripheral blood lymphocytes was used to study the possible clastogenic effects of occupational exposures of workers at a chemical production factory in the State of São Paulo, Brazil, who had been exposed to a variety of chlorinated compounds but mainly carbon tetrachloride, perchloroethylene and hexachlorobenzene. The results were compared with those for 28 control workers who had not been exposed. The presence of micronuclei was investigated in peripheral blood from 41 workers of a group of 85 who were selected from a total of 130 workers in the same company. [The Working Group noted that the basis for the selection of the 85 from 130 and the 41 from 85 was not described.] The 85 exposed workers were men of a median age of 37 years who had worked for a mean of nine years in the company and had a median serum hexachlorobenzene concentration of 4.4 μg/100 mL, with a range of 0.1–16 μg/100 mL. The 28 controls were men working in other companies in the same geographical region and of the same median age, but without detectable serum concentrations of hexachlorobenzene. It was known which subjects in both groups were current smokers. The average frequency of micronucleated lymphocytes was 0.9% (range, 0.6–4.8%) in the exposed workers and 0.25% (range, 0.0–2.8%) in the controls ($p < 0.00001$). In the exposed group, there was no correlation between the occurrence of micronuclei and age, current smoking, length of employment at the factory or hexachlorobenzene concentration in serum. The authors noted that it was not possible to identify a particular factor that might account for the difference in the frequency of micronuclei (da Silva Augusto *et al.*, 1997).

4.5.2   *Experimental systems* (see Table 5 for references)

Hexachlorobenzene did not induce mutations in *Salmonella typhimurium*, but there was a report of a small increase in mutation frequency in exposed *Saccharomyces cerevisiae*. In single studies in non-human mammalian cells, hexachlorobenzene did not induce alkali-labile sites in DNA of rat hepatocytes or chromosomal aberrations in Chinese hamster lung cells. In a study from one laboratory, hexachlorobenzene induced alkali-labile sites in human hepatocytes and micronuclei in rat and human hepatocytes *in vitro*.

Hexachlorobenzene did not induce alkali-labile sites in liver-cell DNA from rats treated *in vivo*, sister chromatid exchange in bone-marrow cells of mice treated *in vivo* or dominant lethal mutations in male rats.

Male C57BL/10ScSn mice received a subcutaneous injection of iron-dextran solution at a dose of 600 mg Fe/kg bw and were then fed a diet containing 0.01% hexachlorobenzene for up to 18 months (see section 3). A total of 23 preoplastic and neoplastic lesions obtained from these mice were analysed for mutations of Ha-*ras* at codon 61, since these often occur at high frequency in the livers of mice treated with carcinogens. Only two mutations were found: an A → T transversion in a focus of altered cells and a C → A transversion in a trabecular-cell carcinoma (Rumsby *et al.*, 1992).

4.6   **Mechanistic considerations**

Neither analysis of tumours arising in hexachlorobenzene-treated mice nor the results of the small number of tests for genetic toxicity support the hypothesis that the induction of genetic damage by hexachlorobenzene plays a role in its carcinogenicity.

Table 5. Genetic and related effects of hexachlorobenzene

Test system	Result[a] Without exogenous metabolic system	Result[a] With exogenous metabolic system	Dose[b] (LED or HID)	Reference
Escherichia coli WP2, WP2 *uvrA*, differential toxicity	–	NT	1000 µg/disc	Siekel *et al.* (1991)
Salmonella typhimurium TA100, TA1535, TA1537, TA98, reverse mutation	–	–	333 µg/plate	Haworth *et al.* (1983)
Salmonella typhimurium TA100, TA1538, TA98, reverse mutation	–	–	1000 µg/plate	Górski *et al.* (1986)
Salmonella typhimurium TA100, TA98, reverse mutation	–	–	500 µg/plate	Siekel *et al.* (1991)
Escherichia coli WP2, WP2*uvrA*, reverse mutation	–	–	500	Siekel *et al.* (1991)
Saccharomyces cerevisiae 632/4, reverse mutation	(+)	NT	100	Guerzoni *et al.* (1976)
DNA single-strand breaks and alkali-labile sites in Sprague-Dawley rat primary hepatocytes *in vitro*	–	NT	160	Canonero *et al.* (1997)
Micronucleus formation, Sprague-Dawley rat hepatocytes *in vitro*	+	NT	91	Canonero *et al.* (1997)
Chromosomal aberrations, Chinese hamster lung cells *in vitro*	–	–	12 000	Ishidate (1988)
DNA single-strand breaks and alkali-labile sites in human primary hepatocytes *in vitro*	(+)	NT	160	Canonero *et al.* (1997)
Micronucleus formation, human primary hepatocytes *in vitro*	+	NT	51	Canonero *et al.* (1997)
Chromosomal aberrations, human lymphocytes *in vitro*	–	NT	29	Siekel *et al.* (1991)
DNA single-strand breaks and alkali-labile sites in rat liver cells *in vivo*	–		300 ip × 1	Górski *et al.* (1986)
Sister chromatid exchange, mouse bone-marrow cells *in vivo*	–		400[c]	Górski *et al.* (1986)
Dominant lethal mutation, male Wistar rats	–		60 po × 10	Khera (1974)
Dominant lethal mutation, male rats	–		221 po × 5	Simon *et al.* (1979)

[a] +, positive; (+), weak positive; –, negative; NT, not tested
[b] LED, lowest effective dose; HID, highest ineffective dose; in-vitro tests, µg/mL; in-vivo tests, mg/kg bw per day; po, orally; ip, intraperitoneal
[c] Route not reported

4.6.1 *Thyroid tumours*

At doses much higher than those used in the bioassays for carcinogenicity, hexachlorobenzene increased the size of the thyroid, decreased the concentration of T4, with a smaller or no decrease in that of T3, and increased the concentration of TSH in rats. No thyroid tumours were reported in rats given much lower doses. The experimental results indicate that hexachlorobenzene induces hypothyroidism in rats through its main metabolite, pentachlorophenol, and through tetrachlorohydroquinone. Displacement of hormones from serum carriers by these metabolites could be a factor in the induction of the observed hypothyroidism. In addition, hexachlorobenzene increases the metabolism of T4 by inducing glucuronosyl transferase and decreases type-1 deiodinase activity. Therefore, the decreased T4 concentrations in serum of rats after exposure to hexachlorobenzene may be due to a combined effect of displacement of T4 from carriers, increased glucuronidation of T4 and enhanced bile flow.

In hamsters, hexachlorobenzene decreased the concentrations of T3 rather than T4 and increased the size of the thyroid; the concentrations of TSH have not been reported. CYP isozymes were induced, but the specific activities that are increased by hexachlorobenzene in hamsters have not been identified. The mechanism of thyroid tumour development in hamsters is probably due to effects similar to those in rats.

4.6.2 *Liver tumours*

Some reports have linked human hepatic porphyria with a risk for liver cancer, but the results vary. The hexachlorobenzene poisoning incident in Turkey demonstrated that hexachlorobenzene can produce porphyria in humans. The acquired porphyria was more frequent and more severe in women, and the effects of the exposure may be exacerbated by estrogens.

The evidence suggests that the production of hepatic tumours by hexachlorobenzene involves biotransformation, oxidative damage, CYP enzyme induction, porphyria, inhibition of UROD and effects on iron metabolism. Hexachlorobenzene produces hepatic porphyria and induces the hepatic CYP isozymes CYP1A1 and CYP1A2 in rodents. There is evidence for a role of the Ah receptor in some but not all of the effects of hexachlorobenzene in the liver. The uroporphyria produced in mice was found to be dependent on expression of CYP1A2, since *Cyp1a2*(–/–) knock-out mice did not develop uroporphyria even when exposed to 3-methylcholanthrene. A pivotal role for inhibition of UROD in the development of hexachlorobenzene-induced porphyria has been shown. Some results suggest that oxidative biotransformation may be related to the porphyrinogenic action of hexachlorobenzene. The results are consistent with the association between CYP1A isozymes and the development of uroporphyria.

Iron accumulation in subcellular organelles such as lysosomes and iron sequestration have been reported in hexachlorobenzene-exposed animals. Iron loading has been found to significantly enhance the effects of hexachlorobenzene. The iron in hepatocyte lysosomes associated with porphyria may result in oxidative damage.

Female rats are more sensitive to the induction of porphyria than males, and mice are less sensitive than rats. Rats and mice also differ in terms of their overall sensitivity to chemical porphyrinogens.

In the absence of definitive evidence, hexachlorobenzene-induced porphyria and the other toxic end-points described above may be involved in the induction of hexachlorobenzene-induced liver tumours, but the mechanism has not been definitively established.

4.6.3   *Kidney tumours*

Hexachlorobenzene induces a male rat-specific α_{2u}-globulin nephropathy that could play a role in the induction of renal tumours in male rats. However, because female rats also develop renal adenomas, other mechanisms must play a role as well.

4.6.4   *Parathyroid tumours*

Pre- and postnatal administration of high doses of hexachlorobenzene increased the incidence of parathyroid adenomas in male and female Sprague-Dawley rats. Short-term (5-week) exposure of Fischer 344 rats to hexachlorobenzene resulted in increased circulating parathyroid hormone and 1,25-dihydroxyvitamin D_3 concentrations, decreased urinary calcium excretion and increased serum alkaline phosphatase activity. It also produced osteosclerosis. Although hexachlorobenzene appears to stimulate the parathyroid, the mechanism of parathyroid tumour development probably involves additional factors, since the parathyroid chief-cell hyperplasia commonly associated with chronic renal failure in rats is not associated with an increased incidence of parathyroid adenomas.

5.   Summary of Data Reported and Evaluation

5.1   Exposure data

Hexachlorobenzene is a chlorinated hydrocarbon which may contain some higher polychlorinated dibenzofurans and dioxins as impurities. It has been used in the manufacture of industrial chemicals, including chlorinated pesticides, and as a fungicide and seed dressing in agriculture. The production and use of hexachlorobenzene have decreased since the 1970s owing to bans and restrictions on its use in many countries, but it still occurs as a by-product of the production of a number of chlorinated solvents and other industrial chemicals. Occupational exposure to hexachlorobenzene has occurred during its production and use in industry and agriculture. Hexachlorobenzene has been detected in many foodstuffs, but dietary intake has probably decreased in recent years.

5.2 Human carcinogenicity data

The risk for breast cancer has been investigated in relation to life-long, accumulated exposure to hexachlorobenzene in nine studies.

Five small case–control studies that included fewer than 50 cases of breast cancer each showed no overall association with the concentration of hexachlorobenzene in contemporary samples of adipose breast tissue. A secondary subgroup analysis in one of the studies revealed a significant association in postmenopausal women with estrogen receptor-positive cancer, based, however, on a small number of cases.

Four large case–control studies of exposure to hexachlorobenzene have been reported, one from Canada and three from the USA. In three of these, the concentration of hexachlorobenzene was measured in biological samples (serum fat or breast fat) from the study subjects, obtained close to the time of breast cancer diagnosis. No consistent increase in the risk for breast cancer was found in women with elevated concentrations of hexachlorobenzene. In the fourth case–control study (from the USA), banked serum samples obtained before the breast cancer diagnosis were used to assess the body burden of hexachlorobenzene. The risk for breast cancer of women whose concentration of hexachlorobenzene was in the upper three quartiles was twice that of those whose samples were in the lower quartile. However, there was no evidence of a dose–response relationship, and the association was limited to women whose blood was collected close to the time of diagnosis of their breast cancer.

One case–control study each of endometrial cancer, pancreatic cancer and hairy-cell leukaemia yielded no notable results with respect to exposure to hexachlorobenzene.

5.3 Animal carcinogenicity data

Hexachlorobenzene was tested for carcinogenicity by oral administration in one study in mice, four studies in rats and one in hamsters. It produced liver-cell tumours in all three species and renal tubular tumours in rats of each sex in one study. After perinatal administration to rats, it increased the incidences of parathyroid adenomas in males and adrenal phaeochromocytomas in females. In hamsters, it also produced liver haemangioendotheliomas and thyroid follicular-cell adenomas. In several studies in which it was given with other compounds, hexachlorobenzene promoted liver carcinogenesis in mice and rats.

5.4 Other relevant data

Hexachlorobenzene is lipophilic, accumulates in humans and is excreted as a cysteine conjugate of pentachlorobenzene. In rats, hexachlorobenzene has been shown to follow several metabolic pathways, which include the formation of pentachloro-benzene, tetrachlorobenzene and tri- and tetrachlorophenol.

Accidental consumption by humans of a large quantity of hexachlorobenzene resulted in porphyria cutanea tarda, liver toxicity, neurological effects and skin changes, which were persistent.

In experimental animals, the effects of treatment with hexachlorobenzene on the thyroid include decreased thyroid hormone concentrations due to increased glucuro-nidation and inhibition of type-1 deiodinase, interference with serum carrier binding of the thyroid hormones and increased thyroid-stimulating hormone concentrations. In the livers of experimental animals, hexachlorobenzene induced cytochrome P450 enzymes and inhibited uroporphyrinogen decarboxylase, iron accumulation and oxidative damage. These effects are believed to be involved in the production of hepatic tumours.

In a poisoning epidemic in Turkey, exposure to hexachlorobenzene via breast milk caused a very high rate of lethality among infants. An increased frequency of pregnancy loss was reported among women exposed to hexachlorobenzene as children. The presence of this compound in breast milk has been associated with altered immune function in Inuits. Hexachlorobenzene was teratogenic in mice, and increased mortality rates were observed among rats and monkeys exposed *in utero*. Effects on steroid hormones have also been reported in exposed female mice.

In a single study of workers exposed to a number of chlorinated solvents, including hexachlorobenzene, an increased frequency of micronucleated lymphocytes was found; there was no association with the concentrations of hexachlorobenzene in blood. Micronuclei were induced by hexachlorobenzene in human and rat primary hepatocytes *in vitro*. Otherwise, there was little evidence that hexachlorobenzene has genetic activity.

5.5 Evaluation

There is *inadequate evidence* in humans for the carcinogenicity of hexachloro-benzene.

There is *sufficient evidence* in experimental animals for the carcinogenicity of hexachlorobenzene.

Overall evaluation

Hexachlorobenzene is *possibly carcinogenic to humans (Group 2B)*.

6. References

Abraham, K., Hille, A., Ende, M. & Helge, H. (1994) Intake and fecal excretion of PCDDs, PCDFs, HCB and PCBs (138, 153, 180) in a breast-fed and a formula-fed infant. *Chemosphere*, **29**, 2279–2286

Agency for Toxic Substances and Disease Registry (1998) *Toxicological Profile for Hexachlorobenzene*, Atlanta, GA

Alawi, M.A. & Ababneh, M. (1991) Residue analysis of chlorinated pesticides in Jordanian human adipose tissue. *Anal. Lett.*, **25**, 1897–1911

Alleman, M.A., Koster, J.F., Wilson, J.H.P., Edixhoven-Bosdijk, A., Slee, R.G., Kroos, M.J. & Eijk, H.G.V. (1985) The involvement of iron and lipid peroxidation in the pathogenesis of HCB induced porphyria. *Biochem. Pharmacol.*, **34**, 161–166

Almeida, M.G., Fanini, S.C., Davino, S.C., Aznar, A.E., Koch, O.R. & Barros, S.B. (1997) Pro- and anti-oxidant parameters in rat liver after short term exposure to hexachlorobenzene. *Hum. exp. Toxicol.*, **16**, 257–261

Alvarez, L., Randi, A., Alvarez, P., Kolliker Frers, R. & Kleiman de Pisarev, D.L. (1999) Effect of hexachlorobenzene on NADPH-generating lipogenic enzymes and L-glycerol-3-phosphate dehydrogenase in brown adipose tissue. *J. endocrinol. Invest.*, **22**, 436–445

Alvarez, L., Randi, A., Alvarez, P., Piroli, G., Chamson-Reig, A., Lux-Lanso, V. & Kleiman de Pisarev, D. (2000) Reproductive effects of hexachlorobenzene in female rats. *J. appl. Toxicol.*, **20**, 81–87

American Conference of Governmental Industrial Hygienists (2000) *TLVs and other Occupational Exposure Values 2000* [CD-ROM], Cincinnati, OH

American Public Health Association/American Water Works Association/Water Environment Federation (1999a) Method 6040B. Closed-loop stripping, gas chromatographic/mass spectrometric analysis. In: *Standard Methods for the Examination of Water and Wastewater*, 20th Ed., Washington DC

American Public Health Association/American Water Works Association/Water Environment Federation (1999b) Method 6410B. Liquid–liquid extraction gas chromatographic/mass spectrometric method. In: *Standard Methods for the Examination of Water and Wastewater*, 20th Ed., Washington DC

Ando, M., Hirano, S. & Itoh, Y. (1985) Transfer of hexachlorobenzene (HCB) from mother to new-born baby through placenta and milk. *Arch. Toxicol.*, **56**, 195–200

Andrews, J.E. & Courtney, K.D. (1986) Hexachlorobenzene-induced renal maldevelopment in CD-1 mice and CD rats. In: Morris, C.R. & Cabral, J.R.P., eds, *Hexachlorobenzene: Proceedings of an International Symposium* (IARC Scientific Publications No. 77), Lyon, IARC*Press*, pp. 381–391

Andrews, J.E., Courtney, K.D. & Donaldson, W.E. (1988) Impairment of calcium homeostasis by hexachlorobenzene (HCB) exposure in Fischer 344 rats. *J. Toxicol. environ. Health*, **23**, 311–320

Andrews, J.E., Courtney, K.D., Stead, A.G. & Donaldson, W.E. (1989) Hexachlorobenzene-induced hyperparathyroidism and osteosclerosis in rats. *Fundam. appl. Toxicol.*, **12**, 242–251

Andrews, J.E., Jackson, L.D., Stead, A.G. & Donaldson, W.E. (1990) Morphometric analysis of osteosclerotic bone resulting from hexachlorobenzene exposure. *J. Toxicol. environ. Health*, **31**, 193–201

AOAC International (2000) *Official Methods of Analysis of AOAC International*, 17th Ed., Gaithersburg, MD [CD-ROM] [Methods 977.19, 980.22, 999.04]

Arnold, D.L. & Krewski, D. (1988) Long-term toxicity of hexachlorobenzene (Letter to the Editor). *Food chem. Toxicol.*, **26**, 169–174

Arnold, D.L., Moodie, C.A., Charbonneau, S.M., Grice, H.C., McGuire, P.F., Bryce, F.R., Collins, B.T., Zawidzka, Z.Z., Krewski, D.R., Nera, E.A. & Munro, C.I. (1985) Long-term toxicity of hexachlorobenzene in the rat and the effect of dietary vitamin A. *Food chem. Toxicol.*, **23**, 779–793

Aronson, K.J., Miller, A.B., Woolcott, C.G., Sterns, E.E., McCready, D.R., Lickley, L.A., Fish, E.B., Hiraki, G.Y., Holloway, C., Ross, T., Hanna, W.H., SenGupta, S.K. & Weber, J.P. (2000) Breast adipose tissue concentrations of polychlorinated biphenyls and other organochlorines and breast cancer risk. *Cancer Epidemiol. Biomarkers Prev.*, **9**, 55–63

Bailey, J., Knauf, V., Mueller, W. & Hobson, W. (1980) Transfer of hexachlorobenzene and polychlorinated biphenyls to nursing infant rhesus monkeys: Enhanced toxicity. *Environ. Res.*, **21**, 190–196

Barnett, J.B., Barfield, L., Walls, R., Joyner, R., Owens, R. & Soderberg, L.S. (1987) The effect of in utero exposure to hexachlorobenzene on the developing immune response of BALB/c mice. *Toxicol. Lett.*, **39**, 263–274

den Besten, C., Bennik, M., Bruggeman, I., Schielen, P., Kuper, F., Brouwer A., Koeman, J.H., Vos, J.G. & van Bladeren, P.J. (1993) The role of oxidative metabolism in hexachlorobenzene-induced porphyria and thyroid hormone homeostasis: A comparison with pentachlorobenzene in a 13-week feeding study. *Toxicol. appl. Pharmacol.*, **119**, 181–194

den Besten, C., Bennik, M., van Iersel, M., Peters, M.A., Teunis, C. & van Bladeren, P.J. (1994) Comparison of the urinary metabolite profiles of hexachlorobenzene and pentachlorobenzene in the rat. *Chem.-biol. Interactions*, **90**, 121–137

Billi de Catabbi, S., Koss, G. & San Martin de Viale, L.C. (1986) Screening for the ability of hexachlorobenzene metabolites to decrease rat liver porphyrinogen carboxylase. *Res. Commun. chem. Pathol. Pharmacol.*, **51**, 325–336

Billi de Catabbi, S., Sterin-Speziale, N., Fernandez, M.C., Minutolo, C., Aldonatti, C. & San Martin de Viale, L. (1997) Time course of hexachlorobenzene-induced alterations of lipid metabolism and their relation to porphyria. *Int. J. Biochem. Cell Biol.*, **29**, 335–344

Billings, W.N. & Bidleman, T.F. (1980) Field comparison of polyurethane foam and Tenax-GC resin for high-volume air sampling of chlorinated hydrocarbons. *Environ. Sci. Technol.*, **14**, 679–683

Bleavins, M.R., Bursian, S.J., Brewster, J.S. & Aulerich, R.J. (1984) Effects of dietary hexachlorobenzene exposure on regional brain biogenic amine concentrations in mink and European ferrets. *J. Toxicol. environ. Health*, **14**, 363–377

Booth, N.H. & McDowell, J.R. (1975) Toxicity of hexachlorobenzene and associated residues in edible animal tissues. *J. Am. vet. med. Assoc.*, **166**, 591–595

Bouthillier, L., Greselin, E., Brodeur, J., Viau, C. & Charbonneau, M. (1991) Male rat specific nephrotoxicity resulting from subchronic administration of hexachlorobenzene. *Toxicol. appl. Pharmacol.*, **110**, 315–326

Bristol, D.W., Crist, H.L., Lewis, R.G., MacLeod, K.E. & Sovocool, G.W. (1982) Chemical analysis of human blood for assessment of environmental exposure to semivolatile organochlorine chemical contaminants. *J. anal. Toxicol.*, **6**, 269–275

Brusick, D.J. (1986) Genotoxicity of hexachlorobenzene and other chlorinated benzenes. In: Morris, C.R. & Cabral, J.R.P., eds, *Hexachlorobenzene: Proceedings of an International Symposium* (IARC Scientific Publications No. 77), Lyon, IARC*Press*, pp. 393–397

Budavari, S., ed. (2000) *The Merck Index*, 12th Ed., Version 12:3, Whitehouse Station, NJ, Merck & Co. & Boca Raton, FL, Chapman & Hall/CRC[CD-ROM]

Burns, J.E. & Miller, F.M. (1975) Hexachlorobenzene contamination: Its effects in a Louisiana population. *Arch. environ. Health*, **30**, 44–48

Burse, W.W., Head, S.L., Korver, M.P., McClure, P.C., Donahue, J.F. & Needham, L.L. (1990) Determination of selected organochlorine pesticides and polychlorinated biphenyls in human serum. *J. anal. Toxicol.*, **14**, 137–142

Cabral, J.R. & Shubik, P. (1986) Carcinogenic activity of hexachlorobenzene in mice and hamsters. In: Morris, C.R. & Cabral, J.R.P., eds, *Hexachlorobenzene: Proceedings of an International Symposium* (IARC Scientific Publications No. 77), Lyon, IARC*Press*, pp. 411–416

Cabral, J.R.P., Shubik, P., Mollner, T. & Raitano, F. (1977) Carcinogenic activity of hexachlorobenzene in hamsters. *Nature*, **269**, 510–511

Cabral, J.R.P., Mollner, T., Raitano, F. & Shubik, P. (1979) Carcinogenesis of hexachlorobenzene in mice. *Int. J. Cancer*, **23**, 47–51

Cabral, R., Hoshiya, T., Hakoi, K., Hasegawa, R. & Ito, N. (1996) Medium-term bioassay for the hepatocarcinogenicity of hexachlorobenzene. *Cancer Lett.*, **100**, 223–226

Cam, C. (1960) [A new epidemic dermatosis of children.] *Ann. Derm. Syph.*, **87**, 393–397 (in French)

Cam, C. & Nigogosyan, G. (1963) Acquired toxic porphyria cutanea tarda due to hexachlorobenzene. Report of 348 cases caused by this fungicide. *J. Am. med. Assoc.*, **183**, 88–91

Canonero, R., Campart, G.B., Mattioli, F., Robbiano, L. & Martelli, A. (1997) Testing of *p*-dichlorobenzene and hexachlorobenzene for their ability to induce DNA damage and micronucleus formation in primary cultures of rat and human hepatocytes. *Mutagenesis*, **12**, 35–39

Cantoni, L., Rizzardini, M., Tacconi, M.T. & Graziani, A. (1987) Comparison of hexachlorobenzene-induced alterations of microsomal membrane composition and monooxygenase activity in male and female rats. *Toxicology*, **45**, 291–305

Carthew, P. & Smith, A.G. (1994) Pathological mechanisms of hepatic tumor formation in rats exposed chronically to dietary hexachlorobenzene. *J. appl. Toxicol.*, **14**, 447–452

Carvalho, F.P., Montenegro-Guillen, S., Villeneuve, J.-P., Barticci, J., Lacayo, M. & Cruz, A. (1999) Chlorinated hydrocarbons in coastal lagoons of the Pacific coast of Nicaragua. *Arch. environ. Contam. Toxicol.*, **36**, 132–139

CIS Information Services (2000) *Directory of World Chemical Producers (Version 2000.1)*, Dallas, TX [CD-ROM]

Cochón, A.C., San Martín de Viale, L.C. & Billi de Catabbi, S.C. (1999) Effects of hexachlorobenzene on phospholipid and porphyrin metabolism in Harderian glands: A time-course study in two strains of rats. *Toxicol. Lett.*, **106**, 129–136

Courtney, K.D. & Andrews, J.E. (1985) Neonatal and maternal body burdens of hexachloro-benzene (HCB) in mice: Gestational exposure and lactational transfer. *Fundam. appl. Toxicol.*, **5**, 265–277

Courtney, K.D., Andrews, J.E. & Svendsgaard, D.J. (1979) Hexachlorobenzene (HCB) deposi-tion in maternal and fetal tissues of rat and mouse. I. Chemical quantification of HCB in tissues. *Environ. Res.*, **19**, 1–13

Courtney, K.D., Andrews, J.E., Grady, M.A. & Ebron, M.T. (1984) Postnatal effects of hexa-chlorobenzene (HCB) on cardiac lactic dehydrogenase (LDH) and creatine kinase (CK) isozymes in CD-1 mice. *Toxicol. Lett.*, **22**, 223–228

Courtney, K.D., Andrews, J.E. & Grady, M.A. (1985) Placental transfer and fetal deposition of hexachlorobenzene in the hamster and guinea pig. *Environ. Res.*, **37**, 239–249

Cripps, D.J., Gocmen, A. & Peters, H.A. (1980) Porphyria turcica. Twenty years after hexa-chlorobenzene intoxication. *Arch. Dermatol.*, **116**, 46–50

Cripps, D.J., Peters, H.A., Gocmen, A. & Dogramici, I. (1984) Porphyria turcica due to hexa-chlorobenzene: A 20 and 30 year follow-up study on 204 patients. *Br. J. Dermatol.*, **111**, 413–422

D'Amour, M. & Charbonneau, M. (1992) Sex-related difference in hepatic glutathione conju-gation of hexachlorobenzene in the rat. *Toxicol. appl. Pharmacol.*, **112**, 229–234

Debets, F.M.H., Hamers, W.J.H.M.B. & Strik, J.J.T.W.A. (1980) Metabolism as a prerequisite for the porphyrinogenic action of polyhalogenated aromatics, with special reference to hexachlorobenzene and polybrominated biphenyls (Firemaster BP-6). *Int. J. Biochem.*, **12**, 1019–1025

Debets, F.M.H., Reinders, J.-H., Debets, A.J.M., Lossbroek, T.G., Strik, J.J.T.W.A. & Koss, G. (1981a) Biotransformation and porphyrinogenic action of hexachlorobenzene and its meta-bolites in a primary liver cell culture. *Toxicology*, **19**, 185–196

Debets, F.M.H., Reinders, J.-H., Koss, G., Seidel, J. & Strik, A. (1981b) Effects of dietary anti-oxidants on the biotransformation and porphyrinogenic action of hexachlorobenzene in two strains of rats. *Chem.-biol. Interactions*, **37**, 77–94

DeLeon, I.R., Maberry, M.A., Overton, E.B., Raschke, C.K., Remele, P.C., Steele, C.F., Warren, V.L. & Laseter, J.L. (1980) Rapid gas chromatographic method for the determi-nation of volatile and semivolatile organochlorine compounds in soil and chemical waste disposal site samples. *J. chromatogr. Sci.*, **18**, 85–88

Deutsche Forschungsgemeinschaft (2000) *List of MAK and BAT Values 1999* (Report No. 36), Weinheim, Wiley-VCH Verlag GmbH, pp. 64, 179

Dewailly, E., Dodin, S., Verreault, R., Ayotte, P., Sauvé, L., Morin, J. & Brisson, J. (1994) High organochlorine body burden in women with oestrogen receptor-positive breast cancer. *J. natl Cancer Inst.*, **86**, 232–234

Dewailly, E., Ayotte, P., Bruneau, S., Gingras, S., Bellels-Isles, M. & Roy, R. (2000) Suscepti-bility to infections and immune status to Inuit infants exposed to organochlorines. *Environ. Health Perspect.*, **108**, 205–211

Dienhart, M.K., Sommer, R.J., Peterson, R.E., Hirshfield, A.N. & Silbergeld, E.K. (2000) Gestational exposure to 2,3,7,8-tetrachlorodibenzo-*p*-dioxin induces developmental defects in the rat vagina. *Toxicol. Sci.*, **56**, 141–149

Dorgan, J.F., Brock, J.W., Rothman, N., Needham, L.L., Miller, R., Stephenson, H.E., Schussler, N. & Taylor, P.R. (1999) Serum organochlorine pesticides and PCBs and breast cancer risk: Results from a prospective analysis (USA). *Cancer Causes Control*, **10**, 1–11

Doss, M., Schermuly, E. & Koss, G. (1976) Hexachlorobenzene porphyria in rats as a model for human chronic hepatic porphyrias. *Ann. clin. Res.*, **8**, 171–181

Driscoll, M.S., Hassett, J.P., Fish, C.L. & Litten, S. (1991) Extraction efficiencies of organochlorine compounds from Niagara River water. *Environ. Sci. Technol.*, **25**, 1432–1439

Engst, R., Macholz, R.M. & Kujawa, M. (1976) The metabolism of hexachlorobenzene (HCB) in rats. *Bull. environ. Contam. Toxicol.*, **16**, 248–252

Environmental Protection Agency (1994a) Method 8121. Chlorinated hydrocarbons by gas chromatography: Capillary column technique. In: *Test Methods for Evaluating Solid Waste — Physical/chemical Methods, Update II* (US EPA No. SW-846), Washington DC, Office of Solid Waste.

Environmental Protection Agency (1994b) Method 8410. Gas chromatography/Fourier transform infrared (GC/FT-IR) spectrometry for semivolatile organics: capillary column. In: *Test Methods for Evaluating Solid Waste — Physical/Chemical Methods*, Update II (US EPA No. SW-846), Washington DC, Office of Solid Waste

Environmental Protection Agency (1995a) Method 505. Analysis of organohalide pesticides and commercial polychlorinated biphenyl (PCB) products in water by microextraction and gas chromatography [Rev. 2.1]. In: *Methods for the Determination of Organic Compounds in Drinking Water*, Supplement III (EPA Report No. EPA-600/R-95-131; US NTIS PB-216616), Cincinnati, OH, Environmental Monitoring Systems Laboratory

Environmental Protection Agency (1995b) Method 508.1. Determination of chlorinated pesticides, herbicides, and organohalides by liquid–solid extraction and electron capture gas chromatography [Rev. 2.0]. In: *Methods for the Determination of Organic Compounds in Drinking Water*, Supplement III (EPA Report No. EPA-600/R-95-131; US NTIS PB-216616), Cincinnati, OH, Environmental Monitoring Systems Laboratory

Environmental Protection Agency (1995c) Method 525.2. Determination of organic compounds in drinking water by liquid–solid extraction and capillary column gas chromatography/mass spectrometry [Rev. 2.0]. In: *Methods for the Determination of Organic Compounds in Drinking Water*, Supplement III (EPA Report No. EPA-600/R-95-131; US NTIS PB-216616), Cincinnati, OH, Environmental Monitoring Systems Laboratory

Environmental Protection Agency (1995d) Method 551.1. Determination of chlorination byproducts, chlorinated solvents, and halogenated pesticides/herbicides in drinking water by liquid–liquid extraction and gas chromatography with electron-capture detection [Rev. 1.0]. In: *Methods for the Determination of Organic Compounds in Drinking Water*, Supplement III (EPA Report No. EPA-600/R-95-131; US NTIS PB-216616), Cincinnati, OH, Environmental Monitoring Systems Laboratory

Environmental Protection Agency (1996a) Method 8081A. Organochlorine pesticides by gas chromatography [Rev. 1]. In: *Test Methods for Evaluating Solid Waste — Physical/ Chemical Methods*, Update III (US EPA No. SW-846), Washington DC, Office of Solid Waste

Environmental Protection Agency (1996b) Method 8270C. Semivolatile organic compounds by gas chromatography/mass spectrometry (GC/MS) [Rev. 3]. In: *Test Methods for Evaluating Solid Waste — Physical/Chemical Methods*, Update III (US EPA No. SW-846), Washington, DC, Office of Solid Waste

Environmental Protection Agency (1996c) Method 8275A. Semivolatile organic compounds (PAHs and PCBs) in soil/sludges and solid wastes using thermal extraction/gas chromatography/mass spectrometry (TE/GS/MS) [Rev. 1]. In: *Test Methods for Evaluating Solid Waste — Physical/Chemical Methods*, Update III (US EPA No. SW-846), Washington, DC, Office of Solid Waste

Environmental Protection Agency (1999a) Method TO-04A. Determination of pesticides and polychlorinated biphenyls in ambient air using high volume polyurethane foam (PUF) sampling followed by gas chromatographic/multidetector detection (GC/MD). In: *Compendium of Methods for the Determination of Toxic Compounds in Ambient Air*, 2nd Ed. (EPA Report No. EPA-625/R-96-010b), Cincinnati, OH, Center for Environmental Research Information

Environmental Protection Agency (1999b) Method TO-10A. Determination of pesticides and polychlorinated biphenyls in ambient air using low volume polyurethane foam (PUF) sampling followed by gas chromatographic/multidetector detection (GC/MD). In: *Compendium of Methods for the Determination of Toxic Compounds in Ambient Air*, 2nd Ed. (EPA Report No. EPA-625/R-96-010b), Cincinnati, OH, Center for Environmental Research Information

Environmental Protection Agency (1999c) Methods for organic chemical analysis of municipal and industrial wastewater. Method 612 — Chlorinated hydrocarbons. *US Code Fed. Regul., Title 40*, Part 136, App. A, pp. 167–178

Environmental Protection Agency (1999d) Methods for organic chemical analysis of municipal and industrial wastewater. Method 625 — Base/neutrals and acids. *US Code Fed. Regul., Title 40*, Part 136, App. A, pp. 202–228

Environmental Protection Agency (1999e) Methods for organic chemical analysis of municipal and industrial wastewater. Method 1625, Revision B — Semivolatile organic compounds by isotope dilution GC/MS. *US Code Fed. Regul., Title 40*, Part 136, App. A, pp. 286–306

Environmental Protection Agency (2000) *1997 Toxics Release Inventory* (EPA 745-F99-002), Washington DC, Office of Pollution Prevention and Toxics

Ertürk, E., Lambrecht, R.W., Peters, H.A., Cripps, D.J., Gocmen, A., Morris, C.R. & Bryan, G.T. (1986) Oncogenicity of hexachlorobenzene. In: Morris, C.R. & Cabral, J.R.P., eds, *Hexachlorobenzene: Proceedings of an International Symposium* (IARC Scientific Publications No. 77), Lyon, IARC*Press*, pp. 417–423

Falck, J., Jr, Ricci, A., Wolff, M.S., Godbold, J. & Deckers, P. (1992) Pesticides and polychlorinated biphenyl residues in human breast lipids and their relation to breast cancer. *Arch. environ. Health*, **47**, 143–146

FAO/UNEP (1997) *Prior Informed Consent Decision Guidance Document: Hexachlorobenzene*, Geneva, Rotterdam Convention on the Prior Informed Consent Procedure for Certain Hazardous Chemicals and Pesticides in International Trade

Feldman, E.S. & Bacon, B.R. (1989) Hepatic mitochondrial oxidative metabolism and lipid peroxidation in experimental hexachlorobenzene-induced porphyria with dietary carbonyl iron overload. *Hepatology*, **9**, 686–692

Food and Drug Administration (1999) Methods 302, 303 and 304. In: Makovi, C.M. & McMahon, B.M., eds, *Pesticide Analytical Manual*, Vol. I: *Multiresidue Methods*, 3rd Rev. Ed., Management Methods Branch, Washington DC

Foster, W.G., Pentick, J.A., McMahon, A. & LeCavalier, P.R. (1992a) Ovarian toxicity of hexachlorobenzene (HCB) in the superovulated female rat. *J. biochem. Toxicol.*, 7, 1–4

Foster, W.G., McMahon, A., Villeneuve, D.C. & Jarrell, J.F. (1992b) Hexachlorobenzene (HCB) suppresses circulating progesterone concentrations during the luteal phase in the cynomolgus monkey. *J. appl. Toxicol.*, 12, 13–17

Foster, W.G., Pentick, J.A., McMahon, A. & Lecavalier, P.R. (1993) Body distribution and endocrine toxicity of hexachlorobenzene (HCB) in the female rat. *J. appl. Toxicol.*, 13, 79–83

Foster, W.G., Mertineit, C., Yagminas, A., McMahon, A. & Lecavalier, P. (1995a) The effects of hexachlorobenzene on circulating levels of adrenal steroids in the ovariectomized rat. *J. biochem. Toxicol.*, 10, 129–135

Foster, W.G., McMahon, A., Younglai, E.V., Jarrell, J.F. & Lecavalier, P. (1995b) Alterations in circulating ovarian steroids in hexachlorobenzene-exposed monkeys. *Reprod. Toxicol.*, 9, 541–548

Foster, W.G., Jarrell, J.F., Younglai, E.V., Wade, M.G., Arnold, D.L. & Jordon, S. (1996) An overview of some reproductive toxicology studies conducted at Health Canada. *Toxicol. ind. Health*, 12, 447–459

Franklin, R.B., Breger, R.K. & Lech, J.J. (1983) Comparative effects of hexachloro- and hexabromobenzene on hepatic monooxygenase activity of male and female rats. *J. Toxicol. environ. Health*, 12, 223–234

Franklin, M.R., Phillips, J.D. & Kushner, J.P. (1997) Cytochrome P450 induction, uroporphyrinogen decarboxylase depression, porphyrin accumulation and excretion, and gender influence in a 3-week rat model of porphyria cutanea tarda. *Toxicol. appl. Pharmacol.*, 147, 289–299

Fries, G.F. & Marrow, G.S. (1976) Hexachlorobenzene retention and excretion by dairy cows. *J. dairy Sci.*, 59, 475–480

Garrison, A.W. & Pellizzari, E.D. (1987) Application of the master analytical scheme to polar organic compounds in drinking water. In: Suffet, I.H. & Malaiyandi, M., eds, *Organic Pollutants in Water: Sampling, Analysis, and Toxicity Testing* (Advances in Chemistry Series No. 214), Washington DC, American Chemical Society, pp. 83–95

Gerhard, I., Daniel, V., Link, S., Monga, B. & Runnebaum, B. (1998) Chlorinated hydrocarbons in women with repeated miscarriages. *Environ. Health Perspectives*, 106, 675–681

Gocmen, A., Peters, H.A., Cripps, D.J., Bryan, G.T. & Morris, C.R. (1989) Hexachlorobenzene episode in Turkey. *Biomed. environ. Sci.*, 2, 36–43

Goerz, G., Vizethum, W., Bolsen, K., Krieg, T. & Lissner, R. (1978) [Hexachlorobenzene (HCB)-induced porphyria in rats. Influence of HCB metabolites on the biosynthesis of haem.] *Arch. dermatol. Res.*, 263, 189–196 (in German)

Goldey, E.S. & Taylor, D.H. (1992) Developmental neurotoxicity following premating maternal exposure to hexachlorobenzene in rats. *Neurotoxicol. Teratol.*, 14, 15–21

Goldstein, J.A., Linko, P., Hahn, M.E., Gasiewicz, T.A. & Yeowell, H.N. (1986) Structure–activity relationships of chlorinated benzenes as inducers of hepatic cytochrome P-450 isoenzymes in the rat. In: Morris, C.R. & Cabral, J.R.P., eds, *Hexachlorobenzene: Proceedings of an International Symposium* (IARC Scientific Publications, No. 77), Lyon, IARC*Press*, pp. 519–526

Górski, T., Górska, E., Górecka, D. & Sikora, M. (1986) Hexachlorobenzene is non-genotoxic in short-term tests. In: Morris, C.R. & Cabral, J.R.P., eds, *Hexachlorobenzene: Proceedings of an International Symposium* (IARC Scientific Publications No. 77), Lyon, IARC*Press*, pp. 399–401

Government of Canada (1993) *Canadian Environmental Protection Act — Priority Substances List Assessment Report: Hexachlorobenzene*, Ottawa, Canada Communication Group Publishing

Graef, V., Golf, S.W. &.Tyrell, C. (1982) Further evidence for the participation of 5β-steroids in the development of a porphyria induced by hexachlorobenzene. *Arch. Toxicol.*, **50**, 233–239

Grant, D.L., Iverson, F., Hatina, G.V. & Villeneuve, D.C. (1974) Effects of hexachlorobenzene on liver porphyrin levels and microsomal enzymes in the rat. *Environ. Physiol. Biochem.*, **4**, 159–165

Grimalt, J.O., Sunyer, J., Moreno, V., Amaral, O.C., Sala, M., Rosell, A., Anto, J.M. & Albaiges, J. (1994) Risk excess of soft-tissue sarcoma and thyroid cancer in a community exposed to airborne organochlorinated compound mixtures with high hexachlorobenzene content. *Int. J. Cancer*, **56**, 200–203

Guerzoni, M.E., Del Cupolo, L. & Ponti, I. (1976) [Mutagenic activity of pesticides.] *Riv. Sci. tecnol. aliment. Nutr. um.*, **6**, 161–165 (in Italian)

Gustafson, D.L., Long, M.E., Thomas, R.S., Benjamin, S.A. & Yang, R.S.H. (2000) Comparative hepatocarcinogenicity of hexachlorobenzene, pentachlorobenzene, 1,2,4,5-tetrachlorobenzene, and 1,4-dichlorobenzene: Application of a medium-term liver focus bioassay and molecular and cellular indices. *Toxicol. Sci.*, **53**, 245–252

Güttes, S., Failing, K., Neumann, K., Kleinstein, J., Georgii, S. & Brunn, H. (1998) Chloroorganic pesticides and polychlorinated biphenyls in breast tissue of women with benign and malignant breast disease. *Arch. environ. Contam. Toxicol.*, **35**, 140–147

Hahn, M.E., Gasiewicz, T.A., Linko, P. & Goldstein, J.A. (1988) The role of the *Ah* locus in hexachlorobenzene-induced porphyria. Studies in congenic C57BL/6J mice. *Biochem. J.*, **254**, 245–254

Hahn, M.E., Goldstein, J.A., Linko, P. & Gasiewicz, T.A. (1989) Interaction of hexachlorobenzene with the receptor for 2,3,7,8-tetrachlorodibenzo-*p*-dioxin *in vitro* and *in vivo*. Evidence that hexachlorobenzene is a weak *Ah* receptor agonist. *Arch. Biochem. Biophys.*, **270**, 344–355

Haworth, S., Lawlor, T., Mortelmans, K., Speck, W. & Zeiger, E. (1983) *Salmonella* mutagenicity test results for 250 chemicals. *Environ. Mutag.*, **5**, 3–142

Hippelein, M., Kaupp, H., Dörr, G. & McLachlan, M.S. (1993) Testing of a sampling system and analytical method for determination of semivolatile organic compounds in ambient air. *Chemosphere*, **26**, 2255–2263

Hogue, C. (2000) Dioxins to be major issue at treaty negotiations. *Chem. Eng. News*, **20 March**, 35

Hoppin, J.A., Tolbert, P.E., Holly, E.A., Brook, J.W., Korrick, S.A., Altshul, L.M., Zhang, R.H., Bracci, P.M., Burse, V.W. & Needham, L.L. (2000) Pancreatic cancer and serum organochlorine levels. *Cancer Epidemiol. Biomarkers Prev.*, **9**, 199-205

Hsu, J.P., Wheeler, H.G. & Schattenberg, H.J. (1988) *Analytical Sampling Methods of the Non-occupational Pesticide Exposure Study (NOPES)* (EPA 600/9/88-0105), Washington DC, Environmental Protection Agency

IARC (1979) *IARC Monographs on the Evaluation of the Carcinogenic Risk of Chemicals to Humans*, Vol. 20, *Some Halogenated Hydrocarbons*, Lyon, IARCPress, pp. 155–178

IARC (1987) *IARC Monographs on the Evaluation of Carcinogenic Risks to Humans*, Suppl. 7, *Overall Evaluations of Carcinogenicity: An Updating of* IARC Monographs *Volumes 1 to 42*, Lyon, IARCPress, pp. 219–220

Iatropoulos, M.J., Milling, A., Müller, W.F., Nohynek, G., Rozman, K., Coulston, F. & Korte, F. (1975) Absorption, transport and organotropism of dichlorobiphenyl (DCB), dieldrin, and hexachlorobenzene (HCB) in rats. *Environ. Res.*, **10**, 384–318

Ishidate, M., Jr (1988) *Data Book of Chromosomal Aberration Test In Vitro*, Amsterdam, Elsevier, p. 221

Jarrell, J.F., McMahon, A., Villeneuve, D., Franklin, C., Singh, A., Valli, V.E. & Bartlet, S. (1993) Hexachlorobenzene toxicity in the monkey primordial germ cell without induced porphyria. *Reprod. Toxicol.*, **7**, 41–47

Jarrell, J., Gocmen, A., Foster, W., Brant, R., Chan, S. & Sevcik, M. (1998) Evaluation of reproductive outcomes in women inadvertently exposed to hexachlorobenzene in southeastern Turkey in the 1950s. *Reprod. Toxicol.*, **12**, 469–476

Jones, R.E. & Chelsky, M. (1986) Further discussion concerning porphyria cutanea tarda and TCDD exposure. *Arch. environ. Health*, **41**, 100–103

Khera, K.S. (1974) Teratogenicity and dominant lethal studies on hexachlorobenzene in rats. *Food Cosmet. Toxicol.*, **12**, 471–477

Kimbrough, R.D. & Linder, R.E. (1974) The toxicity of technical hexachlorobenzene in the Sherman strain rat. A preliminary study. *Res. Commun. chem. Pathol. Pharmacol.*, **8**, 653–664

Kitchin, K.T., Linder, R.E., Scotti, T.M., Walsh, D., Curley, A.O. & Svendsgaard, D. (1982) Offspring mortality and maternal lung pathology in female rats fed hexachlorobenzene. *Toxicology*, **23**, 33–39

Kleiman de Pisarev, D.L., Sancovich, H.A. & Ferramola de Sancovich, A.M. (1989) Enhanced thyroxine metabolism in hexachlorobenzene-intoxicated rats. *J. endocrinol. Invest.*, **12**, 767–772

Kleiman de Pisarev, D.L., Rios de Molina, M.C. & San Martin de Viale, L.C. (1990) Thyroid function and thyroxine metabolism in hexachlorobenzene-induced porphyria. *Biochem. Pharmacol.*, **39**, 817–825

Kleiman de Pisarev, D.L., Ferramola de Sancovich, A.M. & Sancovich, H.A. (1995) Hepatic indices of thyroid status in rats treated with hexachlorobenzene. *J. endocrinol. Invest.*, **18**, 271–276

Knauf, V. & Hobson, W. (1979) Hexachlorobenzene ingestion by female rhesus monkeys: Tissue distribution and clinical symptomatology. *Bull. environ. Contam. Toxicol.*, **21**, 243–248

Koizumi, A. (1991) Experimental evidence for the possible exposure of workers to hexachlorobenzene by skin contamination. *Br. J. ind. Med.*, **48**, 622–628

Kondo, M. & Shimizu, Y. (1986) The effects of ethanol, estrogen and hexachlorobenzene on the activities of hepatic δ-aminolevulinate synthetase, δ-aminolevulinate dehydratase, and uroporphyrinogen decarboxylase in male rats. *Arch. Toxicol.*, **59**, 141–145

Koss, G., Koransky, W. & Steinbach, K. (1976) Studies on the toxicology of hexachlorobenzene. II. Identification and determination of metabolites. *Arch. Toxicol.*, **35**, 107–114

Koss, G., Seubert, S., Seubert, A., Koransky, W. & Ippen, H. (1978) Studies on the toxicology of hexachlorobenzene. III. Observations in a long-term experiment. *Arch. Toxicol.*, **40**, 285–294

Koss, G., Koransky, W. & Steinbach, K. (1979) Studies of the toxicology of hexachlorobenzene. IV. Sulphur-containing metabolites. *Arch. Toxicol.*, **42**, 19–31

Koss, G., Seubert, S., Seubert, A., Seidel, J., Koransky, W. & Ippen, H. (1983) Studies on the toxicology of hexachlorobenzene. V. Different phases of porphyria during and after treatment. *Arch. Toxicol.*, **52**, 13–22

Krishnan, K., Brodeur, J. & Charbonneau, M. (1991) Development of an experimental model for the study of hexachlorobenzene-induced hepatic porphyria in the rat. *Fundam. appl. Toxicol.*, **17**, 433–441

Kuiper-Goodman, T., Grant, D.L., Moodie, C.A., Korsrud, G.O. & Munro, I.C. (1977) Subacute toxicity of hexachlorobenzene in the rat. *Toxicol. appl. Pharmacol.*, **40**, 529–549

Lamparski, L.L., Langhorst, M.L., Nestrick, T.J. & Cutié, S. (1980) Gas–liquid chromatographic determination of chlorinated benzenes and phenols in selected biological matrices. *J. Assoc. off. anal. Chem.*, **63**, 27–32

Langhorst, M.L. & Nestrick, T.J. (1979) Determination of chlorobenzenes in air and biological samples by gas chromatography with photoionization detection. *Anal. Chem.*, **51**, 2018–2025

Lewis, R.G. & MacLeod, K.E. (1982) Portable sampler for pesticides and semivolatile industrial organic chemicals in air. *Anal. Chem.*, **54**, 310–315

Li, S.M.A., Denomme, M.A., Leece, B., Safe, S., Dutton, D., Parkinson, A., Thomas, P.E., Ryan, D., Bandiera, S., Leik, L.M. & Levin, W. (1986) Hexachlorobenzene and substituted pentachlorobenzenes (X-C$_6$Cl$_5$) as inducers of hepatic cytochrome P-450-dependent mono-oxygenases. In: Morris, C.R. & Cabral, J.R.P., eds, *Hexachlorobenzene: Proceedings of an International Symposium* (IARC Scientific Publications, No. 77), Lyon, IARC*Press*, pp. 527–534

Lide, D.R. & Milne, G.W.A. (1996) *Properties of Organic Compounds*, Version 5.0, Boca Raton, FL, CRC Press [CD-ROM]

Lilienthal, H., Benthe, C., Heinzow, B. & Winneke, G. (1996) Impairment of schedule-controlled behavior by pre- and postnatal exposure to hexachlorobenzene in rats. *Arch. Toxicol.*, **70**, 174–181

Liljegren, G., Hardell, L., Lindström, G., Dahl, P. & Magnuson, A. (1998) Case–control study on breast cancer and adipose tissue concentrations of congener specific polychlorinated biphenyls, DDE and hexachlorobenzene. *Eur. J. Cancer Prev.*, **7**, 135–140

Linko, P., Yeowell, H.N., Gasiewicz, T.A. & Goldstein, J.A. (1986) Induction of cytochrome P-450 isoenzymes by hexachlorobenzene in rats and aromatic hydrocarbon (Ah)-responsive mice. *J. biochem. Toxicol.*, **1**, 95–107

Loaiza-Perez, A.I., Seisdedos, M.-T., Kleiman de Pisarev, D.L., Sancovich, H.A., Randi, A.S., Ferramola de Sancovich, A.M. & Santisteban, P. (1999) Hexachlorobenzene, a dioxin-type compound, increases malic enzyme gene transcription through a mechanism involving the thyroid hormone response element. *Endocrinology*, **140**, 4142–4151

Loose, L.D., Pittman, K.A., Benitz, K.-F. & Silkworth, J.B. (1977) Polychlorinated biphenyl and hexachlorobenzene induced humoral immunosuppression. *J. Reticuloendothel. Soc.*, **22**, 253–271

Loose, L.D., Silkworth, J.B., Mudzinski, S.P., Pittman, K.A., Benitz, K.-F. & Mueller, W. (1979) Modification of the immune response by organochlorine xenobiotics. *Drug chem. Toxicol.*, **21**, 111–132

Lopez-Avila, V., Northcutt, R., Onstot, J., Wickham, M. & Billets, S. (1983) Determination of 51 priority organic compounds after extraction from standard reference materials. *Anal. Chem.*, **55**, 881–889

Lunde, G. & Bjorseth, A. (1977) Human blood samples as indicators of occupational exposure to persistent chlorinated hydrocarbons. *Sci. total Environ.*, **8**, 241–246

Lunde, G. & Ofstad, E.B. (1976) Determination of fat-soluble chlorinated compounds in fish. *Fresenius' Z. anal. Chem.*, **282**, 395–399

Manson, M.M. & Smith, A.G. (1984) Effect of hexachlorobenzene on male and female rat hepatic gamma-glutamyl transpeptidase levels. *Cancer Lett.*, **22**, 227–234

Mazzei, E.S. & Mazzei, C.M. (1973) [Intoxication by a fungicide, hexachlorobenzene, contaminating wheat grains.] *Sem. Hôp. Paris*, **49**, 63–67 (in French)

Mehendale, H.M., Fields, M. & Matthews, H.B. (1975) Metabolism and effects of hexachlorobenzene on hepatic microsomal enzymes in the rat. *J. agric. Food Chem.*, **23**, 261–265

Melnikova, L.V., Belyakov, A.A., Smirnova, V.G. & Kurenko, L.T. (1975) [Sanitary-chemical methods for determination of noxious substances encountered in the production of sodium pentachlorophenolate.] *Gig. Tr. prof. Zabol.*, **7**, 37–39 (in Russian)

Mendonça, G.A.S., Eluf-Neto, J., Andrada-Serpa, M.J., Carmo, P.A.O., Barreto, H.H.C., Inomata, O.N.K. & Kussumi, T.A. (1999) Organochlorines and breast cancer: A case–control study in Brazil. *Int. J. Cancer*, **83**, 596–600

Mendoza, C.E., Grant, D.L. & Shields, J.B. (1975) Body burden of hexachlorobenzene in suckling rats and its effects on various organs and on liver porphyrin accumulation. *Environ. physiol. Biochem.*, **5**, 460–464

Mes, J. (1992) Organochlorine residues in human blood and biopsy fat and their relationship. *Bull. environ. Contam. Toxicol.*, **48**, 815–820

Mes, J., Davies, D.J., Doucet, J., Weber, D. & McMullen, E. (1993) Levels of chlorinated hydrocarbon residues in Canadian human breast milk and their relationship to some characteristics of the donors. *Food Addit. Contam.*, **10**, 429–441

Michielsen, C.P.P.C., Bloksma, N., Ultee, A., van Mil, F. & Vos, J.G. (1997) Hexachlorobenzene-induced immunomodulation and skin and lung lesions: A comparison between brown Norway, Lewis, and Wistar rats. *Toxicol. appl. Pharmacol.*, **144**, 12–26

Michielsen, C.P.P.C., Bloksma, N., Klatter, F.A., Rozing, J., Vos, J.G. & van Dijk, J.E. (1999) The role of thymus-dependent T cells in hexachlorobenzene-induced inflammatory skin and lung lesions. *Toxicol. appl. Pharmacol.*, **161**, 180–191

Miskiewicz, A.G. & Gibbs, P.J. (1994) Organochlorine pesticides and hexachlorobenzene in tissues of fish and invertebrates caught near a sewage outfall. *Environ. Pollut.*, **84**, 269–277

Moysich, K.B., Ambrosone, C.B., Vena, J.E., Shields, P.G., Mendola, P., Kostyniak, P., Greizerstein, H ., Graham, S., Marshall, J.R., Schisterman, E.F. & Freudenheim, J.L. (1998) Environmental organochlorine exposure and postmenopausal breast cancer risk. *Cancer Epidemiol. Biomarkers Prev.*, **7**, 181–188

Munch, D.J., Graves, R.L., Maxey, R.A. & Engel, T.M. (1990) Methods development and implementation for the National Pesticide Survey. *Environ. Sci. Technol.*, **24**, 1446–1451

Murray, H.E., Neff, G.S., Hrung, Y. & Giam, C.S. (1980) Determination of benzo(a)pyrene, hexachlorobenzene and pentachlorophenol in oysters from Galveston Bay, Texas. *Bull. environ. Contam. Toxicol.*, **25**, 663–667

Mussalo-Rauhamaa, H., Häsänen, E., Pyysalo, H., Antervo, K., Kauppila, R. & Pantzar, P. (1990) Occurrence of beta-hexachlorocyclohexane in breast cancer patients. *Cancer*, **66**, 2124–2128

Nakashima, Y., Ohsawa, S., Umegaki, K. & Ikegami, S. (1997) Hexachlorobenzene accumulated by dams during pregnancy is transferred to suckling rats during early lactation. *J. Nutr.*, **127**, 648–654

Nam, K.-S. & King, J.W. (1994) Coupled SFE/SFC/GC for the trace analysis of pesticide residues in fatty food samples. *J. high Resol. Chromatogr.*, **17**, 577–582

National Institute for Occupational Safety and Health (2000) *National Occupational Exposure Survey 1981–83*, Cincinnati, OH, US Department of Health and Human Services, Public Health Service

Newsome, W.H. & Ryan, J.J. (1999) Toxaphene and other chlorinated compounds in human milk from northern and southern Canada: A comparison. *Chemosphere*, **39**, 519–526

Newsome, W.H., Davies, D. & Doucet, J. (1995) PCB and organochlorine pesticides in Canadian human milk — 1992. *Chemosphere*, **30**, 2143–2153

Nordström, M., Hardell, L., Lindstrom, G., Wingfors, H., Hardell, K. & Linde, A. (2000) Concentrations of organochlorines related to titers of Epstein-Barr virus early antigen IgG as risk factors for hairy cell leukemia. *Environ. Health Perspectives*, **108**, 441-445

Oehme, M. & Stray, H. (1982) Quantitative determination of ultra-traces of chlorinated compounds in high-volume air samples from the Arctic using polyurethane foam as collection medium. *Fresenius' Z. anal. Chem.*, **311**, 665–673

Oliver, B.G. & Nicol, K.D. (1982) Chlorobenzenes in sediments, water, and selected fish from Lakes Superior, Huron, Erie, and Ontario. *Environ. Sci. Technol.*, **16**, 532-536

van Ommen, B., Adang, A.E., Brader, L., Posthumus, M.A., Muller, F. & van Bladeren, P.J. (1986) The microsomal metabolism of hexachlorobenzene. Origin of the covalent binding to protein. *Biochem. Pharmacol.*, **35**, 3233–3238

van Ommen, B., Hendriks, W., Bessems, J.G.M., Geesink, G., Muller, F. & van Bladeren, P.J. (1989) The relation between the oxidative biotransformation of hexachlorobenzene and its porphyrinogenic activity. *Toxicol. appl. Pharmacol.*, **100**, 517–528

Onuska, F.I. & Terry, K.A. (1993) Extraction of pesticides from sediments using a microwave technique. *Chromatographia*, **36**, 101–104

van Oostdam, J., Gilman, A., Dewailly, E., Usher, P., Wheatley, B., Kuhnlein, H., Neve, S., Walker, J., Tracy, B., Feely, M., Jerome, V. & Kwavnick, B. (1999) Human health implications of environmental contaminants in Arctic Canada: A review. *Sci. total Environ.*., **230**, 1–82

Pereira, M.A., Herren, S.L., Britt, A.L. & Khoury, M.M. (1982) Sex difference in enhancement of GGTase-positive foci by hexachlorobenzene and lindane in rat liver. *Cancer Lett.*, **15**, 95–101

Peters, H.A. (1976) Hexachlorobenzene poisoning in Turkey. *Fed. Proc.*, **35**, 2400–2403

Peters, H.A., Johnson, S.A.M., Cam, S., Oral, S., Müftü, Y. & Ergene, T. (1966) Hexachlorobenzene-induced porphyria: Effect of chelation on the disease, porphyrin and metal metabolism. *Am. J. med. Sci.*, **251**, 314–322

Peters, H.A., Cripps, D.J. & Gocmen, A. (1978) Porphyria 20 years after hexachlorobenzene exposure (Abstract No. PP 10). *Neurology*, **28**, 333

Peters, H.A., Gocmen, A., Cripps, D.J., Bryan, G.T. & Dogramaci, I. (1982) Epidemiology of hexachlorobenzene-induced porphyria in Turkey. *Arch. Neurol.*, **39**, 744–749

Peters, H.A., Gocmen, A., Cripps, D.J., Morris, C.R. & Bryan, G.T. (1986) Porphyria turcica: Hexachlorobenzene-induced porphyria. Neurological manifestations and therapeutic trials of ethylenediaminetetraacetic acid in the acute syndrome. In: Morris, C.R. & Cabral, J.R.P., eds, *Hexachlorobenzene: Proceedings of an International Symposium,* (IARC Scientific Publications, No. 77), Lyon, IARC*Press*, pp. 575–579

Peters, H.A., Cripps, D.J., Gocmen, A., Bryan, G.T., Erturk, E. & Morris, CR. (1987) Turkish epidemic of hexachlorobenzene porphyria. A 30-year study. *Ann. N.Y. Acad. Sci.*, **514**, 183–190

Pylypiw, H.M., Jr (1993) Rapid gas chromatographic method for the multiresidue screening of fruits and vegetables for organochlorine and organophosphate pesticides. *J. AOAC int.*, **76**, 1369–1373

Queiroz, M.L.S., Bincoletto, C., Perlingeiro, R.C., Quadros, M.R. & Souza, C.A. (1998a) Immunoglobulin levels in workers exposed to hexachlorobenzene. *Hum. exp. Toxicol.*, **17**, 172–175

Queiroz, M.L.S., Quadros, M.R., Valadares, M.C. & Silveira, J.P. (1998b) Polymorphonuclear phagocytosis and killing in workers occupationally exposed to hexachlorobenzene. *Immunopharm. Immunotoxicol.*, **20**, 447–454

van Raaij, J.A., van den Berg, K.J., Engel, R., Bragt, P.C. & Notten, W.R. (1991a) Effects of hexachlorobenzene and its metabolites pentachlorophenol and tetrachlorohydroquinone on serum thyroid hormone levels in rats. *Toxicology*, **67**, 107–116

van Raaij, J.A., van den Berg, K.J. & Notten, W.R. (1991b) Hexachlorobenzene and its metabolites pentachlorophenol and tetrachlorohydroquinone: Interaction with thyroxine binding sites of rat thyroid hormone carriers *in vivo* and *in vitro*. *Toxicol. Lett.*, **59**, 101–107

van Raaij, J.A., Frijters, C.M. & van den Berg, K.J. (1993a) Hexachlorobenzene-induced hypothyroidism. Involvement of different mechanisms by parent compound and metabolite. *Biochem. Pharmacol.*, **46**, 1385–1391

van Raaij, J.A., Kaptein, E., Visser, T.J. & van den Berg, K.J. (1993b) Increased glucuronidation of thyroid hormone in hexachlorobenzene-treated rats. *Biochem. Pharmacol.*, **45**, 627–631

Rahman, M.S., Bowadt, S. & Larsen, B. (1993) Dual-column GC analysis of Mediterranean fish for ten organochlorine pesticides and sixty two chlorobiphenyls. *J. high Resol. Chromatogr.*, **16**, 731–735

Randi, A.S., Sancovich, H.A., Feramola de Sancovich, A.M., Loaiza, A., Krawiec, L. & Kleiman de Pisarev, D.L. (1998) Hexachlorobenzene-induced alterations of rat hepatic microsomal membrane function. *Toxicology*, **125**, 83–94

Ray, S., Bailey, M., Paterson, G., Metcalfe, T. & Metcalfe, C. (1998) Comparative levels of organochlorine compounds in flounders from the northeast coast of Newfoundland and an offshore site. *Chemosphere*, **36**, 2201–2210

Renner, G. & Schuster, K.P. (1977) 2,4,5-Trichlorophenol, a new urinary metabolite of hexa-chlorobenzene. *Toxicol. appl. Pharmacol.*, **39**, 355–356

Rietjens, I.M.C.M., Steensma, A., den Besten, C., van Tintelen, G., Haas, J., van Ommen, B. & van Bladeren, P.J. (1995) Comparative biotransformation of hexachlorobenzene and hexa-fluorobenzene in relation to the induction of porphyria. *Eur. J. Pharmacol.*, **293**, 293–299

Rios de Molína, M.C., Wainstok de Calmanovici, R. & San Martin de Viale, L.C. (1980) Inves-tigations on the presence of porphyrinogen carboxylyase inhibitor in the liver of rats intoxicated with hexachlorobenzene. *Int. J. Biochem.*, **12**, 1027–1032

Rizzardini, M. & Smith, A.G. (1982) Sex differences in the metabolism of hexachlorobenzene by rats and the development of porphyria in females. *Biochem. Pharmacol.*, **31**, 3543–3548

Rizzardini, M., Cantoni, L., Villa, P. & Ubezio, P. (1990) Biochemical, morphological and flow-cytometric evaluation of the effects of hexachlorobenzene on rat liver. *Cell Biol. Toxicol.*, **6**, 185–203

Rozman, K., Mueller, W., Coulston, F. & Korte, F. (1977) Long-term feeding study of hexa-chlorobenzene in rhesus monkeys. *Chemosphere*, **6**, 81–84

Rozman, K., Gorski, J.R., Rozman, P. & Parkinson, A. (1986) Reduced serum thyroid hormone levels in hexachlorobenzene-induced porphyria. *Toxicol. Lett.*, **30**, 71–78

Rumsby, P.C., Evans, J.G., Phillimore, H.E., Carthew, P. & Smith, A.G. (1992) Search for Ha-ras codon 61 mutations in liver tumours caused by hexachlorobenzene and Aroclor 1254 in C57BL/10ScSn mice with iron overload. *Carcinogenesis*, **13**, 1917–1920

Sadtler Research Laboratories (1980) *Sadtler Standard Spectra, 1980 Cumulative Molecular Formula Index*, Philadelphia, PA, p. 82

Sala, M., Sunyer, J., Otero, R., Santiago-Silva, M., Camps, C. & Grimalt, J. (1999a) Organo-chlorine in the serum of inhabitants living near an electrochemical factory. *Occup. environ. Med.*, **56**, 152–158

Sala, M., Sunyer, J., Otero, R., Santiago-Silva, M., Ozalla, D., Herrero, C., To-Figueras J., Kogevinas, M., Anto, J.M., Camps, C. & Grimalt, J. (1999b) Health effects of chronic high exposure to hexachlorobenzene in a general population sample. *Arch. environ. Health*, **54**, 102–109

Savela, A., Vuorela, R. & Kauppinen, T. (1999) *ASA 1997* (Katsauksia 140), Helsinki, Finnish Institute of Occupational Health, p. 30 (in Finnish)

Schielen, P., Schoo, W., Tekstra, J., Oostermeijer, H.H.A., Seinen, W. & Bloksma, N. (1993) Autoimmune effects of hexachlorobenzene in the rat. *Toxicol. appl. Pharmacol.*, **122**, 233–243

Schielen, P., den Besten, C., Vos, J.G., van Bladeren, P.J., Seinen, W. & Bloksma, N. (1995) Immune effects of hexachlorobenzene in the rat: Role of metabolism in a 13-week feeding study. *Toxicol. appl. Pharmacol.*, **131**, 37–43

Seidel, V. & Linder, W. (1993) Universal sample enrichment technique for organochlorine pesticides in environmental and biological samples using a redesigned simultaneous steam distillation–solvent extraction apparatus. *Anal. Chem.*, **65**, 3677–3683

Seldén, A.I., Nygren, Y., Westberg, H.B. & Bodin, L.S. (1997) Hexachlorobenzene and octa-chlorostyrene in plasma of aluminium foundry workers using hexachloroethane for degassing. *Occup. environ. Med.*, **54**, 613–618

Seldén, A.I., Floderus, Y., Bodin, L.S., Westberg, H.B. & Thunell, S. (1999) Porphyrin status in aluminum foundry workers exposed to hexachlorobenzene and octachlorostyrene. *Arch. environ. Health*, **54**, 248–253

Shan, T.H., Hopple, J.A. & Foster, G.D. (1994) Alternative tissue analysis method developed for organochlorine contaminants in aquatic organisms. *Bull. environ. Contam. Toxicol.*, **53**, 382–389

Sherwood, R.L., Thomas, P.T., O'Shea, W.J., Bradof, J.N., Ratajczak, H.V., Graham, J.A. & Aranyi, C. (1989) Effects of inhaled hexachlorobenzene aerosols on rat pulmonary host defenses. *Toxicol. ind. Health*, **5**, 451–461

Shirai, T., Miyata, Y., Nakanishi, K., Murasaki, G. & Ito, N. (1978) Hepatocarcinogenicity of polychlorinated terphenyl (PCT) in ICR mice and its enhancement by hexachlorobenzene (HCB). *Cancer Lett.*, **4**, 271–275

Siekel, P., Chalupa, I., Beňo, J., Blaško, M., Novotný, J. & Burian, J. (1991) A genotoxico-logical study of hexachlorobenzene and pentachloroanisole. *Teratog. Carcinog. Mutag.*, **11**, 55–60

da Silva Augusto, L.G., Lieber, S.R., Ruiz, M.A. & de Souza, C.A. (1997) Micronucleus moni-toring to assess human occupational exposure to organochlorides. *Environ. mol. Mutag.*, **29**, 46–52

Simon, G.S., Tardiff, R.G. & Borzelleca, J.F. (1979) Failure of hexachlorobenzene to induce dominant lethal mutations in the rat. *Toxicol. appl. Pharmacol.*, **47**, 415–419

Sims, D.E., Singh, A., Donald, A., Jarrell, J. & Villeneuve, C. (1991) Alteration of primate ovary surface epithelium by exposure to hexachlorobenzene: A quantitative study. *Histol. Histopathol.*, **6**, 525–529

Sinclair, P.R., Gorman, N., Walton, H.S., Bement, W.J., Dalton, T.P., Sinclair, J.F., Smith, A.G. & Nebert, D.W. (2000) CYP1A2 is essential in murine uroporphyria caused by hexa-chlorobenzene and iron. *Toxicol. appl. Pharmacol.*, **162**, 60–67

Smith, A.G. & Cabral, J.R. (1980) Liver-cell tumours in rats fed hexachlorobenzene. *Cancer Lett.*, **11**, 169–172

Smith, A.G. & Francis, J.E. (1983) Synergism of iron and hexachlorobenzene inhibits hepatic uroporphyrinogen decarboxylase in inbred mice. *Biochem. J.*, **214**, 909–913

Smith, A.G., Francis, J.E., Dinsdale, D., Manson, M.M. & Cabral J.R.P. (1985) Hepatocarcino-genicity of hexachlorobenzene in rats and the sex difference in hepatic iron status and development of porphyria. *Carcinogenesis*, **6**, 631–636

Smith, A.G., Wright, A.L. & Cabral, J.R.P. (1986) Influence of hexachlorobenzene on thyroids of male hamsters. In: Morris, C.R. & Cabral, J.R.P., eds, *Hexachlorobenzene: Proceedings of an International Symposium* (IARC Scientific Publications No. 77), Lyon, IARC*Press*, pp. 357–359

Smith, A.G., Dinsdale, D., Cabral, J.R.P. & Wright, A.L. (1987) Goitre and wasting induced in hamsters by hexachlorobenzene. *Arch. Toxicol.*, **60**, 343–349

Smith, A.G., Cabral, J.R.P., Carthew, P., Francis, J.E. & Manson, M.M. (1989) Carcinogenicity of iron in conjunction with a chlorinated environmental chemical, hexachlorobenzene, in C57BL/10ScSn mice. *Int. J. Cancer*, **43**, 92–96

Smith, A.G., Francis, J.E., Green, J.A., Greig, J.B., Wolf, C.R. & Manson, M.M. (1990) Sex-linked hepatic uroporphyria and the induction of cytochromes P450IA in rats caused by hexachlorobenzene and polyhalogenated biphenyls. *Biochem. Pharmacol.*, **40**, 2059–2068

Sopena de Kracoff, Y.E., Ferramola de Sancovich, A.M., Sancovich, H.A. & Kleiman de Pisarev, D.L. (1994) Effect of thyroidectomy and thyroxine on hexachlorobenzene induced porphyria. *J. endocrinol. Invest.*, **17**, 301–305

Stachel, B., Dougherty, R.C., Lahl, U., Schlosser, M. & Zeschmar, B. (1989) Toxic environmental chemicals in human semen: Analytical method and case studies. *Andrologia*, **21**, 282–291

Stanley, J.S. (1986) *Broad Scan Analysis of the FY82 National Human Adipose Tissue Survey Specimens* — Volume I: *Executive summary* (EPA 560/5-86/035). Kansas City, MO, Midwest Research Institute (Prepared for the US Environmental Protection Agency, Office of Toxic Substances, Field Studies Branch)

Stewart, F.P. & Smith, A.G. (1987) Metabolism and covalent binding of hexachlorobenzene by isolated male and female rat hepatocytes. *Biochem. Pharmacol.*, **36**, 2232–2234

Stewart, F.P., Manson, M.M., Cabral, J.R.P. & Smith, A.G. (1989) Hexachlorobenzene as a promoter of diethylnitrosamine-initiated hepatocarcinogenesis in rats and comparison with induction of porphyria. *Carcinogenesis*, **10**, 1225–1230

Stonard, M.D. (1975) Mixed type hepatic microsomal enzyme induction by hexachloro-benzene. *Biochem. Pharmacol.*, **24**, 1959–1963

Sundlof, S.F., Hansen, L.G., Koritz, G.D. & Sundlof, S.M. (1982) The pharmacokinetics of hexachlorobenzene in male beagles. Distribution, excretion, and pharmacokinetic model. *Drug Metab. Disposition*, **10**, 371–381

Thomas, R.S., Gustafson, D.L., Ramsdell, H.S., el-Masri, H.A., Benjamin, S.A. & Yang, R.S. (1998) Enhanced regional expression of glutathione S-transferase P1-1 with colocalized AP-1 and CYP 1A2 induction in chlorobenzene-induced porphyria. *Toxicol. appl. Pharmacol.*, **150**, 22–31

To-Figueras, J., Gómez-Catalán, J., Rodamilans, M. & Corbella, J. (1991) Studies on sex differences in excretion of sulphur derivatives of hexachlorobenzene and pentachloronitro-benzene by rats. *Toxicol. Lett.*, **56**, 87–94

To-Figueras, J., Gómez-Catalán, J.. Rodamilans, M. & Corbella, J. (1992) Sulphur derivative of hexachlorobenzene in human urine. *Hum. exp. Toxicol.*, **11**, 271–273

To-Figueras, J., Barrot, C., Rodamilans, M., Gómez-Catalán, J., Torra, M., Brunet, M., Sabater, F. & Corbella, J. (1995) Accumulation of hexachlorobenzene in humans: A long standing risk. *Hum. exp. Toxicol.*, **14**, 20–23

To-Figueras, J., Sala, M., Otero, R., Barrot, C., Santiago-Silva, M., Rodamilans, M., Herrero, C., Grimalt, J. & Sunyer, J. (1997) Metabolism of hexachlorobenzene in humans: Association between serum levels and urinary metabolites in a highly exposed population. *Environ. Health Perspectives*, **105**, 78–83

den Tonkelaar, E.M., Verschuuren, H.G., Bankovska, J., de Vries, T., Kroes, R. & van Esch, G.J. (1978) Hexachlorobenzene toxicity in pigs. *Toxicol. appl. Pharmacol.*, **43**, 137–145

Trotter, W.J. & Dickerson, R. (1993) Pesticide residues in composited milk collected through the US Pasteurized Milk Network. *J. Assoc. off. anal. Chem. int.*, **76**, 1220–1225

Vandebriel, R.J., Meredith, C., Scott, M.P., Roholl, P.J.M. & van Loveren, H. (1998) Effects of *in vivo* exposure to bis(tri-*n*-butyltin)oxide, hexachlorobenzene, and benzo(*a*)pyrene on cytokine (receptor) mRNA levels in cultured rat splenocytes and on IL-2 receptor protein levels. *Toxicol. appl. Pharmacol.*, **148**, 126–136

Villeneuve, D.C., van Logten, M.J., den Tonkelaar, E.M., Greve, P.A., Vos, J.G., Speijers, G.J.A. & van Esch, G.J. (1977) Effect of food deprivation on low level hexachlorobenzene exposure in rats. *Sci. total Environ.*, **8**, 179–186

Vos, J.G., van Logten, M.J., Kreeftenberg, J.G. & Kruizinga, W. (1979a) Hexachlorobenzene-induced stimulation of the humoral immune response in rats. *Ann. N.Y. Acad. Sci.*, **320**, 535–550

Vos, J.G., van Logten, M.J., Kreeftenberg, J.G., Steerenberg, P.A. & Kruizinga, W. (1979b) Effect of hexachlorobenzene on the immune system of rats following combined pre- and post-natal exposure. *Drug chem. Toxicol.*, **2**, 61–76

Wainstok de Calmanovici, R., Billi de Catabbi, S., Aldonatti, C.A. & San Martin de Viale, L.C. (1986) Effect of desferrioxamine on the development of hexachlorobenzene-induced porphyria. *Biochem Pharmacol.*, **35**, 2399–2405

Wainstok de Calmanovici, R., Billi de Catabbi, S., Aldonatti, C.A. & San Martin de Viale, L.C. (1989) Influence of the strain of rats on the induction of hexachlorobenzene induced porphyria. *Int. J. Biochem.*, **21**, 377–381

Wainstok de Calmanovici, R., Cochón, A.C., Zenklusen, J.C., Aldonatti, C., Cabral, J.R.P. & San Martin de Viale, L.C. (1991) Influence of hepatic tumors caused by diethylnitrosamine on hexachlorobenzene-induced porphyria in rats. *Cancer Lett.*, **58**, 225–232

Waliszewski, S.M. & Szymczynski, G.A. (1985) Inexpensive, precise method for the determination of chlorinated pesticide residues in soil. *J. Chromatogr.*, **321**, 480–483

Watts, R.R., Hodgson, D.W., Christ, H.L. & Moseman, R.F. (1980) Improved method for hexachlorobenzene and mirex determination with hexachlorobenzene confirmation in adipose tissue: Collaborative study. *J. Assoc. off. anal. Chem.*, **63**, 1128-1134

Weiderpass, E., Adami, H.-O., Baron, J.A., Wicklund-Glynn, A., Aune, M., Atuma, S. & Persson, I. (2000) Organochlorines and endometrial cancer risk. *Cancer Epidemiol. Biomarkers Prev.*, **9**, 487–493

WHO (1987) *Pentachlorophenol* (Environmental Health Criteria 71), Geneva, International Programme on Chemical Safety

WHO (1993) *Guidelines for Drinking-water Quality*, 2nd Ed., Vol. 1, *Recommendations*, Geneva, p. 84

WHO (1997) *Hexachlorobenzene* (Environmental Health Criteria 195), Geneva, International Programme on Chemical Safety

WHO (1999) *Inventory of IPCS and Other WHO Pesticide Evaluations and Summary of Toxicological Evaluations Performed by the Joint Meeting on Pesticide Residues [JMPR} through 1999*, 3rd Ed., Geneva, International Programme on Chemical Safety

Yess, N.J., Gundersson, E.L. & Roy, R.R. (1993) US Food and Drug Administration monitoring of pesticide residues in infant foods and adult foods eaten by infants/children. *J. AOAC int.*, **76**, 492–507

Zheng, T., Holford, T.R., Mayne, S.T., Tessari, J., Owens, P.H., Zham, S.H, Zhang, B., Dubrow, R., Ward, B., Carter, D. & Boyle, P. (1999) Environmental exposure to hexachlorobenzene (HCB) and risk of female breast cancer in Connecticut. *Cancer Epidemiol. Biomarkers Prev.*, **8**, 407–411

TOXAPHENE

This substance was considered by previous working groups, in 1978 (IARC, 1979) and 1986 (IARC, 1987). Since that time, new data have become available, and these have been incorporated into the monograph and taken into consideration in the present evaluation.

1. Exposure Data

1.1 Chemical and physical data

1.1.1 *Nomenclature*

Chem. Abstr. Serv. Reg. No.: 8001-35-2
Deleted CAS Reg. Nos: 8022-04-6; 12687-42-2; 12698-98-5; 12770-20-6; 37226-11-2; 56645-28-4
Chem. Abstr. Name: Toxaphene
IUPAC Systematic Name: Toxaphene
Synonyms: Camphechlor; chlorinated camphene; PCC; polychlorocamphene

1.1.2 *Structural and molecular formulae and relative molecular mass*

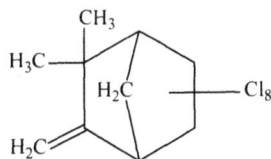

$C_{10}H_{10}Cl_8$ (approximately)   Relative molecular mass: 414 (average)

[Note: Structure representative of the predominant chlorinated camphene compounds present in technical-grade toxaphene]

1.1.3   *Chemical and physical properties of the pure substance*

From Budavari (2000)

(*a*) *Description*: Yellow waxy solid

(*b*) *Melting-point*: 65–90 °C

(*c*) *Solubility*: Very slightly soluble in water (0.003 g/L); freely soluble in aromatic hydrocarbons

(*d*) *Stability*: Dehydrochlorinates in the presence of alkali, prolonged exposure to sunlight and at temperatures of about 155 °C

(*e*) *Octanol/water partition coefficient (P)*: log P, 6.44

1.1.4   *Technical products and impurities*

In the past, toxaphene was available as dust formulations, emulsifiable concentrates, granules and wettable powders (FAO/UNEP, 1999). Trade names for toxaphene include Alltox, Anatox, Camphochlor, Canfeclor, Estonox, Geniphene, Hercules 3956, Kamfochlor, M 5055, Melipax, Motox, PChK, Phenacide, Phenatox, PKhF, Strobane-T, Toxakil, Toxaphen and Toxyphen.

1.1.5   *Analysis*

Methods for the analysis of toxaphene in various media are summarized in Table 1.

1.2   Production

Toxaphene is a very complex, but fairly reproducible mixture of at least 177 C_{10} polychloro derivatives, having an approximate overall empirical formula of $C_{10}H_{10}Cl_8$. Toxaphene is produced by chlorination of camphene to 67–69% chlorine by weight and is made up mainly of compounds of $C_{10}H_8Cl_{10}$, $C_{10}H_{18-n}Cl_n$ (mostly polychlorobornanes) and $C_{10}H_{16-n}Cl_n$ (polychlorobornenes and/or polychlorotricyclenes) with $n = 6$–9 (Budavari, 2000). Annual production of toxaphene in the USA in 1976 was about 19 000 t (Agency for Toxic Substances and Disease Registry, 1998).

Information available in 2000 indicated that toxaphene was manufactured by one company in the USA (CIS Information Services, 2000).

1.3   Use

Toxaphene (chlorinated camphene) was used as a broad-spectrum, nonsystemic contact and stomach insecticide, with some acaricidal action. It was often used in combination with other pesticides. Its primary usage was on agricultural crops, mainly cotton, but also corn, fruit, vegetables and small grains. It has been used as an insecticide to control armyworms, boll weevils, bollworms, cotton aphids, cotton fleahoppers, cotton leafworms, grasshoppers and others. It was also used to control livestock ectoparasites such as lice, flies, ticks, mange and scab mites.

Table 1. Methods for the analysis of toxaphene

Sample matrix	Sample preparation	Assay procedure	Limit of detection	Reference
Air	Collect sample in prefilter and ethylene glycol; dilute with water; extract with hexane; extract; prefilter with hexane; pool extracts before drying; concentrate	GC/ECD	1–10 ng/m^3	Kutz et al. (1976)
	Adsorb onto polyurethane foam; extract with hexane; reduce volume	GC/ECD; GC/MS	1.6 pg/m^3 (11 300 m^3 sample)	Barrie et al. (1993)
	Collect vapours on cellulose ester membrane; desorb with petroleum ether	GC/ECD	0.14 μg/ sample	Eller (1994) [Method 5039]
	Collect vapours on polyurethane foam (low or high volume); extract with 5–10% diethyl ether in hexane	GC/ECD	NR	Environmental Protection Agency (1999a) [Method TO-04A]
Drinking-water	Extract with hexane; inject extract	GC/ECD	1.0 μg/L	Environmental Protection Agency (1995a) [Method 505]
	Extract with dichloromethane; isolate extract; dry; concentrate with methyl tert-butyl ether (capillary column)	GC/ECD	0.03 μg/L	Environmental Protection Agency (1995b) [Method 508.1]
	Extract by passing sample through liquid–solid extractor; elute with dichloromethane; concentrate by evaporation (capillary column)	GC/MS	1.0–1.7 μg/L	Environmental Protection Agency (1995c) [Method 525.2]
Tapwater, groundwater, river water	Isolate compounds from water on C$_{18}$ SPE followed by recovery of adsorbed analytes with supercritical carbon dioxide containing acetone	GC/ion trap MS	7.4 μg/L (w/v)	Ho et al. (1995)
Liquid and solid wastes	Extract with dichloromethane (liquid); hexane:acetone (1:1) or dichloromethane:acetone (1:1) (solid); clean-up	GC/ECD or GC/ELCD	NR	Environmental Protection Agency (1996a) [Method 8081A]

Table 1 (contd)

Sample matrix	Sample preparation	Assay procedure	Limit of detection	Reference
Liquid and solid wastes (contd)	Mix with anhydrous sodium sulfate; extract by Soxhlet or sonication process; clean-up on Florisil or gel-permeation (capillary column)	GC/MS	NR	Environmental Protection Agency (1996b) [Method 8270C]
	Extract with dichloromethane	Tandem MS	5 μg/sample	Hunt *et al.* (1985)
	Extract with dichloromethane; dry; exchange to hexane; clean-up on Florisil	GC/ECD	0.24 μg/L	Environmental Protection Agency (1999b) [Method 608]
	Extract with dichloromethane; dry; concentrate (packed column)	GC/MS	NR	Environmental Protection Agency (1999c) [Method 625]
	Extract with dichloromethane; dry; concentrate; optional clean-up (acetonitrile partition or Florisil)	GC/ECD	NR	Environmental Protection Agency (1993a) [Method 617]
Municipal and industrial wastewater	Adjust to pH 11; extract with dichloromethane; dry; concentrate	GC/MS	NR	APHA/AWWA/WEF (1999a)
	Extract with diethyl ether: hexane or dichloromethane: hexane; concentrate; clean-up by column adsorption chromatography	GC/ECD	NR	APHA/AWWA/WEF (1999b) [Method 6630B]
	Extract with dichloromethane; solvent exchange to hexane; clean-up with magnesia–silica gel; concentrate	GC/ECD	0.24 μg/L	APHA/AWWA/WEF (1999c)

Table 1 (contd)

Sample matrix	Sample preparation	Assay procedure	Limit of detection	Reference
Municipal and industrial waste water, sludges	If solids < 1%, extract with dichloromethane; for non-sludges with solids 1–30%, dilute to 1% and extract with dichloromethane; if solids > 30%, sonicate with dichloro-methane:acetone; for sludges: if solids < 30%, treat as above; if solids > 30%, sonicate with acetonitrile then dichloro-methane. Back-extract with sodium sulfate; concentrate; clean-up	GC/ECD or GC/MCD or GC/ELCD	0.91 µg/L	Environmental Protection Agency (1993b) [Method 1656]
Soil	Add water; extract with methanol:toluene (1:1); concentrate; add methanolic KOH solution and reflux; extract with hexane; clean-up on Florisil	GC/MS and HPLC	50 µg/kg	Crist et al. (1980)
	Soxhlet extract with dichloromethane or sonicate with dichloromethane:acetone (1:1, v/v); clean-up with GPC or SPE	GC/EC-NIMS	100 µg/kg	Brumley et al. (1993)
	Extract with dichloromethane: acetone (1:1) with sonication; remove water with sodium sulfate; solvent exchange to isooctane; clean-up on Florisil	GC/NCIMS	50 µg/kg (w/w)	Onuska et al. (1994)
	Extract with methanol; add aliquot and enzyme conjugate reagent to immobilized antibody; compare colour produced to reference reaction	Immuno-assay	500 µg/kg	Environmental Protection Agency (1996c) [Method 4040]
Sediment and mussel tissue	Extract with hexane; elute from alumina column; concentrate	HPLC followed by GC/FID or GC/ECD	< 1 µg/kg	Petrick et al. (1988)

Table 1 (contd)

Sample matrix	Sample preparation	Assay procedure	Limit of detection	Reference
Pesticide formulations	Extract with methanolic KOH; elute with diethyl ether from Florisil	GC/ECD	1 ng/sample	Gomes (1977)
	Remove solvent (xylene) from pesticide sample by reduced pressure; extract with hexane	GC and GC/TLC	NR	Saleh & Casida (1977)
	Extraction with hexane	TLC	1 µg/sample	Ismail & Bonner (1974)
	Dissolve in hexane and load onto alumina column; elute with hexane, dichloromethane in benzene then methanol	GC/ECD or GC/FID	NR	Seiber et al. (1975)
	Extract with acetone; filter or centrifuge	TLC	NR	AOAC International (2000) [Method 972.05]
Non-fatty foods	Extract with acetone; partition or remove water; clean-up on Florisil; elute with dichloro-methane	GC/ECD or GC/ELCD	NR	Food and Drug Administration (1999) [Method 302]
	Extract with acetonitrile or water:acetonitrile; partition into petroleum ether; clean-up on Florisil	GC/ECD or GC/ELCD	NR	Food and Drug Administration (1999)
Various products	Extract with acetonitrile; filter; add salt to affect phase separation; evaporate to near dryness; reconstitute in benzene	GC/ECD	2 mg/kg	Hsu et al. (1991)
Fruits and vegetables	Extract with acetone; filter extract with petroleum ether:dichloromethane; evaporate solvent; dissolve in acetone	GC/ECD	NR	WHO (1984)
Molasses	Dilute with water; extract with hexane:isopropanol	GC/ECD	0.03 mg/kg	WHO (1984)
Fatty foods	Extract fat; partition into acetonitrile:petroleum ether; clean-up on Florisil	GC/ECD or GC/ELCD	NR	Food and Drug Administration (1999) [Method 304]

Table 1 (contd)

Sample matrix	Sample preparation	Assay procedure	Limit of detection	Reference
Meat	Blend with ethyl acetate; dry (Na_2SO_4) and filter; treat with KOH and heat; extract with hexane; clean-up on Florisil	GC/ECD	NR	Boshoff & Pretorius (1979)
Bovine defibrinated whole blood	Dilute with water; extract with hexane	GC/ECD	0.58 mg/L	Maiorino et al. (1980)
	Add sample to formic acid and shake; extract with hexane; extract with potassium carbonate; reduce volume	GC/ECD	0.47 mg/L	Maiorino et al. (1980)
	Add sample to formic acid; mix and load onto Florisil column; elute with diethyl ether in petroleum ether; reduce volume; wash with hexane	GC/ECD	0.03 mg/L	Maiorino et al. (1980)
Lard	Extract with petroleum ether; centrifuge; remove water with anhydrous Na_2SO_4; reduce volume	GC/ECD	1.4 mg/kg	Head & Burse (1987)
Poultry fat	Render fat; direct analysis	GC/ECD	0.48 mg/kg	Ault & Spurgeon (1984)
Milk fat	Centrifuge; fractionate on Florisil	GC/ECD and GC/MS	< 10 µg/kg (ECD) 7 µg/kg (MS)	Cairns et al. (1981)
Milk and butter	Add to KOH; heat; extract with hexane; centrifuge; clean-up on Florisil	GC/ECD	NR	Boshoff & Pretorius (1979)
Fish (whole)	Blend frozen sample with dry ice and anhydrous Na_2SO_4; extract with hexane:acetone (1:1), followed by methanol	GC/NCIMS	75 pg/sample	Swackhamer et al. (1987)
Fish tissues	Extract with hexane:acetone; extract with hexane:diethyl ether; evaporate; dissolve in hexane; shake with H_2SO_4 to remove lipid	GC/NCIMS	NR	Jansson et al. (1991)

Table 1 (contd)

Sample matrix	Sample preparation	Assay procedure	Limit of detection	Reference
Fish tissues (contd)	Homogenize sample with hexane:acetone (1:2.5) under acid conditions; extract twice more with diethyl ether in hexane; treat with concentrated H_2SO_4, clean-up with GPC and silica gel	GC/NCIMS	NR	Jansson *et al.* (1991)
	Homogenize sample; extract with hexane:acetone; add internal standards; clean-up with GPC and Florisil	GC/HRMS (SIM)	10 µg/kg (wet weight)	Andrews *et al.* (1993)
	Pulverize tissue with anhydrous sodium sulfate; extract with acetone; solvent exchange to hexane; reduce volume; clean-up on Florisil and silica gel	GC/MS (SIM)	0.1 µg/kg	Jarnuzi & Wakimoto (1991)
Human tissues (toxaphene and some metabolites)	Macerate tissue; add anhydrous Na_2SO_4 and acetone; filter; extract with chloroform; add KOH; extract with water; remove water (Na_2SO_4); evaporate; dissolve in acetone	TLC	1 µg/sample	Tewari & Sharma (1977)
Human tissues	Grind sample; extract with dichloromethane:hexane (1:1), reduce volume; clean-up with GPC and Florisil	GC/NCIMS	~ 10 µg/kg	Fowler *et al.* (1993)
Human breast milk	Centrifuge; freeze-dry fat concentrate; dissolve in acetone; re-dissolve in hexane; shake with concentrated H_2SO_4; clean-up with silica gel	GC/ECD and GC/NCIMS	100 µg/L	Vaz & Blomkvist (1985)
Human breast fat	Homogenize; extract with petroleum ether; remove water with anhydrous Na_2SO_4; reduce volume	GC/ECD	NR	Head & Burse (1987)
Stomach washings and urine (toxaphene and some metabolites)	Filter sample; wash with water; add saturated solution of Na_2SO_4; extract with hexane; filter through anhydrous Na_2SO_4; evaporate to dryness; dissolve in acetone	TLC	1 µg/sample	Tewari & Sharma (1977)

Table 1 (contd)

Sample matrix	Sample preparation	Assay procedure	Limit of detection	Reference
Human blood	Add H_2SO_4 to blood sample; extract with hexane:acetone (9:1); centrifuge and evaporate to dryness; dissolve in hexane	GC/ECD or GC/MCD	NR 10–40 µg/L	Griffith & Blanke (1974)
	Add to dilute H_2SO_4 and 10% sodium tungstate solution; filter and wash with water; remove water with Na_2SO_4; extract with hexane; filter through anhydrous Na_2SO_4; evaporate to dryness; dissolve in acetone	TLC	1 µg/sample	Tewari & Sharma (1977)

NR, not reported; APHA/AWWA/WEF, American Public Health Association/American Water Works Association/Water Environment Federation; ECD, electron capture detection; EC-NIMS, electron capture–negative-ion mass spectrometry; ELCD, electrolytic conductivity detection; FID, flame ionization detection; FTIR, Fourier transform infrared spectroscopy; GC, gas chromatography; GPC, gel permeation chromatography; HPLC, high-performance liquid chromatography; HRMS, high-resolution mass spectrometry; MCD, microcoulometry detection; MS, mass spectrometry; NCIMS, negative chemical ionization mass spectrometry; SIM, selected ion monitoring; SPE, solid-phase extraction; TLC, thin-layer chromatography

Introduced in 1948, toxaphene was the most heavily used insecticide in the USA in the 1960s and 1970s, having replaced many of the agricultural applications of the banned DDT (Blair & Hoar Zahn, 1993; Agency for Toxic Substances and Disease Registry, 1998; FAO/UNEP, 1999).

1.4   Occurrence

1.4.1   *Occupational exposure*

The concentrations of toxaphene in the air of manufacturing plants in the former USSR were found to exceed the permissible level of 0.2 mg/m^3 by five to six times. By the end of a work shift, the concentrations on uncovered skin of employees were 30–1000 mg/m^2; covered skin areas had toxaphene concentrations of up to 40 mg/m^2 (Ashirova, 1971).

1.4.2   *Environmental occurrence*

Toxaphene is a persistent pesticide, the use of which has diminished substantially over the past two decades. This compound has low volatility and is only slightly soluble in water. Its biodegradation in soil is very slow, with a half-time measured in decades. Hence, toxaphene persists in the environment and can be expected to accumulate in the sediment long after application has ceased.

The environmental occurrence of toxaphene has been reviewed (IARC, 1979; WHO, 1984; Agency for Toxic Substances and Disease Registry, 1998).

The concentrations in the air in Bermuda and in the USA measured in the 1970s ranged from < 0.02 ng/m³ to 1540 ng/m³ (IARC, 1979). A more recent study in Canada (Shoeib et al., 1999) reported airborne toxaphene concentrations of 0.9–10.1 pg/m³ between 1995 and 1997.

In the 1970s, the concentrations of toxaphene in rainwater in the USA ranged from 44 to 280 ng/L (Munson, 1976). A more recent study in the USA showed concentrations in water ranging from 0.17 ng/L in Lake Ontario to 1.12 ng/L in Lake Superior (Swackhamer et al., 1998).

In the 1970s, the concentrations of toxaphene in soil in the USA were found to range from 7.7 to 33.4 mg/kg (Carey et al., 1976). Soil samples taken in the USA in 1969 had concentrations ranging from 0.1 to 53 mg/kg (Wiersma et al., 1972). More recently, the concentration of toxaphene in Great Lakes sediments were found to be 15 ± 4 (SD) µg/kg dry weight (Swackhamer et al., 1998).

Toxaphene present in sediments can continue to enter the food chain by uptake by small organisms in direct contact with the sediment. The log of the bioaccumulation factor (organism concentration/water concentration) ranged from 5.8 to 7.0 for a series of biota including phytoplankton, zoo plankton, Mysis, Bythotrephes, sculpin and lake trout (Swackhamer et al., 1998).

In the USA, the concentrations in wildlife ranged from 1.7 to 88.9 mg/kg in adult animals (Causey et al., 1972) and from 0.12 to 0.58 mg/kg in pelican eggs (Blus et al., 1975). A study in 1976–86 by the National Contamination Biomonitoring Program in the USA of various freshwater fish across the country showed annual geometric mean concentrations of toxaphene ranging from 0.066 to 0.178 mg/kg (Schmitt et al., 1999). Musial and Uthe (1983) reported that the concentration of toxaphene in Canadian East Coast marine fish tissues was 0.4–1.1 mg/kg on a wet weight basis.

Saleh (1991) reviewed the concentrations of toxaphene in the environment before 1990. Those in birds' eggs ranged from 0.03 (osprey) to 10 (vulture) mg/kg, while the concentrations in adult birds ranged from 0.02 to 4.0 mg/kg on a wet weight basis. The maximum concentration in tertiary consumer species in the Mississippi River (Louisiana, USA), such as herons, was 24.0 mg/kg, indicating substantial biomagnification of toxaphene. The concentrations in bats were ≤ 2 mg/kg. In fish, the concentrations of toxaphene were 5–7 mg/kg in Lake Superior trout, 5–10 mg/kg in Lake Michigan trout, 9 mg/kg in Lake Huron trout, 0.068 mg/kg of lipid in South Atlantic cod, 9 mg/kg of lipid in Arctic char in Sweden and 13 mg/kg of lipid in Atlantic herring from the Baltic Sea. Datta et al. (1999) reported a concentration of 0.154 mg/kg in a trout from Lake Tahoe (USA).

The arithmetic mean concentrations of toxaphene in traditional foods in northern and Arctic Canada, e.g., marine mammal meat and blubber and terrestrial mammal meat and organs ranged from < 0.001 to 3.89 mg/kg wet weight (Chan, 1998). In another study, the concentration of toxaphene in beluga whale blubber ranged from 2.38 to 3.54 mg/kg lipid in females and 4.06 and 15.94 mg/kg in two males. A single fetal specimen contained 3.71 mg/kg, which was comparable to the mother's value of 3.20 mg/kg (Wade *et al.*, 1997).

Concentrations of 2.3–18 mg/L were reported in the milk of cows fed toxaphene-treated hay in Finland (Bateman *et al.*, 1953).

The estimate average dietary intake of toxaphene in the USA during the period 1986–91 ranged from 0.0057 to 0.0224 µg/kg bw per day, with age- and sex-specific differences (Agency for Toxic Substances and Disease Registry, 1998).

The median concentrations in breast milk from various populations in northern and southern Canada in 1986, 1992 and 1996 ranged from 4.94 to 56.4 ng/g of extractable lipid, the concentrations observed in northern Canada being substantially higher than those observed elsewhere (Newsome & Ryan, 1999). In the Nordic countries, the mean toxaphene concentration in 1985 in pooled breast milk was 0.1 mg/kg of milk fat in Uppsala and Stockholm, Sweden, and 1–10 µg/L as a fraction of whole milk in Finland (Saleh, 1991). Adipose tissue samples taken in Finland in 1985 showed toxaphene concentrations of 0.01–0.1 mg/kg, but the result was strongly dependent on the diet.

1.5   Regulations and guidelines

Occupational exposure limits for toxaphene in several countries are presented in Table 2. The use of toxaphene has been banned or product registrations have been cancelled or withdrawn in many countries since 1970, because of concerns about risks to human health and the environment. For example, in the Joint FAO/UNEP Programme for the Operation of Prior Informed Consent for Banned or Severely Restricted Chemicals in International Trade (PIC Programme), more than 19 countries have reported that use of toxaphene had been banned or severely restricted (FAO/UNEP, 1999).

Toxaphene is one of 12 persistent organic pollutants being considered for international action to reduce or eliminate their releases under a global convention (FAO/UNEP, 1999). At negotiations in September 1999, the participating governments agreed to phase out use of toxaphene and two other chlorinated pesticides (aldrin and endrin). As of December 2000, three other chlorinated pesticides had been phased out (chlordane, heptachlor and hexachlorobenzene) (Hogue, 2000).

No maximum residue limit or acceptable daily intake values have been allocated to toxaphene by the FAO/WHO Joint Meeting on Pesticide Residues (FAO/UNEP, 1999).

The Environmental Protection Agency (2000) set a maximum contaminant level for toxaphene in drinking-water of 0.003 mg/L and a 'maximum contaminant level goal' of zero.

Table 2. Occupational exposure limits and guidelines for toxaphene

Country	Year	Concentration (mg/m^3)	Interpretation
Australia	1993	0.5 (sk)	TWA
		1	STEL
Austria	1993	0.5 (sk)	TWA
Belgium	1993	0.5 (sk)	TWA
		1	STEL
Denmark	1993	0.5 (sk)	TWA
Egypt	1993	0.5 (sk)	TWA
Finland	1998	0.5 (sk)	TWA
		1.5	STEL
France	1993	0.5 (sk)	TWA
Germany	2000	carcinogen-2	
Netherlands	1999	0.5 (sk)	TWA
Philippines	1993	0.5 (sk)	TWA
Switzerland	1993	0.5 (sk)	TWA
Thailand	1993	0.5	TWA
Turkey	1993	0.5 (sk)	TWA
USA			
ACGIH (TLV)	2000	0.05 (A3, sk)	TWA
		1	STEL
NIOSH (REL)	1997	(Ca, lfc, sk)	
OSHA (PEL)	1999	0.5 (sk)	TWA

From Ministry of Social Affairs and Health (1998); American Conference of Governmental Industrial Hygienists (ACGIH) (2000); Deutsche Forschungsgemeinschaft (2000)

A3, confirmed animal carcinogen with unknown relevance to humans; Ca, carcinogen; lfc, lowest feasible concentration; carcinogen-2, substances which are considered to be carcinogenic for man because sufficient data from long-term animal studies or limited evidence from animal substantiated by evidence from epidemiological studies indicate that they can make a significant contribution to cancer risk; sk, danger of cutaneous absorption; TWA, time-weighted average; STEL, short-term exposure limit; REL, recommended exposure limit; PEL, permissible exposure limit; NIOSH, National Institute for Occupational Safety and Health; OSHA, Occupational Safety and Health Administration

2.   Studies of Cancer in Humans

2.1   Case–control studies

In a case–control study on non-Hodgkin lymphoma in the USA, cases were identified through the Iowa State Health Registry and surveillance of Minnesota hospital and pathology laboratory records (Cantor *et al.*, 1992). Men were eligible as cases if they had been aged 30 years or more at the time of diagnosis, their lymphoma had been diagnosed between March 1981 and October 1983 in Iowa and between October 1980 and September 1982 in Minnesota and they were resident in the state, excluding, for Minnesota, the cities of Minneapolis, St Paul, Duluth and Rochester. The diagnoses were reviewed by a panel of four experienced regional pathologists. Of the 780 identified patients, 694 (89%) were interviewed, and 622 of the cases were confirmed to be non-Hodgkin lymphoma after the review. The 1245 controls were frequency matched to cases by age, residence and vital status. Living subjects were selected by random-digit dialling (age < 65 years) and from Medicare rosters (age ≥ 65); death certificate files were used to select deceased controls. The response rates for the various groups of controls were 77–79%. Proxy interviews were conducted for deceased or incompetent men (184 cases and 425 controls). A detailed history of farming and pesticide use was obtained by an interviewer from all subjects who had worked on a farm for at least 6 months since the age of 18 by means of a questionnaire to the participating subjects or proxy responders. Odds ratios were estimated by unconditional multiple logistic regression, allowing for the matching variables plus other potential risk factors. The reference category was men who had never worked or lived on a farm as adults (266 cases and 547 controls). Eight patients and 19 controls had ever handled toxaphene as an animal insecticide (odds ratio, 0.8; 95% confidence interval [CI], 0.3–2.0), and 10 patients and 13 controls had used it as crop insecticide (odds ratio, 1.5; 0.6–3.5). When the analysis was limited to those who had handled it prior before 1965, the odds ratio for use on crops was 2.4 (0.7–8.2).

In a study of leukaemia parallel to that of non-Hodgkin lymphoma conducted in Iowa and Minnesota (Cantor *et al.*, 1992) described above, 578 men with leukaemia (340 living and 238 deceased) and 1245 controls (820 living and 425 deceased) were included (Brown *et al.*, 1990). Farmers who reported use of toxaphene on animals had an odds ratio of 1.4 (95% CI, 0.6–3.1), which was higher for those who had handled it at least 20 years before interview (or at least 16 years before diagnosis) (2.6; 0.8–8.8).

3.   Studies of Cancer in Experimental Animals

3.1   Oral administration

Mouse: Groups of 50 male and 50 female B6C3F$_1$ mice, 5 weeks of age, were fed a diet containing 160 or 320 mg/kg toxaphene for 19 weeks and 80 or 160 mg/kg of diet for a further 61 weeks, followed by a toxaphene-free diet for 10–11 weeks. A group of 10 mice of each sex served as matched controls and received normal diet for 90–91 weeks; 50 male and 50 female pooled controls from other experiments were used to provide further control data. Survival was not significantly affected by toxaphene: by 52 weeks, 49/50 males at the low dose and 46/50 at the high dose and 46/50 females at both doses were still alive. The incidences of hepatocellular carcinoma in males were 0/10 matched controls, 4/48 (8%) pooled controls, 34/49 (69%) at the low dose and 45/46 (98%) at the high dose ($p < 0.001$, dose-related response). In females, the incidences were 0/9 matched controls, 0/48 pooled controls, 5/49 (10%) at the low dose and 34/49 (69%) at the high dose ($p < 0.001$, dose-related response). 'Neoplastic nodules' (authors' terminology) of the liver were found in 2/10 (20%) matched control males, 6/49 (12%) males at the low dose, 0/46 males at the high dose, 0/9 matched control females, 13/49 (26%) females at the low dose and 6/49 (12%) females at the high dose (National Cancer Institute, 1979). The liver tumours in this study were re-evaluated by a pathology working group, which reclassified most of the hepatocellular carcinomas as adenomas and the adenomas as hepatocellular foci. This analysis indicated no statistically significant increase in the incidence of carcinomas at any dose, but the incidences of adenomas and total tumours remained statistically significantly increased in both male and female mice at the high dose. The revised incidences of carcinomas in males were 3/48 pooled controls, 8/50 at the low dose and 5/47 at the high dose, and those in females were 0/50 pooled controls, 0/49 at the low dose and 3/47 at the high dose. The revised incidences of adenomas in males were 5/48 pooled controls, 30/50 at the low dose and 42/47 at the high dose, and those in females were 1/50 pooled controls, 11/49 at the low dose and 37/47 at the high dose (Goodman *et al.*, 2000).

A study conducted by Litton Bionetics in 1978, but not published by that organization, was later reviewed by Goodman *et al.* (2000). Groups of 55 male and 55 female B6C3F$_1$ mice [age unspecified] were fed a diet containing 0, 7, 20 or 50 mg/kg toxaphene [purity unspecified] for 18 months, followed by untreated diet for a further 6 months. Survival was not affected by treatment, and no clinical signs were observed. No significant difference in the incidence of liver adenomas or carcinomas was observed between the treated and untreated groups when evaluated separately, although a significant difference was observed in the total number of liver tumours in males at the high dose and controls (18/51 versus 10/53; $p < 0.05$). No such difference was observed in females. [The Working Group noted that the original report was not available and that the slides of liver lesions were not available for reclassification by modern histological criteria].

Rat: Groups of 50 male and 50 female Osborne-Mendel rats, 5 weeks of age, were fed a diet containing toxaphene for 80 weeks and were then observed for 28 (males) or 30 (females) weeks. The dose regimen for high-dose males was 2560 mg/kg of diet for 2 weeks, 1280 mg/kg of diet for 53 weeks and 640 mg/kg of diet for a further 25 weeks; that for high-dose females was 1280 mg/kg of diet for 55 weeks followed by 640 mg/kg of diet for 25 weeks; that for low-dose males was 1280 mg/kg of diet for 2 weeks, 640 mg/kg of diet for 53 weeks and 320 mg/kg of diet for 25 weeks; and that for low-dose females was 640 mg/kg of diet for 55 weeks, followed by 320 mg/kg diet for 25 weeks. Matched control groups of 10 untreated rats of each sex were given toxaphene-free diet for 108–109 weeks; 55 untreated males and 55 untreated females from other bioassays served as pooled controls. Survival was not significantly affected, as 90–92% of rats were alive at week 52 of the study, even at the high dose. The incidences of thyroid follicular-cell tumours (adenomas and carcinomas) were 7/41 (17%) and 9/35 (26%) in male rats at the low and high doses, respectively, in comparison with 1/7 (14%) matched controls and 2/44 (5%) pooled controls. In females, the incidences were 1/43 (2%) at the low dose and 7/42 (17%) at the high dose in comparison with 0/6 (0%) matched controls and 1/46 (2%) pooled controls. In male rats, the incidence of thyroid tumours (adenomas and carcinomas) was dose-related ($p = 0.007$) in comparison with pooled controls. In female rats, the incidence of thyroid follicular-cell adenomas was dose-related in comparison with either matched ($p = 0.022$) or pooled ($p = 0.008$) controls. Follicular-cell carcinomas were found in two males at the high dose, while all the remaining thyroid tumours were follicular-cell adenomas. Hyperplasia of thyroid follicular cells was observed only in treated males (low-dose, 3/41; high-dose, 3/35) and females (low-dose, 5/43; high-dose, 3/42). In female rats, pituitary tumours (mainly chromophobe adenomas) occurred in 15/41 at the low dose and 23/39 at the high dose, the incidence being statistically significantly increased in comparison with either the matched (3/8; $p = 0.046$) or pooled (17/51; $p = 0.012$) controls. In male rats, the incidence of hepatocellular adenomas at the low dose (6/44) was higher than that in pooled controls (1/52; $p = 0.034$), but animals at the high dose did not show a significantly higher incidence (4/45) than that in either control group (National Cancer Institute, 1979).

Hamster: A study conducted by Litton Bionetics in 1978, but not published by that organization, was later reviewed by Goodman *et al.* (2000). Groups of 51 male and 51 female ARS golden Syrian hamsters [age unspecified] were fed diets containing 0, 100, 300 or 1000 mg/kg toxaphene for 21.5 (males) or 18 (females) months. Treatment-related effects were observed only in males and included decreased body weight and the presence of megahepatocytes in the liver at the high dose. Treatment with toxaphene was not associated with tumours of any type. [The Working Group noted that the original report was not available and that the slides of liver lesions were not available for reclassification by modern histological criteria.]

3.2   Administration with known carcinogens

Mouse: To investigate the effects of toxaphene on benzo[*a*]pyrene-induced lung adenoma development, groups of female A/J mice, 9 weeks of age, were fed diets containing 0, 100 or 200 mg/kg toxaphene [purity not specified] in corn oil for 12 or 20 weeks, having been intubated with 0 or 3 mg of benzo[*a*]pyrene on day 7 and day 21 of the experiment. Toxaphene administered for 12 weeks had no effect on the induction of forestomach tumours by benzo[*a*]pyrene although at 200 mg/kg of diet there appeared to be a slight but significant decrease in the number of forestomach tumours per mouse (4.18 ± 0.34 (control group) versus 3.14 ± 0.34; $p < 0.05$) [no significant change in the incidence of tumours as stated by the authors; 100% in all groups]. Toxaphene fed at 100 mg/kg of diet for 12 weeks resulted in a small but significant reduction in the incidence (25% versus 8.1%; p value not given) and number of lung tumours per mouse induced by benzo[*a*]pyrene (1.17 ± 0.11 versus 1.00 ± 0.00; $p < 0.05$). At 200 mg/kg of diet for 20 weeks, toxaphene markedly decreased the incidence of lung tumours (100% versus 67%) and the mean number of lung tumours (7.2 ± 0.8 versus 1.6 ± 0.3; $p < 0.001$) per mouse. Groups fed toxaphene only did not develop lung tumours at either dose (Triolo *et al.*, 1982). [The Working Group noted that the incidences of forestomach tumours at 20 weeks were not reported.]

4.   Other Data Relevant to an Evaluation of Carcinogenicity and its Mechanisms

The chemistry, biochemistry, toxicity and environmental fate of toxaphene have been reviewed (Saleh, 1991).

4.1   Absorption, distribution, metabolism and excretion

4.1.1   *Humans*

Toxaphene has been found in human milk collected in Finland and Sweden (Mussalo-Rauhamaa *et al.*, 1988; Saleh, 1991; see also section 1.4.2). No other information was available to the Working Group on the absorption, distribution metabolism and excretion of toxaphene in humans.

4.1.2   *Experimental systems*

In mice and rats, toxaphene is absorbed through the skin and gastrointestinal tract, at a rate depending on the vehicle used for its administration. Of a single oral dose of 20 mg/kg bw technical-grade [^{36}Cl]toxaphene administered by gavage in 0.5 mL peanut oil/acacia gum to rats, about 52% was excreted within 9 days, with 15% in the urine, mainly as ^{36}Cl ion, and 37% in the faeces (Crowder & Dindal, 1974).

Approximately 3% of an oral dose of [^{14}C]toxaphene was excreted unchanged in the faeces of rats after 14 days. More than 5% of the administered dose was excreted in the urine and faeces as completely dechlorinated metabolites and 27% as partially dechlorinated metabolites; 1.2% of the label was found in expired air, probably as ^{14}CO$_2$. The concentrations of radiolabel associated with toxaphene or its metabolites 14 days after administration of 8.5 mg/kg bw [^{14}C]toxaphene were 0.52 mg/kg in fat, 0.17 mg/kg in kidney, 0.14 mg/L in blood, 0.12 mg/kg in liver and 0.02–0.09 mg/kg each in bone, brain, heart, lung, muscle, spleen and testis. After administration of [^{36}Cl]toxaphene, 50% of the activity was excreted as ^{36}Cl ion in the urine (Ohsawa et al., 1975).

Toxaphene was analysed in tissues 72 h after administration of about 13 mg/kg bw by gavage to female white Leghorn chickens, male rabbits, Swiss-Webster mice, Sprague-Dawley rats, Hartley guinea-pigs, hamsters and long-tailed monkeys (Macaca fascicularis). Analysis of acetone extracts of fat by capillary gas chromatography showed similar peaks in all species. In the faeces, the peaks were similar, except for that of the monkeys, which contained three metabolites of heptachlorobornane: two hexa-chlorobornane isomers and hexachlorobornene (Saleh et al., 1979).

Toxaphene is metabolized not only to reductive dechlorination and dehydro-chlorination products but also to polar hydroxyl and acidic compounds and water-soluble conjugates by the NADPH-dependent mixed-function oxidase system in rats. Thus, male Sprague-Dawley rats given radiolabelled toxaphene and rat liver micro-somal preparations in vitro treated with radiolabelled toxaphene showed the meta-bolites 2-endo,3,3,5,6-exo,8,9,10,10-nonachlorobornane and 2,2,5-endo,6-exo,8,9,10-heptachlorobornane (Chandurkar & Matsumura, 1979a,b).

When pregnant Sprague-Dawley rats were given [^{14}C]toxaphene orally, 28.3% of the activity was excreted in the faeces and 22.0% in the urine within 5 days. The fetuses contained the lowest concentration of radiolabel of all tissues tested at 5 days (28 μg/kg), and maternal fat contained the highest concentration (7476 mg/kg). A comparison of the activity in the fetuses with that in the dams' fat showed slight differences, indicating the presence of more polar compounds (perhaps metabolites) in the fetal tissue (Pollock & Hillstrand, 1982).

Autoradiographic studies in virgin and pregnant albino mice given [^{14}C]toxaphene at 16 mg/kg bw intravenously showed that, after initial accumulation in the liver, brown fat, lung, brain, kidney and corpora lutea, gradual redistribution to the white fat occurred within 4 h. The labelling then decreased rapidly and only very small amounts of radiolabel were present in adipose tissue after 32 days. In the fetus, only the liver and adrenals showed distinct labelling. Specific, persistent accumulation of the label was detected in some zones of the adrenal cortex. In hypolipidaemic mice, less label accumulated initially in the liver and adrenals and more in the kidneys and heart, with much less subsequent distribution to the adipose tissue (Mohammed et al., 1983).

In cultured adrenocortical cells, toxaphene inhibited adrenocorticotrophic hormone-stimulated corticosterone synthesis at a median inhibitory concentration of about 12 μg/mL. When female rats [strain not specified] were given a diet containing 1.2 mg/kg toxaphene for 5 weeks, adrenocorticotrophic hormone-stimulated cortico-sterone synthesis was also found to be decreased in isolated adrenocortical cells (Mohammed *et al.*, 1983, 1985, 1990).

4.2   Toxic effects

4.2.1   *Humans*

The acute lethal dose of toxaphene for humans has been estimated to be 2–7 g/person (Conley, 1952).

A 9-month-old child poisoned with a 2:1 mixture of toxaphene:DDT died after convulsions and respiratory arrest. The ratio of toxaphene:DDT in the brain and liver was 10:1, and that in the kidneys was 3:1 (Haun & Cueto, 1967). Four other cases of acute poisoning in children, three of which were fatal, have been reported (McGee *et al.*, 1952).

4.2.2   *Experimental systems*

In Sherman rats, the oral LD_{50} of technical-grade toxaphene was 90 mg/kg bw for males and 80 mg/kg bw for females (Gaines, 1960). The oral LD_{50} of technical-grade toxaphene was 80 mg/kg bw in male albino Wistar rats fed a protein-deficient diet (3.5% casein), 293 mg/kg bw in those fed a 26% casein diet and 220 mg/kg bw in those fed standard laboratory diet. In rats that died after ingesting toxaphene, renal tubular damage and fatty degeneration of the liver with necrosis were observed (Boyd & Taylor, 1971).

In fasted dogs, the oral LD_{50} of toxaphene was reported to be approximately 25 mg/kg bw (Lackey, 1949). In male mice, the intraperitoneal LD_{50} of technical-grade toxaphene was 42 mg/kg bw. The intraperitoneal LD_{50} values of two toxic fractions were 3.1 and 6.6 mg/kg bw (Khalifa *et al.*, 1974); the first was identified by nuclear magnetic resonance spectroscopy as a mixture of 2,2,5-*endo*, 6-*exo*,8,8,9,10-octa-chlorobornane and 2,2,5-*endo*,6-*exo*, 8,9,9,10-octachlorobornane (Turner *et al.*, 1975) and the second as 2,2,5-*endo*,6-*exo*,8,9,10-heptachlorobornane (Casida *et al.*, 1974).

In Sherman rats fed diets containing 50 or 200 mg/kg toxaphene for 2–9 months, centrilobular hypertrophy of liver cells was observed in 3 of 11 and 6 of 12 animals, respectively (Ortega *et al.*, 1957); however, no effects on liver-cell histology were observed by Clapp *et al.* (1971) in rats fed a diet containing up to 189 mg/kg for 12 weeks.

Administration of a diet containing 5, 50 or 500 mg/kg toxaphene to quail for up to 4 months produced hypertrophy of the thyroid, with increased uptake of ^{131}I and adrenal hypertrophy (Hurst *et al.*, 1974).

Toxaphene fed to female weanling Swiss-Webster mice in the diet at a concentration of 10, 100 or 200 mg/kg for 8 weeks depressed immunoglobulin G antibody formation at the two higher doses, but cell-mediated immune responses were not affected. In another experiment, mature female mice fed diets containing the same amounts of toxaphene were mated 3 weeks after feeding began and were maintained on the diets until 3 weeks after parturition, at which time the pups were weaned onto the control diet. Assays performed on the offspring 8 weeks after birth revealed suppressed antibody formation in the offspring of dams given 100 mg/kg of diet toxaphene and enhanced antibody formation in those of dams given 200 mg/kg of diet. The cell-mediated immune response was suppressed only at the intermediate concentration. The phagocytic capacity of macrophages was significantly reduced in all treated groups, but to a greater extent in the offspring of the mice that consumed toxaphene at 100 mg/kg of diet (Allen *et al.*, 1983).

In estrogen-sensitive MCF7 human breast cancer cells, toxaphene increased cell proliferation only at a concentration of 10 μmol/L and not at lower concentrations. In comparison, estradiol caused proliferation at 10 pmol/L (Soto *et al.*, 1994).

In MCF-7 human breast cancer cells treated with 10 μmol/L toxaphene for 48 h, approximately 60% and 80% inhibition of constitutive and 17β-estradiol-induced estrogen receptor-dependent transactivation, respectively, were observed. The involvement of the estrogen receptor in the ability of toxaphene to block estrogen activity was verified by cotransfection studies with estrogen receptor-negative MDA-MB-231 cells. The interference of toxaphene with the estrogen receptor-mediated responses was confirmed by the observation of significant suppression of endogenously expressed pS2 RNA and decreased secretion of pS2 protein. These results indicate that toxaphene disturbed hormonal signals mediated by the estrogen receptor (Bonefeld Jørgensen *et al.*, 1997).

In transfection experiments, toxaphene antagonized estrogen-related receptor α-1 (ERRα-1) expression of the reporter chloramphenicol acetyltransferase activity in SK-BR-3 breast cancer cells. ERRα-1 is a member of the orphan nuclear receptor family, since its ligand has not been identified. Toxaphene was also found to suppress aromatase activity through an ERRα-1-mediated mechanism (Yang & Chen, 1999).

Toxaphene was active in a variety of in-vitro assay systems with the androgen receptor (Schrader & Cooke, 2000) and estrogen receptors (Yang & Chen, 1999). Toxaphene and two congeners prevalent in humans can stimulate proliferation of MCF7-E3 human breast cancer cells (Stelzer & Chan, 1999), but this result was not found consistently: Arcaro *et al.* (2000) reported that toxaphene was weakly anti-estrogenic in the MCF7 focus assay and that it did not stimulate cell proliferation.

Groups of 10 male and 10 female Sprague-Dawley rats were fed a diet containing 0, 4, 20, 100 or 500 mg/kg toxaphene for 13 weeks, corresponding to intakes of 0.35–45.9 mg/kg bw per day for males and 0.50–63 mg/kg bw per day for females. No clinical signs of toxicity, such as effects on weight gain or food consumption, or deaths were observed, but effects on the liver (see section 4.4.2) were seen in males and females at the highest dietary concentration, at which toxaphene also caused kidney enlargement in male but not female rats and dose-dependent histological changes in the kidney, thyroid and liver. The changes in the liver and thyroid were considered to be adaptative, but the injury in the proximal tubules of the kidney was focally severe. The changes in the thyroid included increased epithelial height with multifocal papillary proliferation and reduced colloid density. These treatment-related changes were observed at concentrations $\geq$ 20 mg/kg of diet in males but only at 500 mg/kg of diet in females, and were considered to be more severe in the males. The kidneys of males at 20 mg/kg of diet had large eosinophilic inclusions in the proximal tubules. In the kidneys of rats at 100 or 500 mg/kg of diet, these inclusions were smaller, more refractive in appearance and more prevalent, occupying 50% of the tubular area. The changes were accompanied by anisokaryosis and focal tubular necrosis. In the females, only mild changes were found (Chu et al., 1986).

Groups of six male and six female beagle dogs were given toxaphene in gelatin capsules at 0, 0.2, 2 or 5 mg/kg bw per day for 13 weeks. Food consumption and growth rate were not affected, and all animals survived the treatment period. No clinical signs of toxicity were observed. The liver:body weight ratio and serum alkaline phosphatase activity were increased in both males and females at the highest dose. Mild-to-moderate, dose-dependent histological changes were observed in the liver and thyroid. The effects in the thyroid were similar to those seen in rats. Toxaphene accumulated in a dose-dependent manner in the fat and liver of both dogs and rats. On the basis of these findings, the no-observed-adverse-effect levels of the pesticide were considered to be 0.35 mg/kg bw per day for rats and 0.2 mg/kg bw per day for dogs (Chu et al., 1986).

Forty male Sprague-Dawley Crl:Cd BR rats were given 100 mg/kg bw per day technical-grade toxaphene in corn oil by gavage for 3 days, at which time the dose was reduced to 75 mg/kg bw per day because of toxicity. The lower dose was administered daily for 25 days. Another group of 40 male rats were given equivalent volumes of corn oil. A blood sample was obtained on days 0, 7, 14 and 28 from each of 10 treated and 10 vehicle-control animals to determine the serum concentrations of thyroid-stimulating hormone (TSH), thyroxine (T4), thriiodothyronine (T3) and reverse T3 (rT3) (see Figure 1 in General Remarks). Significant, time-related increases in serum TSH concentration were found on days 7, 14 and 28, and, at the last two times, the concentration was increased about two- and threefold. The serum concentrations of T3, T4 and rT3 and the thyroid gland weights and the thyroid:brain weight ratios in the treated group were not significantly different from those of controls at any time. The degree of thyroid follicular-cell hypertrophy and intrafollicular hyperplasia increased and the thyroid follicular-cell colloid stores decreased with duration of treatment with toxaphene (Waritz et al., 1996).

The effects of organochlorine pesticide exposure on the chemotactic functions of rhesus monkey (Macaca mulatta) neutrophils and monocytes were investigated with a 48-well chemotaxis chamber. The chemokines interleukin-8 and RANTES (the natural ligand for the CC chemokine receptor 5) were used as the chemoattractants to induce chemotaxis. When the neutrophils and monocytes were treated with hepta-chlor, chlordane or toxaphene for 1 h at 37 °C, inhibition of chemotaxis was seen in all samples at concentrations as low as 10^{-14} to 10^{-5} mol/L. Toxaphene was the least effective of the three compounds in preventing monocytes from migrating toward RANTES (Miyagi *et al.*, 1998).

4.3 Reproductive and developmental effects

4.3.1 *Humans*

No data were available to the Working Group.

4.3.2 *Experimental systems*

Administration of a diet containing 25 mg/kg toxaphene to mice through five generations caused no embryotoxic or teratogenic effects (Keplinger *et al.*, 1968). In a three-generation study of reproductive toxicity, Sprague-Dawley rats received a diet containing either 25 or 100 mg/kg toxaphene; no effects on litter size, pup survival, weanling body weights or reproductive capacity were observed (Kennedy *et al.*, 1973). In a standard, two-generation study of reproductive toxicity in Sprague-Dawley rats, administration of a diet containing toxaphene at a concentration of 0, 4, 20, 100 or 500 mg/kg [estimated intake, 0.29–49 mg/kg bw per day] did not affect litter size, pup weight or weight gain, fertility, gestation or neonatal survival. Toxic effects were seen in adult animals exposed for 2 weeks to the two highest concentrations, and the highest concentration also decreased weight gain, but did not affect food intake. The liver weights of F_0 and F_1 animals were increased. No effects were seen on the reproductive tissues of F_0 animals. Morphological changes were observed in the thyroid, liver and kidney, and groups at all concentrations had reduced follicle size and other histological changes; however, the authors noted the absence of a dose-dependent effect for many of these observations [the data were not adequate to evaluate this conclusion]. Follicular hyperplasia was described in one F_1 female and two F_1 male rats and an adenoma in one F_0 male at the highest concentration (Chu *et al.*, 1988).

Toxaphene was administered by oral intubation to CD-1 mice and CD rats during the period of embryonic organogenesis (days 7–16 of gestation) at a dose of 0, 15, 25 or 35 mg/kg bw per day. The highest dose produced caused maternal mortality in rats (31%) and mice (8%) and an increase in the incidence of encephaloceles among the offspring of the mice. The fetal mortality rate was slightly increased in mice at all three doses. Small decreases in fetal body weight and in the number of sternal and caudal ossification centres were seen in rats, mostly in the group receiving 25 mg/kg bw per day (Chernoff & Carver, 1976).

Sprague-Dawley rats ($n = 25$) were treated with 32 mg/kg bw per day toxaphene by gavage on days 6–15 of gestation. This high dose caused the deaths of 50% of the dams before parturition but was chosen deliberately to test the hypothesis that developmental toxicity would be observed with a compound known to be toxic to the dam. Treatment reduced the weight gain of dams during gestation, although they had gained weight similarly to controls by the time of parturition. Only six of the toxaphene-treated animals delivered litters, in which a significant increase in the incidence of supernumerary ribs were found as compared with controls (Chernoff *et al.*, 1990).

Injection of 1.5 mg/egg toxaphene had no effect on the hatchability rates of the eggs of chickens (Smith *et al.*, 1970). In a similar study, no embryotoxicity was observed in chicken embryos hatched from eggs previously injected with 400 or 500 mg/kg toxaphene in acetone; although when it was dissolved in corn oil embryotoxicity was seen at 300–400 mg/kg (Dunachie & Fletcher, 1969).

Toxaphene did not induce sex reversal in a temperature-dependent test in the slider turtle (*Trachemys scripta elegans*) (Willingham & Crews, 1999).

In a study of the behavioural effects of pre- and postnatal exposure to toxaphene, Holtzman rats were fed a diet providing a dose of 0.05 mg/kg bw per day. Retarded neurodevelopment on days 7–17 and impaired performance in learning and retaining in a symmetrical maze test were found (Olson *et al.*, 1980).

4.4   Effects on enzyme induction or inhibition and gene expression

4.4.1   *Humans*

No data were available to the Working Group.

4.4.2   *Experimental systems*

In early experiments, alterations in serum alkaline phosphatase and acid phosphatase activity, indicating liver damage, were observed in rats fed toxaphene (Grebenyuk, 1970; Gertig & Nowaczyk, 1975). Toxaphene induces various hepatic microsomal enzymes, such as *O*- and *N*-demethylases (Kinoshita *et al.*, 1966) and androgen hydroxylase (Peakall, 1976); it also stimulates estrone metabolism in rats (Welch *et al.*, 1971). Phenobarbital sleeping times were reduced in rats given toxaphene orally by gavage (Schwabe & Wendling, 1967).

Adult male Sprague-Dawley rats were fed diets containing 0, 50, 100, 150 or 200 mg/kg toxaphene for 14 days. There were no signs of toxicity, but the liver weight was significantly increased and the thymus weight was decreased in all treated groups (Trottman & Desaiah, 1980). A similar effect on relative liver weight was found in young (70 g) Sprague-Dawley rats given an intraperitoneal injection of toxaphene at a dose of 0, 5, 25 or 100 mg/kg bw per day for 5 days. All doses increased the liver:body weight ratios, cytochrome P450 (CYP) enzyme activity, aminopyrine demethylation and aldrin epoxidation. The latter activity was increased nearly sevenfold at the highest dose (Pollock *et al.*, 1983).

Groups of 10 male and 10 female Sprague-Dawley rats were fed a diet containing 0, 4, 20, 100 or 500 mg/kg toxaphene for 13 weeks, corresponding to intakes of 0.35–45.9 mg/kg bw per day for males and 0.50–63 mg/kg bw per day for females. The liver:body weight ratio and the activities of hepatic microsomal enzymes (phenobarbital type) were increased in both males and females at the highest dietary concentration (Chu et al., 1986).

The activities of pentobarbital hydroxylase and aniline hydroxylase were significantly enhanced in rats exposed to toxaphene, and that of ethylmorphine-N-demethylase was elevated. Enhanced hydroxylation of pentobarbital was evident from the decreased sleeping time seen after administration of the two compounds. Exposure to toxaphene increased the activities of CYP isozymes, NADPH-cytochrome c-reductase and dehydrogenase in hepatic microsomal fractions (Trottman & Desaiah, 1980). Toxaphene also induced UDP glucuronosyl transferase and aryl hydrocarbon hydroxylase activity in Sprague-Dawley rats given 20 mg/kg bw orally twice a week for 2 weeks (Thunberg et al., 1984).

Male CD-1 mice given 10, 25, 50 or 100 mg/kg bw per day toxaphene by gavage for 7 days also showed increased liver weight, liver:body weight ratio, total hepatic CYP content and cytochrome b_5. No increase in the activity of immunodetectable CYP4A1 was found, in contrast to the high levels of this enzyme found in clofibrate-exposed mice. However, increases in CYP2B activity were found, indicating induction by toxaphene of phenobarbital-inducible CYP enzymes. No DNA adducts were found by ^{32}P-postlabelling methods in this study (Hedli et al., 1998).

Toxaphene at 200 μmol/L stimulated mouse brain protein kinase C activity in the $10^5 \times g$ supernatant of brain tissue to a maximum velocity almost equal to that obtained when the enzyme was maximally stimulated with the skin tumour-promoting phorbol ester, 12-O-tetradecanoylphorbol-13-acetate (Moser & Smart, 1989).

Experiments with CEM×174 cells, a hybrid of human T and B cells, were performed to investigate the effects of the tumour promoter heptachlor and its congeners chlordane and toxaphene (concentration, 10–50 μmol/L) on retinoblastoma (Rb) gene expression. The lowest concentration of toxaphene tested reduced Rb protein levels. Analysis of Rb mRNA revealed no detectable difference over the same concentration range, suggesting that Rb expression is down-regulated at the post-transcriptional level (Rought et al., 1999).

4.5   Genetic and related effects

The genetic toxicity of toxaphene has been reviewed (Saleh, 1991).

4.5.1   Humans

Cultured peripheral blood lymphocytes were examined from eight women working in an area that had been sprayed from aircraft with toxaphene at 2 kg/ha and an unspecified number of control individuals. The incidence of chromosomal aberrations (acentric fragments and chromosomal exchanges) was 13.1% in the exposed group and 1.6% in the controls (Samosh, 1974).

4.5.2 *Experimental systems* (see Table 3 for references)

Toxaphene was shown to induce gene mutations in several studies with *Salmonella typhimurium* strains with and without metabolic activation. It also induced prophage lambda, but not alkali-labile sites in an *Escherichia coli* plasmid assay. It induced reverse mutation in a photoluminescence assay. In cultured mammalian cells, it did not induce gene mutations at the *Hprt* locus or sister chromatid exchange in Chinese hamster lung V79 cells in single studies, whereas it did induce sister chromatid exchange in Chinese hamster lung Don cells and human lymphoid LAZ-007 cells and micronuclei in beluga whale skin fibroblasts. Toxaphene also inhibited gap-junctional intercellular communication in Chinese hamster lung V79 cells and human primary breast cancer cells.

Toxaphene administered to mice *in vivo* did not bind covalently to liver-cell DNA or induce dominant lethal mutation in males.

4.6 Mechanistic considerations

The results of some tests for genotoxicity with toxaphene were positive. Toxaphene is also a well-known inducer of hepatic microsomal enzymes in rodents, especially phenobarbital-type CYP2B and UDP-glucuronosyl transferase. Administration of toxaphene by gavage to male rats at a dose somewhat higher than the thyroid tumorigenic dose but for a shorter time resulted in increased concentrations of TSH and changes in the thyroid gland including hypertrophy, diffuse hyperplasia and decreased colloid. No effects on T4 or T3 were found in this study. These findings are consistent with the hypothesis that thyroid tumours are produced in rats secondary to increased turnover of thyroid hormones and increased trophic stimulation by TSH secondary to induction of UDP-glucuronosyl transferase, resulting in increasing hepatic disposition of thyroid hormone. No definitive conclusion could be reached about the mechanism of tumour production, in view of the results of the assays for genotoxicity.

Toxaphene has been shown to produce hypertrophy of liver cells without effects on their histological appearance, but the relationship of this finding to the production of liver tumours in mice has not been established.

The results of the tests for genetic toxicity conducted with toxaphene do not provide strong evidence that induction of genetic damage is important in its carcinogenicity, but the possibility cannot be excluded. An important gap in the database is the results of a test for chromosomal aberrations in rodent cells *in vitro* or *in vivo*. Deterioration in gap-junctional intercellular communication could play some role in the carcinogenic process.

Table 3. Genetic and related effects of toxaphene

Test system	Result[a] Without exogenous metabolic system	Result[a] With exogenous metabolic system	Dose[b] (LED/HID)	Reference
Escherichia coli WP-2, prophage ë induction	+	+	40[c]	Houk & DeMarini (1987)
Escherichia coli plasmid ColE1 DNA strand breaks or alkali-labile sites	–	NT	100	Griffin & Hill (1978)
Salmonella typhimurium TA100, TA98, reverse mutation	+	+	500 µg/plate	Hooper *et al.* (1979)
Salmonella typhimurium TA100, reverse mutation	+	+	100 µg/plate	Mortelmans *et al.* (1986)
Salmonella typhimurium TA98, reverse mutation	+	+	333 µg/plate	Mortelmans *et al.* (1986)
Salmonella typhimurium TA100, TA98, reverse mutation	+	+	500 µg/plate	Schrader *et al.* (1998)
Salmonella typhimurium TA104, TA97, reverse mutation	(+)	(+)	1000 µg/plate	Schrader *et al.* (1998)
Salmonella typhimurium TA102, reverse mutation	(+)	(+)	10 000 µg/plate	Schrader *et al.* (1998)
Salmonella typhimurium TA1535, TA1537, reverse mutation	–	–	1000 µg/plate	Mortelmans *et al.* (1986)
Vibrio fisheri dim variant, reverse mutation	+	–[d]	3150	Boon *et al.* (1998)
Gene mutation, Chinese hamster lung V79 cells, *Hprt* locus *in vitro*	–	–[d]	10	Schrader *et al.* (1998)
Sister chromatid exchange, Chinese hamster lung V79 cells *in vitro*	–	?[e]	10	Schrader *et al.* (1998)
Sister chromatid exchange, Chinese hamster lung Don cells *in vitro*	+	NT	5	Steinel *et al.* (1990)
Micronucleus formation, beluga whale skin fibroblasts *in vitro*	+	+	0.05	Gauthier *et al.* (1999)
Sister chromatid exchange, human lymphoid LAZ-007 cells	+	+	4	Sobti *et al.* (1983)
Inhibition of intercellular communication, Chinese hamster lung V79 cells *in vitro*	+	NT	3	Trosko *et al.* (1987)
Inhibition of intercellular communication (dye transfer), human primary breast epithelial cells *in vitro*	+	NT	5	Kang *et al.* (1996)

Table 3 (contd)

Test system	Result[a]		Dose[b] (LED/HID)	Reference
	Without exogenous metabolic system	With exogenous metabolic system		
Dominant lethal mutation, ICR/Ha mice *in vivo*	–		180 ip × 1 or 80 po × 5	Epstein *et al.* (1972)
Covalent binding to DNA (^{32}P-postlabelling) male CD-1 (Swiss) mouse liver *in vivo*	–		100 po × 7	Hedli *et al.* (1998)

[a] +, positive; (+), weak positive; –, negative; NT, not tested ; ?, inconclusive

[b] LED, lowest effective dose; HID, highest ineffective dose; in-vitro tests, µg/mL; in-vivo tests, mg/kg bw per day; ip, intraperitoneal; po, orally

[c] With an exogenous metabolic activation system from 9000 × *g* supernatant of rodent liver (S9), active only at ≥ 4-fold higher dose

[d] Metabolic activation provided by co-cultured HepG2 human hepatoma cells

5.   Summary of Data Reported and Evaluation

5.1   Exposure data

Toxaphene is a complex mixture of chlorinated hydrocarbons produced by the chlorination of camphene. Toxaphene was widely used from the late 1940s as an insecticide on crops and to control parasites on livestock. The use of toxaphene is presently banned or restricted in many countries. Occupational exposure to toxaphene has occurred during its production and application. Human exposure to toxaphene is still possible owing to its persistence in the environment and its consequent continuing occurrence in fish, milk and other foodstuffs. In those countries in which its use has been banned, dietary intake has probably decreased in recent years.

5.2   Human carcinogenicity data

One case–control study of non-Hodgkin lymphoma and one of leukaemia not otherwise specified in the same populations showed no significant increase in risk associated with exposure to toxaphene.

5.3   Animal carcinogenicity data

Toxaphene has been tested for carcinogenicity by oral administration in one study in mice and one study in rats. It increased the incidence of hepatocellular adenomas and carcinomas combined in male and female mice. In rats, it produced thyroid follicular-cell adenomas and carcinomas in both males and females and pituitary adenomas in females.

5.4   Other relevant data

Toxaphene is lipid-soluble and accumulates in animals. It is metabolized by dechlorination and excreted into the bile. Toxaphene is a well-known microsomal enzyme inducer that increases phase I and II drug-metabolizing enzymes, consistent with a phenobarbital-like effect. It also increases the size of the thyroid gland and thyroid-stimulating hormone concentrations.

Toxaphene produced hepatotoxicity and immunotoxicity in experimental animals.

No reproductive or developmental effects were seen in three multigeneration studies in rats.

An increased frequency of chromosomal aberrations was observed in the lymphocytes of workers exposed to toxaphene in one study. In mammalian cells *in vivo*, toxaphene did not bind to DNA or produce dominant lethal mutations. *In vitro*, toxaphene was mutagenic to bacteria but did not induce mutations in mammalian cells. It induced micronuclei in the only assay for this end-point performed in mammalian cells.

It also induced sister chromatid exchange and inhibited gap-junctional intercellular communication in cultured mammalian cells.

5.5   Evaluation

There is *inadequate evidence* in humans for the carcinogenicity of toxaphene.

There is *sufficient evidence* in experimental animals for the carcinogenicity of toxaphene.

Overall evaluation

Toxaphene is *possibly carcinogenic to humans (Group 2B).*

6.   References

Agency for Toxic Substances and Disease Registry (1998) *Toxicological Profile for Toxaphene* (Report 95/10; US NTIS PB97-121057), Atlanta GA, Department of Health and Human Services

Allen, A.L., Koller, L.D. & Pollock, G.A. (1983) Effect of toxaphene exposure on immune responses in mice. *J. Toxicol. environ. Health*, **11**, 61–69

American Conference of Governmental Industrial Hygienists (2000) *TLVs and Other Occupational Exposure Values — 2000 CD-ROM*, Cincinnati, OH

American Public Health Association/American Water Works Association/Water Environment Federation (1999a) Method 6410B. Liquid-liquid extraction gas chromatographic/mass spectrometric method. In: *Standard Methods for the Examination of Water and Wastewater*, 20th Ed., Washington DC

American Public Health Association/American Water Works Association/Water Environment Federation (1999b) Method 6630B. Liquid-liquid extraction gas chromatographic method I. In: *Standard Methods for the Examination of Water and Wastewater*, 20th Ed., Washington DC

American Public Health Association/American Water Works Association/Water Environment Federation (1999c) Method 6630C. Liquid-liquid extraction gas chromatographic method II. In: *Standard Methods for the Examination of Water and Wastewater*, 20th Ed., Washington DC

Andrews, P., Newsome, W.H., Boyle, M. & Collins, P. (1993) High resolution selective ion monitoring GC–MS determination of toxaphene in Great Lakes fish. *Chemosphere*, **27**, 1865–1872

AOAC International (2000) *Official Methods of Analysis of AOAC International*, 17th Ed., Gaithersburg, MD [CD-ROM] [Methods 962.05, 962.07, 965.14, 968.04, 970.52, 972.05, 973.15, 973.16, 973.17, 983.21, 990.06]

Arcaro, K.F., Yang, Y., Vakharia, D.D. & Gierthy, J.F. (2000) Toxaphene is antiestrogenic in a human breast-cancer cell assay. *J. Toxicol. environ. Health*, **59**, 197–210

Ashirova, S.A. (1971) [Work hygiene and effectiveness of health measures in the manufacture of chlorinated terpenes.] *Nauch. Tr. Leningrad Gos. Inst. Usoversh. Vrach.*, **98**, 26–30 (in Russian)

Ault, J.A. & Spurgeon, T.E. (1984) Multiresidue gas chromatographic method for determining organochlorine pesticides in poultry fat: Collaborative study. *J. Assoc. off. anal. Chem.*, **67**, 284–289

Barrie, L., Bidleman, T., Dougherty, D., Fellin, P., Grift, N., Muir, D., Rosenberg, B., Stern, G. & Toom, D. (1993) Atmospheric toxaphene in the high Arctic. *Chemosphere*, **27**, 2037–2046

Bateman, G.Q., Biddulph, C., Harris, J.R., Greenwood, D.A. & Harris, L.E. (1953) Transmission studies of milk of dairy cows fed toxaphene-treated hay. *J. agric. Food Chem.*, **1**, 322–324

Blair, A. & Hoar Zahm, S. (1993) Patterns of pesticide use among farmers: Implications for epidemiologic Research. *Epidemiology*, **4**, 55–62

Blus, L.J., Joanen, T., Belisle, A.A. & Prouty, R.M. (1975) The brown pelican and certain environmental pollutants in Louisiana. *Bull. environ. Contam. Toxicol.*, **13**, 646–655

Bonefeld Jørgensen, E.C., Autrup, H. & Hansen, J.C. (1997) Effect of toxaphene on estrogen receptor functions in human breast cancer cells. *Carcinogenesis*, **18**, 1651–1654

Boon, J.P., Sleiderink, H.M., Helle, M.S., Dekker, M., van Schanke, A., Roex, E., Hillebrand, M.T.J., Klamer, H.J.C., Govers, B., Pastor, D., Morse, D., Wester, P.G. & de Boer, J. (1998) The use of a microsomal in vitro assay to study phase I biotransformation of chloro-bornanes (toxaphene®) in marine mammals and birds. *Comp. Biochem. Physiol. Part C*, **121**, 385–403

Boshoff, P.R. & Pretorius, V. (1979) Determination of toxaphene in milk, butter and meat. *Bull. environ. Contam. Toxicol.*, **22**, 405–412

Boyd, E.M. & Taylor, F.I. (1971) Toxaphene toxicity in protein-deficient rats. *Toxicol. appl. Pharmacol.*, **18**, 158–167

Brown, L.M., Blair, A., Gibson, R., Everett, G.D., Cantor, K.P., Schuman, L.M., Burmeister, L.F., Van-Lier, S.F. & Dick, F. (1990) Pesticide exposures and other agricultural risk factors for leukemia among men in Iowa and Minnesota. *Cancer Res.*, **50**, 6585–6591

Brumley, W.C., Brownrigg, C.M. & Grange, A.H. (1993) Determination of toxaphene in soil by electron-capture negative-ion mass-spectrometry after fractionation by high-performance gel-permeation chromatography. *J. Chromatogr.*, **633**, 177–183

Budavari, S., ed. (2000) *The Merck Index*, 12th Ed., Version 12:3, Whitehouse Station, NJ, Merck & Co. & Boca Raton, FL, Chapman & Hall/CRC [CD-ROM]

Cairns, T., Siegmund, E.G. & Froberg, J.E. (1981) Chemical ionization mass spectrometric examination of metabolized toxaphene from milk fat. *Biomed. Mass Spectrom.*, **8**, 569–574

Cantor, K.P., Blair, A., Everett, G., Gibson, R., Burmeister, L.F., Brown, L.M., Schuman, L. & Dick, F.R. (1992) Pesticides and other agricultural risk factors for non-Hodgkin's lymphoma among men in Iowa and Minnesota. *Cancer Res.*, **52**, 2447–2455

Carey, A.E., Wiersma, G.B. & Tai, H. (1976) Pesticide residues in urban soils from 14 United States cities, 1970. *Pestic. Monit. J.*, **10**, 54–60

Casida, J.E., Holmstead, R.L., Khalifa, S., Knox, J.R., Ohsawa, T., Palmer, K.J. & Wong, R.Y. (1974) Toxaphene insecticide: A complex biodegradable mixture. *Science*, **183**, 520–521

Causey, K., McIntyre, S.C., Jr & Richburg, R.W. (1972) Organochlorine insecticide residues in quail, rabbits, and deer from selected Alabama soybean fields. *J. agric. Food Chem.*, **20**, 1205–1209

Chan, H.M. (1998) A database for environmental contaminants in traditional foods in northern and Arctic Canada: Development and applications. *Food. Addit. Contam.*, **15**, 127–134

Chandurkar, P.S. & Matsumura, F. (1979a) Metabolism of toxaphene components in rats. *Arch. environ. Contam. Toxicol.*, **8**, 1–24

Chandurkar, P.S. & Matsumura, F. (1979b) Metabolism of toxicant B and toxicant C of toxaphene in rats. *Bull. environ. Contam. Toxicol.*, **21**, 539–547

Chernoff, N. & Carver, B.D. (1976) Fetal toxicity of toxaphene in rats and mice. *Bull. environ. Contam. Toxicol.*, **15**, 660–664

Chernoff, N., Setzer, R.W., Miller, D.B., Rosen, M.B. & Rogers, J.M. (1990) Effects of chemically induced maternal toxicity on prenatal development in the rat. *Teratology*, **42**, 651–658

Chu, I., Villeneuve, D.C., Sun, C.-W., Secours, V., Procter, B., Arnold, E., Clegg, D., Reynolds, L. & Valli, V.E. (1986) Toxicity of toxaphene in the rat and beagle dog. *Fundam. appl. Toxicol.*, **7**, 406–418

Chu, I., Secours, V., Villeneuve, D.C., Valli, V.E., Nakamura, A., Colin, D., Clegg, D.J. & Arnold, E.P. (1988) Reproduction study of toxaphene in the rat. *J. environ. Sci. Health*, **B23**, 101–126

CIS Information Services (2000) *Directory of World Chemical Producers (Version 2000.1)*, Dallas, TX [CD-ROM]

Clapp, K.L., Nelson, D.M., Bell, J.T. & Rousek, E.J. (1971) Effect of toxaphene on the hepatic cells of rats. In: *Proceedings of Annual Meeting, Western Section, American Society of Animal Science*, Vol. 22, Fresno, CA, Fresno State College, pp. 313–323

Conley, B.E. (1952) Pharmacologic properties of toxaphene, a chlorinated hydrocarbon insecticide. *J. Am. med. Assoc.*, **149**, 1135–1137

Crist, H.L., Harless, R.L., Moseman, R.F. & Callis, M.H. (1980) Application of dehydrochlorination to the determination of toxaphene in soil and identification of the major gas chromatographic peak. *Bull. environ. Contam. Toxicol.*, **24**, 231–237

Crowder, L.A. & Dindal, E.F. (1974) Fate of ^{36}Cl-toxaphene in rats. *Bull. environ. Contam. Toxicol.*, **12**, 320–327

Datta, S., Ohyama, K., Dunlap, D.Y. & Matsumura, F. (1999) Evidence of organochlorine contamination in tissues of salmonids in Lake Tahoe. *Ecotoxicol. environ. Saf.*, **42**, 94–101

Deutsche Forschungsgemeinschaft (2000) *List of MAK and BAT Values 1999* (Report No. 36), Weinheim, Wiley-VCH Verlag GmbH, p. 37

Dunachie, J.F. & Fletcher, W.W. (1969) An investigation of the toxicity of insecticides to birds' eggs using the egg-injection technique. *Ann. appl. Biol.*, **64**, 409–423

Eller, P.M., ed. (1994) Method 5039. In: *NIOSH Manual of Analytical Methods* (DHHS (NIOSH) Publ. No. 94-113), 4th Ed., Cincinnati, OH, National Institute for Occupational Safety and health

Environmental Protection Agency (1993a) Method 617. The determination of organohalide pesticides and PCBs in municipal and industrial wastewater. In: *Methods for the Determination of Nonconventional Pesticides in Municipal and Industrial Wastewater* (EPA Report No. EPA-821/R-93-010-A), Washington DC

Environmental Protection Agency (1993b) Method 1656. The determination of organohalide pesticides in municipal and industrial wastewater. In: *Methods for the Determination of Nonconventional Pesticides in Municipal and Industrial Wastewater* (EPA Report No. EPA-821/R-93-010-A), Washington DC

Environmental Protection Agency (1995a) Method 505. Analysis of organohalide pesticides and commercial polychlorinated biphenyl (PCB) products in water by microextraction and gas chromatography [Rev. 2.1]. In: *Methods for the Determination of Organic Compounds in Drinking Water,* Supplement III (EPA Report No. EPA-600/R-95-131; US NTIS PB-216616), Cincinnati, OH, Environmental Monitoring Systems Laboratory

Environmental Protection Agency (1995b) Method 508.1. Determination of chlorinated pesticides, herbicides, and organohalides by liquid–solid extraction and electron capture gas chromatography [Rev. 2.0]. In: *Methods for the Determination of Organic Compounds in Drinking Water,* Supplement III (EPA Report No. EPA-600/R-95-131; US NTIS PB-216616), Cincinnati, OH, Environmental Monitoring Systems Laboratory

Environmental Protection Agency (1995c) Method 525.2. Determination of organic compounds in drinking water by liquid–solid extraction and capillary column gas chromatography/mass spectrometry [Rev. 2.0]. In: *Methods for the Determination of Organic Compounds in Drinking Water,* Supplement III (EPA Report No. EPA-600/R-95-131; US NTIS PB-216616), Cincinnati, OH, Environmental Monitoring Systems Laboratory

Environmental Protection Agency (1996a) Method 8081A. Organochlorine pesticides by gas chromatography [Rev. 1]. In: *Test Methods for Evaluating Solid Waste — Physical/Chemical Methods* (US EPA No. SW-846), Washington DC, Office of Solid Waste

Environmental Protection Agency (1996b) Method 8270C. Semivolatile organic compounds by gas chromatography/mass spectrometry (GC/MS) [Rev. 3]. In: *Test Methods for Evaluating Solid Waste — Physical/Chemical Methods* (US EPA No. SW-846), Washington DC, Office of Solid Waste

Environmental Protection Agency (1996c) Method 4041. Soil screening for chlordane by immunoassay [Rev. 0]. In: *Test Methods for Evaluating Solid Waste — Physical/Chemical Methods* (US EPA No. SW-846), Washington DC, Office of Solid Waste

Environmental Protection Agency (1999a) Method TO-04A. Determination of pesticides and polychlorinated biphenyls in ambient air using high volume polyurethane foam (PUF) sampling followed by gas chromatographic/multidetector detection (GC/MD). In: *Compendium of Methods for the Determination of Toxic Compounds in Ambient Air*, 2nd Ed. (EPA Report No. EPA-625/R-96-010b), Cincinnati, OH, Center for Environmental Research Information

Environmental Protection Agency (1999b) Methods for organic chemical analysis of municipal and industrial wastewater. Method 608 — Organochlorine pesticides and PCBs. *US Code Fed. Regul., Title 40*, Part 136, App. A, pp. 114–134

Environmental Protection Agency (1999c) Methods for organic chemical analysis of municipal and industrial wastewater. Method 625 — Base/neutrals and acids. *US Code Fed. Regul., Title 40*, Part 136, App. A, pp. 202–228

Environmental Protection Agency (2000) *Drinking Water Standards and Health Advisories* (EPA Report No. EPA-882/B-00-001), Washington DC, Office of Water

Epstein, S.S., Arnold, E., Andrea, J., Bass, W. & Bishop, Y. (1972) Detection of chemical mutagens by the dominant lethal assay in the mouse. *Toxicol. appl. Pharmacol., 23*, 288–325

FAO/UNEP (1999) *Prior Informed Consent Decision Guidance Documents: Binapacryl and Toxaphene*, Rotterdam Convention on the Prior Informed Consent Procedure for Certain Hazardous Chemicals and Pesticides in International Trade, Geneva

Food and Drug Administration (1999) Methods 302, 303 and 304. In: Makovi, C.M. & McMahon, B.M., eds, *Pesticide Analytical Manual*, Vol. I, *Multiresidue Methods*, 3rd Rev. Ed., Management Methods Branch, Washington DC

Fowler, B., Hoover, D. & Hamilton, M.C. (1993) The quantification of toxaphene in environmental samples. *Chemosphere*, **27**, 1891–1905

Gaines, T.B. (1960) The acute toxicity of pesticides to rats. *Toxicol. appl. Pharmacol.*, **2**, 88–99

Gauthier, J.M., Dubeau, H. & Rassart, E. (1999) Induction of micronuclei *in vitro* by organochlorine compounds in beluga whale skin fibroblasts. *Mutat. Res.*, **439**, 87–95

Gertig, H. & Nowaczyk, W. (1975) The influence of carathane and toxaphene on the activity of some enzymes in rat's tissues in the studies *in vivo*. *Pol. J. Pharmacol. Pharm.*, **27**, 357–364

Gomes, E.D. (1977) Determination of toxaphene by basic alcoholic hydrolysis and Florisil separation. *Bull. environ. Contam. Toxicol.*, **17**, 456–462

Goodman, J.I., Brusick, D.J., Busey, W.M., Cohen, S.M., Lamb, J.C. & Starr, T.B. (2000) Reevaluation of the cancer potency factor of toxaphene: Recommendations from a peer review panel. *Toxicol. Sci.*, **55**, 3–16

Grebenyuk, S.S. (1970) [Effect of polychlorocamphene on liver functions.] *Gig. Primen. Toksikol. Pestits. Klin. Otravlenii*, **8**, 166–169 (in Russian)

Griffin, D.E., III & Hill, W.E. (1978) In vitro breakage of plasmid DNA by mutagens and pesticides. *Mutat. Res.*, **52**, 161–169

Griffith, F.D., Jr & Blanke, R.V. (1974) Microcoulometric determination of organochlorine pesticides in human blood. *J. Assoc. off. anal. Chem.*, **57**, 595–603

Haun, E.C. & Cueto, C., Jr (1967) Fatal toxaphene poisoning in a 9-month-old-infant. *Am. J. Dis. Child.*, **113**, 616–618

Head, S.L. & Burse, V.W. (1987) Organochlorine recovery from small adipose samples with the universal trace residue extractor (Unitrex). *Bull. environ. Contam. Toxicol.*, **39**, 848–856

Hedli, C.C., Snyder, R., Kinoshita, F.K. & Steinberg, M. (1998) Investigation of hepatic cytochrome P-450 enzyme induction and DNA adduct formation in male CD1 mice following oral administration of toxaphene. *J. appl. Toxicol.*, **18**, 173–178

Ho, J.S., Tang, P.H., Eichelberg, J.W. & Budde, W.L. (1995) Liquid–solid disk extraction followed by SFE and GC–ion-trap MS for the determination of trace organic pollutants in water. *J. chromatogr. Sci.*, **33**, 1–8

Hogue, C. (2000) Dioxins to be major issue at treaty negotiations. *Chem. Eng. News*, **20 March**, 35

Hooper, N.K., Ames, B.N., Saleh, M.A. & Casida, J.E. (1979) Toxaphene, a complex mixture of polychloroterpenes and a major insecticide, is mutagenic. *Science*, **205**, 591–593

Houk, V.S. & DeMarini, D.M. (1987) Induction of prophage lambda by chlorinated pesticides. *Mutat. Res.*, **182**, 193–201

Hsu, J.P., Schattenberg, H.J. & Garza, M.M. (1991) Fast turnaround multiresidue screen for pesticides in produce? *J. Assoc. off. anal. Chem.*, **74**, 886–892

Hunt, D.F., Shabanowitz, J., Harvey, T.M. & Coates, M. (1985) Scheme for the direct analysis of organics in the environment by tandem mass spectrometry. *Anal. Chem.*, **57**, 525–537

Hurst, J.G., Newcomer, W.S. & Morrison, J.A. (1974) Some effects of DDT, toxaphene and polychlorinated biphenyl on thyroid function in bobwhite quail. *Poultry Sci.*, **53**, 125–133

IARC (1979) *IARC Monographs on the Evaluation of the Carcinogenic Risk of Chemicals to Humans*, Vol. 20, *Some Halogenated Hydrocarbons*, IARC*Press*, Lyon, pp. 327–348

IARC (1987) *IARC Monographs on the Evaluation of Carcinogenic Risks to Humans*, Suppl. 7, *Overall Evaluations of Carcinogenicity: An Updating of IARC Monographs Volumes 1–42*, IARC*Press*, Lyon, p. 72

Ismail, R.J. & Bonner, F.L. (1974) New, improved thin layer chromatography for polychlorinated biphenyls, toxaphene, and chlordane components. *J. Assoc. off. anal. Chem*, **57**, 1026–1032.

Jansson, B., Andersson, R., Asplund, L., Bergman, A., Litzén, K., Nylund, K., Reutergårdh, L., Sellström, U., Uvemo, U.-B., Wahlberg, C. & Wideqvist, U. (1991) Multiresidue method for the gas-chromatographic analysis of some polychlorinated and polybrominated pollutants in biological samples. *Fresenius J. anal. Chem.*, **340**, 439–445

Jarnuzi, G. & Wakimoto, T. (1991) Determination of chlorinated pinene originated from pulp mill. *Analyt. Sci.*, **7** (Suppl.), 1177–1180

Kang, K.-S., Wilson, M.R., Hayashi, T., Chang, C.-C. & Trosko, J.E. (1996) Inhibition of gap junctional intercellular communication in normal human breast epithelial cells after treatment with pesticides, PCBs, and PBBs, alone or in mixtures. *Environ. Health Perspectives*, **104**, 192–200

Kennedy, G.L., Jr, Frawley, J.P. & Calandra, J.C. (1973) Multigeneration reproductive effects of three pesticides in rats. *Toxicol. appl. Pharmacol.*, **25**, 589–596

Keplinger, M.L., Deichmann, W.B. & Sala, F. (1968) Effects of combinations of pesticides on reproduction in mice. *Ind. Med. Surg.*, **37**, 525

Khalifa S., Mon, T.R., Engel, J.L. & Casida, J.E. (1974) Isolation of 2,2,5-*endo*,6-*exo*,8,9,10-heptachlorobornane and an octachloro toxicant from technical toxaphene. *J. agric. Food Chem.*, **22**, 653–657

Kinoshita, F.K., Frawley, J.P. & DuBois, K.P. (1966) Quantitative measurement of induction of hepatic microsomal enzymes by various dietary levels of DDT and toxaphene in rats. *Toxicol. appl. Pharmacol.*, **9**, 505–513

Kutz, F.W., Yobs, A.R. & Yang, H.S.C. (1976) National pesticide monitoring programs. In: Lee, R.I., ed., *Air Pollution from Pesticide and Agricultural Processes*, Cleveland, OH, CRC Press, pp. 95–137 [cited in Agency for Toxic Substances and Disease Registry (1998)]

Lackey, R.W. (1949) Observations on the acute and chronic toxicity of toxaphene in the dog. *J. ind. Hyg. Toxicol.* **31**, 117–120

Maiorino, R.M., Whiting, F.M., Brown, W.H., Reid, B.L. & Stull, J.W. (1980) Quantitative determination of toxaphene in blood by Florisil extraction and gas chromatography. *J. anal. Toxicol.*, **4**, 192–198

McGee, L.C., Reed, H.L. & Fleming, J.P. (1952) Accidental poisoning by toxaphene. Review of toxicology and case reports. *J. Am. med. Assoc.*, **149**, 1124–1126

Ministry of Social Affairs and Health (1998) *Finnish Occupational Exposure Limits 1998. Concentrations Known to be Harmful*, Helsinki

Miyagi, T., Lam, K.M., Chuang, L.F. & Chuang, R.Y. (1998) Suppression of chemokine-induced chemotaxis of monkey neutrophils and monocytes by chlorinated hydrocarbon insecticides. *In Vivo*, **12**, 441–446

Mohammed, A., Andersson, Ö., Biessmann, A. & Slanina, P. (1983) Fate and specific tissue retention of toxaphene in mice. *Arch. Toxicol.*, **54**, 311–321

Mohammed, A., Hallberg, E., Rydström, J. & Slanina, P. (1985) Toxaphene: Accumulation in the adrenal cortex and effect on ACTH-stimulated corticosteroid synthesis in the rat. *Toxicol. Lett.*, **24**, 137–143

Mohammed, A., Eklund, A., Östlund-Lindqvist, A.-M. & Slanina, P. (1990) Tissue accumulation of lipoprotein associated toxaphene in normo- and hypolipidemic mice. *Arch. Toxicol.*, **64**, 38–42

Mortelmans, K., Haworth, S., Lawlor, T., Speck, W., Tainer, B. & Zeiger, E. (1986) *Salmonella* mutagenicity tests: II. Results from the testing of 270 chemicals. *Environ. Mutag.*, **8** (Suppl. 7), 1–119

Moser, G.J. & Smart, R.C. (1989) Hepatic tumor-promoting chlorinated hydrocarbons stimulate protein kinase C activity. *Carcinogenesis*, **10**, 851–856

Munson, R.O. (1976) A note on toxaphene in environmental samples from the Chesapeake Bay region. *Bull. environ. Contam. Toxicol.*, **16**, 491–494

Musial, C.J. & Uthe, J.F. (1983) Widespread occurrence of the pesticide toxaphene in Canadian East Coast marine fish. *Int. J. environ. anal. Chem.*, **14**, 117–126

Mussalo-Rauhamaa, H., Pyysalo, H. & Antervo, K. (1988) Relation between the content of organochlorine compounds in Finnish human milk and characteristics of the mothers. *J. Toxicol. environ. Health*, **25**, 1–19

National Cancer Institute (1979) *Bioassay of Toxaphene for Possible Carcinogenicity* (Technical Report Series No. 37), Bethesda, MD, Department of Health, Education, and Welfare

Newsome, W.H. & Ryan, J.J. (1999) Toxaphene and other chlorinated compounds in human milk from northern and southern Canada: A comparison. *Chemosphere*, **39**, 519–526

Ohsawa, T., Knox, J.R., Khalifa, S. & Casida, J.E. (1975) Metabolic dechlorination of toxaphene in rats. *J. agric. Food Chem.*, **23**, 98–106

Olson, K.L., Matsumura, F. & Boush, G.M. (1980) Behavioral effects on juvenile rats from perinatal exposure to low levels of toxaphene, and its toxic components, toxicant A, and toxicant B. *Arch. environ. Contam. Toxicol.*, **9**, 247–257

Onuska, F.L., Terry, K.A., Seech, A. & Antonic, M. (1994) Determination of toxaphene in soil by electron-capture negative-ion mass spectrometry and capillary column gas chromatography. *J. Chromatogr.*, **A665**, 125–132

Ortega, O., Hayes, W.J., Jr & Durham, W.F. (1957) Pathologic changes in the liver of rats after feeding low levels of various insecticides. *Arch. Pathol.*, **64**, 614–622

Peakall, D.B. (1976) Effects of toxaphene on hepatic enzyme induction and circulating steroid levels in the rat. *Environ. Health Perspect.*, **13**, 117–120

Petrick, G., Schulz, D.E. & Duinker, J.C. (1988) Clean-up of environment samples by high-performance liquid chromatography for analysis of organochlorine compounds by gas chromatography with electron-capture detection. *J. Chromatogr.*, **435**, 241–248

Pollock, G.A. & Hillstrand, R. (1982) The elimination, distribution, and metabolism of ^{14}C-toxaphene in the pregnant rat. *J. environ. Sci. Health*, **B17**, 635–648

Pollock, G.A., Krasnec, J.P. & Niemann, B.R. (1983) Rat hepatic microsomal enzyme induction by pretreatment with toxaphene and toxaphene fractions. *J. Toxicol. environ. Health*, **11**, 355–363

Rought, S.E., Yau, P.M., Chuang, L.F., Doi, R.H. & Chuang, R.Y. (1999) Effect of the chlorinated hydrocarbons heptachlor, chlordane, and toxaphene on retinoblastoma tumor suppressor in human lymphocytes. *Toxicol. Lett.*, **104**, 127–135

Saleh, M.A. (1991) Toxaphene: Chemistry, biochemistry, toxicity and environmental fate. *Rev. environ. Contam. Toxicol.*, **118**, 1–85

Saleh, M.A. & Casida, J.E. (1977) Consistency of toxaphene composition analyzed by open tubular column gas–liquid chromatography. *J. agric. Food Chem.*, **25**, 63–68

Saleh, M.A., Skinner, R.F. & Casida, J.E. (1979) Comparative metabolism of 2,2,5-*endo*,6-*exo*,8,9,10-heptachlorobornane and toxaphene in six mammalian species and chickens. *J. agric. Food Chem.*, **27**, 731–737

Samosh, L.V. (1974) Chromosome aberrations and character of satellite associations after accidental exposure of the human body to polychlorocamphene. *Cytol. Genet.*, **8**, 23–27

Schmitt, C.J., Zajicek, J.L., May, T.W. & Cowman, D.F. (1999) Organochlorine residues and elemental contaminants in US freshwater fish, 1976–1986: National Contaminant Biomonitoring Program. *Rev. environ. Contam. Toxicol.*, **162**, 43–104

Schrader, T.J. & Cooke, G.M. (2000) Examination of selected food additives and organochlorine food contaminants for androgenic activity *in vitro*. *Toxicol. Sci.*, **53**, 278–288

Schrader, T.J., Boyes, B.G., Matula, T.I., Héroux-Metcalf, C., Langlois, I. & Downie, R.H. (1998) In vitro investigation of toxaphene genotoxicity in *S. typhimurium* and Chinese hamster V79 lung fibroblasts. *Mutat. Res.*, **413**, 159–168

Schwabe, U. & Wendling, I. (1967) [Stimulation of drug metabolism by low doses of DDT and other chlorinated hydrocarbon insecticides.] *Arzneimittel-Forsch.*, **17**, 614–618 (in German)

Seiber, J.N., Landrum, P.F., Madden, S.C., Nugent, K.D. & Winterlin, W.L. (1975) Isolation and gas chromatographic characterization of some toxaphene components. *J. Chromatogr.*, **114**, 361–368

Shoeib, M., Brice, K.A. & Hoff, R.M. (1999) Airborne concentrations of toxaphene congeners at Point Petre (Ontario) using gas-chromatography–electron capture negative ion mass spectrometry (GC–ECNIMS). *Chemosphere*, **39**, 849–871

Smith, S.I., Weber, C.W. & Reid, B.L. (1970) The effect of injection of chlorinated hydrocarbon pesticides on hatchability of eggs. *Toxicol. appl. Pharmacol.*, **16**, 179–185

Sobti, R.C., Krishan, A. & Davies, J. (1983) Cytokinetic and cytogenetic effect of agricultural chemicals on human lymphoid cells in vitro. II. Organochlorine pesticides. *Arch. Toxicol.*, **52**, 221–231

Soto, A.M., Chung, K.L. & Sonnenschein, C. (1994) The pesticides endosulfan, toxaphene, and dieldrin have estrogenic effects on human estrogen-sensitive cells. *Environ. Health Perspectives*, **102**, 380–383

Steinel, H.H., Arlauskas, A. & Baker, R.S.U. (1990) SCE induction and cell-cycle delay by toxaphene. *Mutat. Res.*, **230**, 29–33

Stelzer, A. & Chan, H.M. (1999) The relative estrogenic activity of technical toxaphene mixture and two individual congeners. *Toxicology*, **138**, 69–80

Swackhamer, D.L., Charles, M.J. & Hites, R.A. (1987) Quantitation of toxaphene in environmental samples using negative ion chemical ionization mass spectrometry. *Anal. Chem.*, **59**, 913–917

Swackhamer, D.L., Pearson, R.F. & Schlotter, S.P. (1998) Toxaphene in the Great Lakes. *Chemosphere*, **37**, 2545–2561

Tewari, S.N. & Sharma, J.C. (1977) Isolation and determination of chlorinated organic pesticides by thin-layer chromatography and the application to toxicological analysis. *J. Chromatogr.*, **131**, 275–284

Thunberg, T., Ahlborg, U.G. & Wahlstrom, B. (1984) Comparison between the effects of 2,3,7,8-tetrachlorodibenzo-*p*-dioxin and six other compounds on the vitamin A storage, the UDP-glucuronosyltransferase and the aryl hydrocarbon hydroxylase activity in the rat liver. *Arch. Toxicol.*, **55**, 16–19

Triolo, A.J., Lang, W.R., Coon, J.M., Lindstrom, D. & Herr, D.L. (1982) Effect of the insecticides toxaphene and carbaryl on induction of lung tumors by benzo[*a*]pyrene in the mouse. *J. Toxicol. environ. Health*, **9**, 637–649

Trosko, J.E., Jone, C. & Chang, C.C. (1987) Inhibition of gap junctional-mediated intercellular communication *in vitro* by aldrin, dieldrin, and toxaphene: A possible cellular mechanism for their tumor-promoting and neurotoxic effects. *Mol. Toxicol.*, **1**, 83–93

Trottman, C.H. & Desaiah, D. (1980) Induction of rat hepatic microsomal enzymes by toxaphene pretreatment. *J. environ. Sci. Health*, **B15**, 121–134

Turner, W.V., Khalifa, S. & Casida, J.E (1975) Toxaphene toxicant A. Mixture of 2,2,5-*endo*,6-*exo*,8,8,9,10-octachlorobornane and 2,2,5-*endo*,6-*exo*,8,9,9,10-octachlorobornane. *J. agric. Food Chem.*, **23**, 991–994

Vaz, R. & Blomkvist, G. (1985) Traces of toxaphene components in Swedish breast milk analyzed by capillary GC using ECD, electron impact and negative ion chemical ionization MS. *Chemosphere*, **14**, 223–231

Wade, T.L., Chambers, L., Gardinali, P.R., Sericano, J.L., Jackson, T.J., Tarpley, R.J. & Suydam, R. (1997) Toxaphene, PCB, DDT, and chlordane analyses of beluga whale blubber. *Chemosphere*, **34**, 1351–1357

Waritz, R.S., Steinberg, M., Kinoshita, F.K., Kelly, C.M. & Richter, W.R. (1996) Thyroid function and thyroid tumors in toxaphene-treated rats. *Regul. Toxicol. Pharmacol.*, **24**, 184–192

Welch, R.M., Levin, W., Kuntzman, R., Jacobson, M. & Conney, A.H. (1971) Effect of halogenated hydrocarbon insecticides on the metabolism and uterotropic action of estrogens in rats and mice. *Toxicol. appl. Pharmacol.*, **19**, 234–246

Wiersma, G.B., Tai, H. & Sand, P.F. (1972) Pesticide residues in soil from eight cities — 1969. *Pestic. Monit. J.*, **6**, 126–129

Willingham, E. & Crews, D. (1999) Sex reversal effects of environmentally relevant xenobiotic concentrations on the red-eared slider turtle, a species with temperature-dependent sex determination. *Gen. Comp. Endocrinol.*, **113**, 429–435

WHO (1984) *Camphechlor* (Environmental Health Criteria No. 45), Geneva

Yang, C. & Chen, S. (1999) Two organochlorine pesticides, toxaphene and chlordane, are antagonists for estrogen-related receptor α-1 orphan receptor. *Cancer Res.*, **59**, 4519–4524

FOOD AND COSMETICS AGENT

KOJIC ACID

1. Exposure Data

1.1 Chemical and physical data

1.1.1 *Nomenclature*

Chem. Abstr. Serv. Reg. No.: 501-30-4
Deleted CAS Reg. No.: 123712-78-7
Chem. Abstr. Name: 5-Hydroxy-2-(hydroxymethyl)-4H-pyran-4-one
IUPAC Systematic Name: Kojic acid
Synonym: 5-Hydroxy-2-(hydroxymethyl)-4-pyrone; 2-hydroxymethyl-5-hydroxy-γ-pyrone

1.1.2 *Structural and molecular formulae and relative molecular mass*

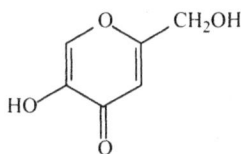

$C_6H_6O_4$ Relative molecular mass: 142.11

1.1.3 *Chemical and physical properties of the pure substance*

(*a*) *Description*: Prismatic needles from acetone (Lide & Milne, 1996; Budavari, 2000)
(*b*) *Melting-point*: 153.5 °C (Lide & Milne, 1996)
(*c*) *Spectroscopy data*: Infrared [prism (6381), grating (18126)], ultraviolet (1761), nuclear magnetic resonance [proton (10454)] and mass spectral data have been reported (Sadtler Research Laboratories, 1980; Lide & Milne, 1996).

(*d*) *Solubility*: Soluble in water (43.85 g/L; Dialog Corp., 2000), acetone, chloroform, diethyl ether, ethanol, ethyl acetate and pyridine; slightly soluble in benzene (Lide & Milne, 1996; Budavari, 2000)

(*e*) *Dissociation constants*: pK_a, 7.90, 8.03 (Budavari, 2000)

1.1.4   *Technical products and impurities*

Kojic acid is commercially available at a purity greater than 98.0% and as a solution for spraying (TCI America, 2000; Tokyo Kasei Kogyo Co., 2000). Impurities may include heavy metals (10 mg/kg max.) and arsenic (4 mg/kg max.) (Jarchem Industries, 2000).

1.1.5   *Analysis*

Methods for the analysis of kojic acid in commercial foods, flavouring compounds, cosmetic products and microorganisms have been reported. These methods include voltammetry, spectrophotometry, column chromatography with ultraviolet detection, thin-layer chromatography, gas chromatography with or without flame ionization, electron capture or mass spectrometry detection, and high-performance liquid chromatography with photodiode-array or ultraviolet detection (Owens *et al.*, 1970; Scott *et al.*, 1970; Kawate *et al.*, 1972; Qureshi *et al.*, 1979; Tanigaki *et al.*, 1980; Yang *et al.*, 1980; Manabe *et al.*, 1984; Dobias *et al.*, 1985; Frisvad, 1987; Frisvad & Thrane, 1987; Manabe *et al.*, 1988; Goto *et al.*, 1990; Karita *et al.*, 1991; Shih & Zen, 1999; Kimura *et al.*, 2000).

1.2   Production

Kojic acid is a natural antibiotic agent obtained from koji malt (*Aspergillus oryzae*). Koji malt has been used for the production of miso, soya sauce and sake in Japan for a long time (Budavari, 2000; Jarchem Industries, 2000).

Information available in 2000 indicated that kojic acid was manufactured by two companies in China and one company each in Japan, Switzerland and the USA (CIS Information Services, 2000).

1.3   Use

Kojic acid can act as a tyrosinase inhibitor (to inhibit melanin formation), an antioxidant, a bacteriostat, a metal chelating agent and an intermediate in synthesis. Applications of kojic acid include the prevention of discolouration of crustacea, meat and fresh vegetables, as a preservative, as an antioxidant for fats and oils, in cosmetics (skin whitening or depigmenting agent), in the preparation of derivative esters (i.e. kojic oleate, kojic stearate), in adhesives, in chelate-forming resins and as a plant growth-regulating agent to increase production, early maturing and increase sweetness (Cabanes *et al.*, 1994; Chemos Group, 2000; Jarchem Industries, 2000).

Kojic acid has been used in flavourings at 0.2% to add luster, to prevent discolouration on vegetables at 1.0%, in flour production at 0.1%, in meat production at 0.2%, in syrup at 0.05% and as a whitening agent in cosmetics at 0.5–1.0% (Chemos Group, 2000).

1.4   Occurrence

1.4.1   *Occupational exposure*

No data were available to the Working Group.

1.4.2   *Environmental occurrence*

Kojic acid is a natural product that has been isolated from various strains of micro-organisms such as *Penicillium*, *Aspergillus* and *Gluconoacetobacter* (Novotny *et al.*, 1999).

1.5   Regulations and guidelines

No data were available to the Working Group.

2.   Studies of Cancer in Humans

No data were available to the Working Group.

3.   Studies of Cancer in Experimental Animals

3.1   Oral administration

Mouse: Groups of 65 male and 65 female B6C3F$_1$ mice, 6 weeks of age, were fed diets containing 0 (control), 1.5 or 3.0% kojic acid [purity unspecified] for 20 months. The survival rates at 18 months were 67% in control males, 56% in males given 1.5% and 76% in males given 3.0% kojic acid in the diet; 91% in female controls, 87% in females given 1.5% and 91% in females given 3.0% kojic acid in the diet. Thyroid follicular-cell adenomas were found in 34/52 (65%) and 46/53 (87%) males given 1.5 and 3.0% kojic acid, respectively, which were significantly higher than the control value of 1/48 (2%). In females, the incidences were 1/52 (2%), 4/51 (8%) and 39/49 (80%) at 0, 1.5 and 3.0% kojic acid, respectively. The increased incidences were statistically significant ($p < 0.01$) in males at both concentrations and in females at the higher dietary concentration. In groups of 10–14 mice that were given normal diet 30 days before termination of the study, the incidence of adenomas was significantly decreased in the males at both the low and high concentration (Fujimoto *et al.*, 1998). [The Working Group noted the rapid and substantial reduction in tumour incidence, at least in male mice, after only 1 month of withdrawal of the test compound.]

3.2   Administration with known carcinogens

Rat: In a study of the time course of thyroid proliferative lesions, male Fischer 344 rats, 6 weeks of age, were initiated with a subcutaneous injection of 2800 mg/kg bw *N*-nitrosobis(2-hydroxypropyl)amine (NBHPA) and 1 week later were promoted with kojic acid in the diet at a concentration of 0%, 2% or 4%. The animals were examined after 1, 2, 4, 8 and 12 weeks of treatment. Increased thyroid gland weights and diffuse follicular-cell hypertrophy (apparent from week 1) were observed in the kojic acid-treated rats. The incidences of thyroid follicular-cell adenomas were 0 with NBHPA alone, 60% with NBHPA plus 2% kojic acid and 20% with NBHPA plus 4% kojic acid at 4 weeks; 0 with NBHPA alone, 100% with NBHPA plus 2% kojic acid and 40% with NBHPA plus 4% kojic acid at 8 weeks; and 0 with NBHPA alone, 80% with NBHPA plus 2% kojic acid and 75% with NBHPA plus 4% kojic acid at 12 weeks. The multiplicity of thyroid tumours in rats treated with 4% kojic acid (0.2 ± 0.5 after 4 weeks, 0.4 ± 0.6 after 8 weeks and 1.0 ± 0.8 after 12 weeks) was lower than that of rats treated with 2% kojic acid (1.2 ± 1.3 after 4 weeks, 2.0 ± 0.7 after 8 weeks and 1.8 ± 0.8 after 12 weeks), perhaps owing to the marked decrease in dietary intake at the higher concentration (Tamura *et al.*, 1999a).

Two groups of 8–10 male Fischer 344 rats, 6 weeks of age, were given a single subcutaneous injection of 2800 mg/kg bw NBHPA, followed 1 week later by basal diet alone or basal diet containing 2% kojic acid. Half the rats were killed after 4 weeks and the remainder after 12 weeks. Thyroid follicular-cell hyperplasia and adenomas were observed in 4/5 and 3/5 rats given NBHPA plus kojic acid at week 4, respectively. At week 12, these lesions were observed in all rats given the two compounds. Animals given kojic acid alone showed marked diffuse hypertrophy of follicular epithelial cells at weeks 4 and 20 (Mitsumori *et al.*, 1999).

4.   Other Data Relevant to an Evaluation of Carcinogenicity and its Mechanisms

4.1   Absorption, distribution, metabolism and excretion

No data were available to the Working Group.

4.2 Toxic effects

4.2.1 *Humans*

The skin-whitening effect of kojic acid involves the formation of an enzyme complex that inhibits tyrosine hydroxylase and blocks the synthesis of 3,4-dihydroxy-phenylalanine. The commonest adverse effect after topical application of skin depigmenting agents is skin irritation and contact allergy. Patch testing of 220 female patients with suspected cosmetic-related contact dermatitis showed five who reacted to kojic acid (Nakagawa *et al.*, 1995). Another case of contact sensitization was reported by Serra-Baldrich *et al.* (1998).

4.2.2 *Experimental systems*

In the study described in section 3.1 (Fujimoto *et al.*, 1998), B6C3F$_1$ mice, aged 6 weeks at the start of the experiment, were given diets containing kojic acid at a concentration of 0, 1.5 or 3.0% for 20 months. At sacrifice, the thyroid gland weights were found to be increased, and diffuse hyperplasia was found, the effects being more severe in males than in females. Serum was collected from five animals per group at 6, 12 and 20 months for measurement of triiodothyronine (T3) and thyroid-stimulating hormone (TSH). At 6 months, the T3 concentration was significantly decreased in males and females at the higher dietary concentrations and in females also at the lower concentration, whereas the serum concentration of TSH was increased. Thereafter, the T3 concentration remained low, but there was no consistent change in TSH.

In the study described in section 3.2 (Mitsumori *et al.*, 1999), male Fischer 344 rats were initiated with NBHPA and 1 week later were given a diet containing kojic acid at a concentration of 0 or 2% for 12 weeks. Serum T3 and thyroxine (T4) concentrations were decreased and those of TSH markedly increased in kojic acid-treated rats at weeks 4 and 12. The weights of the thyroid gland of these animals were increased, and marked diffuse follicular-cell hypertrophy was observed at 4 weeks in four of five rats. No changes were seen in thyroid-related hormone concentrations or in the thyroid glands of rats that received NBHPA alone or no treatment.

In the study described in section 3.2 (Tamura *et al.*, 1999a), changes in serum thyroid hormone concentrations were studied in male Fischer 344 rats initiated with NBHPA and promoted with kojic acid. The serum concentrations of T3 and T4 were significantly reduced and those of TSH were increased, and increased thyroid gland weights were observed in the kojic acid-treated rats.

In a further study on the effect of kojic acid on thyroid iodine uptake and iodine organification, male Fischer 344 rats were given diets containing kojic acid at a concentration of 0.008, 0.03, 0.125, 0.5 or 2% for 4 weeks. ^{125}I uptake was significantly decreased in the groups receiving 0.03% or more, and organification was significantly reduced at 2% kojic acid. Thyroid gland weights were increased at concentrations $\geq 0.5\%$, and decreased colloid and follicular-cell hypertrophy were observed at concentrations $\geq 0.03\%$. The serum concentrations of T3 and T4 were significantly reduced and those of TSH markedly increased, but only in the group at 2% kojic acid. The finding that TSH concentrations were not significantly increased at lower concentrations was attributed to a possible role of TSH receptor autoregulation under conditions of low iodine or inhibition of iodine organification (Tamura *et al.*, 1999b).

In order to study the effect of kojic acid on thyroid gland function during development of thyroid hyperplasia, Fischer 344 rats were given a diet containing 2% kojic acid for 4 weeks. The serum concentrations of T3 and T4 were decreased, with a marked increase in TSH concentration, and iodine uptake into the thyroid gland was markedly decreased. The authors concluded that kojic acid interrupts thyroid gland function primarily by inhibiting iodine uptake (Fujimoto *et al.*, 1999).

4.3   Reproductive and prenatal effects

4.3.1   *Humans*

No data were available to the Working Group.

4.3.2   *Experimental systems*

Seven mated female Sprague-Dawley rats, weighing 140–160g, were dosed orally with 50 µg/rat per day kojic acid dissolved in 0.1 mL propylene glycol on days 1–5 of gestation (positive vaginal smear = day 1) and compared with a similar group of vehicle-treated controls. Laparotomy to count the number of corpora lutea and implants was performed on day 8, and the animals were allowed to litter. One dam treated with kojic acid died before term. There was no effect on corpora lutea count, but a 50% reduction in the number of implantation sites ($p < 0.02$) was seen, and the litter size was reduced to a mean of 2.71 pups ($p < 0.001$), of which only 0.71 ($p < 0.001$) were alive at birth, compared with 6.57 (all alive) in the controls (Choudhary *et al.*, 1992).

Eight proven fertile male Sprague-Dawley rats weighing 150–200 g were given orally 50 µg/rat per day kojic acid dissolved in 0.1 mL propylene glycol orally for 21 days and compared with vehicle-treated controls. Each male was mated with two proven fertile females on days 16–21, and vaginal smears were examined for sperm to confirm the day of mating. Laparotomy to count the number of corpora lutea and implants was performed on day 8, and the animals were allowed to litter. The males were killed on day 22, epididymal spermatozoa were examined for number, morphology and viability, and the testes were examined histologically. The testis and epididymal weights were slightly ($p < 0.05$) reduced, but no interference with spermatogenesis was seen. Six of the males mated successfully with a total of eight females. There was a reduction in the number of implantation sites in the females mated with kojic acid-treated males, to a mean of 4.62 compared with 7.87 ($p < 0.05$) in controls. The litter size was also reduced, to 3.64 (only 1.79 viable) compared with 5.94 (all viable) in controls. Cannibalism 2–3 days after littering was also observed (Choudhary *et al.*, 1994).

4.4 Effects on enzyme induction or inhibition and gene expression

Kojic acid does not appear to induce hepatic microsomal enzymes. The activity of T4-UDP glucuronosyltransferase was not significantly increased in Fischer 344 rats treated for 4 weeks with kojic acid at 2% in the diet (Mitsumori *et al.*, 1999).

4.5 Genetic and related effects

4.5.1 *Humans*

No data were available to the Working Group.

4.5.2 *Experimental systems* (see Table 1 for references)

In most of the experiments reported, but not all, kojic acid induced mutations in *Salmonella typhimurium* TA100, TA1535 and TA98 both without and with an exogenous metabolic system; it was not mutagenic to TA1537. It did not induce a response in the *Escherichia coli* SOS-repair test. Kojic acid did not induce gene mutations in Chinese hamster lung V79 cells, but did induce sister chromatid exchange and chromosomal aberrations in Chinese hamster ovary cells *in vitro*, both in the presence and absence of an exogenous metabolic system. Kojic acid did not induce dominant lethal mutations in mice.

4.6 Mechanistic considerations

Kojic acid is a directly acting genotoxin. It is also a potent goitrogen in rodents, causing decreased serum thyroid hormone concentrations, increased thyroid-stimulating hormone concentrations, increased thyroid gland weights and diffuse follicular-cell hypertrophy and/or hyperplasia. Kojic acid inhibits iodine uptake by the thyroid and inhibits iodine organification at high doses. The antithyroid effects of kojic acid are therefore the probable mechanism by which it produces thyroid gland tumours; however, a role of genotoxicity cannot be excluded in the light of the positive findings.

5. Summary of Data Reported and Evaluation

5.1 Exposure data

Kojic acid is a natural product, which is used as a food additive and preservative, in cosmetics as a skin-whitening agent, as a plant growth regulator and as a chemical intermediate.

Table 1. Genetic and related effects of kojic acid

Test system	Result[a]		Dose[b] (LED/HID)	Reference
	Without exogenous metabolic system	With exogenous metabolic system		
Escherichia coli K12, SOS repair, forward mutation	–	NT	NR	Auffray & Boutibonnes (1986)
Salmonella typhimurium TA100, reverse mutation	+	+	1000 µg/plate	Bjeldanes & Chew (1979)
Salmonella typhimurium TA100, TA1535, TA98, reverse mutation	+	+	2000 µg/plate	Shibuya et al. (1982)
Salmonella typhimurium TA100, reverse mutation	+	(+)	1000 µg/plate	Wei et al. (1991)
Salmonella typhimurium TA98, reverse mutation	+	+[c]	100 µg/plate	Wei et al. (1991)
Salmonella typhimurium TA98, reverse mutation	–	+	0.5 µg/plate	Wehner et al. (1978)
Salmonella typhimurium TA100, TA1535, TA1537, reverse mutation	–	–	500 µg/plate	Wehner et al. (1978)
Salmonella typhimurium TA1537, reverse mutation	–	–	4000 µg/plate	Shibuya et al. (1982)
Salmonella typhimurium TA98, reverse mutation	–	–	10 000 µg/plate	Bjeldanes & Chew (1979)
Gene mutation, Chinese hamster lung V79 cells, 6-TG resistance *in vitro*	–	NT	3000	Shibuya et al. (1982)
Sister chromatid exchange, Chinese hamster ovary cells *in vitro*	+	+	3000	Wei et al. (1991)
Chromosomal aberrations, Chinese hamster ovary cells *in vitro*	+	+	3000	Wei et al. (1991)
Dominant lethal mutation, C57BL/6×DBA/2 mice *in vivo*	–		700 po × 5	Shibuya et al. (1982)

[a] +, positive; (+), weak positive; –, negative; NT, not tested

[b] LED, lowest effective dose; HID, highest ineffective dose; in-vitro tests, µg/mL; in-vivo tests, mg/kg bw per day; po, orally; NR, not reported

[c] With metabolic activation, a positive response was seen only at a $\geq$ 20-fold higher dose.

5.2   Human carcinogenicity data

No data were available to the Working Group.

5.3   Animal carcinogenicity data

Kojic acid was tested by oral administration in one study in mice. It produced thyroid follicular-cell adenomas in both males and females. In two initiation–promotion studies in rats, kojic acid promoted thyroid follicular-cell carcinogenesis initiated by *N*-nitrosobis(2-hydroxypropyl)amine.

5.4   Other relevant data

No data were available on the absorption, distribution, metabolism or excretion of kojic acid.

Kojic acid is a potent goitrogen in rodents, in which treatment results in decreased serum thyroid hormone concentrations, increased thyroid-stimulating hormone secretion, increased thyroid gland weights and diffuse follicular-cell hypertrophy and/or hyperplasia.

Kojic acid inhibited iodine uptake by the thyroid and inhibited iodine organification at high doses.

No data were available on the genetic and related effects of kojic acid in humans. Kojic acid did not induce dominant lethal mutations in mice. In the presence and absence of metabolic activation, it induced sister chromatid exchange and chromosomal aberrations, but not mutations, in hamster cells in culture. Kojic acid was mutagenic in bacteria in the presence and absence of metabolic activation. The overall data indicate that kojic acid is genotoxic *in vitro*.

5.5   Evaluation

There is *inadequate evidence* in humans for the carcinogenicity of kojic acid.

There is *limited evidence* in experimental animals for the carcinogenicity of kojic acid.

Overall evaluation

Kojic acid is *not classifiable as to its carcinogenicity to humans (Group 3)*.

6. References

Auffray, Y. & Boutibonnes, P. (1986) Evaluation of the genotoxic activity of some mycotoxins using *Escherichia coli* in the SOS spot test. *Mutat. Res.*, **171**, 79–82

Bjeldanes, L.F. & Chew, H. (1979) Mutagenicity of 1,2-dicarbonyl compounds: Maltol, kojic acid, diacetyl and related substances. *Mutat. Res.*, **67**, 367–371

Budavari, S., ed. (2000) *The Merck Index*, 12th Ed., Version 12:3, Whitehouse Station, NJ, Merck & Co. & Boca Raton, FL, Chapman & Hall/CRC [CD-ROM]

Cabanes, J., Chazarra, S. & Garcia-Carmona, F. (1994) Kojic acid, a cosmetic skin whitening agent, is a slow-binding inhibitor of catecholase activity of tyrosinase. *J. Pharm. Pharmacol.*, **46**, 982–985

Chemos Group (2000) *Data Sheet: Kojic Acid*, Prague [http://www.chemos-group.com]

Choudhary, D.N., Sahay, G.R. & Singh, J.N. (1992) Effect of some mycotoxins on reproduction in pregnant albino rats. *J. Food Sci. Technol.*, **29**, 264–265

Choudhary, D.N., Sahay, G.R. & Singh, J.N. (1994) Antifertility and cannibalistic properties of some mycotoxins in albino rats. *J. Food Sci. Technol.*, **31**, 497–499

CIS Information Services (2000) *Directory of World Chemical Producers (Version 2000.1)*, Dallas, TX [CD-ROM]

Dialog Corp. (2000) *Beilstein Online (File 390)*, Cary, NC

Dobias, J., Brtko, J. & Nemec, P. (1985) [Quantitative determination of kojic acid in fungal fermentation broth using diffusion in agar plates and spectrophotometry.] *Kvasný Prum.*, **31**, 260–262 (in Slovenian)

Frisvad, J.C. (1987) High-performance liquid chromatographic determination of profiles of mycotoxins and other secondary metabolites. *J. Chromatogr.*, **392**, 333–347

Frisvad, J.C. & Thrane, U. (1987) Standardized high-performance liquid chromatography of 182 mycotoxins and other fungal metabolites based on alkylphenone retention indices and UV-VIS spectra (diode array detection). *J. Chromatogr.*, **404**, 195–214

Fujimoto, N., Watanabe, H., Nakatani, T., Roy, G. & Ito, A. (1998) Induction of thyroid tumours in (C57BL/6N × C3H/N)F$_1$ mice by oral administration of kojic acid. *Food chem. Toxicol.*, **36**, 697–703

Fujimoto, N., Onodera, H., Mitsumori, K., Tamura, T., Maruyama, S. & Ito A. (1999) Changes in thyroid function during development of thyroid hyperplasia induced by kojic acid in F344 rats. *Carcinogenesis*, **20**, 1567–1571

Goto, T., Matsui, M. & Kitsuwa, T. (1990) Analysis of *Aspergillus* mycotoxins by gas chromatography using fused silica capillary column. *Proc. Jpn. Assoc. Mycotoxicol.*, **31**, 43–47

Jarchem Industries (2000) *Technical Information Sheet: Kojic Acid*, Newark, NJ

Karita, S., Umehara, Y., Yano, Y., Hamachi, M. & Nunokawa, Y. (1991) [Determination of kojic acid in rice koji by Bio Gel P-2 column chromatography.] *Nippon Jozo Kyokaishi (J. Brew. Soc. Jpn.)*, **86**, 884–885 (in Japanese)

Kawate, S., Koike, M. & Fukuo, T. (1972) Spectrophotometric determination of kojic acid. *Technol. Rep. Kansai Univ.*, **13**, 67–79

Kimura, K., Hirokado, M., Yasuda, K. & Nishijima, M. (2000) [Determination of kojic acid in various commercial foods by HPLC.] *Shokuhin Eiseigaku Zasshi*, **41**, 70–73 (in Japanese)

Lide, D.R. & Milne, G.W.A. (1996) *Properties of Organic Compounds*, Version 5.0, Boca Raton, FL, CRC Press [CD-ROM]

Manabe, M., Shinshi, E., Goto, T., Misawa, Y., Tanaka, K. & Matsuura, S. (1984) [Fluorescent compound in fermented foods. VI. High-performance liquid chromatographic analysis of kojic acid.] *Nippon Shoyu Kenkyusho Zasshi*, **10**, 146–150 (in Japanese)

Manabe, M., Shinshi, E., Goto, T., Tanaka, K. & Misawa, Y. (1988) [Fluorescent constituents in fermented foods. VIII. Gas–liquid chromatographic analytical system for kojic acid.] *Nippon Shoyu Kenkyusho Zasshi*, **14**, 183–186 (in Japanese)

Mitsumori, K., Onodera, H., Takahashi, M., Funakoshi, T., Tamura, T., Yasuhara, K., Takegawa, K. & Takahashi, M. (1999) Promoting effects of kojic acid due to serum TSH elevation resulting from reduced serum thyroid hormone levels on development of thyroid proliferative lesions in rats initiated with *N*-bis(2-hydroxypropyl)nitrosamine. *Carcinogenesis*, **20**, 173–176

Nakagawa, M., Kawai, K. & Kawai, K. (1995) Contact allergy to kojic acid in skin care products. *Contact Derm.*, **32**, 9–13

Novotny, L., Rauko, P., Abdel-Hamid, M. & Váchalková, A. (1999) Kojic acid — A new leading molecule for a preparation of compounds with an anti-neoplastic potential. *Neoplasma*, **46**, 89–92

Owens, R.G., Welty, R.E. & Lucas, G.B. (1970) Gas chromatographic analysis of the mycotoxins kojic acid, terreic acid, and terrein. *Anal. Biochem.*, **35**, 249–258

Qureshi, A.A., Prentice, N. & Burger, W.C. (1979) Separation of potential flavoring compounds by high-performance liquid chromatography. *J. Chromatogr.*, **170**, 343–353

Sadtler Research Laboratories (1980) *Sadtler Standard Spectra, 1980 Cumulative Molecular Formula Index*, Philadelphia, PA, p. 100

Scott, P.M., Lawrence, J.W. & van Walbeek, W. (1970) Detection of mycotoxins by thin-layer chromatography: Application to screening of fungal extracts. *Appl. Microbiol.*, **20**, 839–842

Serra-Baldrich, E., Tribó, M.J. & Camarasa, J.G. (1998) Allergic contact dermatitis from kojic acid. *Contact Derm.*, **39**, 86–87

Shibuya, T., Murota, T., Sakamoto, K., Iwahara, S. & Ikeno, M. (1982) Mutagenicity and dominant lethal test of kojic acid. *J. toxicol. Sci.*, **7**, 255–262

Shih, Y. & Zen, J.-M. (1999) Voltammetric determination of kojic acid in cosmetic bleaching products using a disposable screen-printed carbon electrode. *Electroanalysis*, **11**, 229–233

Tamura, T., Mitsumori, K., Onodera, H., Takahashi, M., Funakoshi, T., Yasuhara, K., Takegawa, K., Takagi, H. & Hirose, M. (1999a) Time course observation of thyroid proliferative lesions and serum levels of related hormones in rats treated with kojic acid after DHPN initiation. *J. toxicol. Sci.*, **24**, 145–155

Tamura, T., Mitsumori, K., Onodera, H., Fujimoto, N., Yasuhara, K., Takegawa, K. & Takahashi, M. (1999b) Inhibition of thyroid iodine uptake and organification in rats treated with kojic acid. *Toxicol. Sci.*, **47**, 170–175

Tanigaki, H., Obata, H. & Tokuyama, T. (1980) The determination of kojic acid using the stopped-flow method. *Bull. chem. Soc. Jpn.*, **53**, 3195–3197

TCI America (2000) *Product Information: Kojic Acid*, Portland, OR

Tokyo Kasei Kogyo Co. (2000) *Product Information: Kojic Acid*, Tokyo

Wehner, F.C., Thiel, P.G., Van Rensburg, S.J. & Demasius, I.P.C. (1978) Mutagenicity to *Salmonella typhimurium* of some *Aspergillus* and *Penicillium* mycotoxins. *Mutat. Res.*, **58**, 193–203

Wei, C.I., Huang, T.S., Fernando, S.Y. & Chung, K.T. (1991) Mutagenicity studies of kojic acid. *Toxicol. Lett.*, **59**, 213–220

Yang, S.S., Wei, C.B. & Chou, C.C. (1980) [Kojic acid of fermented foods produced in Taiwan.] *Kuo Li T'ai-wan Ta Hsueh Nung Hsueh Yuan Yen Chiu Pao Kao*, **20**, 25–34 (in Chinese)

HAIR DYE

2,4-DIAMINOANISOLE AND ITS SALTS

This substance was considered by previous working groups, in 1977 (IARC, 1978), 1981 (IARC, 1982) and 1987 (IARC, 1987). Since that time, new data have become available, and these have been incorporated into the monograph and taken into consideration in the present evaluation.

1. Exposure Data

1.1 Chemical and physical data

1.1.1 *Nomenclature*

2,4-Diaminoanisole

Chem. Abstr. Serv. Reg. No.: 615-05-4
Chem. Abstr. Name: 4-Methoxy-1,3-benzenediamine
IUPAC Systematic Name: 4-Methoxy-*meta*-phenylenediamine
Synonyms: 3-Amino-4-methoxyaniline; C.I. 76050; C.I. Oxidation Base 12; 1,3-diamino-4-methoxybenzene; 4-methoxy-1,3-phenylenediamine; *para*-methoxy-meta-phenylenediamine

2,4-Diaminoanisole sulfate

Chem. Abstr. Serv. Reg. No.: 39156-41-7
Chem. Abstr. Name: 4-Methoxy-1,3-benzenediamine, sulfate
IUPAC Systematic Name: 4-Methoxy-*meta*-phenylenediamine, sulfate
Synonyms: CI 76051; CI oxidation base 12A; 2,4-DAA sulfate; 2,4-diaminoanisole, hydrogen sulfate; 2,4-diaminoanisole sulphate; 1,3-diamino-4-methoxybenzene sulphate; 2,4-diamino-1-methoxybenzene sulphate; 4-methoxy-1,3-benzenediamine sulfate (1:1); 4-methoxy-1,3-benzenediamine sulphate; 4-methoxy-*meta*-phenylene-diamine sulfate; *para*-methoxy-*meta*-phenylenediamine sulphate; 4-methoxy-*meta*-phenylenediammonium sulphate

2,4-Diaminoanisole dihydrochloride

Chem. Abstr. Serv. Reg. No.: 614-94-8
Chem. Abstr. Name: 4-Methoxy-1,3-benzenediamine, dihydrochloride
IUPAC Systematic Name: 4-Methoxy-*meta*-phenylenediamine, dihydrochloride
Synonyms: 2,4-Diaminoanisole hydrochloride

1.1.2   *Structural and molecular formulae and relative molecular masses*

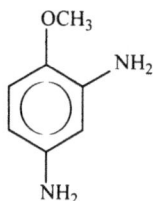

$C_7H_{10}N_2O$ Relative molecular mass: 138.17

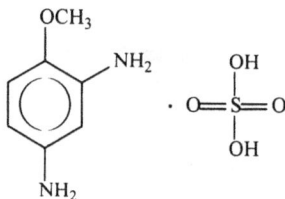

$C_7H_{10}N_2O.H_2SO_4$ Relative molecular mass: 236.25

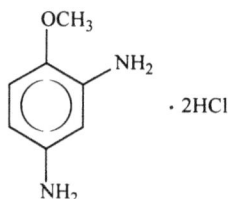

$C_7H_{10}N_2O.2HCl$ Relative molecular mass: 211.07

1.1.3   *Chemical and physical properties of the pure substances*

2,4-Diaminoanisole

(a) *Description*: Needles from diethyl ether (Budavari, 2000)
(b) *Melting-point*: 67.5 °C (Lide & Milne, 1996)
(c) *Spectroscopy data*: Infrared [prism (2971), grating (15399)], ultraviolet (855) and nuclear magnetic resonance [proton (10617)], and mass spectral data have been reported (Sadtler Research Laboratories, 1980; Lide & Milne, 1996).

(d) *Solubility*: Soluble in diethyl ether and ethanol (Lide & Milne, 1996)

(e) *Stability*: Darkens on exposure to light (Budavari, 2000)

2,4-Diaminoanisole sulfate

(a) *Description*: Off-white to violet powder (Budavari, 2000)

(b) *Solubility*: Soluble in water and ethanol (Budavari, 2000)

(c) *Spectroscopy data*: Infrared [prism/grating (51021)], ultraviolet (26381) and nuclear magnetic resonance [proton (23809)] data have been reported (Sadtler Research Laboratories, 1980).

2,4-Diaminoanisole dihydrochloride

(a) *Description*: Crystalline powder (TCI America, 2000)

(b) *Solubility*: Soluble in water (TCI America, 2000)

1.1.4 *Technical products and impurities*

Trade names for 2,4-diaminoanisole include Furro L, Pelagol DA, Pelagol Grey L and Pelagol L.

Trade names for 2,4-diaminoanisole sulfate include BASF Ursol SLA, Durafur Brown MN, Fouramine BA, Fourrine 76, Fourrine SLA, Furro SLA, Nako TSA, Pelagol BA, Pelagol Grey, Pelagol Grey SLA, Pelagol SLA, Renal SLA, Ursol SLA and Zoba SLE.

1.1.5 *Analysis*

Methods for the analysis of aromatic amines, including 2,4-diaminoanisole, in inks of ball-point and fibre-tip pens and watercolour paints, oxidative hair dyes, dyestuff mixtures and in paper, coloured textiles and leather products have been reported. These methods include differential pulse voltammetry, gas chromatography–mass spectrometry with mass ion detection, thin-layer chromatography, high-performance thin-layer chromatography and high-performance liquid chromatography with ultraviolet, diode-array or mass spectrometry detection (Bernabei *et al.*, 1980; Johansson *et al.*, 1981; Liem & Rooselaar, 1981; Mancini *et al.*, 1981; Gottschalck & Machens, 1982; Ohshima *et al.*, 1982; Hoogewijs & Massart, 1983; Sardas *et al.*, 1985; Andrisano *et al.*, 1994, 1995; Friedrichs *et al.*, 1995; Verdú *et al.*, 1996; Winkeler, 1996; Bürgi *et al.*, 1997; Verdú *et al.*, 1997; Anon., 1998a,b; Bürgi *et al.*, 1998; Chen *et al.*, 1998; Mayer *et al.*, 1998; Planelles *et al.*, 1998; Štancer & Jeretin, 1998; Tomaselli *et al.*, 1998; Wang & Chen, 1998; Cioni *et al.*, 1999; Kellert *et al.*, 1999; Planelles *et al.*, 1999; Sinha & Kumar, 1999; Xiao *et al.*, 1999; Yang *et al.*, 2000).

1.2   Production

2,4-Diaminoanisole was first prepared in 1913 by the reduction of 2,4-dinitro-anisole with iron and acetic acid (Richter, 1933; Budavari, 2000).

Information available in 2000 indicated that 2,4-diaminoanisole sulfate was manufactured by one company in China (CIS Information Services, 2000).

1.3   Use

2,4-Diaminoanisole and its sulfate salt have been used in the preparation of dyes, especially hair and fur dyes, as an intermediate in the production of C.I. Basic Brown 2 and as a corrosion inhibitor for steel (Budavari, 2000). It was used extensively in permanent, oxidative hair dyes until the late 1970s (IARC, 1993).

1.4   Occurrence

1.4.1   *Occupational exposure*

According to the 1981–83 National Occupational Exposure Survey (National Institute for Occupational Safety and Health, 2000), about 23 000 workers in the USA were potentially exposed to 2,4-diaminoanisole or its sulfate salt. They were all hair-dressers or cosmetologists. The National Institute for Occupational Safety and Health (1978) estimated in the 1970s that as many as 400 000 workers were potentially exposed to 2,4-diaminoanisole in the USA. Hairdressers and cosmetologists comprised most of this group; a relatively small number of fur dyers were probably exposed to higher concentrations. According to the Finnish Register of Employees Exposed to Carcinogens, no workers were exposed to 2,4-diaminoanisole in Finland in 1997 (Savela *et al.*, 1999).

1.4.2   *Environmental occurrence*

No data were available to the Working Group.

1.5   Regulations and guidelines

No occupational exposure limits for 2,4-diaminoanisole have been established. It is classified as a carcinogen in several countries including Finland, Germany, Sweden, Switzerland and the USA (American Conference of Governmental Industrial Hygienists, 2000; Deutsche Forschungsgemeinschaft, 2000; UNEP, 2000).

The former European Community (now the European Union) stated that, effective in 1978, '2,4-diaminoanisole (and its salts) must not form part of the composition of cosmetic products; and Member States should prohibit the marketing of cosmetic products containing 2,4-diaminoanisole (and its salts)' (UNEP, 2000).

2.   Studies of Cancer in Humans

Although hairdressers and barbers and similar occupational groups as well as users of hair dyes may be exposed to 2,4-diaminoanisole, exposure to this compound itself has not been evaluated in epidemiological studies of cancer risk. The evidence for a carcinogenic risk of occupational and personal exposure to hair dyes was reviewed in a previous *IARC Monographs* volume (IARC, 1993). The risks for haematopoietic neoplasms and lymphomas were addressed in two recent papers (Correa *et al.*, 2000a,b).

3.   Studies of Cancer in Experimental Animals

3.1   Oral administration

Mouse: Groups of 50 male and 50 female B6C3F$_1$ mice, 6 weeks of age, were fed diets containing 1200 or 2400 mg/kg diet technical-grade 2,4-diaminoanisole sulfate (of indeterminate purity, with at least one impurity detected by thin-layer chromatography) for 78 weeks and were observed for a further 18–19 weeks. Groups of 50 animals of each sex served as matched controls for each concentration group. The mean body-weight gains of treated and control animals were similar throughout the study, and the survival rates were comparable among treated and control mice: by the end of the study, 84, 78, 92 and 82% of males and 74, 76, 76 and 78% of females were still alive in the low-concentration control, high-concentration control, low-concentration and high-concentration groups, respectively. Among the males, follicular-cell adenomas of the thyroid were seen in 1/47 low-concentration controls, 0/40 high-concentration controls, 0/46 at the low concentration and 11/45 at the high concentration ($p < 0.001$); one male at the low concentration had a follicular-cell carcinoma. Follicular-cell hyperplasia was found in 12/45 males at the high concentration. Among the females, follicular-cell adenomas were found in 0/43 low-concentration controls, 0/41 high-concentration controls, 0/42 at the low concentration and 6/45 at the high concentration ($p = 0.017$); follicular-cell carcinomas were found in 2/45 at the high concentration; and follicular-cell adenomas and carcinomas combined were found in 8/45 at the high concentration ($p = 0.004$). Thyroid hyperplasia occurred in 11/42 females at the low concentration (National Cancer Institute, 1978). [The Working Group noted that no explanation was provided for having matched controls for each concentration group.]

Rat: Groups of 50 male and 50 female Fischer 344 rats, 6 weeks of age, were fed diets containing technical-grade 2,4-diaminoanisole sulfate (same sample as used above) at a concentration of 5000 mg/kg for 78 weeks or 1250 mg/kg of diet for 10 weeks and 1200 mg/kg of diet for 68 weeks, followed by a 29-week observation period. Groups of 50 (49 for the high-concentration male controls) animals of each sex served as matched controls for each concentration group. The mean body-weight gains of male and female rats at the high concentration were lower than those of controls throughout most of the study. The mortality rates of the treated and control male rats were similar by the end of the study: 54, 61, 60 and 54% of the animals were still alive in the low- and high-concentration control and treated groups, respectively. The female rats showed a significantly accelerated mortality rate, in particular at the high dietary concentration of the chemical, with 46, 74, 58 and 44% of the animals alive in low- and high-concentration control and low- and high-concentration treated groups, respectively. Malignant thyroid follicular-cell tumours were found in 2/35 low-concentration male controls, 0/48 high-concentration male controls, 2/47 at the low concentration and 17/49 at the high concentration ($p = 0.001$) and in 2/38 low-concentration female controls, 1/45 high-concentration female controls, 1/46 at the low concentration and 10/49 at the high concentration ($p = 0.006$). Eight males and three females at the high concentration but none of the controls had multiple follicular-cell tumours. The incidence of tumours of thyroid C-cell origin (adenomas or carcinomas) was significantly increased in male rats, with 1/35 in low-concentration male controls, 1/48 in high-concentration male controls, 4/47 in males at the low concentration and 10/49 at the high concentration ($p = 0.004$), but not in female rats. In males, squamous-cell carcinomas, basal-cell carcinomas or sebaceous adenocarcinomas of the skin were found in 0/36 low-concentration controls, 0/48 high-concentration controls, 2/48 at the low concentration and 7/49 at the high concentration ($p = 0.007$). Preputial or clitoral gland adenomas, papillomas or carcinomas were found in 0/36 low-concentration control males, 0/48 high-concentration control males, 2/48 at the low concentration, 8/49 at the high concentration ($p < 0.003$) and in 0/39 low-concentration female controls, 3/50 high-concentration female controls, 5/49 at the low concentration ($p = 0.049$) and 8/49 at the high concentration. In the Zymbal gland, squamous-cell carcinomas or sebaceous adenocarcinomas were found in 0/36 low-concentration male controls, 0/48 high-concentration male controls, 1/48 at the low concentration and 8/49 at the high concentration ($p = 0.003$); and sebaceous adenocarcinomas were found in 0/39 low-concentration female controls, 0/50 high-concentration female controls, 0/49 at the low concentration and 7/49 at the high concentration ($p = 0.006$) (National Cancer Institute, 1978). [The Working Group noted that no explanation was provided for having matched controls for each concentration group.]

Groups of 40–60 female Fischer 344 rats, 6 weeks of age, were fed a diet containing 2,4-diaminoanisole sulfate [purity not stated] at a concentration of 0 (control), 1200, 2400 or 5000 mg/kg for up to 82–86 weeks. Another 15 rats were fed a diet containing 5000 mg/kg for 10 weeks and were observed up to about 87 weeks. The mean body weights of rats at the high concentration were lower than those of controls. By 87–94 weeks, follicular-cell adenomas or carcinomas of the thyroid were found in 0/37 controls, 0/47 at the low concentration, 2/33 at the intermediate concentration and 28/40 at the high concentration (21 with adenomas and seven with carcinomas) and in 1/12 rats treated for 10 weeks. Mammary adenocarcinomas were found in 0/37 controls, 0/47 at the low concentration, 5/33 at the intermediate concentration and 3/40 at the high concentration; mammary adenomas were found in only 1/33 rats at the intermediate concentration and 1/47 at the low concentration. Carcinomas (squamous- or sebaceous-cell or mixed) of the clitoral gland were found in 0/37 controls, 8/47 at the low concentration, 15/33 at the intermediate concentration, 9/40 at the high concentration and 1/12 rats treated for 10 weeks (Evarts & Brown, 1980). [The Working Group noted that no statistical analysis was provided.]

3.2 Skin application

Two studies, one in mice (Burnett *et al.*, 1975) and one in rats (Kinkel & Holzmann, 1973), in which 2,4-diaminoanisole sulfate was applied by skin painting, could not be evaluated because the test agent represented a mixture of compounds as a hair-dye formulation.

3.3 Administration with known carcinogens or modifying factors

Rat: In an evaluation of the promoting effect of 2,4-diaminoanisole sulfate on thyroid carcinogenesis, groups of 21 male Wistar rats, 7 weeks of age, were given an intraperitoneal injection of 2.1 g/kg bw N-nitrosobis(2-hydroxypropyl)amine (NBHPA) in water at the start of the study followed by a diet containing 0.5% 2,4-diaminoanisole sulfate for 19 weeks; other groups either received the intraperitoneal injection of NBHPA with no 2,4-diaminoanisole sulfate, the diet containing 2,4-diaminoanisole sulfate with no NBHPA or a control diet. The total observation period was 20 weeks. 2,4-Diaminoanisole sulfate alone did not cause thyroid tumours, but NBHPA alone caused thyroid follicular-cell adenomas in 6/21 (28%) rats and carcinomas in 1/21 (4%) rats. The combination of NBHPA and 2,4-diaminoanisole sulfate increased the incidence of thyroid adenomas to 20/21 (95%) and that of carcinomas to 9/21 (42%) ($p < 0.05$; χ^2 test). The incidence of hyperplasia of the thyroid follicular epithelium was also increased in the group given the combination (Kitahori *et al.*, 1989).

In a study to assess the synergistic effect of three thyroid carcinogens, 2,4-diaminoanisole sulfate, N,N'-diethylthiourea (see monograph in this volume) and 4,4'-thiodianiline, groups of 20–21 male Fischer 344/Crj rats, 6 weeks of age, were fed a diet containing 610 mg/kg 2,4-diaminoanisole sulfate for 52 weeks alone or in combination with 200 mg/kg N,N'-diethylthiourea and 46 mg/kg 4,4'-thiodianiline. After 52 weeks of treatment, the rats were killed, necropsied and evaluated for tumour incidences. 2,4-Diaminoanisole sulfate alone did not induce thyroid tumours but significantly ($p < 0.01$) increased the incidences of thyroid follicular-cell tumours caused by the combination of the other two agents. 2,4-Diaminoanisole sulfate did not induce liver tumours or lung tumours but may have increased the incidences of these tumours produced by 4,4'-thiodianiline (Hasegawa *et al.*, 1991). [From the study design, the Working Group concluded that it was not possible to assess the synergistic effect of 2,4-diaminoanisole sulfate, if any, on the incidence of thyroid gland tumours induced by N,N'-diethylthio-urea and/or 4,4′-thiodianiline.]

4.   Other Data Relevant to an Evaluation of Carcinogenicity and Its Mechanisms

4.1   Absorption, distribution, metabolism and excretion

4.1.1   *Humans*

After application of [^{14}C]2,4-diaminoanisole at 4 μg/cm^2 (3–15 cm^2 per individual [exact number of individuals not given]) to the ventral forearm of male volunteers for 24 h, the skin penetration was estimated to be 3.9 ± 0.9%, as determined by excretion of radiolabel in the urine (Marzulli *et al.*, 1981).

4.1.2   *Experimental systems*

After application of [^{14}C]2,4-diaminoanisole at 4 μg/cm^2 (3–15 cm^2 per animal [exact number of animals not given]) to the abdomen of male and female rhesus monkeys (*Macaca mulatta*) for 24 h, the skin penetration was estimated to be 4.7 ± 4.3%, as determined by excretion of radiolabel in the urine (Marzulli *et al.*, 1981). Dermal absorption of [^{14}C]2,4-diaminoanisole from three hair-dye formulations containing 0.6–1.8% by female Sprague-Dawley rats varied from 0.26 to 1.1% of the administered dose (Hofer & Hruby, 1983).

After intraperitoneal injection of 50 mg/kg bw [^{14}C]2,4-diaminoanisole to rats, 85% of the radiolabel was excreted in the urine and 9% in the faeces after 48 h. The major metabolites were 4-acetylamino-2-aminoanisole, 2,4-diacetylaminoanisole and 2,4-diacetylaminophenol, and were excreted in the urine both free and as glucuronides and sulfates (Grantham *et al.*, 1979). After administration by gavage of [^{14}C]2,4-diamino-anisole [dose not specified] to 18 male and female Sprague-Dawley rats, 49.9 ± 6.9 and 52.1 ± 4.8% of the applied dose were recovered in the urine and faeces, respectively, over 5 days. As 5.6 ± 1.7% of the orally administered radiolabel was eliminated in the bile within 3 h, the radiolabel found in the faeces might have originated from absorbed material (Hofer & Hruby, 1983).

The metabolism and covalent binding of [^{14}C]2,4-diaminoanisole to cellular macro-molecules *in vitro* and *in vivo* were shown to be cytochrome P450-dependent. Incubation of rat liver and kidney microsomes with radiolabelled 2,4-diaminoanisole in the presence of NADPH and oxygen led to the formation of products that were bound covalently to microsomal protein. Inhibitors of cytochrome P450 enzymes *in vivo* and *in vitro* decreased the binding; pretreatment with phenobarbital increased binding; and pretreatment with β-naphthoflavone had no effect. More [^{14}C-ring]-labelled than [^{14}C-methyl]-labelled 2,4-diaminoanisole was bound; when the hydrogens in the methyl group were replaced by deuterium, both the binding and the mutagenicity of 2,4-diaminoanisole increased. Liver microsomes catalysed irreversible binding to endogenous microsomal RNA; no binding to purified calf thymus DNA was detected (Dybing *et al.*, 1979a). When 10–200 mg/kg bw [^{3}H]2,4-diaminoanisole were injected into rats, the label was bound covalently to liver and kidney proteins. No covalent binding to hepatic RNA or DNA was detected (Dybing *et al.*, 1979b).

4.1.3   *Comparison of animals and humans*

The amount of 2,4-diaminoanisole absorbed after dermal application is of the same order of magnitude in humans, monkeys and rats. No data were available on metabolism in humans to allow a comparison with data from experiments with rats.

4.2   Toxic effects

4.2.1   *Humans*

No data were available to the Working Group.

4.2.1   *Experimental systems*

The oral LD$_{50}$ of 2,4-diaminoanisole sulfate in an oil-in-water emulsion in rats was > 4000 mg/kg bw; the intraperitoneal LD$_{50}$ of a solution in dimethyl sulfoxide was 372 mg/kg bw (Burnett *et al.*, 1977).

Male and female B6C3F$_1$ mice and Fischer 344 rats were fed diets containing 0.075–0.58% 2,4-diaminoanisole sulfate for 4 weeks, followed by a 2-week observation period. One male rat each at 0.075, 0.125 and 0.58% and one male mouse at the highest dietary concentration died. No gross abnormalities were noted in either rats or mice (National Cancer Institute, 1978).

In a study of the effects of 2,4-diaminoanisole sulfate on thyroid function, groups of 15 male Wistar rats were given the compound in the diet at a concentration of 0.5% or were painted daily with a 5% solution on a 5 × 4-cm area of dorsal skin for up to 6 weeks. Five rats from each group were killed at weeks 1, 3 and 6. The mean thyroid weight of rats fed 2,4-diaminoanisole sulfate was significantly increased (60%) from week 1, and was markedly greater (2.5-fold) than the control value at week 6. In the group treated in the diet, the mean serum concentration of thyroid-stimulating hormone was markedly higher than that in the control group at weeks 1 and 3 (10- and 16-fold, respectively), but was only slightly elevated (2.5-fold) at week 6. Similarly, reductions in the serum concentrations of thyroxine and triiodothyronine noted at earlier times were less pronounced at week 6. In contrast to dietary administration, cutaneous application of 2,4-diaminoanisole sulfate did not have a significant effect on thyroid organ weight or function (Kitahori *et al.*, 1989).

In an experiment in which groups of five male Iva:Siv50 rats were treated with 2,4-diaminoanisole sulfate at a dietary concentration of 0.25% for up to 8 weeks, the serum concentration of thyroid-stimulating hormone was increased by 68% after 1 week and that of triiodothyronine was decreased at weeks 1, 2, 4 and 8 (Zbinden, 1988).

4.3   Reproductive and prenatal effects

4.3.1   *Humans*

No information was available on persons exposed to 2,4-diaminoanisole alone. The evidence for reproductive disorders due to exposure of hairdressers to chemicals was evaluated from a literature review for the years 1985–93. Associations with menstrual disorders and spontaneous abortions were found in some epidemiological studies on hairdressers, but no association was found in other studies. It was concluded that there is little evidence for an increased incidence of reproductive disorders among hairdressers. None of the evidence related specifically to 2,4-diaminoanisole (Kersemaekers *et al.*, 1995).

4.3.2   *Experimental systems*

No studies were available in which 2,4-diaminoanisole was tested alone.

Three commercially available hair-dye formulations, containing 0.02, 2 or 4% 2,4-diaminoanisole sulfate and several aromatic amine derivatives among their constituents, were tested for teratogenicity in groups of 20 mated female Charles River CD rats. Each formulation was mixed with an equal volume of hydrogen peroxide and applied topically to a shaved site on the dorsoscapular region at a dose of 2 mL/kg bw on days 1, 4, 7, 10, 13, 16 and 19 of gestation. The dams were killed on day 20 of gestation. There was no significant increase in the incidence of soft-tissue anomalies in the living fetuses, but minor skeletal changes were seen in nine of 169 live fetuses in three of 20 litters of dams given the formulation containing the highest concentration of 2,4-diaminoanisole sulfate (4%). On comparison with the three negative control groups, this finding was found to be statistically significant ($p < 0.05$ to $p < 0.01$) but was considered by the authors not to be biologically significant (Burnett *et al.*, 1976).

4.4   Effects on enzyme induction/inhibition and gene expression

No data were available to the Working Group.

4.5   Genetic and related effects

4.5.1   *Humans*

No data were available to the Working Group.

4.5.2   *Experimental systems* (see Table 1 for references)

The results obtained with 2,4-diaminoanisole sulfate trihydrate and with 2,4-diami-noanisole dihydrochloride are listed separately, but this distinction is not made in the summary of the results given below.

(a)   *DNA damage*

2,4-Diaminoanisole induced DNA double-strand breaks in primary rat hepatocytes in culture and in liver cells of rats. No change in DNA viscosity was seen in liver cells of rats that received 2,4-diaminoanisole by intraperitoneal injection. DNA damage was produced in liver and brain, but not stomach, colon, kidney, bladder, lung or bone-marrow cells of mice as measured in the Comet assay.

2,4-Diaminoanisole induced unscheduled DNA synthesis in HeLa cells with and without S9.

(b)   *Mutation and allied effects*

2,4-Diaminoanisole caused frameshift mutations in *Salmonella typhimurium* in the presence of exogenous metabolic activation from liver microsomes from uninduced and induced mice, rats and rabbits and from humans. It produced gene mutations and chromosomal aberrations in rodent cells *in vitro*.

2,4-Diaminoanisole was metabolized to mutagenic products by ram seminal vesicle microsomes or purified prostaglandin H synthase (Robertson *et al.*, 1983; Sarkar *et al.*, 1992). The reaction product of 2,4-diaminoanisole and hydrogen peroxide was mutagenic in *Salmonella* in the presence and absence of an exogenous metabolic activation system (Watanabe *et al.*, 1989).

2,4-Diaminoanisole induced mutation and mitotic recombination in *Saccharomyces cerevisiae*. It was not mutagenic to *Neurospora crassa* in a single study.

2,4-Diaminoanisole did not transform Syrian hamster embryo cells in culture in a single study.

Urine of phenobarbital-induced rats treated with 2,4-diaminoanisole was mutagenic in the presence, but not the absence, of rat liver microsomes. If rats were treated with β-naphthoflavone, methylcholanthrene, or 2,3,7,8-tetrachlorodibenzo-*para*-dioxin, the mutagenicity of their urine in the presence of microsomes was decreased. Treatment of the urine with β-glucuronidase increased mutagenic activity in the presence and absence of liver microsomes (Reddy *et al.*, 1980).

2,4-Diaminoanisole produced sex-linked recessive lethal mutations, but not somatic cell recombination, in *Drosophila melanogaster*. It produced sister chromatid exchanges, but not micronuclei, in mouse bone-marrow cells. It did not produce dominant lethal mutations in rats or altered sperm morphology in mice.

Table 1. Genetic and related effects of 2,4-diaminoanisole, its sulfate trihydrate and its dihydrochloride

Test system	Result[a]		Dose[b] (LED/HID)	Reference
	Without exogenous metabolic system	With exogenous metabolic system		
2,4-Diaminoanisole				
Salmonella typhimurium TA100, TA1535, TA1537, reverse mutation	−	−	500 µg/plate	Bruce & Heddle (1979)
Salmonella typhimurium TA100, reverse mutation	NT	−	60	de Giovanni-Donnelly (1981)
Salmonella typhimurium TA100, reverse mutation	NT	+	10 µg/plate	Parodi et al. (1981)
Salmonella typhimurium TA100, TA102, TA98, reverse mutation	NT	(+)[c]	13.26	Sarkar et al. (1992)
Salmonella typhimurium TA1537, reverse mutation	−	+	3	Prival et al. (1980)
Salmonella typhimurium TA98, reverse mutation	(+)	+	3	Prival et al. (1980)
Salmonella typhimurium TA1538, reverse mutation	NT	+	10	Ames et al. (1975); Dybing & Aune (1977); Dybing et al. (1979a)
Salmonella typhimurium TA1538, reverse mutation	NT	+	5	Dybing & Thorgeirsson (1977); Aune & Dybing (1979)
Salmonella typhimurium TA1538, reverse mutation	NT	+	1.4	Aune et al. (1980a)
Salmonella typhimurium TA1538, TA98, reverse mutation	−	+	10	de Giovanni-Donnelly (1981)
Salmonella typhimurium TA1538, reverse mutation	NT	+	60 µg/plate	Mohn et al. (1982)
Salmonella typhimurium TA98, reverse mutation	−	+	19 µg/plate	Yoshikawa et al. (1977)
Salmonella typhimurium TA98, reverse mutation	−	+	20 µg/plate	Bruce & Heddle (1979)
Salmonella typhimurium TA98, reverse mutation	NT	+	10 µg/plate	Aune et al. (1980b)
Salmonella typhimurium TA98, reverse mutation	NT	+	1.25 µg/plate	Parodi et al. (1981)
Salmonella typhimurium TA98, reverse mutation	−	+[d]	50 µg/plate	Maack et al. (1986)
Neurospora crassa, forward mutation, spot test, ad-3 locus	−	NT	400 µg/plate	Ong (1978)
Gene mutation, Chinese hamster V79 cells, Hprt locus in vitro	−	−	552	Fassina et al. (1990)

Table 1 (contd)

Test system	Result[b]		Dose[c] (LED/HID)	Reference
	Without exogenous metabolic system	With exogenous metabolic system		
Cell transformation, Syrian hamster embryo cells, focus assay	–	NT	50	Pienta & Kawalek (1981)
Unscheduled DNA synthesis, human HeLa cells in vitro	+	+	138	Loprieno et al. (1983)
Gene mutation, mouse lymphoma L5178Y cells in vitro, Tk locus	+	NT	19	Palmer et al. (1977)
DNA damage, Sprague-Dawley rat liver cells treated in vivo (alkaline elution assay)	+[e]		91.2 ip × 1	Parodi et al. (1981)
DNA damage, Sprague-Dawley rat liver cells treated in vivo (DNA viscosity)	–		50 ip × 1	Brambilla et al. (1985)
Sister chromatid exchange, male mouse bone-marrow cells in vivo	+		12 ip × 1	Parodi et al. (1983)
Micronucleus formation, rat bone-marrow cells in vivo	–		500 po × 2	Hossack & Richardson (1977)
Micronucleus formation, (C57BL/6 × C3H/He)F$_1$ mouse bone-marrow cells in vivo	–		500 ip × 5	Bruce & Heddle (1979)
Dominant lethal mutation, rats in vivo	–		20 ip × 3/week; 8 weeks	Burnett et al. (1977)
Sperm morphology, (C57BL/6 × C3H/He)F$_1$ mice in vivo	–		500 ip × 5	Bruce & Heddle (1979)
2,4-Diaminoanisole sulfate trihydrate				
Salmonella typhimurium TA100, reverse mutation	–	(+)	333 µg/plate	Dunkel et al. (1985)
Salmonella typhimurium TA100, reverse mutation	–	+	100 µg/plate	Zeiger et al. (1988)
Salmonella typhimurium TA97, reverse mutation	(+)	+	33 µg/plate	Zeiger et al. (1988)
Salmonella typhimurium TA1535, reverse mutation	–	–	10 000 µg/plate	Dunkel et al. (1985)
Salmonella typhimurium TA1535, reverse mutation	–	–	3333 µg/plate	Zeiger et al. (1988)
Salmonella typhimurium TA1537, reverse mutation	–	+	10 µg/plate	Dunkel et al. (1985)
Salmonella typhimurium TA1538, reverse mutation	NT	+[f]	0.87 µg/plate	Robertson et al. (1983)

Table 1 (contd)

Test system	Result[b] Without exogenous metabolic system	Result[b] With exogenous metabolic system	Dose[c] (LED/HID)	Reference
Salmonella typhimurium TA1538, reverse mutation	−	+	1 µg/plate	Dunkel *et al.* (1985)
Salmonella typhimurium TA98, reverse mutation	−	+	3.3 µg/plate	Dunkel *et al.* (1985)
Salmonella typhimurium TA98, reverse mutation	−	+	10 µg/plate	Reddy *et al.* (1980)
Salmonella typhimurium TA98, reverse mutation	+	+	1 µg/plate	Zeiger *et al.* (1988)
Escherichia coli WP2 *uvrA*, reverse mutation	−	−	10 000 µg/plate	Dunkel *et al.* (1985)
Saccharomyces cerevisiae, mitotic recombination (growing cells)	+	NT	500	Mayer & Goin (1980)
Drosophila melanogaster, somatic recombination (w/w⁺ locus)	−		118 feed	Rodriguez-Arnaiz & Hernández Aranda (1994)
Drosophila melanogaster, sex-linked recessive lethal mutations	+		1180 feed	Blijleven (1977)
DNA strand breaks, rat hepatocytes *in vitro* (alkaline elution)	+	NT	708	Storer *et al.* (1996)
Gene mutation, mouse lymphoma L5178Y cells, *Tk* locus *in vitro*	+	+	2	Mitchell *et al.* (1988)
Gene mutation, mouse lymphoma L5178Y cells, *Tk* locus *in vitro*	+	+	3.9	Myhr & Caspary (1988)
Chromosomal aberrations, Chinese hamster lung fibroblasts *in vitro*	+	NT	60	Ishidate (1988)
Urine from rats (50 mg/kg ip × 1), *Salmonella typhimurium* TA98 mutagenicity[g]	−	+	25 µL urine/plate	Reddy *et al.* (1980)
Dominant lethal mutation, Holtzman albino rats *in vivo*	−		40 ip × 3/week; 10 weeks	Sheu & Green (1979)
2,4-Diaminoanisole dihydrochloride				
Salmonella typhimurium TA100, TA1535, reverse mutation	NT	−	1000 µg/plate	Shahin *et al.* (1980)
Salmonella typhimurium TA1537, TA97, reverse mutation	NT	+	50 µg/plate	Shahin *et al.* (1980, 1983, 1985)
Salmonella typhimurium TA1538, TA98, reverse mutation	NT	+	10 µg/plate	Shahin *et al.* (1980)

Table 1 (contd)

Test system	Result[b] Without exogenous metabolic system	Result[b] With exogenous metabolic system	Dose[c] (LED/HID)	Reference
Salmonella typhimurium TA98, reverse mutation	–	+	10 µg/plate	Venitt *et al.* (1984)
Salmonella typhimurium TA1538, reverse mutation	–	+	10 µg/plate	Loprieno *et al.* (1982)
Salmonella typhimurium TA98, reverse mutation (fluctuation test)	NT	+	0.33	Venitt *et al.* (1984)
Salmonella typhimurium TA98, reverse mutation	NT	+	2.5 µg/plate	Loprieno *et al.* (1982)
Salmonella typhimurium TA98, reverse mutation	–	+	10 µg/plate	Watanabe *et al.* (1989)
Salmonella typhimurium TA98, reverse mutation (in the presence of H_2O_2)	+	+	0.03 µg/plate	Watanabe *et al.* (1989)
Saccharomyces cerevisiae D4, mitotic gene conversion	–	+	1055[h]	Loprieno *et al.* (1982)
Schizosaccharomyces pombe, forward mutation *ade* locus	+	+	528	Loprieno *et al.* (1982)
Drosophila melanogaster, sex-linked recessive lethal mutations	+		3165 feed	Blijleven (1982)
Gene mutation, Chinese hamster V79 cells, *Hprt* locus *in vitro*	+	–	844[i]	Loprieno *et al.* (1982)
Chromosomal aberrations, Chinese hamster ovary (CHO) cells *in vitro*	+	+	50	Darroudi *et al.* (1982)
Unscheduled DNA synthesis, human HeLa cells *in vitro*	+	+	176	Loprieno *et al.* (1983)
DNA strand breaks, ddY mice (liver and brain) *in vivo* (Comet assay)	+		200 po × 1	Sasaki *et al.* (1999)
Micronucleus formation, male mouse bone-marrow cells *in vivo*	–		60 ip × 1	Morita *et al.* (1997)
Urine from rats (100 mg/kg bw po or ip), mutation in *Salmonella typhimurium* TA1538, TA98	–	+	100 µL urine/plate	Shahin *et al.* (1980)
Urine from rats (120 mg on skin), mutation in *Salmonella typhimurium* TA1538, TA98	–	+	100 µL urine/plate	Shahin *et al.* (1980)

Table 1 (contd)

Test system	Result[b]		Dose[c] (LED/HID)	Reference
	Without exogenous metabolic system	With exogenous metabolic system		
Urine from rats (100 mg/kg bw po or ip), mutation in *Salmonella typhimurium* TA100	–	–	300 μL urine/ plate	Shahin *et al.* (1980)
Urine from rats (120 mg on skin), mutation in *Salmonella typhimurium* TA100	–	–	300 μL urine/ plate	Shahin *et al.* (1980)

[a] +, positive; (+), weak positive; –, negative; NT, not tested

[b] LED, lowest effective dose; HID, highest ineffective dose; in-vitro tests, μg/mL; in-vivo tests, mg/kg bw per day; ip, intraperitoneal; po, oral

[c] Activation with prostaglandin H synthase

[d] Extracts from mammary tissue of lactating rats and human mammary tumour cell lines

[e] At 4 h after treatment; increase not significant at 24 h

[f] Positive with an exogenous metabolic activation system from a 9000 × g supernatant of rat liver (S9) and, at 10-fold higher dose, with ram seminal vesicle microsomes

[g] Test carried out with 2,4-diaminoanisole disulfate

[h] A threefold higher concentration was negative in the absence of metabolic activation.

[i] 1055 μg/mL was negative in the presence of metabolic activation.

4.6   Mechanistic considerations

2,4-Diaminoanisole is metabolically activated to covalently protein-bound products in rat liver and kidney, but no covalent binding to hepatic DNA was detected. The data on genotoxicity indicate that 2,4-diaminoanisole is genotoxic.

Short-term oral treatment of rats with high doses of diaminoanisole sulfate leads to the development of thyroid tumours and concomitant alterations in thyroid hormone function. The serum concentrations of thyroid-stimulating hormone were elevated and those of thyroxine and triiodothyronine were lowered during the first few weeks after the beginning of treatment. These alterations in hormone concentrations tended to normalize after 6 weeks. The alterations in thyroid hormone homeostasis are presumed to be involved in the induction of thyroid tumours by 2,4-diaminoanisole, but a genotoxic mechanism cannot be excluded.

5.   Summary of Data Reported and Evaluation

5.1   Exposure data

2,4-Diaminoanisole is an aromatic amine which was used extensively in hair dyes and in the dyeing of furs until the late 1970s.

5.2   Human carcinogenicity data

Although epidemiological studies have been conducted on professional and personal users of hair dyes, none made specific mention of 2,4-diaminoanisole.

5.3   Animal carcinogenicity data

2,4-Diaminoanisole sulfate was tested by dietary administration in one experiment in mice and in two experiments in one strain of rats. Thyroid gland adenomas or carcinomas were induced in mice and rats. Tumours of the skin and of the preputial, clitoral and Zymbal glands were also induced in rats. 2,4-Diaminoanisole sulfate was tested for its promoting effects by dietary administration in two strains of rats. In one study in rats, it promoted thyroid gland tumours induced by N-nitrosobis(2-hydroxy-propyl)amine.

5.4   Other relevant data

About 2–4% of a dermal dose of 2,4-diaminoanisole is absorbed by humans, monkeys and rats. The compound is completely absorbed after oral administration to rats, extensively metabolized to free and conjugated acetylated and oxidized products and thereafter excreted in equal percentages of the applied dose in urine and faeces. The substance is metabolically activated to covalently protein-bound products in rat liver and kidney, but no covalent binding to hepatic DNA was detected. Short-term administration of high oral doses to rats induced thyroid enlargement (goitre) and alterations in thyroid hormone homeostasis.

2,4-Diaminoanisole is genotoxic *in vitro*, producing gene mutations and chromosomal damage. It was mutagenic in bacteria in the presence or absence of a microsomal fraction from the livers of uninduced rats, mice, rabbits or humans. It produced chromosomal aberrations and sister chromatid exchange in rodent cells *in vitro*, mitotic recombination in yeast and mutations in insects. The results of most tests in mammals *in vivo* were negative.

5.5   Evaluation

There is *inadequate evidence* in humans for the carcinogenicity of 2,4-diaminoanisole.

There is *sufficient evidence* in experimental animals for the carcinogenicity of 2,4-diaminoanisole.

Overall evaluation

2,4-Diaminoanisole is *possibly carcinogenic to humans (Group 2B)*.

6.   References

American Conference of Governmental Industrial Hygienists (2000) *TLVs and other Occupational Exposure Values — 2000 CD-ROM*, Cincinnati, OH

Ames, B.N., Kammen, H.O. & Yamasaki, E. (1975) Hair dyes are mutagenic: Identification of a variety of mutagenic ingredients. *Proc. natl Acad. Sci. USA*, **72**, 2423–2427

Andrisano, V., Gotti, R., DiPietra, A.M. & Cavrini, V. (1994) Analysis of basic hair dyes by HPLC with on-line post-column photochemical derivatisation. *Chromatographia*, **39**, 138–145

Andrisano, V., Cavrini, V., Summer, P. & Passuti, S. (1995) Determination of impurities in oxidation hair dyes as raw materials by liquid chromatography (HPLC). *Int. J. Cosmet. Sci.*, **17**, 53–60

Anon. (1998a) Method for the detection of certain azo colorants in dyed leather. *J. Soc. Leather Technol. Chem.*, **82**, 251–258

Anon. (1998b) Method for the detection of certain azo colorants in dyestuff mixtures. *J. Soc. Leather Technol. Chem.*, **82**, 259–264

Aune, T. & Dybing, E. (1979) Mutagenic activation of 2,4-diaminoanisole and 2-aminofluorene *in vitro* by liver and kidney fractions from aromatic hydrocarbon responsive and nonresponsive mice. *Biochem. Pharmacol.*, **28**, 2791–2797

Aune, T., Dybing, E. & Nelson, S.D. (1980a) Mutagenic activation of 2,4-diaminoanisole and 2-aminofluorene by isolated rat liver nuclei and microsomes. *Chem.-biol. Interactions*, **31**, 35–49

Aune, T., Dybing, E. & Thorgeirsson, S.S. (1980b) Developmental pattern of 3-methylcholan-threne-inducible mutagenic activation of *N*-2-fluorenylacetamide, 2-fluorenamine, and 2,4-diaminoanisole in the rabbit. *J. natl Cancer Inst.*, **64**, 765–769

Bernabei, M.T., Ferioli, V., Gamberini, G. & Cameroni, R. (1980) [Use of HPLC and IR in the separation and determination of amines, aminophenols, and phenols in hair dyes]. *Atti Soc. nat. Mat. Modena*, **111**, 35–44 (in Italian)

Blijleven, W.G.H. (1977) Mutagenicity of four hair dyes in *Drosophila melanogaster*. *Mutat. Res.*, **48**, 181–186

Blijleven, W.G.H. (1982) Mutagenicity of 2-(2′,4′-diaminophenoxy)ethanol in *Drosophila melanogaster*. *Mutat. Res.*, **102**, 347–349

Brambilla, G., Carlo, P., Finollo, R. & Ledda, A. (1985) Viscometric detection of liver DNA fragmentation in rats treated with ten aromatic amines. Discrepancies with results provided by the alkaline elution technique. *Carcinogenesis*, **6**, 1285–1288

Bruce, W.R. & Heddle, J.A. (1979) The mutagenic activity of 61 agents as determined by the micronucleus, *Salmonella*, and sperm abnormality assays. *Can. J. Genet. Cytol.*, **21**, 319–334

Budavari, S., ed. (2000) *The Merck Index*, 12th Ed., Version 12:3, Whitehouse Station, NJ, Merck & Co. & Boca Raton, FL, Chapman & Hall/CRC [CD-ROM]

Bürgi, C., Bollhalder, R. & Otz, T. (1997) HPLC method for the determination of aromatic amines released from water colours under physiological conditions. *Mitt. geb. Lebensm. Hyg.*, **88**, 305–320

Bürgi, C., Bollhalder, R., Hohl, C., Schlegel, U. & Herrmann, A. (1998) HPLC method for the determination of aromatic amines released from inks of ballpoint and fiber-tip pens under physiological conditions. *Mitt. geb. Lebensm. Hyg.*, **89**, 177–187

Burnett, C., Lanman, B., Giovacchini, R., Wolcott, G., Scala, R. & Keplinger, M. (1975) Long-term toxicity studies on oxidation hair dyes. *Food Cosmet. Toxicol.*, **13**, 353–357

Burnett, C., Goldenthal, E.I., Harris, S.B., Wazeter, F.X., Strausburg, J., Kapp, R. & Voelker, R. (1976) Teratology and percutaneous toxicity studies on hair dyes. *J. Toxicol. environ. Health*, **1**, 1027–1040

Burnett, C., Loehr, R. & Corbett, J. (1977) Dominant lethal mutagenicity study on hair dyes. *J. Toxicol. environ. Health*, **2**, 657–662

Chen, X., Zhen, Z. & Shi, X. (1998) [Determination of prohibited azo dyes in leather and textile materials by HPLC.] *Fenxi Ceshi Xuebao*, **17**, 50–53 (in Chinese)

Cioni, F., Bartolucci, G., Pieraccini, G., Meloni, S. & Moneti, G. (1999) Development of a solid phase microextraction method for detection of the use of banned azo dyes in coloured textiles and leather. *Rapid Commun. Mass Spectrom.*, **13**, 1833–1837

CIS Information Services (2000) *Directory of World Chemical Producers* (Version 2000.1), Dallas, TX [CD-ROM]

Correa, A., Jackson, L., Mohan, A., Perry, H. & Helzlsouer, K. (2000a) Use of hair dyes, hematopoietic neoplasms, and lymphomas: A literature review. I. Leukemias and myelo-dysplastic syndromes. *Cancer Invest.*, **18**, 366–380

Correa, A., Jackson, L., Mohan, A., Perry, H. & Helzlsouer, K. (2000b) Use of hair dyes, hematopoietic neoplasms, and lymphomas: A literature review. II. Lymphomas and multiple myeloma. *Cancer Invest.*, **18**, 467–479

Darroudi, F., van Kesteren-van Leeuwen, A.C. & Natarajan, A.T. (1982) Test for induction of chromosomal aberrations in Chinese hamster ovary cells (in vitro) by 2-(2',4'-diamino-phenoxy)ethanol. *Mutat. Res.*, **102**, 351–355

Deutsche Forschungsgemeinschaft (2000) *List of MAK and BAT Values 2000* (Report No. 36), Weinheim, Wiley-VCH Verlag GmbH, p. 45

Dunkel, V.C., Zeiger, E., Brusick, D., McCoy, E., McGregor, D., Mortelmans, K., Rosenkranz, H.S. & Simmon, V.F. (1985) Reproducibility of microbial mutagenicity assays. II. Testing of carcinogens and noncarcinogens in *Salmonella typhimurium* and *Escherichia coli*. *Environ. Mutag.*, **7** (Suppl. 5), 1–248

Dybing E. & Aune, T. (1977) Hexachlorobenzene induction of 2,4-diaminoanisole muta-genicity in vitro. *Acta pharmacol. toxicol.*, **40**, 575–583

Dybing, E. & Thorgeirsson, S.S. (1977) Metabolic activation of 2,4-diaminoanisole, a hair-dye component. I. Role of cytochrome P-450 metabolism in mutagenicity *in vitro*. *Biochem. Pharmacol.*, **26**, 729–734

Dybing, E., Aune, T. & Nelson, S.D. (1979a) Metabolic activation of 2,4-diaminoanisole, a hair-dye component. II. Role of cytochrome P-450 metabolism in irreversible binding *in vitro*. *Biochem. Pharmacol.*, **28**, 43–50

Dybing, E., Aune, T. & Nelson, S.D. (1979b) Metabolic activation of 2,4-diaminoanisole, a hair-dye component. III. Role of cytochrome P-450 metabolism in irreversible binding *in vivo*. *Biochem. Pharmacol.*, **28**, 51–55

Evarts, R.P. & Brown, C.A. (1980) 2,4-Diaminoanisole sulfate: Early effect on thyroid gland morphology and late effect on glandular tissue of Fischer 344 rats. *J. natl Cancer Inst.*, **65**, 197–204

Fassina, G., Abbondandolo, A., Mariani, L., Taningher, M. & Parodi, S. (1990) Mutagenicity in V79 cells does not correlate with carcinogenicity in small rodents for 12 aromatic amines. *J. Toxicol. environ. Health*, **29**, 109–130

Friedrichs, K., Winkeler, H.-D. & Prior, G. (1995) [Determination of carcinogenic amines from azo dyes by GC/MS analysis]. *GIT Fachz. Lab.*, **39**, 901–902, 905–910 (in German)

de Giovanni-Donnelly, R. (1981) The comparative response of *Salmonella typhimurium* strains TA1538, TA98 and TA100 to various hair-dye components. *Mutat. Res.*, **91**, 21–25

Gottschalck, H. & Machens, R. (1982) [Identification and quantitative determination of oxidation dyes in hair dyes and hair tints.] *J. Soc. Cosmet. Chem.*, **33**, 97–114 (in German)

Grantham, P.H., Benjamin, T., Tahan, L.C., Roller, P.P., Miller, J.R. & Weisburger, E.K. (1979) Metabolism of the dyestuff intermediate 2,4-diaminoanisole in the rat. *Xenobiotica*, **9**, 333–341

Hasegawa, R., Shirai, T., Hakoi, K., Wada, S., Yamaguchi, K. & Takayama, S. (1991) Synergistic enhancement of thyroid tumor induction by 2,4-diaminoanisole sulfate, *N,N'*-diethylthiourea and 4,4'-thiodianiline in male F344 rats. *Carcinogenesis*, **12**, 1515–1518

Hofer, H. & Hruby, E. (1983) Skin penetration by 2,4-diaminoanisole in the rat. *Food chem. Toxicol.*, **21**, 331–334

Hoogewijs, G. & Massart, D.L. (1983) Development of a standardized analysis strategy for basic drugs, using ion-pair extraction and high-performance liquid chromatography. Part V. Separation and determination of aminophenols and phenylenediamine derivatives in hair dye products. *J. Pharm. belg.*, **38**, 76–80

Hossack, D.J.N. & Richardson, J.C. (1977) Examination of the potential mutagenicity of hair dye constituents using the micronucleus test. *Experientia*, **33**, 377–378

IARC (1978) *IARC Monographs on the Evaluation of the Carcinogenic Risk of Chemicals to Man*, Vol. 16, *Some Aromatic Amines and Related Nitro Compounds — Hair Dyes, Colouring Agents and Miscellaneous Industrial Chemicals*, Lyon, IARCPress, pp. 51–62

IARC (1982) *IARC Monographs on the Evaluation of the Carcinogenic Risk of Chemicals to Humans*, Vol. 27, *Some Aromatic Amines, Anthraquinones and Nitroso Compounds, and Inorganic Fluorides Used in Drinking-water and Dental Preparations*, Lyon, IARCPress, pp. 103–117

IARC (1987) *IARC Monographs on the Evaluation of Carcinogenic Risks to Humans*, Suppl. 7, *Overall Evaluations of Carcinogenicity: An Updating of* IARC Monographs *Volumes 1 to 42*, Lyon, IARCPress, p. 61

IARC (1993) *IARC Monographs on the Evaluation of Carcinogenic Risks to Humans*, Vol. 57, *Occupational Exposures of Hairdressers and Barbers and Personal Use of Hair Colourants; Some Hair Dyes, Cosmetic Colourants, Industrial Dyestuffs and Aromatic Amines*, Lyon, IARCPress, pp. 43–118

Ishidate, M., Jr, ed. (1988) *Data Book of Chromosomal Aberration Test In Vitro*, Amsterdam, Life-Science Information Center

Johansson, K., Rappe, C., Lindberg, W. & Nygren, M. (1981) Method 13. Determination of aromatic diamines in hair dyes using liquid chromatography. In: Egan, H., Fishbein, L., Castegnaro, M., O'Neill, I.K. & Bartsch, H., eds, *Environmental Carcinogens. Selected Methods of Analysis*, Vol. 4, *Some Aromatic Amines and Azo Dyes in the General and Industrial Environment* (IARC Scientific Publication No. 40), Lyon, IARCPress, pp. 243–247

Kellert, H.-J., Maier, R. & Delor, B. (1999) [Determination of aromatic amines from azo dyes.] *Leder Häute Markt*, **5**, 25–32 (in German)

Kersemaekers, W.M., Roeleveld, N. & Zielhuis, G.A. (1995) Reproductive disorders due to chemical exposure among hairdressers. *Scand. J. Work Environ. Health*, **21**, 325–334

Kinkel, H.J. & Holzmann, S. (1973) Study of long-term percutaneous toxicity and carcinogenicity of hair dyes (oxidizing dyes) in rats. *Food Cosmet. Toxicol.*, **11**, 641–648

Kitahori, Y., Ohshima, M., Matsuki, H., Konishi, N., Hashimoto, H., Minami, S., Thamavit, W. & Hiasa, Y. (1989) Promoting effect of 2,4-diaminoanisole sulfate on rat thyroid carcinogenesis. *Cancer Lett.*, **45**, 115–121

Lide, D.R. & Milne, G.W.A. (1996) *Properties of Organic Compounds*, Version 5.0, Boca Raton, FL, CRC Press [CD-ROM]

Liem, D.H. & Rooselaar, J. (1981) HPLC of oxidation hair colors. *Mitt. geb. Lebensmitt. Hyg.*, **72**, 164–176

Loprieno, N., Barale, R., Mariani, L. & Zaccaro, L. (1982) Mutagenic studies on the hair dye 2-(2',4'-diaminophenoxy)ethanol with different genetic systems. *Mutat. Res.*, **102**, 331–346

Loprieno, N., Mariani, L. & Rusciano, D. (1983) Lack of genotoxic properties of the hair-dye component N-methyl-amino-2-nitro-4-N',N'-bis-(2-hydroxyethyl)aminobenzene, in mammalian cells *in vitro*, and in yeasts. *Mutat. Res.*, **116**, 161–168

Maack, C.A., Silva, M.H., Petrakis, N.L., Lee, R.E. & Lyon, M. (1986) Procarcinogen activation by rat and human mammary extracts. *Carcinogenesis*, **7**, 899–905

Mancini, G., Polesi, R., Cantarini, R., Sarrocco, G. & Salvetti, E. (1981) [Study on the presence of banned dyes in hair coloring materials.] *Boll. Chim. Farm.*, **120**, 708–714 (in Italian)

Marzulli, F.N., Anjo, D.M. & Maibach, H.I. (1981) *In vivo* skin penetration studies of 2,4-toluenediamine, 2,4-diaminoanisole, 2-nitro-*p*-phenylenediamine, *p*-dioxane and *N*-nitrosodiethanolamine in cosmetics. *Food Cosmet. Toxicol.*, **19**, 743–747

Mayer, V.W. & Goin, C.J. (1980) Induction of mitotic recombination by certain hair-dye chemicals in *Saccharomyces cerevisiae*. *Mutat. Res.*, **78**, 243–252

Mayer, M., Kesners, P. & Mandel, F. (1998) [Determination of carcinogenic azo-dyes by HPLC/MS analysis.] *GIT Spez. Chromatogr.*, **18**, 20–23 (in German)

Mitchell, A.D., Rudd, C.J. & Caspary, W.J. (1988) Evaluation of the L5178Y mouse lymphoma cell mutagenesis assay: Intralaboratory results for sixty-three coded chemicals tested at SRI International. *Environ. mol. Mutag.*, **12** (Suppl. 13), 37–101

Mohn, G., Bouter, S. & de Knijff, P. (1982) Mutagenic activity of 2-(2',4'-diaminophenoxy)-ethanol in strains TA1538 and TA98 of *Salmonella typhimurium*. *Mutat. Res.*, **102**, 313–318

Morita, T., Asano, N., Awogi, T., Sasaki, Y.F., Sato, S., Shimada, H., Sutou, S., Suzuki, T., Wakata, A., Sofuni, T. & Hayashi, M. (1997) Evaluation of the rodent micronucleus assay in the screening of IARC carcinogens (Groups 1, 2A and 2B). The summary report of the 6th collaborative study by CSGMT/JEMS.MMS. *Mutat. Res.*, **389**, 3–122

Myhr, B.C. & Caspary, W.J. (1988) Evaluation of the L5178Y mouse lymphoma cell mutagenesis assay: Intralaboratory results for sixty-three coded chemicals tested at Litton Bionetics, Inc. *Environ. mol. Mutag.*, **12** (Suppl. 13), 103–194

National Cancer Institute (1978) *Bioassay of 2,4-Diaminoanisole Sulfate for Possible Carcinogenicity* (Tech. Rep. Ser. No. 84; DHEW Publ. No. (NIH) 78-1334), Washington DC, Government Printing Office

National Institute for Occupational Safety and Health (1978) *2,4-Diaminoanisole (4-Methoxy-m-phenylenediamine) in Hair and Fur Dyes* (Current Intelligence Bulletin 19; DHEW (NIOSH) Publ. No. 78-111), Rockville, MD

National Institute for Occupational Safety and Health (2000) *National Occupational Exposure Survey 1981–83*, Cincinnati, OH, Department of Health and Human Services, Public Health Service

Ohshima, H., Yamada, S., Noda, N., Hayakawa, J., Uno, K. & Narafu, T. (1982) [Analysis of hair dyes. I. Determination of hair dye ingredients in oxidative hair dyes by thin layer densitometry.] *Eisei Kagaku*, **28**, 330–334 (in Japanese)

Ong, T.-M. (1978) Use of the spot, plate and suspension test systems for the detection of the mutagenicity of environmental agents and chemical carcinogens in *Neurospora crassa*. *Mutat. Res.*, **53**, 297–308

Palmer, K.A., Denunzio, A. & Green, S. (1977) The mutagenic assay of some hair dye components using the thymidine kinase locus of L5178Y mouse lymphoma cells. *J. environ. Pathol. Toxicol.*, **1**, 87–91

Parodi, S., Taningher, M., Russo, P., Pala, M., Tamaro, M. & Monti-Bragadin, C. (1981) DNA-damaging activity *in vivo* and bacterial mutagenicity of sixteen aromatic amines and azo-derivatives, as related quantitatively to their carcinogenicity. *Carcinogenesis*, **2**, 1317–1326

Parodi, S., Zunino, A., Ottaggio, L., De Ferrari, M. & Santi, L. (1983) Lack of correlation between the capability of inducing sister-chromatid exchanges *in vivo* and carcinogenic potency, for 16 aromatic amines and azo derivatives. *Mutat. Res.*, **108**, 225–238

Pienta, R.J. & Kawalek, J.C. (1981) Transformation of hamster embryo cells by aromatic amines. *Natl Cancer Inst. Monogr.*, **58**, 243–251

Planelles, F., Verdú, E., Campello, D., Grane, N. & Santiago, J.M. (1998) Determination of carcinogenic amines in azo dyes. *J. Soc. Leather Technol. Chem.*, **83**, 45–52

Planelles, F., Verdú, E., Campello, D., Grane, N. & Santiago, J.M. (1999) Determination of carcinogenic amines in dyed leathers. *J. Soc. Leather Technol. Chem.*, **83**, 125–134

Prival, M.J., Mitchell, V.D. & Gomez, Y.P. (1980) Mutagenicity of a new hair dye ingredient: 4-Ethoxy-*m*-phenylenediamine. *Science*, **207**, 907–908

Reddy, T.V., Benjamin, T., Grantham, P.H., Weisburger, E.K. & Thorgeirsson, S.S. (1980) Mutagenicity of urine from rats after administration of 2,4-diaminoanisole. *Mutat. Res.*, **79**, 307–317

Richter, F., ed. (1933) *Beilsteins Handbuch der Organischen Chemie*, 4th ed., 1st Suppl., Vol. 13, Syst. No. 1854, Berlin, Springer, p. 204 (in German)

Robertson, I.G.C., Sivarajah, K., Eling, T.E. & Zeiger, E. (1983) Activation of some aromatic amines to mutagenic products by prostaglandin endoperoxide synthetase. *Cancer Res.*, **43**, 476–480

Rodriguez-Arnaiz, R. & Hernández Aranda, J. (1994) Activity of aromatic amines in the eye: *w/w+* somatic assay of *Drosophila melanogaster*. *Environ. mol. Mutag.*, **24**, 75–79

Sadtler Research Laboratories (1980) *Sadtler Standard Spectra, 1980 Cumulative Molecular Formula Index*, Philadelphia, PA, p. 170

Sardas, S., Sener, B. & Karakaya, A.E. (1985) High-performance liquid chromatographic analysis of hair dye ingredients. *J. Fac. Pharm. Gazi*, **2**, 51–57

Sarkar, F.H., Radcliff, G. & Callewaert, D.M. (1992) Purified prostaglandin synthase activates aromatic amines to derivatives that are mutagenic to *Salmonella typhimurium*. *Mutat. Res.*, **282**, 273–281

Sasaki, Y. F., Fujukawa, K., Ishida, K., Kawamura, N., Nishikawa, Y., Ohta, S., Satoh, M., Madarame, H., Ueno, S., Susa, N., Matsusaka, N. & Tsuda, S. (1999) The alkaline single cell gel electrophoresis assay with mouse multiple organs: Results with 30 aromatic amines evaluated by the IARC and the US NTP. *Mutat. Res.*, **440**, 1–18 (see Erratum: *Mutat. Res.*, **444**, 249–255)

Savela, A., Vuorela, R. & Kauppinen, T. (1999) *ASA 1997* (Katsauksia 140), Helsinki, Finnish Institute of Occupational Health, p. 30 (in Finnish)

Shahin, M.M., Rouers, D., Bugaut, A. & Kalopissis, G. (1980) Structure–activity relationships within a series of 2,4-diaminoalkoxybenzene compounds. *Mutat. Res.*, **79**, 289–306

Shahin, M.M., Chopy, C., Mayet, M.J. & Lequesne, N. (1983) Mutagenicity of structurally related aromatic amines in the *Salmonella*/mammalian microsome test with various S-9 fractions. *Food chem. Toxicol.*, **21**, 615–619

Shahin, M.M., Chopy, C. & Lequesne, N. (1985) Comparisons of mutation induction by six monocyclic aromatic amines in *Salmonella typhimurium* tester strains TA97, TA1537, and TA1538. *Environ. Mutag.*, **7**, 535–546

Sheu, C.-J.W. & Green, S. (1979) Dominant lethal assay of some hair-dye components in random-bred male rats. *Mutat. Res.*, **68**, 85–98

Sinha, A.P. & Kumar, R. (1999) Standardization of TLC method for identification of carcinogenic aryl amines in coloured textile and leather products. *Asian J. Chem.*, **11**, 1549–1552

Štancer, A. & Jeretin, B. (1998) [Aromatic amines in consumer goods and their determination by HPLC with a diode array detector (DAD).] In: Glavic, P. & Brodnjak-Voncina, D., eds, *Zbornik Referatov Posvetovanja Slovenski Kemijski Dnevi*, Maribor, Slovenia, Fakulteta za Kemijo in Kemijsko Tehnologijo Univerze v Mariboru, pp. 35–43 (in Slovenian)

Storer, R.D., McKelvey, T.W., Kraynak, A.R., Elia, M.C., Barnum, J.E., Harmon, L.S., Nichols, W.W. & DeLuca, J.G. (1996) Revalidation of the in vitro alkaline elution/rat hepatocyte assay for DNA damage: Improved criteria for assessment of cytotoxicity and genotoxicity and results for 81 compounds. *Mutat. Res.*, **368**, 59–101

TCI America (2000) *Certificate of Analysis: 2,4-Diaminoanisole Dihydrochloride* (Stock No. D0074), Portland, OR

Tomaselli, M., Cozzolino, A., Stasio, A. & Castiello, G. (1998) [Methods for analysis of azo dyes.] *Cuoio Pelli Mater. concianti*, **74**, 231–245 (in Italian)

UNEP (2000) *UNEP Chemicals (IRPTC) Data Bank Legal File, Recommendations and Legal Mechanisms*, Geneva, World Health Organization [http://dbserver.irptc.unep.ch: 8887/irptc/owa/lg.get_search]

Venitt, S., Crofton-Sleigh, C. & Osborne, M.R. (1984) The hair-dye reagent 2-(2′,4′-diaminophenoxy)ethanol is mutagenic to *Salmonella typhimurium*. *Mutat. Res.*, **135**, 31–47

Verdú, E., Planelles, F., Campello, D., Grané, N. & Santiago, J.M. (1996) [Identification of arylamines using gas chromatography–mass spectrometry.] *Bol. Téc. Asoc. Quim. Esp. Ind. Cuero*, **47**, 60–69, 72–74 (in Spanish)

Verdú, E., Planelles, F., Campello, D., Grané, N. & Santiago, J.M. (1997) [Determination of aromatic amines by HPLC (I).] *Tec. Lab.*, **19**, 752–761 (in Spanish)

Wang, L.-H. & Chen, Z.-S. (1998) Determination of phenylenediamines in oxidative hair dyes by differential pulse voltammetry. *J. Chin. chem. Soc.*, **45**, 53–58

Watanabe, T., Hirayama, T. & Fukui, S. (1989) Phenazine derivatives as the mutagenic reaction product from *o*- or *m*-phenylenediamine derivatives with hydrogen peroxide. *Mutat. Res.*, **227**, 135–145

Winkeler, H.D. (1996) [Determination of carcinogenic aromatic amines by HPLC/DAD-analysis.] *GIT Spez. Chromatogr.*, **16**, 6–8, 10–11 (in German)

Xiao, Q., Zheng, J. & Zhai, C. (1999) [Application of characteristic mass ion detection method in GC–MS determination of forbidden azo-dyes.] *Fenxi Ceshi Xuebao*, **18**, 32–35 (in Chinese)

Yang, Y., Liang, M. & Xiao, Q. (2000) [Determination of aromatic amines in colored leather by high performance liquid chromatography.] *Fenxi Huaxue*, **28**, 77–79 (in Chinese)

Yoshikawa, K., Uchino, H., Tateno, N. & Kurata, H. (1977) [Mutagenic activities of the samples prepared with raw material of hair dye.] *Eisei Shikensho Hokuku*, **95**, 15–24 (in Japanese)

Zbinden, G. (1988) Evaluation of thyroid gland activity by hormone assays and flow cytometry in rats. *Exp. Cell Biol.*, **56**, 196–200

Zeiger, E., Anderson, B., Haworth, S., Lawlor, T. & Mortelmans, K. (1988) *Salmonella* mutagenicity tests. IV. Results from the testing of 300 chemicals. *Environ. mol. Mutag.*, **11** (Suppl. 12), 1–158

INDUSTRIAL CHEMICALS

N,N'-DIETHYLTHIOUREA

1. Exposure Data

1.1   Chemical and physical data

1.1.1   *Nomenclature*

Chem. Abstr. Serv. Reg. No.: 105-55-5
Deleted CAS Reg. No.: 27598-95-4
Chem. Abstr. Name: *N,N'*-Diethylthiourea
IUPAC Systematic Name: 1,3-Diethyl-2-thiourea
Synonyms: *N,N'*-Diethylthiocarbamide; 1,3-diethylthiourea

1.1.2   *Structural and molecular formulae and relative molecular mass*

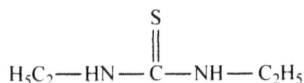

$$H_5C_2-HN-\overset{\overset{\displaystyle S}{\|}}{C}-NH-C_2H_5$$

C$_5$H$_{12}$N$_2$S   Relative molecular mass: 132.23

1.1.3   *Chemical and physical properties of the pure substance*

(*a*) *Description*: White solid (R.T. Vanderbilt Co., 1997)
(*b*) *Boiling-point*: Decomposes (Lide & Milne, 1996)
(*c*) *Melting-point*: 78 °C (Lide & Milne, 1996)
(*d*) *Spectroscopy data*: Infrared [proton (3661), grating (28294)], ultraviolet, nuclear magnetic resonance [proton (190), C-13 (5207)] and mass spectral data have been reported (Sadtler Research Laboratories, 1980; Lide & Milne, 1996).
(*e*) *Solubility*: Very slightly soluble in water; soluble in ethanol; very soluble in diethyl ether; slightly soluble in carbon tetrachloride (Lide & Milne, 1996; R.T. Vanderbilt Co, 1997; Dialog Corp., 2000)

1.1.4   *Technical products and impurities*

Trade names for *N,N'*-diethylthiourea include Accel EUR, Nocceler EUR, Pennzone E, Thiate H and U 15030.

1.1.5   *Analysis*

A method for the isolation, identification and determination of thioureas, including *N,N'*-diethylthiourea, in rat plasma by high-performance liquid chromatography (HPLC) with ultraviolet detection has been reported (Kobayashi *et al.*, 1981). Analysis of lubricating oil additives for *N,N'*-diethylthiourea by HPLC (Musha *et al.*, 1985) and determination with iodine monochloride or by redox titration (Murthy *et al.*, 1979; Verma, 1979) have also been reported.

1.2   Production

N,N'-Diethylthiourea can be made from ethylamine and carbon disulfide (Ohm, 1997).

Information available in 2000 indicated that *N,N'*-diethylthiourea was manufactured by three companies each in France and Japan and one company each in the Netherlands, the United Kingdom and the USA (CIS Information Systems, 2000).

1.3   Use

N,N'-Diethylthiourea is used mainly in the rubber industry as an accelerator for the vulcanization of several types of rubber with reactive cross-linking sites, including polychloroprene (neoprene), ethylene–propylene–diene and chlorobutyl rubber. The suggested concentration ranges from 0.5 to 1.0 %. Chlorinated rubber derivatives are used, among other applications, as resins in some paints (IARC, 1989). The use of thioureas is decreasing, and they are supplied preferably as polymer-bound granulates, which effectively prevent exposure to and inhalation of thiourea dust (Engels, 1993; Ohm, 1997; R.T. Vanderbilt Co., 1997).

1.4   Occurrence

1.4.1   *Occupational exposure*

According to the 1981–83 National Occupational Exposure Survey (National Institute for Occupational Safety and Health, 2000), only about 230 painters or paint-spraying machine workers in the USA were potentially exposed to *N,N'*-diethyl-thiourea. According to the Finnish Register of Employees Exposed to Carcinogens, 13 workers including laboratory workers and surface treatment workers were exposed in Finland in 1997 (Savela *et al.*, 1999).

1.4.2 *Environmental occurrence*

No data were available to the Working Group.

1.5 Regulations and guidelines

No data were available to the Working Group.

2. Studies of Cancer in Humans

Although workers in the rubber industry may be exposed to *N,N'*-diethylthiourea, no specific mention of this compound was found in epidemiological studies of the cancer risk of these populations.

3. Studies of Cancer in Experimental Animals

3.1 Oral administration

Mouse: Groups of 50 male and 50 female B6C3F$_1$ mice, 6 weeks of age, were fed diets containing 125 or 250 mg/kg *N,N'*-diethylthiourea (> 99% pure) for 103 weeks. A control group of 19 males and 20 females was available. The mice were killed at 104 weeks and evaluated for neoplasms. A dose-related depression of mean body weight was observed in both male and female mice after week 30. The survival rate was comparable in treated and control groups, being 79–94% for males and 60–70% for females. There were no significant increases in the incidences of neoplasms, including thyroid follicular-cell neoplasms, associated with the administration of *N,N'*-diethyl-thiourea in males or females. However, there was a significant ($p < 0.01$) decrease in the incidence of combined hepatocellular adenomas and carcinomas in male mice treated at the higher concentration, which may have been related to the depression in body weight (National Cancer Institute, 1979).

Rat: Groups of 50 male and 50 female Fischer 344 rats, 6 weeks of age, were fed diets containing 125 or 250 mg/kg *N,N'*-diethylthiourea (> 99% pure) for 103 weeks. A group of 20 males and 20 females served as controls. The rats were killed at 104 weeks and evaluated for neoplasms. No evidence of a change in mean body weight was observed in either male or female rats, and the survival rates were comparable in treated and control groups, being 80–82% for males and 84–90% for females. The incidences of thyroid follicular-cell adenomas were 0/18, 0/45 and 6/48 males and 0/18, 4/46 and 9/46 females at 0, 125 or 250 mg/kg of diet, respectively. The incidences of thyroid follicular-cell carcinomas were 0/18, 1/45 and 11/45 males and 0/18, 1/46 and 8/46 females in these groups, respectively. The incidences of follicular-cell adenomas and carcinomas combined were 0/18, 1/45 and 15/48 males and 0/18, 4/46 and 17/46 females, that in males and in females at the highest concentration being significantly ($p < 0.05$; Fisher exact test) higher than in the respective control groups. There was no significant increase in the incidence of tumours at other sites in male or female rats (National Cancer Institute, 1979).

3.2 Administration with known carcinogens or modifying factors

Rat: In a study to assess the synergistic effect of three thyroid carcinogens, 2,4-diaminoanisole sulfate, *N,N'*-diethylthiourea and 4,4'-thiodianiline, groups of 20–21 male Fischer 344/Crj rats, 6 weeks of age, were fed a diet containing 200 mg/kg *N,N'*-diethylthiourea for 52 weeks alone or in combination with 2,4-diaminoanisole sulfate at 610 mg/kg and 4,4'-thiodianiline at 46 mg/kg of diet. After 52 weeks of treatment, the rats were killed, necropsied and evaluated for tumour incidences. *N,N'*-Diethylthiourea induced thyroid follicular-cell carcinoma in 1/21 (5%) rats and significantly ($p < 0.01$) increased the incidence of thyroid follicular-cell carcinomas produced by 4,4'-thiodianiline. *N,N'*-Diethylthiourea did not induce liver tumours or lung tumours after 52 weeks, but may have increased the incidences of these tumours caused by 4,4'-thiodianiline (Hasegawa *et al.*, 1991). [From the study design, the Working Group considered that it was not possible to assess the synergistic effect of *N,N'*-diethylthiourea, if any, on the incidence of thyroid follicular-cell carcinomas induced by 4,4'-thiodianiline.]

4. Other Data Relevant to an Evaluation of Carcinogenicity and its Mechanisms

4.1 Absorption, distribution, metabolism and excretion

No data were available to the Working Group.

4.2 Toxic effects

4.2.1 *Humans*

A 27-year-old man developed contact dermatitis to *N,N'*-diethylthiourea used to vulcanize a wet suit (Adams, 1982).

Contact dermatitis followed by depigmentation was reported in a 50-year-old man exposed to *N,N'*-diethylthiourea in a rubber attachment for a sleep apnoea device (Reynaerts *et al.*, 1998).

4.2.2   *Experimental systems*

No data were available to the Working Group.

4.3   Reproductive and developmental effects

No data were available to the Working Group.

4.4   Effects on enzyme induction/inhibition and gene expression

4.4.1   *Humans*

No data were available to the Working Group.

4.4.2   *Experimental systems*

Male Sprague-Dawley rat microsomal systems were used to assess the induction of microsomal epoxide hydrolase and glutathione *S*-transferase A2 mRNAs. Treatment with an oral dose of *N,N'*-diethylthiourea at 160 mg/kg bw increased (by 7–10-fold) the mRNA levels of both enzymes at 24 h. The microsomal epoxide hydrolase and gluta-thione *S*-transferase A2 protein contents were induced approximately threefold after 3 days of oral treatment with 0.6 mmol/kg bw [80 mg/kg bw] per day *N,N'*-diethylthiourea (Kim *et al.*, 1999).

4.5   Genetic and related effects

4.5.1   *Humans*

No data were available to the Working Group.

4.5.2   *Experimental systems* (see Table 1 for references)

N,N'-Diethylthiourea was not mutagenic to *Salmonella typhimurium* in an assay with preincubation with or without metabolic activation. It was mutagenic in mouse lymphoma L5178Y cells without metabolic activation. Sex-linked recessive lethal mutations were not produced in treated male *Drosophila melanogaster*. *N,N'*-Diethyl-thiourea transformed Syrian hamster embryo cells in culture.

4.6   Mechanistic considerations

No information was available on the mechanism of action of *N,N'*-diethylthiourea.

Table 1. Genetic and related effects of N,N'-diethylthiourea

Test system	Result[a]		Dose[b] (LED/HID)	Reference
	Without exogenous metabolic system	With exogenous metabolic system		
Salmonella typhimurium TA100, TA1535, TA1537, TA98, reverse mutation	–	–	10 000 µg/plate	Mortelmans *et al.* (1986)
Drosophila melanogaster, sex-linked recessive lethal mutation	–		3000 ppm feed	Valencia *et al.* (1985)
Drosophila melanogaster, sex-linked recessive lethal mutation	–		10 000 ppm inj	Valencia *et al.* (1985)
Gene mutation, mouse lymphoma L5178Y cells *in vitro*	+	NT	1500	McGregor *et al.* (1988)
Cell transformation, Syrian hamster embryo cells *in vitro*	+	NT	150	LeBoeuf *et al.* (1996)

[a] +, positive; –, negative; NT, not tested
[b] LED, lowest effective dose; HID, highest ineffective dose; in-vitro tests, µg/mL; inj, injection

5. Summary of Data Reported and Evaluation

5.1   Exposure data

N,N'-Diethylthiourea is used in the manufacture of some types of rubber and paint.

5.2   Human carcinogenicity data

No data were available to the Working Group.

5.3 Animal carcinogenicity data

N,N'-Diethylthiourea was tested for carcinogenicity by dietary administration in one experiment each in mice and rats. Thyroid follicular-cell adenomas and carcinomas were induced in rats of each sex, but no increase in the incidence of tumours at any site was seen in mice.

5.4   Other relevant data

No data were available on the absorption, distribution, metabolism or excretion of *N,N'*-diethylthiourea. The only toxic effect seen in humans was contact dermatitis. No data were available on the reproductive or developmental effects of this compound.

N,N'-Diethylthiourea did not cause mutation in bacteria or insects. In single studies, it showed mutagenic activity in mouse lymphoma cells, in the absence of metabolic activation, and it transformed hamster embryo cells in culture.

5.5   Evaluation

There is *inadequate evidence* in humans for the carcinogenicity of *N,N'*-diethylthiourea.

There is *limited evidence* in experimental animals for the carcinogenicity of *N,N'*-diethylthiourea.

Overall evaluation

N,N'-Diethylthiourea is *not classifiable as to its carcinogenicity to humans (Group 3)*.

6. References

Adams, R.M. (1982) Contact allergic dermatitis due to diethylthiourea in a wet suit. *Contact Derm.*, **8**, 277–278

CIS Information Services (2000) *Directory of World Chemical Producers (Version 2000.1)*, Dallas, TX [CD-ROM]

Dialog Corp. (2000) *Beilstein Online (File 390)*, Cary NC

Engels, H.W. (1993) *Rubber, 4. Chemicals and additives (Part 1)*. In: Elvers, B., Hawkins, S., Russey, W. & Schulz, G., eds, *Ullmann's Encyclopedia of Industrial Chemistry, Vol. A23*, 5th rev. Ed., New York, VCH Publishers, pp. 365–380

Hasegawa, R., Shirai, T., Hakoi, K., Wada, S., Yamaguchi, K. & Takayama, S. (1991) Synergistic enhancement of thyroid tumor induction by 2,4-diaminoanisole sulfate, N,N'-diethylthiourea and 4,4'-thiodianiline in male F344 rats. *Carcinogenesis*, **12**, 1515–1518

IARC (1989) *IARC Monographs on the Evaluation of Carcinogenic Risks to Humans*, Vol. 47, *Some Organic Solvents, Resin Monomers and Related Compounds, Pigments and Occupational Exposures in Paint Manufacture and Painting*, Lyon, IARC*Press*, p. 332

Kim, S.G., Kim, H.J. & Yang, C.H. (1999) Thioureas differentially induce rat hepatic microsomal epoxide hydrolase and rGSTA2 irrespective of their oxygen radical scavenging effect: Effects on toxicant-induced liver injury. *Chem.-biol. Interactions*, **117**, 117–134

Kobayashi, H., Matano, O. & Goto, S. (1981) Simultaneous quantitation of thioureas in rat plasma by high-performance liquid chromatography. *J. Chromatogr.*, **207**, 281–285

LeBoeuf, R.A., Kerckaert, G.A., Aardema, M.J., Gibson, D.P., Brauninger, R. & Isfort, R.J. (1996) The pH 6.7 Syrian hamster embryo cell transformation assay for assessing the carcinogenic potential of chemicals. *Mutat. Res.*, **356**, 85–127

Lide, D.R. & Milne, G.W.A. (1996) *Properties of Organic Compounds, Version 5.0*, Boca Raton, FL, CRC Press [CD-ROM]

McGregor, D.B., Brown, A., Cattanach, P., Edwards, I., McBride, D., Riach, C. & Caspary, W.J. (1988) Responses of the L5178Y tk+/tk− mouse lymphoma cell forward mutation assay: III. 72 coded chemicals. *Environ. mol. Mutag.*, **12**, 85–154

Mortelmans, K., Haworth, S., Lawlor, T., Speck, W., Tainer, B. & Zeiger, E. (1986) Salmonella mutagenicity tests: II. Results from the testing of 270 chemicals. *Environ. Mutag.*, **8** (Suppl. 7), 1–119

Murthy, N.K., Prasad, G.U. & Rao, K.R. (1979) Determination of thiourea and some of its organic derivatives with sodium vanadate, hexacyanoferrate(III), cerium(IV) sulfate, manganese(III), and manganese(IV). *Talanta*, **26**, 1049–1051

Musha, K., Nagata, C. & Tanaka, S. (1985) [Rapid analysis of lubricating oil additives by normal-phase and adsorption high performance liquid chromatography.] *Bunseki Kagaku*, **34**, T40–T44 (in Japanese)

National Cancer Institute (1979) *Bioassay of N,N'-Diethylthiourea for Possible Carcinogenicity* (NCI Carcinogenesis Technical Report No. 149), Washington DC, Department of Health, Education, and Welfare

National Institute for Occupational Safety and Health (2000) *National Occupational Exposure Survey 1981–83*, Cincinnati, OH, Department of Health and Human Services, Public Health Service

Ohm, R.F. (1997) Rubber chemicals. In: Kroschwitz, J.I. & Howe-Grant, M., eds, *Kirk-Othmer Encyclopedia of Chemical Technology*, 4th Ed., Vol. 21, New York, John Wiley & Sons, pp. 460–481

Reynaerts, A., Bruze, M., Erikstam, U. & Goossens, A. (1998) Allergic contact dermatitis from a medical device, followed by depigmentation. *Contact Derm.*, **39**, 204–205

R.T. Vanderbilt Co. (1997) *Specification Sheet: Thiate® H (1,3-diethylthiourea)*, Norwalk, CT

Sadtler Research Laboratories (1980) *Sadtler Standard Spectra, 1980 Cumulative Molecular Formula Index*, Philadelphia, PA, p. 78

Savela, A., Vuorela, R. & Kauppinen, T. (1999) *ASA 1997* (Katsauksia 140), Helsinki, Finnish Institute of Occupational Health, p. 30 (in Finnish)

Valencia, R., Mason, J.M., Woodruff, R.C. & Zimmering, S. (1985) Chemical mutagenesis testing in Drosophila. III. Results of 48 coded compounds tested for the National Toxicology Program. *Environ. Mutag.*, **7**, 325–348

Verma, K.K. (1979) Determination of alkyl thioureas, isothiocyanates and amines with iodine monochloride. *Bull. chem. Soc. Jpn.*, **52**, 2155–2156

ETHYLENETHIOUREA

This substance was considered by previous working groups, in 1974 (IARC, 1974) and 1987 (IARC, 1987). Since that time, new data have become available, and these have been incorporated into the monograph and taken into consideration in the present evaluation.

1.   Exposure Data

1.1   Chemical and physical data

1.1.1   *Nomenclature*

Chem. Abstr. Serv. Reg. No.: 96-45-7
Deleted CAS Reg. Nos: 96-46-8; 12261-94-8; 26856-29-1; 71836-04-9; 90613-75-5
Chem. Abstr. Name: 2-Imidazolidinethione
IUPAC Systematic Name: Imidazoline-2-thiol
Synonyms: 4,5-Dihydroimidazole-2(3*H*)-thione;   4,5-dihydro-2-mercaptoimidazole; *N,N'*-1,2-ethanediylthiourea; ethylenethiocarbamide; ethylene thiourea; 1,3-ethylenethiourea; 1,3-ethylene-2-thiourea; *N,N'*-ethylenethiourea; ETU; imidazolidinethione; 2-imidazoline-2-thiol; 2-mercapto-4,5-dihydroimidazole; mercaptoimidazoline; 2-mercaptoimidazoline; 2-mercapto-2-imidazoline; tetrahydro-2*H*-imidazole-2-thione; 2-thioimidazolidine

1.1.2   *Structural and molecular formulae and relative molecular mass*

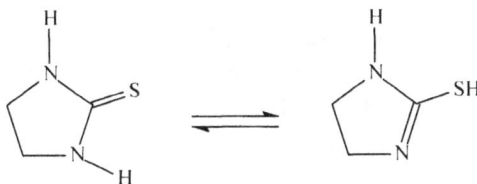

$C_3H_6N_2S$

Relative molecular mass: 102.16

1.1.3   *Chemical and physical properties of the pure substance*

(a) *Description*: Needles or prisms from alcohol (Lide & Milne, 1996; Budavari, 2000)

(b) *Melting-point*: 203 °C (Lide & Milne, 1996)

(c) *Spectroscopy data*: Infrared [prism (5619, 6556), grating (18092)], ultraviolet (4571), nuclear magnetic resonance [proton (7058), C-13 (5213)] and mass spectral data have been reported (Sadtler Research Laboratories, 1980; Lide & Milne, 1996).

(d) *Solubility*: Soluble in water (20 g/L at 30 °C), ethanol, methanol, ethylene glycol and pyridine; slightly soluble in dimethyl sulfoxide; insoluble in acetone, benzene, chloroform, diethyl ether and ligroin (Lide & Milne, 1996; Budavari, 2000)

1.1.4   *Technical products and impurities*

Trade names for ethylenethiourea include Accel 22, Accel 22S, Akrochem ETU-22, END 75, ETC, Mercazin I, NA-22, Nocceler 22, Pennac CRA, Rhenogran ETU, Robac 22, Rodanin S 62, Sanceller 22, Sanceller 22C, Sanceller 22S, Soxinol 22, Thiate N, Vulkacit NPV/C and Warecure C.

1.1.5   *Analysis*

Methods for the analysis of ethylenethiourea in fresh, baked or frozen food commodities (fruit, vegetables, canned goods, soups), beverages (milk, beer, juice), water (finished drinking-, surface, ground-, river), cigarette smoke condensate, blood serum, urine and formulated fungicides have been reported. The methods include thin-layer chromatography with liquid scintillation counting, micellar electrokinetic capillary chromatography, spectrophotometry, gas chromatography with flame photometric, electron capture, nitrogen–phosphorus or negative-ion chemical-ionization mass spectrometry detection, liquid chromatography with mass spectrometry or ultraviolet detection, high-performance liquid chromatography (HPLC) with amperometric, chemiluminescent nitrogen, diode-array or electrochemical detection, and reversed-phase HPLC with ultraviolet detection (Autio, 1983; Prince, 1985; Sonobe & Tanaka, 1986; Krause & Wang, 1988; Kurttio *et al.*, 1988; Longbottom *et al.*, 1993; van der Poll *et al.*, 1993; Walash *et al.*, 1993; Beneventi *et al.*, 1994; Maruyama, 1994; Meiring & de Jong, 1994; Ahmad *et al.*, 1995; Dubey *et al.*, 1997; Lo & Hsiao, 1997; Neicheva *et al.*, 1997; do Nascimento *et al.*, 1997; Fujinari, 1998; AOAC International, 1999a,b; Knio *et al.*, 2000; Picó *et al.*, 2000). Earlier methods for the determination of ethylenethiourea residues have been reviewed (Bottomley *et al.*, 1985).

1.2   Production

Ethylenethiourea can be made from ethylenediamine and carbon disulfide (Ohm, 1997).

Information available in 2000 indicated that ethylenethiourea was manufactured by three companies each in China, France and Japan, two companies in Germany and one company each in Brazil, India, Italy, the Netherlands and Switzerland (CIS Information Services, 2000).

1.3   Use

Ethylenethiourea is used mainly in the rubber industry as an accelerator for the vulcanization of polychloroprene (neoprene) and other rubbers. The use of thioureas is decreasing, and it is supplied preferably as polymer-bound granulates, which effectively prevent exposure to and inhalation of thiourea dust (Engels, 1993; Ohm, 1997; Budavari, 2000).

1.4   Occurrence

Ethylenethiourea is an environmental degradation product, a metabolite and an impurity in ethylenebisdithiocarbamate fungicides such as mancozeb, maneb and zineb. Mancozeb and maneb have a wide range of approved uses on agricultural and horticultural crops in many countries. Ethylenebisdithiocarbamate residues in foods are readily converted to ethylenethiourea during storage (Kurttio et al., 1990) and when processing includes a heating step (cooking or industrial processing) (FAO/WHO, 1993a; IPCS/INCHEM, 1993; Aprea et al., 1996; Budavari, 2000).

1.4.1   Occupational exposure

According to the 1981–83 National Occupational Exposure Survey (National Institute for Occupational Safety and Health, 2000), about 10 700 workers in the USA were potentially exposed to ethylenethiourea. Exposure occurred mainly during the manufacture of fabricated metal products (5000 exposed), the manufacture of machinery (3300) and in rubber mills (2300). The occupational groups exposed included grinding, abrading, buffing and polishing machine operators (2700 exposed), metal-plating-machine operators (1900) and moulding- and casting-machine operators (1300). Farmers, who may have been exposed to ethylenethiourea through the use of ethylenebisdithiocarbamate fungicides, were not included in the survey. According to the Finnish Register of Employees Exposed to Carcinogens, 47 chemical process workers and cleaners were exposed to ethylenethiourea in Finland in 1997. Most Finnish farmers are self-employed and therefore not covered by this register (Savela et al., 1999).

The average concentration of ethylenethiourea in the breathing zone was 0.14 µg/m³ for Finnish potato-field workers and 0.60 µg/m³ for pine nursery workers during spraying of an ethylenebisdithiocarbamate, maneb. Higher short-term concentrations (0.87 µg/m³ and 1.81 µg/m³ respectively) were measured during weighing of the pesticide. The average concentration of ethylenethiourea in the urine was 1.5 µg/L for potato-field workers and 0.9 µg/L for pine nursery workers 3 h after exposure (Savolainen *et al.*, 1989). In another study in Finland on potato-farmers spraying maneb or mancozeb, 0.004–3.3 µg/m³ were found in the breathing zone of farmers and 0.006–0.8 µg/m³ in tractor cabins. The urine samples contained < 0.2–11.8 µg/L ethylenethiourea (Kurttio *et al.*, 1990).

The concentration of ethylenethiourea in a rubber mill in the USA ranged from not detected to 1100 µg/m³ when ethylenethiourea was used in a dry powder form as an accelerator for curing neoprene rubber. When the powder was replaced by a 75% dispersion in a rubber binder, the concentration of ethylenethiourea in the air dropped to not detected to 29 µg/m³ (Salisbury & Lybarger, 1977).

1.4.2 *Environmental occurrence*

Within a Food and Drug Administration monitoring programme in the USA, 864 samples of baby foods were monitored for pesticide residues. Ethylenethiourea residues were detected in 65 samples at concentrations ranging from traces to 0.06 mg/kg (Yess *et al.*, 1993).

In 1989–90 in the USA, a large survey of food items (approximately 300 samples each of 19 raw and processed commodities) was conducted for dithiocarbamate and ethylenethiourea residues. No measurable residues of ethylenethiourea (limit of detection, 0.001 mg/kg) were found in 82% of the samples. All of the concentrations detected were < 0.1 mg/kg (FAO/WHO, 1993a).

Ethylenethiourea was not detected (< 0.005 mg/kg) in any of 100 commercial grape juice samples in the USA taken from producers using grapes from areas where dithiocarbamate fungicides were used (FAO/WHO, 1993a).

As part of a study of new analytical techniques, Walash *et al.* (1993) reported that the disappearance of maneb and zineb sprayed on cucumbers and tomatoes grown in a greenhouse followed first-order kinetics.

In 1988 and 1989, the concentrations of residues of ethylenebisdithiocarbamate, chlorothalonil and anilazine on raw, unwashed, unpeeled processing tomatoes in field experiments represented 16–25% of those tolerated by the Environmental Protection Agency in the USA. The concentrations of ethylenethiourea were at or below detection limit (< 0.01 mg/L) in tomato juice processed from field-grown tomatoes in both years (Precheur *et al.*, 1992).

The efficiency of vegetable washing was evaluated by measuring the concentrations of residues of ethylenethiourea in canned products. Collard and spinach retained more carbamate residues in the field than other green vegetables. Spinach retained more residues than the other leafy green vegetables, regardless of the washing treatment. With the exception of mustard, neither mild nor strong detergent removed significantly more epicuticular waxes in leafy green vegetables than did water (Gonzalez *et al.*, 1990).

Urinary ethylenethiourea concentrations were measured in the populations of several urban and rural regions in Italy in 1994 and 1995. Measurable concentrations were found in an average of 24% of the urban population (range, 0.8–8.3; mean, 2.7 μg/g of creatinine) and 37% of the rural population (range, 0.9–61.4; mean, 9.1 μg/g creatinine). The concentrations were increased by smoking and wine-drinking. The estimated intake of ethylenethiourea from several food commodities (mean values in μg/day per capita ± SD) were: wine, 6.03 ± 4.62; vegetables, 18.53 ± 40.16; whole fruit, 155.33 ± 122.41; and fruit pulp, 31.07 ± 24.48 (Aprea *et al.*, 1996).

As zineb, maneb and mancozeb are used as fungicides in vineyards (IARC, 1976), trace concentrations of ethylenethiourea can occur in wine (Cabras *et al.*, 1987). For example, 5–10 μg/L ethylenethiourea were found in all of 10 local wine samples in Italy (Aprea *et al.*, 1996).

Ethylenethiourea may occur also in cigarette smoke. The condensate of four of 12 brands of cigarettes contained 8–27 ng/cigarette of ethylenethiourea, owing to the use of ethylenebisdithiocarbamate on tobacco crops (Autio, 1983).

1.5   Regulations and guidelines

In Germany, ethylenethiourea is classified as 3B ('substances for which in-vitro or animal studies have yielded evidence of carcinogenic effects that is not sufficient for classification of the substance in one of the other categories. Further studies are required before a final decision can be made. A MAK value can be established provided no genotoxic effects have been detected') (Deutsche Forschungsgemeinschaft, 2000). Finland, France, Sweden and the USA (National Institute for Occupational Safety and Health) list ethylenethiourea as a carcinogen; Finland has set a time-weighted average occupational exposure limit of 0.2 mg/m^3 and a short-term exposure limit of 0.6 mg/m^3 for ethylenethiourea (American Conference of Governmental Industrial Hygienists, 2000).

Ethylenethiourea was reviewed in conjunction with the ethylenebisdithiocarbamates by the Joint FAO/WHO Meeting on Pesticide Residues several times between 1963 and 1993. In 1993, the Joint Meeting established an acceptable daily intake for ethylenethiourea of 0–0.004 mg/kg bw (FAO/WHO, 1993b; WHO, 1999).

2. Studies of Cancer in Humans

2.1   Cohort study

A list of 1929 workers at several large rubber manufacturing firms where ethylene-thiourea was used and at a firm producing ethylenethiourea in England was drawn up from employment records (Smith, 1976). According to the records of the Birmingham Cancer Registry for the period 1957–71, none of the workers developed thyroid cancer. [The Working Group noted that the lack of details on methods, including the number of expected cases, makes it difficult to assess the relevance of this finding.]

Although workers in the rubber industry and pesticide applicators may be exposed to ethylenethiourea, no specific mention of this compound was found in epidemiological studies of the cancer risks of these populations.

3. Studies of Cancer in Experimental Animals

3.1   Oral administration

Mouse: In a preliminary report of a screening study, groups of 18 male and 18 female hybrid mice of the $(C57BL/6 \times C3H/Anf)F_1$ $(B6C3F_1)$ and $(C57BL/6 \times AKR)F_1$ $(B6AKF_1)$ strains, 7 days of age, were given doses of 0 (control) or 215 mg/kg bw commercial-grade ethylenethiourea [purity not specified] daily in 0.5% gelatin in water by gavage for 3 weeks. The dose determined at 7 days of age was not adjusted for body weight. The mice were weaned at 4 weeks of age, and the chemical without vehicle was mixed into the diet at a concentration of 0 (control) or 646 mg/kg and provided *ad libitum* from 4 weeks to approximately 18 months. The concentration of the compound in the diet was calculated from the weight and food consumption of the 4-week-old mice to be approximately the maximum tolerated dose on a mg/kg bw basis. The same concentration was maintained throughout the duration of the study up to 82–83 weeks of age. The incidence of 'hepatomas' was 14/16 (male) and 18/18 (female) in treated $B6C3F_1$ mice and 18/18 (male) and 9/16 (female) in treated $B6AKF_1$ mice, with incidences in the pooled control groups of 8/79 (male) and 0/87 (female) for the $B6C3F_1$ mice and 5/90 (male) and 1/82 (female) for the $B6AKF_1$ mice. The increases in incidences of hepatomas in male and female mice of both strains were statistically significant ($p < 0.01$) (Innes *et al.*, 1969).

The carcinogenic potential of ethylenethiourea was evaluated during and after perinatal exposure (*in utero* and throughout suckling). Female C57BL/6 mice, 10–11 weeks of age (F_0 generation), were fed a diet containing 0, 33, 110 or 330 mg/kg ethylene-thiourea for 1 week before breeding. After mating with previously unexposed male C3H/HeN mice, all the females were continued on the diets containing ethylenethiourea. On day 7 *post partum*, the litters (F_1 generation) were standardized to a maximum of eight, weaned on day 28 and separated by sex. Up to 8 weeks of age, the litters were exposed to ethylenethiourea at the same concentrations in the diet as those given to their dams; at approximately 8 weeks of age, the pups were divided into groups of 50 animals per sex and exposed to the adult concentrations of 0, 330 and 1000 mg/kg of diet for 2 years. The F_0:F_1 treatments were thus 0:0, 0:330, 0:1000, 330:0, 330:330, 330:1000, 33:100 and 110:330 mg/kg of diet. The tumour incidences in the various groups are shown in Table 1. Significant ($p < 0.01$) increases were found in the incidences of liver tumours in males and females at 330 mg/kg of diet, with or without perinatal exposure. Significant ($p < 0.01$) increases in the incidences of thyroid follicular-cell tumours were observed in females at 330 mg/kg of diet with perinatal exposure and in males and females at 1000 mg/kg of diet with or without perinatal exposure. Significant ($p < 0.01$) increases in the incidences of anterior pituitary tumours were observed in females at 330:330 and 330:1000 mg/kg of diet and in F_1 males and F_1 females at 0:1000 mg/kg of diet. The incidences of tumours were generally similar with and without perinatal exposure, except that the incidences of thyroid and anterior pituitary tumours in the females were higher after perinatal exposure (Chhabra et al., 1992; National Toxicology Program, 1992).

Table 1. Incidences of neoplasms in B6C3F$_1$ mice exposed to ethylenethiourea in the diet with or without perinatal exposure

Concentration of ethylenethiourea (F_0:F_1) (mg/kg of diet)	Hepatocellular adenoma and carcinoma combined		Thyroid follicular-cell adenoma and carcinoma combined		Anterior pituitary adenoma and carcinoma combined	
	Males	Females	Males	Females	Males	Females
Adult exposure only						
0:0	20/49	4/50	1/50	0/50	0/44	11/47
0:330	32/50*	44/50**	1/49	2/50	0/42	19/49
0:1000	46/50**	48/50**	29/50**	38/50**	8/41**	26/49**
Perinatal and adult exposure						
33:100	9/33	4/28	1/47	1/29	0/28	2/28
110:330	26/47	46/50**	1/47	5/50*	0/41	14/48
330:330	34/49*	46/50**	2/48	10/49**	0/45	26/47**
330:1000	47/49**	49/50**	35/49**	38/50**	4/39	24/47**
Perinatal exposure only						
330:0	13/49	5/49	1/46	1/49	0/42	11/48

From Chhabra et al. (1992); National Toxicology Program (1992). Incidences are numbers of lesions observed/number of animals
* $p < 0.05$ versus 0:0 group (logistic regression test)
** $p < 0.01$ versus 0:0 group (logistic regression test)

Rat: Groups of 26 male and 26 female Sprague-Dawley (Crl:CD®) rats, 5–6 weeks of age, were fed diets containing 175 or 350 mg/kg technical-grade ethylenethiourea (97% pure) for 18 months. Five rats per dose group were killed and necropsied at 18 months, and the remaining rats at the two concentrations were continued on control diet for up to a further 6 months, for a total of up to 24 months. Thyroid (follicular or papillary) carcinomas were observed in 0/30 and 0/30 male and female controls, 2/26 and 2/26 males and females at the lower concentration and 15/26 and 6/26 males and females at the higher concentration, respectively (Ulland *et al.*, 1972; Weisburger *et al.*, 1981).

Groups of 11–13 male and 9–12 female Sprague-Dawley (Crl:CD®) rats, approximately 5 weeks of age, were given diets containing 0 (control), 5, 25, 125, 250 or 500 mg/kg ethylenethiourea [purity not specified] *ad libitum* for up to 12 months and were evaluated for histological changes. Thyroid follicular-cell adenocarcinomas were observed in 3/13 males at 250 mg/kg of diet and 10/13 males and 5/12 females at 500 mg/kg of diet at 12 months. No neoplastic changes were found in the other groups, including the controls (Graham *et al.*, 1973). In a second study, which was a continuation of the previous one, the carcinogenic potential of the same concentrations when given for 12–24 months was evaluated. When the results for male and female rats were combined, the incidences of thyroid tumours (adenomas and adenocarcinomas/carcinomas) were 4/72 controls, 37/69 rats at 250 mg/kg of diet and 65/70 rats at 500 mg/kg of diet. A few thyroid tumours occurred in other groups of 72–75 rats, including that given no ethylenethiourea (Graham *et al.*, 1975).

Five groups of 20 male and 20 female rats [strain or stock and age not specified] were fed diets containing ethylenethiourea at 0 (control), 5,17, 60 or 200 mg/kg for 24 months. There was a strong negative association between food consumption and body-weight gain and dietary concentration, the decreases in food consumption and body-weight gain being > 10% at the two higher concentrations. The incidences of thyroid tumours were 0, 0, 5.9, 42.1 ($p < 0.01$) and 82.4% ($p < 0.001$) in males and 5.3, 6.3, 18.8, 22.2 and 56.3% ($p < 0.001$) in females at 0, 5, 17, 60 and 200 mg/kg of diet ethylenethiourea, respectively (Gak *et al.*, 1976).

Female Fischer 344 rats, 10–11 weeks of age (F_0 generation), were fed a diet containing 0, 9, 30 or 90 mg/kg ethylenethiourea for 1 week before breeding. After mating with previously unexposed male Fischer 344 rats, all the females were continued on their previous diets. On day 4 *post partum*, the litters (F_1 generation) were standardized to a maximum of eight and weaned on day 28. The pups continued to be exposed at the concentrations given to their dams until they were 8 weeks of age. The pups were separated by sex at weaning, and at approximately 8 weeks of age were divided into groups of 50 animals per sex and exposed to the adult dietary concentrations of 0, 25, 83 and 250 mg/kg for 2 years. The $F_0:F_1$ treatments were thus 0:0 (control), 0:83, 0:250, 90:0, 90:83, 9:250, 30:83, and 9:25 mg/kg of diet. The incidences of thyroid tumours in the various groups are shown in Table 2. Significant increases in the incidences of thyroid follicular-cell tumours were observed in males at 83 and 250 mg/kg of diet, with or

Table 2. Incidences of thyroid follicular-cell adenoma and carcinoma combined in Fischer 344 rats exposed to ethylenethiourea in the diet with or without perinatal exposure

Concentration of ethylenethiourea ($F_0:F_1$) (mg/kg of diet)	No. of lesions observed/number of animals	
	Males	Females
Adult exposure only		
0:0	1/49	3/50
0:83	12/46*	7/44
0:250	37/50*	30/49*
Perinatal and adult exposures		
9:25	3/46	1/49
30:83	14/47*	6/47
90:83	13/50*	9/47
90:250	48/50*	37/50*
Perinatal exposure only		
90:0	4/49	3/50

From Chhabra *et al.* (1992); National Toxicology Program (1992)

* $p < 0.01$ versus 0:0 group (logistic regression test)

without perinatal exposure, and in females at 250 mg/kg of diet, with or without perinatal exposure when compared with their respective control groups. Marginally significant ($p < 0.05$) increases in the incidence of Zymbal gland tumours were observed in males (5/50) at 90:250 mg/kg of diet and in only 1/50 control males. The incidences of tumours were generally similar with and without perinatal exposure, except that the incidences of thyroid tumours were higher with perinatal exposure at the higher concentrations (Chhabra *et al.*, 1992; National Toxicology Program, 1992).

Hamster: Five groups of 20 male and 20 female hamsters [strain or stock and age not specified] were fed diets containing ethylenethiourea at 0 (control), 5, 17, 60 or 200 mg/kg for 20 months. There was a strong negative association between food consumption and body-weight gain and dietary concentration, the decreases in food consumption and body-weight gain being > 10% at the two higher concentrations. No carcinogenic effects were observed (Gak *et al.*, 1976).

3.2   Administration with known carcinogens and modifying factors

Mouse: Groups of 30 male and 30 female ICR mice, 5 weeks of age, were given a prescribed amount of ethylenethiourea (obtained from commercial sources and purified by recrystallization twice from 1:1 ethanol:water or methanol) and/or sodium nitrite by gavage at a dosage volume of 0.1 mL/10 g bw distilled water. The doses of ethylene-thiourea/sodium nitrite were 0/0 (control), 100/0, 0/70, 25/17.5, 50/35 or 100/70 mg/kg bw per week. The animals were treated once a week for 10 weeks, and the study was terminated 18 months after the first administration. Significant increases ($p < 0.05$) in the incidences of tumours at various sites, including the lung, forestomach and uterus (see Table 3), were observed with the combinations of 50/35 and 100/70 mg/kg bw per week (Yoshida *et al.*, 1993).

Table 3. Tumour incidences in ICR mice treated with ethylenethiourea and sodium nitrite

| Neoplasm | Tumour incidence per dose group (mg/kg bw per week) | | | | | |
| | Males | | | Females[a] | | |
	0/0	50/35	100/70	0/0	50/35	100/70
Lymphoma	3/30	8/30	13/30*	6/30	12/30	19/30*
Lung (adenoma/adenocarcinoma)[a]	9/30	22/30*	25/30*	3/30	16/30*	21/30*
Forestomach (squamous papilloma/ carcinoma)	0/30	4/30	12/30*	0/30	2/30	8/30*
Harderian gland (adenoma)	3/30	2/30	9/30	0/30	3/30	7/30*
Uterus (adenocarcinoma)				0/30	3/30	6/30*

From Yoshida *et al.* (1993)
* Significantly different from controls ($p < 0.05$)
[a] A significantly increased incidence (12/30) of lung tumours was also observed with the 25/17.5 combination in females

The uterine adenocarcinomas induced in the above study prompted two further studies.

Groups of female ICR mice, 5 weeks of age, were given distilled water (40 mice) or a combination of 100 mg/kg bw ethylenethiourea (purity, > 95%) and 70 mg/kg bw sodium nitrite (purity, > 98%) by gavage (90 mice) in distilled water once a week for up to 6 months. The experiment was terminated at 12 months. Small groups of control and treated mice were killed sequentially between 1 and 12 months of the study. Significantly higher incidences ($p < 0.05$) of endometrial adenocarcinomas (17/40) and stromal polyps (23/40) were observed in treated mice after 10–12 months than in control mice (0/13 adenocarcinomas and 2/13 stromal polyps) (Yoshida *et al.*, 1994).

Groups of 20 female ICR mice, aged 1, 6 and 12 months, were given the same treatment as described above for 6 months, followed by a withdrawal period of 3 months, at which time all surviving mice were necropsied. Age-matched control groups of 10 mice per group were gavaged with distilled water for 6 months. All mice were evaluated for uterine lesions. The incidences of endometrial adenocarcinoma were 1/20, 8/20 and 4/20 in treated 1-, 6- and 12-month-old mice, respectively, with none in age-matched control groups, but the incidence was significantly ($p < 0.05$) higher only in the 6-month-old group. The incidences of endometrial stromal polyps were 5/20, 13/20 ($p < 0.05$) and 10/20 in the treated 1-, 6- and 12-month-old mice, with 0/10, 1/10 and 2/10 in the respective age-matched control groups. The authors concluded that adult mice are more susceptible than young or old mice to induction of endometrial adenocarcinoma by the reaction product of ethylenethiourea and sodium nitrite, N-nitrosoethylenethiourea (Yoshida et al., 1996).

Rat: The initiating and promoting effects of oral administration of ethylenethiourea and sodium nitrite were investigated in female Donryu rats, which are predisposed to a high incidence of endometrial adenocarcinomas (approximately 35% by 120 weeks of age; Nagaoka et al., 1990) probably due to a high oestrogen:progesterone ratio (imbalance). Groups of 21–37 female Donryu rats, 10 weeks of age, were treated as follows: group 1 received a single intrauterine injection of polyethylene glycol, followed by oral gavage with distilled water at weekly intervals from weeks 11 to 51 of age (vehicle control); group 2 received a single intrauterine injection of 15 mg/kg bw N-ethyl-N-nitrosourea (ENU) in polyethylene glycol; group 3 received a single intrauterine injection of polyethylene glycol followed by oral gavage with a combination of 80 mg/kg bw ethylenethiourea and 50 mg/kg bw sodium nitrite in water at weekly intervals from week 11 to 51 of age; and group 4 received a single intrauterine injection of 15 mg/kg bw ENU followed by oral gavage with a combination of 80 mg/kg bw ethylenethiourea and 50 mg/kg bw sodium nitrite in water at weekly intervals from week 11 to 51 of age. The study was terminated at 52 weeks of age, and the tissues were evaluated for histological changes. The incidences of endometrial adenocarcinomas were 0/21, 6/21 ($p < 0.01$; significantly different from group 1), 4/31 and 21/37 ($p < 0.001$; significantly different from groups 1 and 3) in groups 1–4, respectively, suggesting that concurrent administration of ethylenethiourea and sodium nitrite promoted ENU-initiated endometrial adenocarcinoma (Nishiyama et al., 1998).

4. Other Data Relevant to an Evaluation of Carcinogenicity and its Mechanisms

4.1 Absorption, distribution, metabolism and excretion

4.1.1 *Humans*

Urinary excretion of ethylenethiourea was monitored in non-smoking male volunteers given a diet with no detectable ethylenethiourea except in wine (8.8 μg/L) for 8 days. An average of 48.3% of the ethylenethiourea ingested from wine was excreted unmodified in the urine (Aprea *et al.*, 1997).

4.1.2 *Experimental systems*

Imidazoline, ethylene urea, 4-imidazolin-2-one(imidazolone) and unchanged ethylenethiourea were identified in the 24-h urine of male Sprague-Dawley rats after oral administration of 4 mg/kg bw [^{14}C]ethylenethiourea. In two female cats given the same dose, a half-time of 3.5 h was determined, and ethylenethiourea, ethylene urea and S-methyl ethylenethiourea were present in the 24-h urine. S-Methyl ethylene-thiourea comprised 64% of the total radiolabel in urine. In-vitro metabolism by cat and rat liver microsomes also produced ethylene urea, imidazoline and other unidentified compounds. When cat liver supernatant contained S-adenosyl methionine, S-methyl ethylenethiourea was produced (Iverson *et al.*, 1980). Using microsomes from male Sprague-Dawley rats, Decker and Doerge (1991) showed that, under normal physio-logical conditions, the reactive species from flavin-monooxygenase and cytochrome P450 metabolism of ethylenethiourea are sequestered by endogenous glutathione. The main metabolite of [^{14}C]ethylenethiourea, formed *in vivo* after treatment of male NMRI mice with an oral dose of 67 mg/kg bw or *in vitro* with mouse liver micro-somes, was 2-imidazolin-2-yl sulfenate (Savolainen & Pyysalo, 1979). A metabolite of ethylenethiourea detected in female rat plasma was identified as 1-methylthiourea (Kobayashi *et al.*, 1982).

After ethylenethiourea was administered once orally at 200 mg/kg bw to Wistar rats on day 12 of gestation, the concentration in maternal plasma and amniotic fluid peaked at about 2 h and disappeared within 48 h. In the embryos, the concentration peaked after only 30 min and disappeared within 48 h (Iwase *et al.*, 1996). In pregnant Wistar rats given a single oral dose of 240 mg/kg bw [^{14}C]ethylenethiourea, maternal blood maintained peak radiolabel concentrations for 2 h; the distribution was equal among maternal tissues but lower in embryos. Twenty-four hours after treatment, the radiolabel had been cleared and 72.8% had been excreted in the urine. The elution patterns suggested very little metabolism of the parent compound (Ruddick *et al.*, 1975). When Wistar rats were given 100 mg/kg bw [^{14}C]ethylenethiourea orally on day 12 of gestation, the compound was readily absorbed, the concentration reaching a maximum in maternal blood within 2 h. Ethylenethiourea was distributed throughout the maternal system and the embryo. Accumulation was noted in the thyroid. The major elimination route was the urine (Kato *et al.*, 1976). Swiss mice and Wistar rats were treated by gavage on gestational day 15 with 240 mg/kg bw [^{14}C]ethylenethiourea (mice) or [^{35}S]ethylenethiourea (rats). The maternal and fetal concentrations of ethylenethiourea in tissues were similar in the two species 3 h after treatment, but the mice eliminated ethylenethiourea more rapidly, with a half-time of 5.5 h in mice and 9.4 h in rats (Ruddick *et al.*, 1977).

Two female rhesus monkeys (*Macaca mulatta*) and four Sprague-Dawley rats were given [^{14}C]ethylenethiourea at 40 mg/kg bw by gastric intubation, and excretion was monitored for 48 h. The major excretion route was urine. The amount retained in tissues at 48 h was much higher in the two monkeys (21 and 28%) than in the rats (1%) (Allen *et al.*, 1978).

4.2   Toxic effects

4.2.1   *Humans*

A 53-year-old woman reported allergic contact dermatitis after exposure to ethylene-thiourea used as a rubber additive (Bruze & Fregert, 1983).

A group of 49 male workers without protective equipment used backpack sprayers to apply ethylenebisdithiocarbamate fungicides in which ethylenethiourea was found as a contaminant and metabolic product. They were found to have a marginal increase in the serum concentration of thyroid-stimulating hormone but no change in that of thyroxine (T4) (Steenland *et al.*, 1997).

Over a period of 3 years, five workers involved in mixing ethylenethiourea into monomer rubber showed decreased serum concentrations (by approximately 20%) of T4. One had an increased concentration of thyroid-stimulating hormone on two occasions [about 10-fold], but he was found to have premyxoedema (Smith, 1984).

4.2.2   *Experimental systems*

Osborne-Mendel rats were fed diets containing ethylenethiourea at a concentration of of 50, 100, 500 or 750 mg/kg for 30, 60, 90 or 120 days. Rats at the two higher concentrations showed decreased body weight and hyperplasia of the thyroid at all times. The thyroid:body weight ratios were increased at concentrations of 100, 500 and 750 mg/kg of diet at 30 and 60 days, at the two higher concentrations at 90 days and at all concentrations at 120 days. Decreased iodine uptake was measured 24 h after injection at concentrations of 100, 500 and 750 mg/kg of diet at all times (Graham & Hansen, 1972).

Male Sprague-Dawley rats given diets containing 125 or 625 mg/kg ethylene-thiourea for up to 90 days had decreased serum concentrations of triiodothyronine and T4 [by 65% and 60%, respectively] and, at 625 mg/kg of diet, decreased iodide uptake [by 35%] in the thyroid (Freudenthal *et al.*, 1977). Male Sprague-Dawley rats given ethylenethiourea in drinking-water at 500 mg/L for 4 months had altered hepatic morphology, increased smooth endoplasmic reticulum, decreased rough endoplasmic reticulum and relocation of microbodies and mitochondria to the periphery of the smooth endoplasmic reticulum (Moller *et al.*, 1986). When male and female Sprague-Dawley rats were given ethylenethiourea in the diet for 7 weeks and then removed to control diet, the increases in relative and absolute thyroid weights (at 75 and 100 mg/kg of diet) and the decrease in T4 blood concentration (at 150 mg/kg bw) were partially reversed (Arnold *et al.*, 1983).

Male Wistar rats given ethylenethiourea in the drinking-water at 100–300 mg/L [corresponding to 10.6–23.4 mg/kg bw per day] for 28 days showed reduced secretion of T4 and triiodothyronine and a 10-fold increase in the secretion of thyroid-stimulating hormone over that in controls. Ultrastructural changes were also found in the thyroid, with an increased number of myelin bodies, dilatation of the rough endoplasmic reticulum and increased vacuolization in the epithelial cells of thyroid follicles (Kurttio *et al.*, 1986). Alterations in renal proximal tubule epithelial cells were seen in male Wistar rats given a high concentration of ethylenethiourea in the drinking-water (300 mg/L) for 28 days. Continuous oral administration had only minor effects on renal function (Kurttio *et al.*, 1991).

Both male and female Charles River rats showed decreased body weight and body-weight gain when fed diets containing 250 or 500 mg/kg ethylenethiourea for 2–12 months. The body weight of the female rats was also decreased at 125 mg/kg of diet. Iodine uptake was decreased in male rats after 12 months at 500 mg/kg of diet. Females had an initial decrease in iodine uptake at a dose of 125 or 500 mg/kg of diet at 6 months, but by 12 months the uptake had increased even on diets containing 125, 250 or 500 mg/kg (Graham *et al.*, 1973).

Sprague-Dawley rats were given ethylenethiourea as a single intraperitoneal injection of 2.5 or 250 mg/kg bw, by gavage for 3 days at 5 or 250 mg/kg bw per day or in the diet for 3 weeks at 5 or 250 mg/kg of diet. The livers of the animals were morphologically normal, and no changes in hepatic RNA synthesis occurred (Austin & Moyer, 1979).

Chinese hamster ovary cells transfected with the human thyroid peroxidase (*TPO*) gene were exposed to ethylenethiourea. The oxidative activity of the enzyme was inhibited at 50 μmol/L ethylenethiourea, and its iodinating activity was blocked at 5 μmol/L (Marinovich *et al.*, 1997).

In vitro, ethylenethiourea inhibited thyroid peroxidase, the enzyme that catalyses the iodination and coupling of the tyrosine residues needed for the synthesis of triiodothyronine and T4, by interacting with the iodinated enzyme intermediate. Once the ethylenethiourea was depleted, normal enzymatic activity returned (Doerge & Takazawa, 1989).

4.3   Reproductive and developmental effects

4.3.1   *Humans*

A retrospective study of women who had been employed in the manufacture of rubber containing ethylenethiourea was reported (Smith, 1976). The potential participants were all 699 women of child-bearing age who had left employment at the factory between 1963 and 1971. Of these, 255 who had given birth to 420 children were traced. Of these women, 59 had been employed in the rubber plant at the time of their first pregnancy, and none had given birth to an abnormal child. Of the 420 children, 11 had malformations. Three of these had been born before the employment of their mother and eight had been born more than 1 year after their mothers' employment.

4.3.2   *Experimental systems*

The teratogenicity of ethylenethiourea has been reviewed (Khera, 1987).

(*a*)   *General developmental toxicity*

As reported in an abstract, rats [strain and group size not specified] were given 0, 10, 20, 40 or 80 mg/kg bw per day ethylenethiourea by gavage either from 21 days before gestation to day 15 or on days 6–15 or 7–20 of gestation. A variety of malformations was observed, with minimal effects noted at the lowest dose. Rabbits similarly exposed on days 7–20 of gestation were reported to have an increased incidence of resorptions and decreased brain weight at 80 mg/kg bw per day (Khera, 1973).

The teratogenic effects of ethylenethiourea were evaluated in groups of 12–29 Sprague-Dawley rats, 31–33 CD-1 mice, 15–19 golden hamsters and three to five Hartley guinea-pigs exposed daily by oral gavage on days 7–21, 7–16, 5–10 and 7–25 of gestation, respectively, to a dose of 0, 5, 10, 20, 30, 40 or 80 mg/kg bw per day, 0, 100 or 200 mg/kg bw per day, 0, 75, 150 or 300 mg/kg bw per day and 0, 50 or 100 mg/kg bw per day, respectively. The fetuses were examined at the end of gestation for external, internal and skeletal malformations. Ethylenethiourea was toxic to the pregnant rats at 80 mg/kg bw per day, while a variety of malformations (e.g., hydrocephalus, encephalocoele, cleft palate, kyphosis and limb and digital defects) were observed at doses ≥ 20 mg/kg bw per day; fetal body weights were reduced at doses as low as 10 mg/kg bw per day. In mice, the maternal liver weights were increased at the two highest doses; the only significant fetal effect was an increased incidence of supernumerary ribs at 200 mg/kg bw per day. No significant maternal or fetal effects were seen in hamsters or guinea-pigs. Other groups of 11–13 rats received 0, 20, 25 or 30 mg/kg bw per day ethylenethiourea on gestation day 7; they delivered their offspring, and exposure was continued until lactation day 15. The offspring were tested for a variety of indicators of reflex development, and the motor activity of males was recorded in an open-field device for 4 min over 2 consecutive days at 6 weeks of age. There were no effects on litter size at birth, but 6/13 litters of dams at the highest dose failed to nurse, and 40%

of the surviving offspring had developed hydrocephaly by day 45. There were no treatment-related effects on the offspring body weights, startle or righting reflex development or eye opening, but there was a dose-related increase in defaecation in the open-field test on days 1 and 2 and in activity on day 2 (Chernoff *et al.*, 1979).

In a screening assay for developmental toxicity, 600 mg/kg bw ethylenethiourea were given by oral gavage to 35 CD-1 mice on days 7–14 of gestation, and the growth and viability of the offspring were evaluated after birth for 3 days and compared with those of a group of 45 untreated controls. A significant increase in the frequency of litters that were completely resorbed was found, but there were no effects on postnatal growth or viability (Plasterer *et al.*, 1985).

Groups of 20–23 Sprague-Dawley rats were given 0, 15, 25 or 35 mg/kg bw per day ethylenethiourea by oral gavage on gestation days 6–20. There were no signs of maternal toxicity at any dose. The fetal body weights were reduced at the highest dose, which also caused malformations such as cranial meningocoele and meningorrhoea, severe hind limb talipes and short and/or kinky tails. Rats at the two higher doses had higher incidences of dilated brain ventricles and hydroureter than controls (Saillenfait *et al.*, 1991).

Six thioureas, including ethylenethiourea, were evaluated for embryotoxicity by injection onto the heart of 3-day-old white Leghorn chicken embryos. The median effective dose of ethylenethiourea for total embryotoxicity (dead and malformed) was 4.5 μmol [460 μg]/egg; it was the least potent of the thioureas tested (Korhonen *et al.*, 1982).

Ethylenethiourea was added at a concentration of 20, 30, 40 or 50 μg/mL to cultures of *Daphnia magna* eggs. No eggs hatched at the highest dose, and hatchability was reduced by about 20% at 30 and 40 μg/mL. The incidence of morphological anomalies of the carapace was significantly increased at 20, 30 and 40 μg/mL (Ohta *et al.*, 1998).

(b)   Phase specificity

The stage-dependence of the teratogenic effects of ethylenethiourea was demonstrated in Wistar rats exposed by gavage to 40–480 mg/kg bw on one of days 6–21 of gestation. The earliest teratogenic effects were seen after treatment on day 10, and included failure of coccygeal growth, spina bifida, ectopic genitalia and nephrosis. The incidence of defects peaked after exposure on days 12–15, but effects such as hydranencephaly, hydronephrosis and subcutaneous oedema were seen after exposure as late as day 21 (Ruddick & Khera, 1975).

Ethylenethiourea was given orally to Wistar rats at a single dose of 1–50 mg/kg bw in aqueous suspension on day 17, 18, 19 or 20 of gestation. The incidence of stillbirths was increased at doses of 30 and 50 mg/kg bw on day 18, 19 or 20. Regardless of the age at exposure, doses as low as 10 mg/kg bw were associated with reduced offspring viability due to hydrocephaly (Lewerenz & Bleyl, 1980).

Ethylenethiourea has been used as a prototype teratogen to study postnatal functional development of the kidney. Prenatal exposure of Sprague-Dawley rats to

0–160 mg/kg bw ethylenethiourea on day 11 of gestation produced dose-related increases in the incidence of enlarged renal pelvis in the fetuses on day 21 of gestation. Further studies were conducted to explore the postnatal consequences on renal development and function after exposure to 0, 20, 40 or 60 mg/kg bw on day 11 of gestation. The incidence of hydronephrosis after birth was lower than anticipated from the study of prenatal exposure, probably as a result of increased postnatal mortality. The severity of the hydronephrosis, however, increased with postnatal age. The hydonephrotic animals had impaired concentrating ability, but cortical function (proximal tubule transport) was unaffected. Rats exposed to ethylenethiourea prenatally had grossly normal kidneys but showed suppressed electrolyte clearance early in life. The latter effect was no longer apparent by postnatal day 27 (Daston et al., 1988).

The effect of prenatal exposure to ethylenethiourea on the development of the posterior gut was studied in 28 Wistar-Imamichi rats treated with 100, 125, 150 or 200 mg/kg bw ethylenethiourea by intragastric administration on day 11 of gestation. Another four pregnant rats were available as controls. Fetuses were examined on day 20 of gestation. The dose-related malformations included absent or kinked tails, spina bifida and myeloschisis. The incidences of malformations were significantly higher in male than female fetuses. Histological examination of 57 fetuses exposed to 125 mg/kg bw revealed an incidence of anorectal malformations in 92% of males and 41% of females (Hirai & Kuwabara, 1990).

The phase specificity of ethylenethiourea was studied in Sprague-Dawley rats exposed by oral gavage to 0, 60, 120 or 240 mg/kg bw on one day of gestation between days 8 and 19. The number of litters per group was not specified, but there were 113 females in the experiment and 717 fetuses (16–86 per group). Fetuses were examined on day 20 for soft-tissue anomalies by histological procedures. A high rate of mortality was seen after exposure on days 8–10. Exposure to the two higher doses resulted in a variety of central nervous system malformations (e.g., spinal raphism, exencephaly, hydranencephaly and hydrocephaly) after exposure on one of days 11–18 of gestation, and the specific malformations showed phase sensitivity. Thus, short tail was observed after exposure on one of days 11–14, spinal raphism after exposure on day 11, exencephaly after exposure on day 12 or 13, microencepahly after exposure on day 14 and hydranencephaly after exposure on day 15 or 16 (Hung et al., 1986). The effects of ethylenethiourea on prenatal brain development were further studied in 20 pregnant Sprague-Dawley rats that were exposed to 60, 120, 240 or 360 mg/kg bw ethylenethiourea by gavage on day 11 of gestation (Hung, 1992). A total of 155 fetuses from the treated groups and 38 fetuses from three controls were examined on day 20 of gestation. Dose-related incidences of malformations, which reached 100% at the highest dose, were observed. The most prominent defects included omphalocoele, lumbosacral myeloschisis and imperforate anus. No malformations were observed in the fetuses of control dams. The author noted that the effects were consistent with an early alteration of mesodermal development (Hung et al., 1986).

To study the effect of ethylenethiourea on neural tube development, nine groups of 66 pregnant Long Evans rats received a single intragastric administration of ethylene-thiourea on one of days 11–19 of gestation. Each group was further divided into three groups that were given 80, 120 or 160 mg/kg bw ethylenethiourea. A control group of 11 females was available. Fetuses were examined on gestation day 20. Fetal mortality was highest (21%) after treatment on day 11 and was not significantly increased with treatment after day 13. Regardless of the day of treatment, 100% of the fetuses were malformed, except after treatment on day 19, when no malformations were observed. The malformations shifted from myeloschisis with treatment on day 11 to abnormally enlarged head on days 12 and 13 to hydranencephaly and hydrocephalus on days 14–18. Histological examination of the fetuses with myeloschisis indicated hyper-trophy of neural tissue, especially in the hindbrain and lower spinal chord. The tissue hypertrophy and rosette formation indicated reparative action in regions of the neural tube where extensive cellular degeneration and necrosis had been reported previously (Sato *et al.*, 1985).

(c)   *Mode of action* in vitro

The direct effect of ethylenethiourea on rodent embryo development was studied in whole-embryo cultures. Addition of 40–200 µg/mL ethylenethiourea to 10-day-old Sprague-Dawley rat embryos and culturing for 48 h *in vitro* resulted in dose-related inhibition of growth and differentiation and increased incidences of malformations. The authors attributed the findings to altered osmotic fluid balance in the embryo, as the osmolality of the exocoelomic fluid was reduced after 48 h in culture (Daston *et al.*, 1987).

The development of 10-day-old Sprague-Dawley rat embryos exposed *in vitro* to ethylenethiourea by direct addition of 0–2.0 mmol/L (0–204 µg/mL) ethylenethiourea to the growth medium of whole-embryo culture or exposed *in utero* to 0, 60 or 120 mg/kg bw ethylenethiourea by oral gavage was examined to assess the similarity of the two approaches in inducing central nervous system defects (Khera, 1989). In culture, the embryos showed hydrocephalus after 26 h of exposure to 1.5 or 2.0 mmol/L ethylene-thiourea. No hydrocephaly was observed in embryos exposed *in vivo*. The lack of consistency in results obtained *in vitro* and *in vivo* may be due to differences in kinetics and in the critical period of exposure. It has been pointed out that the concentrations and the areas under the curve of concentration–time used *in vitro* are substantially higher than those obtained for teratogenic exposures *in vivo* (Daston, 1990).

The sensitivity of comparably staged Sprague-Dawley rats (gestation day 10.5) and CD-1 mice (gestation day 8.5) in whole-embryo culture was evaluated after a 48-h expo-sure to ethylenethiourea (at 0, 80, 120 or 160 µg/mL for rats and at 0, 80, 160, 240 or 320 µg/mL for mice). The teratogenic effects were qualitatively similar in the two species and were characterized by excessive accumulation of fluid in structures, particu-larly in the neural tube, but the potency was approximately twice as great in rats. When an exogenous metabolic activation system from a $9000 \times g$ supernatant of liver from

Arochlor 1254-induced rats and mice (S9 mix) was added to the treatment protocol, rat S9 had virtually no effect on the embryonic effects typical of ethylenethiourea, but these were virtually eliminated by mouse S9 in both species. Of note, however, was that addition of mouse S9 and ethylenethiourea to mouse embryos in culture resulted in the induction of abnormalities (mainly open neural tube) not seen in rat or mouse embryos exposed *in vitro* to ethylenethiourea alone, or in mouse embryos exposed *in vivo* (Daston *et al.*, 1989).

The effects were studied of direct addition of ethylenethiourea to 11-day-old Wistar-Imamichi rat embryos cultured for 48 h and to midbrain and limb bud cells removed from 11-day-old embryos. Malformations in cultured embryos were observed at concentrations ≥ 30 μg/mL ethylenethiourea. Consistent with the predilection for neural tube defects over limb defects, when the cells were exposed to ethylenethiourea in culture, the median concentration for inhibition of differentiation of midbrain cells was 2.3- and > 14-fold lower than that for limb bud cells on days 11 and 12 of gestation, respectively (Tsuchiya *et al.*, 1991a).

Ethylenethiourea was added at 0, 10 or 30 μg/mL to 11.5-day-old Wistar-Imamichi rat embryos in whole-embryo culture for 17 h, and the embryos were then grown in control media for another 29 h. Dose-related morphological anomalies were found that were largely prevented by the addition of an S9 mix from rats induced with pheno-barbital and 5,6-benzoflavon (Iwase *et al.*, 1997).

Using micromass cultures of midbrain or limb bud cells from 10-day-old JcL/ICR mice or 11-, 12- or 13-day-old Wistar-Imamichi rats exposed either directly to ethylene-thiourea in culture (0–600 μg/mL) or using serum of rats and mice treated *in vivo* (collected 2 h after exposure to 200 mg/kg bw), it was demonstrated that the species difference is at least partially intrinsic to the embryo. That is, the concentration of ethylenethiourea required to affect midbrain cell cultures from 10-day-old mouse embryos directly was 11-fold greater than that required for cultures from 12- and 13-day-old rat embryos. In addition, rat, but not mouse, midbrain cell differentiation was affected when serum from treated rats or mice was used in the culture medium. In the rat cell culture, the midbrain was affected more than limb bud cells, in parallel with effects noted in embryos treated *in vivo*. The concentration of ethylenethiourea in rat sera was only twofold higher than that in mouse sera. The study indicates that the species difference is likely to be due to differences in both kinetics and dynamics between rats and mice (Tsuchiya *et al.*, 1991b).

(d)   Altered thyroid function

A teratogenic dose (40 mg/kg bw per day) of ethylenethiourea was given by gavage once daily on days 7–15 of gestation to hypothyroid and euthyroid Charles River rats, and the fetuses were examined on day 20 of gestation. Additional euthyroid groups received subcutaneous injections of ethylenethiourea with or without thyroxine (5 μg/0.1 mL per 100 g bw/day) on days 7–15 of gestation. Hypothyroidism was induced by surgical removal of the thyroparathyroid gland at 75 days of age, 3 weeks before breeding. As expected, the serum concentration of T4 was reduced by this surgery (2.3 versus 6.2 µg/mL). The endogenous concentrations of T4 were further reduced by ethylenethiourea in the thyroparathyroidectomized groups (1.4 versus 2.3 µg/mL, compared with 4.8 versus 5.9 µg/mL in the sham-operated controls). Malformations were present in 100% of the fetuses regardless of thyroid status, although some different malformations (e.g., oedema, micrognathia, cleft palate and micromelia) were seen in the thyroparathyroidectomized females given ethylenethiourea. The only increase in the incidence of malformations in control groups was a 10.3% incidence in the thyroparathyroidectomized animals not treated with ethylenethiourea. The results did not support a role of altered thyroid function in ethylenethiourea-induced teratogenesis in rats (Lu & Staples, 1978).

The teratogenic potential of ethylenethiourea was compared with that of the thyroid antagonist methimazole (see monograph in this volume) in rat embryo cultures. Exposure of 9.5-day-old Wistar rat embryos to ethylenethiourea at a concentration of 50 µmol/L to 1 mmol/L for 48 h resulted in dose-related reductions in embryonic growth and differentiation; the effects were significant at concentrations of 500 µmol/L and 1 mmol/L. The commonest anomaly was abnormal development of the caudal region of the neural tube. While some similarities in embryonic responses were noted, reductions and swellings of the caudal region in many embryos exposed to ethylenethiourea was not seen in embryos exposed to methimazole, and other effects seen in methimazole-exposed embryos were not seen in ethylenethiourea-treated embryos (Stanisstreet *et al.*, 1990).

(e)   Other aspects of developmental toxicity

In order to study the potential of nitrites to activate ethylenethiourea by nitrosation, the teratogenic effects of ethylenethiourea were studied in SLC-ICR mice exposed to either ethylenethiourea alone or ethylenethiourea in combination with sodium nitrite. The authors hypothesized that ethylenethiourea would react with nitrite at the low pH in the stomach and form a reactive *N*-nitroso compound. Ethylenethiourea was administered by oral gavage at 400 mg/kg bw with or without 200 mg/kg bw sodium nitrite on day 6, 8, 10 or 12 of gestation. There were 12–29 dams in each group, and the fetuses were examined on gestation day 18. When nitrite was administered 2 h after treatment with ethylenethiourea, no teratogenic effects were seen in mouse embryos. Concomitant treatment on day 6 was most effective for induction of fetal death and growth retardation, while various malformations were present after exposure on day 6, 8 or 10. Exposure on day 12 did not adversely effect embryonic development. In particular, treatment on day 6 or 8 caused abnormal lobation of the left and right lung, respectively. Some of the observed defects resembled those observed in ethylenethiourea-treated rats (Teramoto *et al.*, 1980).

The role of altered hepatic function in ethylenethiourea-induced teratogenicity was studied in Swiss-Webster mice that received 0, 1600, 2000 or 2400 mg/kg bw ethylenethiourea by oral gavage on day 12 of gestation. The modulating treatments included phenobarbital (at 60 mg/kg bw per day by subcutaneous injection on days 7–10 of gestation), SKF-525A (at 40 mg/kg bw by intraperitoneal injection on day 12) and 3-methylcholanthrene (at 20 mg/kg bw per day on days 10–12). Ethylenethiourea alone induced dose-related incidences of hindpaw ectrodactyly and syndactyly and low incidences of cleft palate and hindpaw polydactyly. The incidence of defects was altered only by 3-methylcholanthrene, which reduced the incidences of hindpaw ectrodactyly, syndactyly and cleft palate at the two higher doses of ethylenethiourea (Khera, 1984).

Histological changes to the central nervous system were studied after exposure of Wistar rats to 0, 15 or 30 mg/kg bw ethylenethiourea by oral gavage on day 13 of gestation. Four to six females per dose were killed 12, 24, 48 and 72 h after exposure. Other dams were allowed to litter, and their offspring were followed to postnatal day 80. Within 12 h of receiving the higher dose, karyorrhexis was evident in the germinal layer of the basal lamina of the central nervous system, extending from the spinal cord to the telencephalon. By 48 h, rosettes were present in the neuroepithelium and there was extensive disorganization of the germinal and mantle layers. Similar, but less severe responses were seen at the lower dose. During the postnatal phase, 50% of the offspring of dams at the higher dose had died by 80 days after birth, and hydrocephaly was invariably present. There were no postnatal effects at the lower dose (Khera & Tryphonas, 1985).

4.4 Effects on enzyme induction or inhibition and gene expression

4.4.1 Humans

No data were available to the Working Group.

4.4.2 Experimental systems

Male WIST rats and male RIEMS/A mice were given oral doses of ethylenethiourea on 3 consecutive days. At a dose of 75 mg/kg bw per day, decreased activities of cytochrome P450 enzymes and aniline hydroxylase were noted in the rats 3 days after treatment. Aminopyrine N-demethylase activity was reduced to 60–70% of control values 24 h after treatment with doses of 50 and 75 mg/kg bw per day. In mice, the activity of cytochrome P450 enzymes was increased 24 h after treatment with doses of ethylenethiourea ranging from 50 to 1000 mg/kg bw per day, and aniline hydroxylase activity was increased at doses of 100–1000 mg/kg bw per day. No change in aminopyrine-N-demethylase activity was seen (Lewerenz & Plass, 1984).

After a single oral dose of 50–600 mg/kg bw ethylenethiourea, male Swiss mice showed an increase (up to 2.4-fold) in microsomal aniline hydroxylase activity, which returned to control levels within 4 days after treatment. Treatment with actinomycin D, a transcription inhibitor, completely prevented the increase in enzyme activity when given by intraperitoneal injection 1 h before and 5 h after ethylenethiourea (Meneguz & Michalek, 1986).

In a study with microsomes from male and female Swiss-Webster mice, ethylene-thiourea was shown to be preferentially metabolized by flavin-dependent monooxy-genases, with binding of ethylenethiourea metabolites to liver microsomes (Hui *et al.*, 1988).

4.5   Genetic and related effects

The genotoxicity of ethylenethiourea has been reviewed (Dearfield, 1994; Elia *et al.*, 1995; Houeto *et al.*, 1995).

4.5.1   *Humans*

The frequency of sister chromatid exchange was increased in peripheral lymphocytes of pesticide applicators who had presumably been exposed to ethylene-thiourea as a metabolite of ethylenebisthiocarbamate fungicides. In the same study, the exposed individuals also had a higher frequency of chromosomal translocations than controls but not of other types of chromosomal damage (Steenland *et al.*, 1997).

4.5.2   *Experimental systems* (see Table 4 for references)

(*a*)   *DNA damage*

Ethylenethiourea did not induce SOS repair in *Salmonella typhimurium* or *Esche-richia coli*. It induced λ phage in *Escherichia coli*. It was weakly active in the *E. coli polA* test for differential toxicity only in liquid suspension; it caused differential toxi-city in one *E. coli rec* assay and equivocal results in two assays in *Bacillus subtilis rec*.

Ethylenethiourea induced DNA damage in the yeast *Saccharomyces cerevisiae*, as measured by differential survival of repair-deficient strains.

(*b*)   *Mutation and allied effects* in vitro

Ethylenethiourea was not mutagenic in *S. typhimurium* with or without metabolic activation, except in a few base-pair substitution or frameshift strains with metabolic activation. No mutation was induced in *E. coli*, except for a weak response in one study. In mouse or rat host-mediated assays, no mutations were induced in *S. typhimurium* G46 or TA1950, but a positive response was seen in *S. typhimurium* TA1530 in mice.

Ethylenethiourea did not induce forward mutation in *Schizosaccharomyces pombe*, but it induced reverse mutation in *Saccharomyces cerevisiae*. It induced mitotic gene conversion in one study but not in others, and induced intrachromosomal recombination and aneuploidy in yeast. Ethylenethiourea marginally induced petite mutants in yeast.

There is disagreement in the literature with regard to the mutagenicity of ethylene-thiourea at the *Tk* locus in mouse lymphoma L5178Y cells. It was not mutagenic at multiple loci in Chinese hamster ovary cells with or without S9. Ethylenethiourea did

Table 4 Genetic and related effects of ethylenethiourea

Test system	Result[a]		Dose[b] (LED/HID)	Reference
	Without exogenous metabolic system	With exogenous metabolic system		
Escherichia coli, λ phage induction	NT	+	10 000	Thomson (1981)
Escherichia coli, SOS repair (Chromotest), forward mutation	–	–	NR	Quillardet et al. (1985)
Salmonella typhimurium, SOS repair (Vitotox) test		NT	NR	van der Lelie et al. (1997)
Escherichia coli pol A, differential toxicity (liquid suspension test)	(+)	–	NR	Rosenkranz et al. (1981)
Escherichia coli pol A, lexA, recA, differential toxicity	–	–	NR	Green (1981)
Escherichia coli pol A, lexA, recA, differential toxicity			1000	Tweats (1981)
Escherichia coli rec assay, differential toxicity (spot test)	NT	+	NR	Ichinotsubo et al. (1981a)
Bacillus subtilis rec assay, differential toxicity	(+)		2 mg/disc	Kada (1981)
Bacillus subtilis rec assay, differential toxicity	–	NT	4 mg/disc	Teramoto et al. (1977)
Salmonella typhimurium, forward mutation, aza resistance	NT	–	100	Skopek et al. (1981)
Salmonella typhimurium TA100, reverse mutation	–	–	20 000 µg/plate	Teramoto et al. (1977)
Salmonella typhimurium TA100, TA1535, TA1538, TA98, reverse mutation	NT	+	20 µg/plate	Anderson & Styles (1978)
Salmonella typhimurium TA100, TA1535, TA1537, TA1538, TA98, reverse mutation	–	–	2000 µg/plate	Brooks & Dean (1981); Rowland & Severn (1981)
Salmonella typhimurium TA100, TA98, reverse mutation	–	–	500 µg/plate	Venitt & Crofton-Sleigh (1981)
Salmonella typhimurium TA100, TA98, reverse mutation	–	–	500	Hubbard et al. (1981)
Salmonella typhimurium TA100, reverse mutation	–	–	NR	Ichinotsubo et al. (1981b)
Salmonella typhimurium TA98, reverse mutation	–	+	NR	Ichinotsubo et al. (1981b)
Salmonella typhimurium TA100, TA98, reverse mutation	–	–	5000 µg/plate	MacDonald (1981); Franekic et al. (1994)
Salmonella typhimurium TA100, TA1537, TA98, reverse mutation	–	–	NR	Nagao & Takahashi (1981)

Table 4 (contd)

Test system	Result[a] Without exogenous metabolic system	Result[a] With exogenous metabolic system	Dose[b] (LED/HID)	Reference
Salmonella typhimurium TA100, TA1535, TA1537, TA1538, TA98, reverse mutation	–	–	2500 µg/plate	Trueman (1981)
Salmonella typhimurium TA100, TA98, reverse mutation	–	–	100 µg/plate	Kanamaru et al. (1984)
Salmonella typhimurium TA100, TA1535, TA1537, TA1538, TA98, reverse mutation	–	–	1000 µg/plate	Falck et al. (1985)
Salmonella typhimurium TA100, TA1537, TA98, reverse mutation	–	–	10 000 µg/plate	Mortelmans et al. (1986)
Salmonella typhimurium TA102, TA104, reverse mutation	–		50 µg/plate	Franekic et al. (1994)
Salmonella typhimurium TA1530, reverse mutation	+	NT	40 000 µg/plate	Schüpbach & Hummler (1977)
Salmonella typhimurium TA1535, reverse mutation	+	–	5000 µg/plate	Teramoto et al. (1977)
Salmonella typhimurium TA1535, TA1537, TA98, reverse mutation	–	–	1000	Gatehouse (1981)
Salmonella typhimurium TA100, TA1535, TA1537, TA1538, TA98, reverse mutation	–	–	5000 µg/plate	Richold & Jones (1981)
Salmonella typhimurium TA1535, reverse mutation	?	+	1000 µg/plate	Simmon & Shepherd (1981)
Salmonella typhimurium TA1535, reverse mutation	+	+	5000 µg/plate	Moriya et al. (1983)
Salmonella typhimurium TA1535, reverse mutation	(+)	(+)	3333 µg/plate	Mortelmans et al. (1986)
Salmonella typhimurium TA1537, TA1538, reverse mutation	–	–	10 000 µg/plate	Teramoto et al. (1977)
Salmonella typhimurium TA1537, reverse mutation	–	–	2000 µg/plate	MacDonald (1981)
Salmonella typhimurium TA100, TA1537, TA1538, TA98, reverse mutation	–	–	5000 µg/plate	Simmon & Shepherd (1981); Moriya et al. (1983)
Salmonella typhimurium TA98, reverse mutation	–	+	100 µg/plate	Garner et al. (1981)
Salmonella typhimurium G46, reverse mutation (spot test)	+	NT	100	Seiler (1974)

Table 4 (contd)

Test system	Result[a] Without exogenous metabolic system	With exogenous metabolic system	Dose[b] (LED/HID)	Reference
Salmonella typhimurium G46, reverse mutation	–	NT	80 000 µg/plate	Schüpbach & Hummler (1977)
Salmonella typhimurium G46, reverse mutation	–	–	10 000 µg/plate	Teramoto et al. (1977)
Salmonella typhimurium TA1531, TA1532, TA1964, reverse mutation (spot test)	–	NT	NR	Schüpbach & Hummler (1977)
Salmonella typhimurium TA92, reverse mutation	–	–	2000 µg/plate	Brooks & Dean (1981)
Salmonella typhimurium TA1950, reverse mutation	+	NT	10 000 µg/plate	Autio et al. (1982)
Salmonella typhimurium TA1950, reverse mutation (spot test)	+	NT	5 mg/disc	Autio et al. (1982)
Escherichia coli K-12/343/113, forward or reverse mutation	–	(+)	0.2 mg/mL	Mohn et al. (1981)
Escherichia coli WP2 hcr, reverse mutation	–		10 000 µg/plate	Teramoto et al. (1977)
Escherichia coli WP2 uvrA, reverse mutation	–	–	1000	Gatehouse (1981); Falck et al. (1985)
Escherichia coli WP2 uvrA, WP2, reverse mutation	–	–	NR	Matsushima et al. (1981)
Escherichia coli WP2 uvrA, reverse mutation	–	–	1000 µg/plate	Falck et al. (1985)
Escherichia coli WP2 uvrA pKM101, reverse mutation	–	–	500 µg/plate	Venitt & Crofton-Sleigh (1981)
Escherichia coli WP2 pKM101, reverse mutation	–	–	100 µg/plate	Venitt & Crofton-Sleigh (1981)
Escherichia coli WP2 hcr, reverse mutation	–	–	5000 µg/plate	Moriya et al. (1983)
Saccharomyces cerevisiae, repair-deficient strain, differential toxicity	+	+	300	Sharp & Parry (1981a)
Saccharomyces cerevisiae D6, petite mutations	(+)	NT	1000	Wilkie & Gooneskera (1980)
Saccharomyces cerevisiae D4, mitotic gene conversion	–	–	333 µg/plate	Jagannath et al. (1981)

Table 4 (contd)

Test system	Result[a] Without exogenous metabolic system	With exogenous metabolic system	Dose[b] (LED/HID)	Reference
Saccharomyces cerevisiae T$_1$ and T$_2$, mitotic crossing-over	−	−	1000	Kassinova *et al.* (1981)
Saccharomyces cerevisiae JD1, mitotic gene conversion	+	NT	50	Sharp & Parry (1981b)
Saccharomyces cerevisiae D7, mitotic gene conversion	−	−	2 mg/mL	Zimmermann & Scheel (1981)
Saccharomyces cerevisiae RS112, intrachromosomal recombination	+	NT	20 mg/mL	Schiestl *et al.* (1989)
Saccharomyces cerevisiae D6 (stationary phase cells), mitotic aneuploidy	+	NT	500	Parry & Sharp (1981)
Saccharomyces cerevisiae, chromosome loss	+	NT	400	Franekic *et al.* (1994)
Saccharomyces cerevisiae, reverse mutation	+	−	88.9	Mehta & von Borstel (1981)
Schizosaccharomyces pombe, forward mutation	−	−	1	Loprieno (1981)
Aspergillus nidulans 35, forward mutation	−	NT	11 860	Crebelli *et al.* (1986)
Aspergillus nidulans P$_1$, mitotic malsegregation	+	NT	4000	Crebelli *et al.* (1986)
Shallot root tips, micronucleus formation	+	NT	2.5	Franekic *et al.* (1994)
Shallot root tips, chromosomal aberrations	+	NT	2.5	Franekic *et al.* (1994)
Drosophila melanogaster, somatic recombination, *w/w*$^+$ locus	−		51.1 mg/kg feed	Vogel & Nivard (1993)
Drosophila melanogaster, somatic recombination, *w/w*$^+$ locus	+		51.1 mg/kg feed	Rodriguez-Arnaiz (1997)
Drosophila melanogaster, sex-linked recessive lethal mutation	−		250 mg/kg feed	Valencia & Houtchens (1981)
Drosophila melanogaster, sex-linked recessive lethal mutation	−		4900 mg/kg inj	Woodruff *et al.* (1985)
Drosophila melanogaster, sex-linked recessive lethal mutation	−		12 500 mg/kg feed	Woodruff *et al.* (1985)

Table 4 (contd)

Test system	Result[a] Without exogenous metabolic system	With exogenous metabolic system	Dose[b] (LED/HID)	Reference
Drosophila melanogaster, sex-linked recessive lethal mutation	–		5100 mg/kg feed	Mason *et al.* (1992)
Gene mutation, Chinese hamster ovary cells, resistance to 8-azaadenine, 6-thioguanine, ouabain octahydrate, 5-fluoro-deoxyuridine, *in vitro*	–	–	2000	Carver *et al.* (1981)
Gene mutation, *Tk* locus, mouse lymphoma L5178Y cells *in vitro*	–	–	3000	Jotz & Mitchell (1981)
Gene mutation, *Tk* locus, mouse lymphoma L5178Y cells *in vitro*	–	+	1800	McGregor *et al.* (1988)
Sister chromatid exchange, Chinese hamster ovary cells *in vitro*	–	–	1000	Evans & Mitchell (1981)
Sister chromatid exchange, Chinese hamster ovary cells *in vitro*	–	–	5000	Natarajan & van Kesteren-van Leeuwen (1981)
Sister chromatid exchange, Chinese hamster ovary cells *in vitro*	–	–	100	Perry & Thomson (1981)
Sister chromatid exchange, Chinese hamster ovary cells *in vitro*	–	–	5000	National Toxicology Program (1992)
Cell transformation, BALB/c-3T3 mouse cells	(+)	NT	NR	Matthews *et al.* (1993)
Cell transformation, BHK-21 mouse cells	+	+	NR	Daniel & Dehnel (1981)
Cell transformation, BHK-21 mouse cells	+	NT	0.2	Styles (1981)
Cell transformation, SA7/Syrian hamster embryo cells	(+)	NT	1000	Hatch *et al.* (1986)
Micronucleus formation, Syrian hamster embryo cells *in vitro*	–	NT	NR	Fritzenschaf *et al.* (1993)
Chromosomal aberrations, Chinese hamster DON cells *in vitro*	?c	NT	3200	Teramoto *et al.* (1977)
Chromosomal aberrations, Chinese hamster ovary cells *in vitro*	?c	?c	5000	Natarajan & van Kesteren-van Leeuwen (1981)
Chromosomal aberrations, Chinese hamster ovary cells *in vitro*	–	–	10 000	National Toxicology Program (1992)
Chromosomal aberrations, rat liver RL1 cells *in vitro*	–	NT	200	Dean (1981)

Table 4 (contd)

Test system	Result[a] Without exogenous metabolic system	Result[a] With exogenous metabolic system	Dose[b] (LED/HID)	Reference
Host-mediated assay, *Salmonella typhimurium* G46 in Swiss albino mice	–		6000 mg/kg bw; im × 1	Schüpbach & Hummler (1977)
Host-mediated assay, *Salmonella typhimurium* TA1530 in Swiss albino mice	+		6000 mg/kg bw; im × 1	Schüpbach & Hummler (1977)
Host mediated assay, *Salmonella typhimurium* TA1950 in male NMRI mice	–		5 po × 1	Autio et al. (1982)
Host-mediated assay, *Salmonella typhimurium* G46 in JCR-ICR mice and Wistar rats	–		400 po × 3	Teramoto et al. (1997)
DNA damage (Comet assay), male CD-1 mouse liver, kidney, lung and spleen *in vivo*	+		2000 ip × 1	Sasaki et al. (1997)
DNA damage (Comet assay), male CD-1 mouse bone marrow *in vivo*	–		2000 ip × 1	Sasaki et al. (1997)
Sister chromatid exchange, male CBA/J mouse bone-marrow cells *in vivo*	–		1000 ip × 1	Paika et al. (1981)
Micronucleus formation, female ICR mouse bone-marrow cells *in vivo*	–		450 ip × 2	Seiler (1973)
Micronucleus formation, mouse bone-marrow cells *in vivo*	–		6000 po × 2	Schüpbach & Hummler (1977)
Micronucleus formation, male ICR mouse bone-marrow cells *in vivo*	(+)		880 ip × 1	Kirkhart (1981)
Micronucleus formation, B6C3F$_1$ mouse bone-marrow cells *in vivo*			1400 ip × 2[d]	Salamone et al. (1981)
Micronucleus formation, CD-1 mouse bone-marrow cells *in vivo*	–		880 ip × 2	Tsuchimoto & Matter (1981)
Micronucleus formation, CD-1 mouse peripheral blood and bone-marrow cells *in vivo*	–		2500 ip × 2	Morita et al. (1997)
Chromosomal aberrations, male and female Wistar rat bone-marrow cells *in vivo*	–		400 po × 2	Teramoto et al. (1977)
Dominant lethal mutation, Swiss albino mice *in vivo*	–		3500 po × 1	Schüpbach & Hummler (1977)

Table 4 (contd)

Test system	Result[a]		Dose[b] (LED/HID)	Reference
	Without exogenous metabolic system	With exogenous metabolic system		
Dominant lethal mutation, JCL-ICR mice *in vivo*	—		600 po × 5	Teramoto *et al.* (1977)
Dominant lethal mutation, C3H/HeCr mice *in vivo*	—		150 po × 5	Teramoto *et al.* (1978)
Inhibition of DNA synthesis, mouse testis *in vivo*	—		100 ip × 1	Seiler (1977)
Sperm morphology, (CBA × BALB/c)F₁ mice *in vivo*	—		2000 ip × 5	Topham (1981)
Sperm morphology, B6C3F₁/CRL mice *in vivo*	—		2655 ip × 5	Wyrobek *et al.* (1981)

[a] +, positive; (+), weak positive; −, negative; NT, not tested; ?, inconclusive

[b] LED, lowest effective dose; HID, highest ineffective dose; in-vitro tests, μg/mL; in-vivo tests, mg/kg bw/day; ip, intraperitoneal; po, oral; im, intramuscular; inj, injection

[c] No dose–response relationship

[d] Dose is 80% of LD₅₀ (as reported by Tsuchimoto & Matter, 1981)

not induce chromosomal aberrations or sister chromatid exchange in cultured Chinese hamster cells or a rat liver cell line or micronuclei in Syrian hamster embryo cells.

Ethylenethiourea transformed BHK-21 cells in culture and had weak transforming activity on BALB/c-3T3 cells.

(c) Mutation and allied effects in vivo

DNA damage, as measured in the Comet assay, was induced in liver, kidney, lung and spleen, but not bone-marrow cells of mice given an intraperitoneal injection of ethylenethiourea.

Chromosomal aberrations were not induced in rat bone-marrow cells after oral administration, and no sister chromatid exchange was induced in mouse bone-marrow cells after intraperitoneal injection. Micronucleus formation was not induced in mouse blood or bone-marrow cells after intraperitoneal or oral administration.

Ethylenethiourea did not induce dominant lethal mutations or sperm abnormalities or inhibit testicular DNA synthesis in male mice.

In *Drosophila melanogaster*, sex-linked recessive lethal mutations were not induced, but somatic recombination was induced at the w/w^+ locus in one of two studies.

Micronuclei and chromosomal aberrations were induced by ethylenethiourea in shallot root tips.

4.6 Mechanistic considerations

Ethylenethiourea is not genotoxic.

The available data indicate that thyroid hormone imbalance plays a role in the development of follicular-cell neoplasia caused by ethylenethiourea in rats and mice.
- Ethylenethiourea is considered not to be genotoxic because of its lack of activity in appropriate tests in bacteria, mammalian cells *in vitro* and mice and rats treated *in vivo.*
- Ethylenethiourea alters thyroid hormone homeostasis in rats treated with doses spanning the range that induced thyroid tumours in this species.
- Ethylenethiourea produces thyroid gland enlargement (goitre) in rats and follicular-cell hypertrophy and hyperplasia in rats and mice. The mechanism is based on interference with thyroid peroxidase.

On the basis of this information, which meets the criteria laid out in the IARC consensus report (Capen *et al.*, 1999), ethylenethiourea would be expected not to be carcinogenic to humans exposed to concentrations that do not lead to alterations in thyroid hormone homeostasis.

The hyperplasia induced by ethylenethiourea in the thyroid gland is diffuse, in analogy with the morphological changes induced by stimulation of thyroid-stimulating hormone, rather than only multifocal, as would be induced by a genotoxic thyroid carcinogen (Hard, 1998). In view of the lack of genotoxicity, the liver tumours in mice and the benign pituitary tumours in mice were considered not to be produced by a geno-toxic mechanism.

5.   Summary of Data Reported and Evaluation

5.1   Exposure data

Ethylenethiourea is used as a vulcanization accelerator in the rubber industry. It is a degradation product of and an impurity in ethylenebisdithiocarbamate fungicides, and field workers may be exposed to ethylenethiourea while applying these fungicides. The general population may be exposed to low concentrations of residues of ethylenethiourea in foods.

5.2   Human carcinogenicity data

The available data were inadequate to evaluate the carcinogenicity of ethylenethiourea to humans.

5.3   Animal carcinogenicity data

Ethylenethiourea was tested for carcinogenicity by oral administration in two studies in three strains of mice, with perinatal exposure in one study. It was also tested in five studies in rats by oral administration, with perinatal exposure in one study. In mice, it produced thyroid follicular-cell tumours and tumours of the liver and anterior pituitary gland. In rats, it consistently produced thyroid follicular-cell adenomas and carcinomas. Ethylenethiourea did not cause neoplasms in one strain of hamsters.

5.4   Other relevant data

Ethylenethiourea caused thyroid gland enlargement (goitre) in rats and mice as a result of diffuse hypertrophy and hyperplasia of thyroid follicular cells. Administration of ethylenethiourea under bioassay conditions that caused predominantly benign follicular-cell tumours resulted in alteration of thyroid hormone homeostasis, including increased secretion of thyroid-stimulating hormone. The underlying mechanism of the changes induced by ethylenethiourea is interference with the functioning of thyroid peroxidase activity. This is considered to be the basis for its tumorigenic activity in experimental animals.

One retrospective study of pregnancy outcomes in women employed in the manufacture of rubber containing ethylenethiourea showed no exposure-related effects. Ethylenethiourea was teratogenic in rats, but not in mice, hamsters or guinea-pigs. The central nervous system was particularly vulnerable in rats. The available data suggest that both toxicokinetics and embryo sensitivity are components of the species-specificity of the teratogenicity of ethylenethiourea. Furthermore, effects on thyroid function do not appear to be involved.

Ethylenethiourea was not genotoxic in appropriate tests in bacteria and cultured mammalian cells or in rodents *in vivo*. Ethylenethiourea induced chromosomal recombination and aneuploidy in yeast and cell transformation in mammalian cells.

5.5   Evaluation

There is *inadequate evidence* in humans for the carcinogenicity of ethylenethiourea.

There is *sufficient evidence* in experimental animals for the carcinogenicity of ethylenethiourea.

Overall evaluation

Ethylenethiourea is *not classifiable as to its carcinogenicity to humans (Group 3)*.

In making its evaluation, the Working Group concluded that ethylenethiourea produces thyroid tumours in mice and rats by a non-genotoxic mechanism, which involves interference with the functioning of thyroid peroxidase resulting in a reduction in circulating thyroid hormone concentrations and increased secretion of thyroid-stimulating hormone. Consequently, ethylenethiourea would not be expected to produce thyroid cancer in humans exposed to concentrations that do not alter thyroid hormone homeostasis.

An additional consideration of the Working Group, based on the lack of genotoxicity of ethylenethiourea, was that the liver tumours and benign pituitary tumours in mice were also produced by a non-genotoxic mechanism.

Evidence from epidemiological studies and from toxicological studies in experimental animals provide compelling evidence that rodents are substantially more sensitive than humans to the development of thyroid tumours in response to thyroid hormone imbalance.

6.   References

Ahmad, N., Guo, L., Mandarakas, P. & Appleby, S. (1995) Determination of dithiocarbamate and its breakdown product ethylenethiourea in fruits and vegetables. *J. AOAC int.*, **78**, 1238–1243

Allen, J.R., Van Miller, J.P. & Seymour, J.L. (1978) Absorption, tissue distribution and excretion of ^{14}C ethylenethiourea by the rhesus monkey and rat. *Res. Commun. chem. Pathol. Pharmacol.*, **20**, 109–115

American Conference of Governmental Industrial Hygienists (2000) *TLVs and Other Occupational Exposure Values — 2000 CD-ROM*, Cincinnati, OH

Anderson, D. & Styles, J.A. (1978) The bacterial mutation test. *Br. J. Cancer*, **37**, 924–930

AOAC International (1999a) AOAC Official Method 978.16. Ethylenethiourea. Pesticide residues. In: *Official Methods of Analysis of AOAC International*, 16th Ed., 5th rev., Gaithersburg, MD [CD-ROM]

AOAC International (1999b) AOAC Official Method 992.31. Ethylene thiourea (ETU). Residues in water. In: *Official Methods of Analysis of AOAC International*, 16th Ed., 5th Rev., Gaithersburg, MD [CD-ROM]

Aprea, C., Betha, A., Catenacci, G., Lotti, A., Minoia, C., Passini, W., Pavan, I., Saverio Robustelli della Cuna, F., Roggi, C., Ruggeri, R., Soave, C., Sciarra, G., Vannini, P. & Vitalone, V. (1996) Reference values of urinary ethylenethiourea in four regions of Italy (multicentric study). *Sci. total Environ.*, **192**, 83–93

Aprea, C., Betta, A., Catenacci, G., Colli, A., Lotti, A., Minoia, C., Olivieri, P., Passini, V., Pavan, I., Roggi, C., Ruggeri, R., Sciarra, G., Turci, R., Vannini, P. & Vitalone, V. (1997) Urinary excretion of ethylenethiourea in five volunteers on a controlled diet (multicentric study). *Sci. total Environ.*, **203**, 167–179

Arnold, D.L., Krewski, D.R., Junkins, D.B., McGuire, P.F., Moodie, C.A. & Munro, I.C. (1983) Reversibility of ethylenethiourea-induced thyroid lesions. *Toxicol. appl. Pharmacol.*, **67**, 264–273

Austin, G.E. & Moyer, G.H. (1979) Hepatic RNA synthesis in rats treated with ethylene thiourea. *Res. Commun. chem. Pathol. Pharmacol.*, **23**, 639–642

Autio, K. (1983) Determination of ethylenethiourea (ETU) [imidazolidine-2-thione] as a volatile *N,N'*-dimethyl derivative by GLC-MS and GLC-NPSD. Determination of ETU residues in berries and cigarette-smoke condensate. *Finn. chem. Lett.*, **4**, 10–14

Autio, K., von Wright, A. & Pyysalo, H. (1982) The effect of oxidation of the sulfur atom on the mutagenicity of ethylenethiourea. *Mutat. Res.*, **106**, 27–31

Beneventi, G., Barbieri, C., Del Carlo, G., Dondi, C. & Forti, S. (1994) [Pesticides in wine: Simultaneous determination of ethylenethiourea (ETU), propylenethiourea (PTU), fungicides and insecticides by SPE extraction with a C18 cartridge.] *Ind. Bev.*, **23**, 317–323 (in Italian)

Bottomley, P., Hoodless, R.A. & Smart, N.A. (1985) Review of methods for the determination of ethylenethiourea (imidazolidine-2-thione) residues. *Residue Rev.*, **95**, 45–89

Brooks, T.M. & Dean, B.J. (1981) Mutagenic activity of 42 coded compounds in the *Salmonella*/microsome assay with preincubation. *Prog. Mutat. Res.*, **1**, 261–270

Bruze, A. & Fregert, S. (1983) Allergic contact dermatitis from ethylene thiourea. *Contact Derm.*, **9**, 208–212

Budavari, S., ed. (2000) *The Merck Index*, 12th Ed., Version 12:3, Whitehouse Station, NJ, Merck & Co. & Boca Raton, FL, Chapman & Hall/CRC [CD-ROM]

Cabras, P., Menoni, M. & Pirisi, F.M. (1987) Pesticide fate from vine to wine. *Rev. Environ. Contam. Toxicol.*, **99**, 83–117

Capen, C.C., Dybing, E., Rice, J.M. & Wilbourn, J.D., eds (1999) *Species Differences in Thyroid, Kidney and Urinary Bladder Carcinogenesis* (IARC Scientific Publications No. 147), Lyon, IARC*Press*

Carver, J.H., Salazar, E.P., Knize, M.G. & Wandres, D.L. (1981) Mutation induction at multiple gene loci in Chinese hamster cells: The genetic activity of 15 coded carcinogens and noncarcinogens. *Prog. Mutat. Res.*, **1**, 594–601

Chernoff, N., Kavlock, R.J., Rogers, E.H., Carver, B.D. & Murray, S. (1979) Perinatal toxicity of maneb, ethylene thiourea, and ethylenebisisothiocyanate sulfide in rodents. *J. Toxicol. environ. Health*, **5**, 821–834

Chhabra, R.S., Eustis, S., Haseman, J.K., Kurtz, P.J. & Carlton, B.D. (1992) Comparative carcinogenicity of ethylene thiourea with or without perinatal exposure in rats and mice. *Fundam. appl. Toxicol.*, **18**, 405–417

CIS Information Services (2000) *Directory of World Chemical Producers (Version 2000.1)*, Dallas, TX [CD-ROM]

Crebelli, R., Bellincampi, D., Conti, G., Conti, L., Morpurgo, G. & Carere, A. (1986) A comparative study on selected chemical carcinogens for chromosome malsegregation, mitotic crossing-over and forward mutation induction in *Aspergillus nidulans*. *Mutat. Res.*, **172**, 139–149

Daniel, M.R. & Dehnel, J.M. (1981) Cell transformation test with baby hamster kidney cells. *Prog. Mutat. Res.*, **1**, 626–637

Daston, G.P. (1990) Ethylenethiourea: In vivo/in vitro comparisons of teratogenicity. *Teratology*, **41**, 475–476

Daston, G.P., Ebron, M.T., Carver, B. & Stefanadis, J.G. (1987) In vitro teratogenicity of ethylenethiourea in the rat. *Teratology*, **35**, 239–245

Daston, G.P., Rehnberg, B.F., Carver, B. & Kavlock, R.J. (1988) Functional teratogens of the rat kidney. II. Nitrofen and ethylenethiourea. *Fundam. appl. Toxicol.*, **11**, 401–415

Daston, G.P., Yonker, J.E., Powers, J.F. & Heitmeyer, S.A. (1989) Difference in teratogenic potency of ethylenethiourea in rats and mice: Relative contribution of embryonic and maternal factors. *Teratology*, **40**, 555–566

Dean, B.J. (1981) Activity of 27 coded compounds in the RL_1 chromosome assay. *Prog. Mutat. Res.*, **1**, 570–579

Dearfield, K.L. (1994) Ethylene thiourea (ETU). A review of the genetic toxicity studies. *Mutat. Res.*, **317**, 111–132

Decker, C.J. & Doerge, D.R. (1991) Rat hepatic microsomal metabolism of ethylenethiourea. Contributions of the flavin-containing monooxygenase and cytochrome P-450 isozymes. *Chem. Res. Toxicol.*, **4**, 482–489

Deutsche Forschungsgemeinschaft (2000) *List of MAK and BAT Values 2000* (Report No. 36), Weinheim, Wiley-VCH Verlag GmbH, p. 60

Doerge, D.R. & Takazawa, R.S. (1989) Mechanism of thyroid peroxidase inhibition by ethylenethiourea. *Chem. Res. Toxicol.*, **3**, 98–101

Dubey, J.K., Heberer, T. & Stan, H.-J. (1997) Determination of ethylenethiourea in food commodities by a two-step derivatization method and gas chromatography with electron-capture and nitrogen–phosphorus detection. *J. Chromatogr.*, **A765**, 31–38

Elia, M.C., Arce, G., Hurt, S.S., O'Neill, P.J. & Scribner, H.E. (1995) The genetic toxicology of ethylenethiourea: A case study concerning the evaluation of a chemical's genotoxic potential. *Mutat. Res.*, **341**, 141–149

Engels, H.W. (1993) Rubber, 4. Chemicals and additives (Part 1). In: Elvers, B., Hawkins, S., Russey, W. & Schulz, G., eds, *Ullmann's Encyclopedia of Industrial Chemistry*, Vol. A23, 5th rev. Ed., New York, VCH Publishers, pp. 365–380

Evans, E.L. & Mitchell, A.D. (1981) Effects of 20 coded chemicals in sister chromatid exchange frequencies in cultured Chinese hamster ovary cells. *Prog. Mutat. Res.*, **1**, 538–550

Falck, K., Partanen, P., Sorsa, M., Souvaniemi, O. & Vainio, H. (1985) Mutascreen®, an automated bacterial mutagenicity assay. *Mutat. Res.*, **150**, 119–125

FAO/WHO (1993a) *Ethylenethiourea, ETU* (108), *Pesticide residues in food — 1993. Report of the Joint Meeting of the FAO Panel of Experts on Pesticide Residues in Food and the Environment and a WHO Expert Group on Pesticide Residues* (FAO Plant Production and Protection Paper, 122), Rome

FAO/WHO (1993b) *Ethylenethiourea*. JMPR Evaluation 1993 Toxicology [http://www.inchem.org/documents/jmpr/jmpmono/v93pr08.htm]

Franekic, J., Bratulic, N., Pavlica, M. & Papeš, D. (1994) Genotoxicity of dithiocarbamates and their metabolites. *Mutat. Res.*, **325**, 65–74

Freudenthal, R.I., Kerchner, G., Persing, R. & Baron, R.L. (1977) Dietary subacute toxicity of ethylene thiourea in the laboratory rat. *J. environ. Pathol. Toxicol.*, **1**, 147–161

Fritzenschaf, H., Kohlpoth, M., Rusche, B. & Schiffmann, D. (1993) Testing of known carcinogens and noncarcinogens in the Syrian hamster embryo (SHE) micronucleus test *in vitro*; correlations with in vivo micronucleus formation and cell transformation. *Mutat. Res.*, **319**, 47–53

Fujinari, E.M. (1998) High performance liquid chromatography–chemiluminescent nitrogen detection: HPLC–CLND. *Dev. Food Sci.*, **39**, 431–466

Gak, J.C., Graillot, C. & Truhaut, R. (1976) [Differences in hamsters and rats regarding the effects of long-term administration of ethylene thiourea.] *Eur. J. Toxicol.*, **9**, 303–312 (in French)

Garner, R.C., Welch, A. & Pickering, C. (1981) Mutagenic activity of 42 coded compounds in the *Salmonella*/microsome assay. *Prog. Mutat. Res.*, **1**, 280–284

Gatehouse, D. (1981) Mutagenic activity of 42 coded compounds in the 'Microtiter' fluctuation test. *Prog. Mutat. Res.*, **1**, 376–386

Gonzalez, A.R., Mauromoustakos, A., Elkins, E.R. & Kims, E.S. (1990) Removal of carbamate residues from leafy greens with water and detergent solutions. *J. environ. Sci. Health*, **A25**, 1009–1017

Graham, S.L. & Hansen, W.H. (1972) Effects of short-term administration of ethylenethiourea upon thyroid function of the rat. *Bull. environ. Contam. Toxicol.*, **7**, 19–25

Graham, S.L., Hansen, W.H., Davis, K.J. & Perry, C.H. (1973) Effects of one-year administration of ethylenethiourea upon the thyroid of the rat. *J. agric. Food Chem.*, **21**, 324–329

Graham, S.L., Davis, K.J., Hansen, W.H. & Graham, C.H. (1975) Effects of prolonged ethylene thiourea ingestion on the thyroid of the rat. *Food Cosmet. Toxicol.*, **13**, 493–499

Green, M.H.L. (1981) A differential killing test using an improved repair-deficient strain of *Escherichia coli. Prog. Mutat. Res.*, **1**, 183–194

Hard, G.C. (1998) Recent developments in the investigation of thyroid regulation and thyroid carcinogenesis. *Environ. Health Perspectives*, **106**, 427–436

Hatch, G.G., Anderson, T.M., Lubet, R.A., Kouri, R.E., Putman, D.L., Cameron, J.W., Nims, R.W., Most, B., Spalding, J.W., Tennant, R.W. & Schechtman, L.M. (1986) Chemical enhancement of SA7 virus transformation of hamster embryo cells: Evaluation by interlaboratory testing of diverse chemicals. *Environ. Mutag.*, **8**, 515–531

Hirai, Y. & Kuwabara, N. (1990) Transplacentally induced anorectal malformations in rats. *J. pediatr. Surg.*, **25**, 812–816

Houeto, P., Bindoula, G. & Hoffman, J.R. (1995) Ethylenebisdithiocarbamates and ethylene-thiourea: Possible human health hazards. *Environ. Health Perspectives*, **103**, 568–573

Hubbard, S.A., Green, M.H.L., Bridges, B.A., Wain, A.J. & Bridges, J.W. (1981) Fluctuation tests with S9 and hepatocyte activation. *Prog. Mutat. Res.*, **1**, 361–370

Hui, Q.Y., Armstrong, C., Laver, G. & Iverson, F. (1988) Monooxygenase-mediated metabolism and binding of ethylene thiourea to mouse liver microsomal protein. *Toxicol. Lett.*, **41**, 231–237

Hung, C.-F. (1992) Experimentally induced axial dysraphism and anorectal malformation in male rat fetuses by intragastric administration of ethylenethiourea. *J. Formosan med. Assoc.*, **91**, 1166–1169

Hung, C.-F., Lee, K.-R. & Lee, C.-S. (1986) Experimental production of congenital malformation of the central nervous system in rat fetuses by single dose intragastric administration of ethylenethiourea. *Proc. natl Sci. Counc. Republ. China B.*, **10**, 127–136

IARC (1974) *IARC Monographs on the Evaluation of Carcinogenic Risk of Chemicals to Man*, Vol. 7, *Some Anti-thyroid and Related Substances, Nitrofurans and Industrial Chemicals*, Lyon, IARCPress, pp. 45–52

IARC (1987) *IARC Monographs on the Evaluation of Carcinogenic Risks to Humans*, Suppl. 7, *Overall Evaluations of Carcinogenicity: An Updating of* IARC Monographs *Volumes 1 to 42*, Lyon, IARCPress, pp. 207–208

Ichinotsubo, D., Mower, H. & Mandel, M. (1981a) Testing of a series of paired compounds (carcinogen and noncarcinogenic structural analog) by DNA repair-deficient *E. coli* strains. *Prog. Mutat. Res.*, **1**, 195–198

Ichinotsubo, D., Mower, H. & Mandel, M. (1981b) Mutagen testing of a series of paired compounds with the Ames *Salmonella* testing system. *Prog. Mutat. Res.*, **1**, 298–301

Innes, J.R.M., Ulland, B.M., Valerio, M.G., Petrucelli, L., Fishbein, L., Hart, E.R., Pallota, A.J., Bates., R.R., Falk, H. L., Gart, J.J., Klein, M., Mitchell, I. & Peters, J. (1969) Bioassay of pesticides and industrial chemicals for tumorigenicity in mice: A preliminary note. *J. natl Cancer Inst.*, **42**, 1101–1114

IPCS/INCHEM (1993) *Joint Meeting on Pesticide Residue — Monographs and evaluations. Ethylene thiourea* [http://www.inchem.org/aboutjmpr.html]

Iverson, F., Khera, K.S. & Hierlihy, S.L. (1980) In vivo and in vitro metabolism of ethylene-thiourea in the rat and the cat. *Toxicol. appl. Pharmacol.*, **52**, 16–21

Iwase, T., Yamamoto, M., Shirai, M., Akahori, F., Masaoka, T., Takizawa, T., Arishima, K. & Eguchi, Y. (1996) Time course of ethylene thiourea in maternal plasma, amniotic fluid and embryos in rats following single oral dosing. *J. vet. med. Sci.*, **58**, 1235–1236

Iwase, T., Yamamoto, M., Shirai, S., Akahori, F., Masaoka, T., Takizawa, T., Arishima, K. & Eguchi, Y. (1997) Effect of ethylene thiourea on cultured rat embryos in the presence of hepatic microsomal fraction. *J. vet. Med. Sci.*, **59**, 59–61

Jagannath, D.R., Vultaggio, D.M. & Brusick, D.J. (1981) Genetic activity of 42 coded compounds in the mitotic gene conversion assay using *Saccharomyces cerevisiae* strain *D4*. *Prog. Mutat. Res.*, **1**, 456–467

Jotz, M.M. & Mitchell, A. D. (1981) Effects of 20 coded chemicals on the forward mutation frequency at the thymidine kinase locus in L5178Y mouse lymphoma cells. *Prog. Mutat. Res.*, **1**, 580–593

Kada, T. (1981) The DNA-damaging activity of 42 coded compounds in the rec-assay. *Prog. Mutat. Res.*, **1**, 175–182

Kanamaru, M., Suzuki, H., Yamaguchi, M. & Furukawa, H. (1984) [Mutagenicity of pesticides and their catabolites.] *Jpn. J. agric. Med.*, **33**, 203–210 (in Japanese)

Kassinova, G.V., Kovaltsova, S.V., Marfin, S.V. & Zakharov, I.A. (1981) Activity of 40 coded compounds in differential inhibition and mitotic crossing-over assays in yeast. *Prog. Mutat. Res.*, **1**, 434–455

Kato, Y., Odanaka, Y., Teramoto, S. & Matano, O. (1976) Metabolic fate of ethylenethiourea in pregnant rats. *Bull. environ. Contam. Toxicol.*, **16**, 546–555

Khera, K.S. (1973) Teratogenic effects of ethylenethiourea in rats and rabbits (Abstract). *Toxicol. appl. Pharmacol.*, **26**, 455–456

Khera, K.S. (1984) Ethylenethiourea-induced hindpaw deformities in mice and effects of metabolic modifiers on their occurrence. *J. Toxicol. environ. Health*, **13**, 747–756

Khera, K.S. (1987) Ethylenethiourea: A review of teratogenicity and distribution studies and an assessment of reproduction risk. *CRC crit. Rev. Toxicol.*, **18**, 129–139

Khera, K.S. (1989) Ethylenethiourea-induced hydrocephalus *in vivo* and *in vitro* with a note on the use of a constant gaseous atmosphere for rat embryo cultures. *Teratology*, **39**, 277–285

Khera, K.S. & Tryphonas, L. (1985) Nerve cell degeneration and progeny survival following ethylenethiourea treatment during pregnancy in rats. *Neurotoxicology*, **6**, 97–102

Kirkhart, B. (1981) Micronucleus test on 21 compounds. *Prog. Mutat. Res.*, **1**, 698–704

Knio, K.M., Saad, A. & Dagher, S. (2000) The fate and persistence of zineb, maneb and ethylenethiourea on fresh and processed tomatoes. *Food Addit. Contam.*, **17**, 393–398

Kobayashi, H., Kaneda, M. & Teramoto, S. (1982) Identification of 1-methylthiourea as the metabolite of ethylenethiourea in rats by high-performance liquid chromatography. *Toxicol. Lett.*, **12**, 109–113

Korhonen, A., Hemminki, K. & Vainio, H. (1982) Embryotoxicity of industrial chemicals on the chicken embryo: Thiourea derivatives. *Acta pharmacol. toxicol.*, **51**, 38–44

Krause, R.T. & Wang, Y. (1988) Liquid-chromatographic — Electrochemical technique for determination of ethylenethiourea [imidazolidine-2-thione] residues. *J. Liq. Chromatogr.*, **11**, 349–362

Kurttio, P., Savolainen, K., Tuominen, R., Kosma, V.M., Naukkarinen, A., Männistö, P. & Collan, Y. (1986) Ethylenethiourea and nabam induced alterations of function and morphology of thyroid gland in rats. *Arch. Toxicol.*, **Suppl. 9**, 339–344

Kurttio, P., Vartiainen, T. & Savolainen, K. (1988) A high-performance liquid chromatographic method for the determination of ethylenethiourea in urine and on filters. *Anal. chim. Acta*, **212**, 297–301

Kurttio, P., Vartiainen, T. & Savolainen, K. (1990) Environmental and biological monitoring of exposure to ethylenebisdithiocarbamate fungicides and ethylenethiourea. *Br. J. ind. Med.*, **47**, 203–206

Kurttio, P., Savolainen, K., Naukkarinen, A., Kosma, V.-M., Tuomisto, L., Penttilä, I. & Jolkkonen, J. (1991) Urinary excretion of ethylenethiourea and kidney morphology in rats after continuous oral exposure to nabam or ethylenethiourea. *Arch. Toxicol.*, **65**, 381–385

van der Lelie, D., Regniers, L., Borremans, B., Provoost, A. & Verschaeve, L. (1997) The VITOTOX® test, an SOS bioluminescence *Salmonella typhimurium* test to measure genotoxicity kinetics. *Mutat. Res.*, **389**, 279–290

Lewerenz, H.J. & Bleyl, D.W.R. (1980) Postnatal effects of oral administration of ethylene-thiourea to rats during late pregnancy. *Arch. Toxicol.*, **Suppl. 4**, 292–295

Lewerenz , H.J. & Plass, R. (1984) Contrasting effects of ethylenethiourea on hepatic mono-oxygenases in rats and mice. *Arch. Toxicol.*, **56**, 92–95

Lide, D.R. & Milne, G.W.A. (1996) *Properties of Organic Compounds*, Version 5.0, Boca Raton, FL, CRC Press [CD-ROM]

Lo, C.-C. & Hsiao, Y.-M. (1997) Comparison of micellar electrokinetic capillary chromato-graphic method with high-performance liquid chromatographic method for the determination of imidazolidine-2-thione (ethylenethiourea) in formulated products. *J. agric. Food Chem.*, **45**, 3118–3122

Longbottom, J.E., Edgell, K.W., Erb, E.J. & Lopez-Avila, V. (1993) Gas chromatographic/ nitrogen–phosphorus detection method for determination of ethylene thiourea in finished drinking waters: Collaborative study. *J. Assoc. off. anal. Chem. int.*, **76**, 1113–1120

Loprieno, N. (1981) Screening of coded carcinogenic/noncarcinogenic chemicals by a forward-mutation system with the yeast *Schizosaccharomyces pombe*. *Prog. Mutat. Res.*, **1**, 424–433

Lu, M.-H. & Staples, R.E. (1978) Teratogenicity of ethylenethiourea and thyroid function in the rat. *Teratology*, **17**, 171–178

MacDonald, D.J. (1981) *Salmonella*/microsome tests on 42 coded chemicals. *Prog. Mutat. Res.*, **1**, 285–297

Marinovich, M., Guizzetti, M., Ghilardi, F., Viviani, B., Corsini, E. & Galli, C.L. (1997) Thyroid peroxidase as toxicity target for dithiocarbamates. *Arch. Toxicol.*, **71**, 508–512

Maruyama, M. (1994) Residue analysis of ethylenethiourea in vegetables by high-performance liquid chromatography with amperometric detection. *Fresenius' J. anal. Chem.*, **348**, 324–326

Mason, J.M., Valencia, R. & Zimmering, S. (1992) Chemical mutagenesis testing in *Droso-phila*: VIII. Reexamination of equivocal results. *Environ. mol. Mutag.*, **19**, 227–234

Matsushima, T., Takamoto, Y., Shirai, A., Sawamura, M. & Sugimura, T. (1981) Reverse muta-tion test on 42 coded compounds with the *E. coli* WP2 system. *Prog. Mutat. Res.*, **1**, 387–395

Matthews, E.J., Spalding, J.W. & Tennant, R.W. (1993) Transformation of BALB/c-3T3 cells: V. Transformation responses of 168 chemicals compared with mutagenicity in Salmonella and carcinogenicity in rodent bioassays. *Environ. Health Perspectives*, **101** (Suppl. 2), 347–482

McGregor, D.B., Brown, A., Cattanach, P., Edwards, I., McBride, D., Riach, C. & Caspary, W.J. (1988) Responses of the L5178Y tk$^+$/tk$^-$ mouse lymphoma cell forward mutation assay: III. 72 coded chemicals. *Environ. mol. Mutag.*, **12**, 85–154

Mehta, R.D. & von Borstel, R.C. (1981) Mutagenic activity of 42 encoded compounds in the haploid yeast reversion assay, strain XV185-14C. *Prog. Mutat. Res.*, **1**, 414–423

Meiring, H.D. & de Jong, A.P.J.M. (1994) Determination of ethylenethiourea in water by single-step extractive derivatization and gas chromatography–negative ion chemical ionization mass spectrometry. *J. Chromatogr.*, **A683**, 157–165

Meneguz, A. & Michalek, H. (1986) Induction of hepatic microsomal mixed function oxidase system by ethylenethiourea in mice. *Arch. Toxicol.*, **Suppl. 9**, 346–350

Mohn, G.R., Vogels-Bouter, S. & van der Horst-van der Zon, J. (1981) Studies on the mutagenic activity of 20 coded compounds in liquid tests using the multipurpose strain *Escherichia coli* K-12/343/113 and derivatives. *Prog. Mutat. Res.*, **1**, 396–413

Moller, P.C., Chang, J.P. & Partridge, L.R. (1986) The effects of ethylene thiourea administration upon rat liver cells. *J. environ. Pathol. Toxicol. Oncol.*, **6**, 127–142

Morita, T., Asano, N., Awogi, T., Sasaki, Y.F., Sato, S., Shimada, H., Sutou, S., Suzuki, T., Wakata, A., Sofuni, T. & Hayashi, M. (1997) Evaluation of the rodent micronucleus assay in the screening of IARC carcinogens (Groups 1, 2A and 2B). The summary report of the 6th collaborative study by CSGMT/JEMS.MMS. *Mutat. Res.*, **389**, 3–122

Moriya, M., Ohta, T., Watanabe, K., Miyazawa, T., Kato, K. & Shirasu, Y. (1983) Further mutagenicity studies on pesticides in bacterial reversion assay systems. *Mutat. Res.*, **116**, 185–216

Mortelmans, K., Haworth, S., Lawlor, T., Speck, W., Tainer, B. & Zeiger, E. (1986) *Salmonella* mutagenicity tests: II. Results from the testing of 270 chemicals. *Environ. Mutag.*, **8** (Suppl. 7), 1–119

Nagao, M. & Takahashi, Y. (1981) Mutagenic activity of 42 coded compounds in the *Salmonella*/microsome assay. *Prog. Mutat. Res.*, **1**, 302–313

Nagaoka, T., Onodera, H., Matsushima, Y., Todate, A., Shibutani, M., Ogasawara, H. & Maekawa, A. (1990) Spontaneous uterine adenocarcinomas in aged rats and their relation to endocrine imbalance. *J. Cancer Res. clin. Oncol.*, **116**, 623–628

do Nascimento, P.C., Bohrer, D., Garcia, S. & Ritzel, A.F. (1997) Liquid chromatography with ultraviolet absorbance detection of ethylenethiourea in blood serum after microwave irradiation as an auxiliary cleanup step. *Analyst*, **122**, 733–735

Natarajan, A.T. & van Kesteren-van Leeuwen, A.C. (1981) Mutagenic activity of 20 coded compounds in chromosome aberrations/sister chromatid exchanges assay using Chinese hamster ovary (CHO) cells. *Prog. Mutat. Res.*, **1**, 551–559

National Institute for Occupational Safety and Health (2000) *National Occupational Exposure Survey 1981–83*, Cincinnati, OH, Department of Health and Human Services, Public Health Service

National Toxicology Program (1992) *Toxicology and Carcinogenesis Studies of Ethylene Thiourea (CAS No. 96-45-7) in F344/N Rats and B6C3F₁ Mice (Feed Studies)* (NTP Technical Report 388), Bethesda, MD

Neicheva, A., Vasileva-Aleksandrova, P., Ivanov, K. & Nikolova, M. (1997) [Determination of ethylenethiourea in plant products using high-performance liquid chromatography.] *Anal. Lab.*, **6**, 43–48 (in Bulgarian)

Nishiyama, K., Ando-Iu, J., Nishimura, S., Takahashi, M., Yoshida, M., Sasahara, K., Miyajima, K. & Maekawa, A. (1998) Initiating and promoting effects of concurrent oral administration of ethylenethiourea and sodium nitrite on uterine endometrial adenocarcinoma development in Donryu rats. *In Vivo*, **12**, 363–368

Ohm, R.F. (1997) Rubber chemicals. In: Kroschwitz, J.I. & Howe-Grant, M., eds, *Kirk-Othmer Encyclopedia of Chemical Technology*, 4th Ed., Vol. 21, New York, John Wiley & Sons, pp. 460–481

Ohta, T., Tokishita, S., Shiga, Y., Hanazato, T. & Yamagata, H. (1998) An assay system for detecting environmental toxicants with cultured cladoceran eggs *in vitro*: Malformations induced by ethylenethiourea. *Environ. Res.*, **77**, 43–48

Paika, I.J., Beauchesne, M.T., Randall, M., Schreck, R.R. & Latt, S.A. (1981) In vivo SCE analysis of 20 coded compounds. *Prog. Mutat. Res.*, **1**, 673–681

Parry, J.M. & Sharp, D.C, (1981) Induction of mitotic aneuploidy in the yeast strain D6 by 42 coded compounds. *Prog. Mutat. Res.*, **1**, 468–480

Perry, P.E. & Thomson, E.J. (1981) Evaluation of the sister chromatid exchange method in mammalian cells as a screening system for carcinogens. *Prog. Mutat. Res.*, **1**, 560–569

Picó, Y., Font, G., Moltó, J.C. & Mañes, J. (2000) Pesticide residue determination in fruit and vegetables by liquid chromatography–mass spectrometry. *J. Chromatogr.*, **A882**, 153–173

Plasterer, M.R., Bradshaw, W.S., Booth, G.M. & Carter, M.W. (1985) Developmental toxicity of nine selected compounds following prenatal exposure in the mouse: Naphthalene, *p*-nitrophenol, sodium selenite, dimethyl phthalate, ethylenethiourea, and four glycol ether derivatives. *J. Toxicol. environ. Health*, **15**, 25–38

van der Poll, J.M., Versluis-de Haan, G.G. & de Wilde, O. (1993) Determination of ethylene-thiourea in water samples by gas chromatography with alkali flame ionization detection and mass spectrometric confirmation. *J. Chromatogr.*, **643**, 163–168

Precheur, R.J., Bennett, M.A., Riedel, R.M., Wiese, K.L. & Dudek, J. (1992) Management of fungicide residues on processing tomatoes. *Plant Dis.*, **76**, 700–702

Prince, J.L. (1985) Analysis of ethylenethiourea in urine by high-performance liquid chromato-graphy. *J. agric. Food Chem.*, **33**, 93–94

Quillardet, P., de Bellecombe, C. & Hofnung, M. (1985) The SOS Chromotest, a colorimetric bacterial assay for genotoxins: Validation study with 83 compounds. *Mutat. Res.*, **147**, 79–95

Richold, M. & Jones, E. (1981) Mutagenic activity of 42 coded compounds in the *Salmonella*/ microsome assay. *Prog. Mutat. Res.*, **1**, 314–322

Rodriguez-Arnaiz, R. (1997) Genotoxic activation of hydrazine, two dialkylhydrazines, thio-urea and ethylene thiourea in the somatic w/w^+ assay of *Drosophila melanogaster*. *Mutat. Res.*, **395**, 229–242

Rosenkranz, H.S., Hyman, J. & Leifer, Z. (1981) DNA polymerase deficient assay. *Prog. Mutat. Res.*, **1**, 210–218

Rowland, I. & Severn, B. (1981) Mutagenicity of carcinogens and noncarcinogens in the *Salmo-nella*/microsome test. *Prog. Mutat. Res.*, **1**, 323–332

Ruddick, J.A. & Khera, K.S. (1975) Pattern of anomalies following single oral doses of ethylene thiourea to pregnant rats. *Teratology*, **12**, 277–281

Ruddick, J.A., Williams, D.T., Hierlighy, L. & Khera, K.S. (1975) [14C]Ethylenethiourea: Distribution, excretion, and metabolism in pregnant rats. *Teratology*, **13**, 35–40

Ruddick, J.A., Newsome, W.H. & Iverson, F. (1977) A comparison of the distribution, meta-bolism and excretion of ethylenethiourea in the pregnant mouse and rat. *Teratology*, **16**, 159–162

Sadtler Research Laboratories (1980) *Sadtler Standard Spectra, 1980 Cumulative Molecular Formula Index*, Philadelphia, PA, p. 20

Saillenfait, A.M., Sabate, J.P., Langonne, I. & de Ceaurriz, J. (1991) Difference in the develop-mental toxicity of ethylenethiourea and three *N,N'*-substituted thiourea derivatives in rats. *Fundam. appl. Toxicol.*, **17**, 399–408

Salamone, M.F., Heddle, J.A. & Katz, M. (1981) Mutagenic activity of 41 compounds in the in vivo micronucleus assay. *Prog. Mutat. Res.*, **1**, 686–697

Salisbury, S.A. & Lybarger, J. (1977) *Health Hazard Evaluation Determination, St. Clair Rubber Company, Marysville, MI* (Report No. 77-67-499), Cincinnati, OH, National Insti-tute for Occupational Safety and Health

Sasaki, Y.F., Izumiyama, F., Nishidate, E., Matsusaka, N. & Tsuda, S. (1997) Detection of rodent liver carcinogen genotoxicity by the alkaline single-cell gel electrophoresis (Comet) assay in multiple mouse organs (liver, lung, spleen, kidney, and bone marrow). *Mutat. Res.*, **391**, 201–214

Sato, S., Nakagata, N., Hung, C.-F., Wada, M., Shimoji, T. & Ishii, S. (1985) Transplacental induction of myeloschisis associated with hindbrain crowding and other malformations in the central nervous system in Long-Evans rats. *Child. nerv. Syst.*, **1**, 137–144

Savela, A., Vuorela, R. & Kauppinen, T. (1999) *ASA 1997* (Katsauksia 140), Helsinki, Finnish Institute of Occupational Health, p. 30 (in Finnish)

Savolainen, K. & Pyysalo, H. (1979) Identification of the main metabolite of ethylenethiourea in mice. *J. agric. Food Chem.*, **27**, 1177–1181

Savolainen, K., Kurttio, P., Vartiainen, T. & Kangas, J. (1989) Ethylenethiourea as an indicator of exposure to ethylenebisdithiocarbamate fungicides. *Arch. Toxicol.*, **Suppl. 13**, 120–123

Schiestl, R.H., Gietz, R.D., Mehta, R.D. & Hastings, P.J. (1989) Carcinogens induce intra-chromosomal recombination in yeast. *Carcinogenesis*, **10**, 1445–1455

Schüpbach, M. & Hummler, H. (1977) A comparative study on the mutagenicity of ethylene-thiourea in bacterial and mammalian test systems. *Mutat. Res.*, **56**, 111–120

Seiler, J.P. (1973) In vivo mutagenic interaction of nitrite and ethylenethiourea. *Experientia*, **31**, 214–215

Seiler, J.P. (1974) Ethylenethiourea (ETU), a carcinogenic and mutagenic metabolite of ethylenebis-dithiocarbamate. *Mutat. Res.*, **26**, 189–191

Seiler, J.P. (1977) Inhibition of testicular DNA synthesis by chemical mutagens and carcinogens. Preliminary results in the validation of a novel short term test. *Mutat. Res.*, **46**, 305–310

Sharp, D.C. & Parry, J.M. (1981a) Use of repair-deficient strains of yeast to assay the activity of 40 coded compounds. *Prog. Mutat. Res.*, **1**, 502–516

Sharp, D.C. & Parry, J.M. (1981b) Induction of mitotic gene conversion by 41 coded compounds using the yeast culture *JD1*. *Prog. Mutat. Res.*, **1**, 491–501

Simmon, V.F. & Shepherd, G.F. (1981) Mutagenic activity of 42 coded compounds in the *Salmonella*/microsome assay. *Prog. Mutat. Res.*, **1**, 333–342

Skopek, T.R., Andon, B.M., Kaden, D.A. & Thilly, W.G. (1981) Mutagenic activity of 42 coded compounds using 8-azaguanine resistance as a genetic marker in *Salmonella typhimurium*. *Prog. Mutat. Res.*, **1**, 371–375

Smith, D. (1976) Ethylene thiourea: A study of possible teratogenicity and thyroid carcinogenicity. *J. soc. occup. Med.*, **26**, 92–94

Smith, D. (1984) Ethylene thiourea: Thyroid function in two groups of exposed workers. *Br. J. ind. Med.*, **41**, 362–366

Sonobe, H. & Tanaka, T. (1986) Simultaneous determination of ethylenethiourea [imidazolidine-2-thione] and propylenethiourea [3-methylimidazolidine-2-thione] in beer. *Brew. Dig.*, **61**, 15–17

Stanisstreet, M., Herbert, L.C. & Pharoah, P.O.D. (1990) Effects of thyroid antagonists on rat embryos cultured in vitro. *Teratology*, **41**, 721–729

Steenland, K., Cedillo, L., Tucker, J., Hines, C., Sorensen, K., Deddens, J. & Cruz, V. (1997) Thyroid hormones and cytogenetic outcomes in backpack sprayers using ethylenebis-(dithiocarbamate) (EBDC) fungicides in Mexico. *Environ. Health Perspectives*, **105**, 1126–1130

Styles, J.A. (1981) Activity of 42 coded compounds in the BHK-21 cell transformation test. *Prog. Mutat. Res.*, **1**, 638–646

Teramoto, S., Moriya, M., Kato, K., Tezuka, H., Nakamura, S., Shingu, A. & Shirasu, Y. (1977) Mutagenicity testing on ethylenethiourea. *Mutat. Res.*, **56**, 121–129

Teramoto, S., Shingu, A. & Shirasu, Y. (1978) Induction of dominant-lethal mutations after administration of ethylenethiourea with nitrite or of *N*-nitroso-ethylenethiourea in mice. *Mutat. Res.*, **56**, 335–340

Teramoto, S., Saito, R. & Shirasu, Y. (1980) Teratogenic effects of combined administration of ethylenethiourea and nitrite in mice. *Teratology*, **21**, 71–78

Thomson, J.A. (1981) Mutagenic activity of 42 coded compounds in the lambda induction assay. *Prog. Mutat. Res.*, **1**, 224–235

Topham, J.C. (1981) Evaluation of some chemicals by the sperm morphology assay. *Prog. Mutat. Res.*, **1**, 718–720

Trueman, R.W. (1981) Activity of 42 coded compounds in the *Salmonella* reverse mutation test. *Prog. Mutat. Res.*, **1**, 343–350

Tsuchimoto, T. & Matter, B.E. (1981) Activity of coded compounds in the micronucleus test. *Prog. Mutat. Res.*, **1**, 705–711

Tsuchiya, T., Takahashi, A., Asada, S., Takakubo, F., Ohsumi-Yamashita, N. & Eto, K. (1991a) Comparative studies of embryotoxic action of ethylenethiourea in rat whole embryo and embryonic cell culture. *Teratology*, **43**, 319–324

Tsuchiya, T., Nakamura, A., Iio, T. & Takahashi, A. (1991b) Species differences between rats and mice in the teratogenic action of ethylenethiourea: *In vivo/in vitro* tests and teratogenic activity of sera using an embryonic cell differentiation system. *Toxicol. appl. Pharmacol.*, **109**, 1–6

Tweats, D.J. (1981) Activity of 42 coded compounds in a differential killing test using *Escherichia coli* strains WP2, WP67 (*uvrA polA*), and CM871 (*uvrA lexA rec A*). *Prog. Mutat. Res.*, **1**, 199–209

Ulland, B.M., Weisburger, J.H., Weisburger, E.K., Rice, J.M. & Cypher, R. (1972) Thyroid cancer in rats from ethylene thiourea intake. *J. natl Cancer Inst.*, **49**, 583–584

Valencia, R. & Houtchens, K. (1981) Mutagenic activity of 10 coded compounds in the *Drosophila* sex-linked recessive lethal test. *Prog. Mutat. Res.*, **1**, 651–659

Venitt, S. & Crofton-Sleigh, C. (1981) Mutagenicity of 42 coded compounds in a bacterial assay using *Escherichia coli* and *Salmonella typhimurium*. *Prog. Mutat. Res.*, **1**, 351–360

Vogel, E.W. & Nivard, M.J.M. (1993) Performance of 181 chemicals in a Drosophila assay predominantly monitoring interchromosomal mitotic recombination. *Mutagenesis*, **8**, 57–81

Walash, M.I., Belal, F., Metwally, M.E. & Hefnawy, M.M. (1993) Spectrophotometric determination of maneb, zineb and their decomposition products in some vegetables and its application to kinetic studies after greenhouse treatment. *Food Chem.*, **47**, 411–416

Weisburger, E.K., Ulland, B.M., Nam, J.-M., Gart, J.J. & Weisburger, J.H. (1981) Carcinogenicity tests of certain environmental and industrial chemicals. *J. natl Cancer Inst.*, **67**, 75–88

WHO (1999) *Meeting on Pesticide Residues. Summary of Toxicological Evaluations Performed by the Joint FAO/WHO (JMPR)*, Geneva, International Programme on Chemical Safety

Wilkie, D. & Gooneskera, S. (1980) The yeast mitochondrial system in carcinogen testing. *Chem. Ind.*, 21, 847–850

Woodruff, R.C., Mason, J.M., Valencia, R. & Zimmering, S. (1985) Chemical mutagenesis testing in *Drosophila*: V. Results of 53 coded compounds tested for the National Toxicology Program. *Environ. Mutag.*, **7**, 677–702

Wyrobek, A., Gordon, L. & Watchmaker, G. (1981) Effect of 17 chemical agents including 6 carcinogen/noncarcinogen pairs on sperm shape abnormalities in mice. *Prog. Mutat. Res.*, **1**, 712–717

Yess, N.J., Gunderson, E.L. & Roy, R.R. (1993) US Food and Drug Administration monitoring of pesticide residues in infant foods and adult foods eaten by infants/children. *J. Assoc. off. anal. Chem.*, **76**, 492–507

Yoshida, A., Harada, T. & Maita, K. (1993) Tumor induction by concurrent oral administration of ethylenethiourea and sodium nitrite in mice. *Toxicol. Pathol.*, **21**, 303–310

Yoshida, A., Harada, T., Hayashi, S.M., Mori, I., Miyajima, Y. & Maita, K. (1994) Endometrial carcinogenesis induced by concurrent oral administration of ethylenethiourea and sodium nitrite in mice. *Carcinogenesis*, **15**, 2311–2318

Yoshida, A., Harada, T., Kitazawa, T., Yoshida, T., Kinoshita, M. & Maita, K. (1996) Effect of age on endometrial carcinogenesis induced by concurrent oral administration of ethylenethiourea and sodium nitrite in mice. *Exp. Toxicol. Pathol.*, **48**, 289–298

Zimmermann, F.K. & Scheel, I. (1981) Induction of mitotic gene conversion in strain *D7* of *Saccharomyces cerevisiae* by 42 coded chemicals. *Prog. Mutat. Res.*, **1**, 481–490

THIOUREA

This substance was considered by previous working groups, in 1974 (IARC, 1974) and 1987 (IARC, 1987). Since that time, new data have become available, and these have been incorporated into the monograph and taken into consideration in the present evaluation.

1. Exposure Data

1.1 Chemical and physical data

1.1.1 *Nomenclature*

Chem. Abstr. Serv. Reg. No.: 62-56-6
Chem. Abstr. Name: Thiourea
IUPAC Systematic Name: Thiourea
Synonyms: Isothiourea; pseudothiourea; thiocarbamide; 2-thiopseudourea; β-thiopseudourea; 2-thiourea; THU

1.1.2 *Structural and molecular formulae and relative molecular mass*

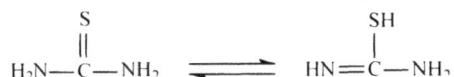

CH$_4$N$_2$S   Relative molecular mass: 76.12

1.1.3 *Chemical and physical properties of the pure substance*

(*a*) *Description*: White solid which crystallizes in a rhombic bipyramidal structure (Mertschenk & Beck, 1995; Lide & Milne, 1996)
(*b*) *Melting-point*: 182 °C (Lide & Milne, 1996)
(*c*) *Spectroscopy data*: Infrared [prism (3962), grating (8315)], ultraviolet (3292), nuclear magnetic resonance [proton (12880), C-13 (6809)] and mass spectral

data have been reported (Sadtler Research Laboratories, 1980; Lide & Milne, 1996).

(d) *Solubility*: Soluble in water (140 g/L at 20 °C) and ethanol; insoluble in diethyl ether (Mertschenk & Beck, 1995; Lide & Milne, 1996)

1.1.4   *Technical products and impurities*

Thiourea is commercially available in Germany with the following typical specifications: purity, ≥ 99.0%; water, ≤ 0.30%; ash, ≤ 0.10%; thiocyanate (rhodanide), ≤ 0.15%; other nitrogen-containing compounds, ≤ 0.5%; and iron, ≤ 10 mg/kg. Special grades with higher purity are also available (Mertschenk & Beck, 1995).

Trade names for thiourea include TsizP 34.

1.1.5   *Analysis*

Methods for the analysis of thiourea in citrus fruit juices and peels, urine, wine, wastewater, magnetic film plating solutions, copper electrolyte solutions and zinc electroplating solutions have been reported. The methods include colorimetry, ultraviolet spectrophotometry, direct ultraviolet reflectance spectrometry, atmospheric-pressure chemical ionization mass spectrometry, gas chromatography, high-performance liquid chromatography (HPLC) with ultraviolet detection, reversed-phase HPLC with ultraviolet detection, periodate titration, potentiometric titration with an ion-selective electrode, anodic and cathodic stripping voltammetry, cathodic polarization potentiometry, chemiluminescence spectroscopy, flow-injection amperometry, flow-injection fluorimetry, micellar electrokinetic capillary chromatography and atomic absorption spectrometry (Mandrou *et al.*, 1977a,b; Toyoda *et al.*, 1979; Akintonwa, 1985; Bian, 1985; Grigorova & Wright, 1986; Kiryushov *et al.*, 1986; Zejnilovic & Jovanovic, 1986; Xu *et al.*, 1987; Sastry *et al.*, 1988; Abdalla & Al-Swaidan, 1989; Berestetskii & Tulyupa, 1989; Zhou *et al.*, 1990; Komljenovic & Radic, 1991; Budnikov *et al.*, 1992; Chemezova & Khlynova, 1992; Kiryushov, 1992; Lebedev *et al.*, 1992; Yao *et al.*, 1992; He *et al.*, 1994; Lee *et al.*, 1994; Pérez-Ruiz *et al.*, 1995; Shao, 1995; Wang, 1996a,b; Anisimova *et al.*, 1997; Huang *et al.*, 1997; Raffaelli *et al.*, 1997; Duan *et al.*, 1998; Kato *et al.*, 1998; Xu & Tang, 1998; AOAC International, 1999; He *et al.*, 1999; Hida *et al.*, 1999).

1.2   Production

Thiourea was first prepared by thermal rearrangement of ammonium thiocyanate at approximately 150 °C. As this is an equilibrium reaction and separation of the two substances is quite difficult, better methods of preparation were investigated. Production of thiourea is now carried out by treating technical-grade calcium cyanamide with hydrogen sulfide or one of its precursors, e.g., ammonium sulfide or calcium hydrogen sulfide. In Germany, thiourea is produced in a closed system by reaction of calcium cyanamide with hydrogen sulfide. The quantity of thiourea produced worldwide in 1995 was estimated to be 10 000 t/year (Mertschenk & Beck, 1995; Budavari, 2000).

Information available in 2000 indicated that thiourea was manufactured by 44 companies in China, three companies each in Japan and Mexico, two companies each in Germany and Italy and one company each in India, Poland, the Russian Federation, Spain, Taiwan, the Ukraine and Uzbekistan (CIS Information Services, 2000a).

Information available in 2000 indicated that thiourea was used in the formulation of pharmaceuticals by six companies in Italy, two companies in Switzerland and one company in Germany (CIS Information Services, 2000b).

1.3   Use

Thiourea has a wide range of uses, such as for producing and modifying textile and dyeing auxiliaries, in the production and modification of synthetic resins, in image reproduction, in the production of pharmaceuticals (sulfathiazoles, thiouracils, tetramisole and cephalosporins), in the production of industrial cleaning agents (e.g., for photographic tanks and metal surfaces in general), for engraving metal surfaces, as an isomerization catalyst in the conversion of maleic to fumaric acid, in copper refining electrolysis, in electroplating (e.g., of copper) and as an antioxidant (e.g., in biochemistry). Other uses are as a vulcanization accelerator, an additive for slurry explosives, as a viscosity stabilizer for polymer solutions (e.g., in drilling muds) and as a mobility buffer in petroleum extraction. The removal of mercury from wastewater by chlorine–alkali electrolysis and gold and silver extraction from minerals are also uses of economic importance (Mertschenk & Beck, 1995; Budavari, 2000). Thiourea was investigated as an anti-thyroid drug in the 1940s (Winkler *et al.*, 1947). It is used only as an excipient in drugs in Italy and in Portugal (Instituto Nacional de Farmacia e do Medicamento, 2000; Ministry of Health, 2000).

Thiourea is used in four main ways: as an intermediate in the production of thiourea dioxide for wool and textile processing (30%), in ore leaching (25%), in diazo papers (15%) and as a catalyst in fumaric acid synthesis (10%); the remainder has smaller areas of use (Mertschenk & Beck, 1995). Thiourea is registered as a veterinary agent in Ireland and Sweden.

1.4   Occurrence

1.4.1   *Occupational exposure*

According to the 1981–83 National Occupational Exposure Survey (National Institute for Occupational Safety and Health, 2000), about 38 000 workers in the USA were potentially exposed to thiourea. Occupational exposure occurred, e.g., in the metal product industry (7900 exposed), chemical industry (6000), machinery except electrical industry (3500), electric and electronic equipment production (3500), instrument production (3500), health services (3100), transportation equipment (2600), business services (1800) and lumber and wood product mills (1000). The most commonly exposed occupational group was that of machine operators (8000 workers). According to the Finnish Register of Employees Exposed to Carcinogens, about 100 laboratory workers, nurses or surface treatment workers were exposed to thiourea in Finland in 1997 (Savela *et al.*, 1999).

1.4.2   *Environmental occurrence*

No data were available to the Working Group.

1.5   Regulations and guidelines

Thiourea is classified as a suspected carcinogen in Germany and the European Union and as a carcinogen in Finland (1993), France (1993), Japan (1999) and Sweden (1993); the Netherlands recommended in 1999 an occupational exposure limit of 0.5 mg/m^3 with a skin notation; and the Russian Federation in 1993 imposed a short-term exposure limit of 0.3 mg/m^3 (Mertschenk & Beck, 1995; American Conference of Governmental Industrial Hygienists, 2000; Deutsche Forschungsgemeinschaft, 2000).

2.   Studies of Cancer in Humans

No data were available to the Working Group.

3.   Studies of Cancer in Experimental Animals

Since the first evaluation of thiourea (IARC, 1974), there have been a few studies on its carcinogenicity in animals, but none representing a conventional carcinogenicity bioassay meeting present-day standards. A selection of the most relevant studies from the previous monograph were therefore summarized or re-analysed in greater depth. Studies on the carcinogenicity of anti-thyroid chemicals, including thiourea, in experimental animals have been reviewed (Paynter *et al.*, 1988).

3.1   Oral administration

Mouse: Of four studies in several strains of mice conducted prior to 1952 in which various concentrations of thiourea were administered in the diet or drinking-water for various times ranging from 7 months to life, none reported an increased incidence of thyroid tumours; however, some reported thyroid hyperplasia (Gorbman, 1947; Dalton *et al.*, 1948; Vasquez-Lopez, 1949; Casas & Koppisch, 1952). One representative study is described below.

Groups of 31 strain A, 43 C57 and 17 strain I mice [sex unspecified], 1–3 months of age, were fed a diet containing thiourea [purity not specified] at a concentration of 2% for various periods up to 81 weeks [the numbers of animals examined at each time were not given]. The survival rate at necropsy was 58% for strain A, 66% for C57 and 71% for strain I mice. The author reported that thyroid hyperplasia was seen from 40 days of treatment, developing into cystic or nodular lesions from 150 days. Seven strain A mice out of 22 that lived longer than 300 days of treatment had nodules of 'thyroid-like tissue' in the lungs. [It was not clear whether all of these mice were fed thiourea, as the study also included thiouracil-treated groups.] The author considered the thyroid and pulmonary lesions to be non-malignant (Gorbman, 1947).

Rat: Groups of 10 male and 10 female albino rats (New Zealand strain of *Rattus norvegicus*) and 10 male Wistar rats, 8 weeks of age, were given drinking-water containing thiourea [purity not specified] at a concentration of 0.25% for up to 23.5 months. The survival rate for 12 months or longer was 90% for the albino males, 80% for albino females and 80% for male Wistar rats. Thyroid follicular-cell tumours occurred in 8/10 albino male, 8/10 albino female and 6/10 male Wistar rats. The tumour diagnoses included thyroid adenoma, carcinoma and fetal adenoma [authors' terminology]. The incidences of thyroid carcinomas in these groups were 4/10 albino males, 3/10 albino females and 0/10 male Wistar rats. Two of the thyroid carcinomas in the albino rats [sex not specified] metastasized to the lung (Purves & Griesbach, 1947). [The Working Group noted the lack of control groups.]

Groups of 18 albino rats [identified as Osborne-Mendel by Deichmann *et al.* (1967); sex not specified], 21 days of age, were given a diet of ground commercial rat biscuits containing thiourea [purity not specified] at a concentration of 0 (control), 100, 250, 500, 1000, 2500, 5000 or 10 000 mg/kg for 2 years. All rats at concentrations ≥ 2500 mg/kg of diet died before 17 months. Of the 29 treated rats that survived for 2 years, 14 had hepatocellular adenomas [group distribution not stated], with none in 18 controls. Only one treated rat that survived less than 17 months developed a liver tumour [group not stated]. The incidence of spontaneous hepatic tumours in other control groups in the same laboratory was cited as 1%. Thyroid (follicular-cell) hyperplasia was observed, ranging in severity from moderate at 1000 mg/kg of diet to marked at 10 000 mg/kg of diet, but no thyroid tumours were reported (Fitzhugh & Nelson, 1948). [The Working Group noted the small group sizes, the poor survival and the lack of detail provided in this report.]

Groups of 12 and 19 male random-bred albino (Hebrew University strain) rats, weighing approximately 100 g [age not specified], were given drinking-water containing thiourea [purity not specified] at a concentration of 0 (control) or 0.2% for up to 26 months. Epidermoid carcinomas of the external auditory duct or meibomian glands of the eyelids were diagnosed in 17/19 treated rats in contrast to 0/12 control rats.

In a companion study, 16 male rats of the same strain were given intraperitoneal injections of about 3.4–4 mL of a 10% aqueous solution of thiourea three times per week for 6 months, followed by 0.2% thiourea in the drinking-water for up to 22 months. Similar tumours were produced in 10/16 rats (Rosin & Ungar, 1957). A subsequent study from the same laboratory, in which the same strain of rat was given 0.2% thiourea in the drinking-water for 14–23 months, showed squamous-cell carcinomas of the Zymbal gland and/or meibomian gland in 7/8 survivors (Ungar & Rosin, 1960). [The Working Group noted that the rats used in the last study were survivors of tumour transplantation studies in which the intrascapular implant was considered to have failed.]

In a study of the synergistic effects of various carcinogens, groups of 30 male and 30 female Osborne-Mendel rats were fed a diet containing 0 (control) or 80 mg/kg thiourea [purity not stated] from weaning for 104 weeks. Treatment had no effect on the mortality rate, the cumulative rate for the experiment being 65% for males and 60% for females. There was no difference between control and treated groups in tumour incidence at any site examined, including the liver (1/60 in controls and 0/60 in treated rats) (Radomski et al., 1965). [The Working Group noted that the concentration of thiourea used, which produced no liver tumours, was only 20% less than the dose that produced a 60% liver tumour incidence in the same rat strain in the study of Fitzhugh and Nelson (1948).]

As part of another study of the synergistic effects of combinations of carcinogens on tumorigenesis, groups of 30 male and 30 female Osborne-Mendel rats were fed 50 mg/kg diet thiourea (purity, 100%) from weaning for 26 months. A control group of 30 males and 30 females fed basal diet was terminated at 25 months. After 24 months, the survival rate of rats receiving thiourea was 51%. There was no increase in tumour incidence at any of the organ sites examined, including the liver, in which there were no tumours observed in either control or treated groups (Deichmann et al., 1967).

3.2   Administration with known carcinogens

The studies described below were published since the previous evaluation.

Rat: Thiourea was tested in an initiation–promotion model of liver carcinogenesis in which *N*-nitrosodiethylamine (NDEA) was used as the initiating agent and Clophen A 50 (a technical-grade mixture of polychlorinated biphenyls) as the promoting agent. In the initiating arm, groups of four to six male and female Sprague-Dawley rats, 21–26 days of age, received an oral dose of 200 or 500 mg/kg bw per day thiourea (purity, 99.9%) in 2 mL water by gavage on three consecutive days, followed 6 days later by oral gavage with Clophen A 50 at a dose of 10 mg/kg bw per day in 2 mL olive oil for 11 consecutive weeks. Another four groups received either thiourea, Clophen A 50 or olive oil alone at the same doses. In the promoting arm, two groups of four to six males and females received a single oral gavage dose of 8 mg/kg bw NDEA (purity, 99%), followed 1 week later by thiourea in the drinking-water at a concentration of 0.2% for 51 days. Two additional groups of female rats received 0.05% or 0.1% thiourea in the drinking-water for 70 days starting 1 week after NDEA treatment. Another two groups of male and female rats received NDEA alone. After 12 weeks, the livers were scored for preneoplastic foci identified by ATPase deficiency. Thiourea did not enhance the incidence of foci of hepatocellular alteration when given either as an initiator or a promoter (Oesterle & Deml, 1988).

Groups of 30 male Fischer 344 rats, 5 weeks of age, received a single subcutaneous injection of 2 g/kg bw *N*-nitrosobis(2-hydroxypropyl)amine (NBHPA), followed 1 week later either by thiourea at a concentration of 0.1% in the drinking-water for 19 weeks or basal diet and water alone. Five animals from each group were killed at various intervals up to the end of the study. From four weeks onwards, thyroid follicular-cell adenomas occurred in 5/20 rats receiving NBHPA plus thiourea, in contrast to 0/20 receiving NBHPA alone (Shimo *et al.*, 1994a).

Groups of 10 or 15 male Fischer 344 rats, 5 weeks of age, received a single subcutaneous injection of 1.5 g/kg bw NBHPA, followed 1 week later by thiourea in the drinking-water at a concentration of 0, 0.05 or 0.1% for 20 weeks. A group of 19 control rats received basal diet and distilled water alone. The incidences of thyroid follicular-cell tumours were increased at both doses of thiourea ($p < 0.01$), with 5/10 rats bearing tumours after receiving NBHPA plus 0.05% or 0.1% thiourea, in contrast to 0/15 with NBHPA only and 0/19 untreated controls. All tumours but one (a carcinoma) were thyroid adenomas (Onodera *et al.*, 1994).

Groups of 20 and 15 male Fischer 344 rats, 6 weeks of age, received a single subcutaneous injection of 2 g/kg bw NBHPA, followed 1 week later by thiourea at a concentration of 0 or 0.1% in the drinking-water for 19 weeks. The study was terminated at 20 weeks. Administration of thiourea increased the incidence ($p < 0.01$) of thyroid follicular-cell adenomas, in 10/15 animals given NBHPA plus thiourea and 0/20 given NBHPA only. Thiourea did not promote the induction of hepatocellular tumours to a statistically significant degree (Shimo *et al.*, 1994b).

A group of 15 male Fischer 344 rats, 6 weeks of age, received a single subcutaneous injection of 2.8 g/kg bw NBHPA, followed by thiourea at a concentration of 0.2% in the drinking-water for 19 weeks. The study was terminated at 20 weeks. Administration of thiourea increased the incidence of thyroid follicular-cell neoplasms: of the animals given NBHPA plus thiourea, 10/15 had tumours with an adenomatous growth pattern and 6/15 with a solid growth pattern; no tumours were seen in five rats treated with NBHPA alone (Mitsumori *et al.*, 1996).

Groups of 10 male Fischer 344 rats, 6 weeks of age, received a single subcutaneous injection of 2.8 g/kg bw NBHPA, followed 1 week later either by thiourea at a concentration of 0.2% in the drinking-water for 10 weeks or basal diet and water alone. Administration of thiourea increased the incidence ($p < 0.01$) of thyroid follicular-cell tumours, which were seen in 10/10 rats given NBHPA plus thiourea and 1/10 given NBHPA only (Takegawa *et al.*, 1997).

4.   Other Data Relevant to an Evaluation of Carcinogenicity and its Mechanisms

4.1   Absorption, distribution, metabolism and excretion

4.1.1   *Humans*

Thiourea is absorbed from the gastrointestinal tract. A single oral dose of 100 mg of thiourea was almost completely eliminated from the blood within 24 h; 15% was broken down in the intestine and 30–50% in other tissues and body fluids, the remainder (approximately 30%) being excreted as thiourea in the urine (Williams & Kay, 1947).

4.1.2   *Experimental systems*

Thiourea is absorbed from the gastrointestinal tract in rats. In rats given 5 mg by intravenous injection, 30% of the thiourea was recovered from the carcasses after 3 h and only traces after 25 h (Williams & Kay, 1947).

In homogenized liver preparations from female Holtzman rats, 28–35% of added thiourea was metabolized within 3 h. The pathway for the breakdown of thiourea was suggested to be as follows: uracil; β-ureidopropionic acid, which was further metabolized to β-alanine; ammonia and carbon dioxide (Spector & Shideman, 1959).

Thiourea is transferred across the placenta in rabbits and dogs (Shepard, 1963).

Autoradiographic analysis of pregnant NMRI mice given about 0.05 mg of [^{14}C]-thiourea by intravenous injection at a late stage of gestation [gestational age not specified] revealed accumulation of radiolabel in the fetal thyroid (Slanina *et al.*, 1973).

[^{14}C]Thiourea administered by intraperitoneal injection bound to liver, kidney and lung protein in male Sprague-Dawley rats (Hollinger *et al.*, 1974) and was found to be uniformly distributed in alveolar walls 24 h after dosing (Hollinger *et al.*, 1976).

4.2   Toxic effects

4.2.1   *Humans*

No data were available to the Working Group.

4.2.2   *Experimental systems*

Male Fischer 344 rats, 4 weeks of age, were given drinking-water containing 0.1 or 0.05% thiourea for 1 week. Dose-dependent decreases were found in the serum concentrations of triiodothyronine [by 60% and 15%, respectively] and thyroxine (T4) [by 85% and 45%, respectively]. A single subcutaneous dose of 1500 mg/kg bw NBHPA given to another group of rats, followed 1 week later by 0.1 or 0.05% thiourea in the drinking-water for 20 weeks, caused thyroid follicular-cell proliferative lesions and decreased serum T4 concentrations (by < 20%). The concentration of T3 was unchanged, and that of thyroid-stimulating hormone (TSH) was increased by 40% at the higher concentration only (Onodera *et al.*, 1994).

Male Fischer 344 rats, 4 weeks of age, were given 0.1% thiourea in the drinking-water for 19 weeks starting 1 week after they had received a single subcutaneous injection of 2000 mg/kg bw NBHPA. Groups of rats were sacrificed at weeks 1, 2, 4, 8, 12 and 16. In comparison with the serum T4 concentration after treatment with NBHPA alone, that in rats given thiourea was decreased by approximately 60% at week 1 and remained significantly reduced throughout the experiment. The serum TSH concentration was elevated; it peaked at 4 weeks (20-fold increase) and returned to normal at 12 weeks. Thyroid weights were significantly increased in a treatment duration-dependent manner. Hyperplasia was noted at 2 weeks and adenomas at 4 weeks, both of which increased with length of treatment. Proliferation was greatest when the TSH concentrations were elevated (Shimo *et al.*, 1994a).

Starting 1 week after initial treatment with NBHPA (2800 mg/kg bw) by subcutaneous injection, male Fischer 344 rats were given 0.2% thiourea in the drinking-water for 10 weeks. The treated animals had decreased body weights, increased thyroid weights [fivefold], decreased T4 concentrations [25%] and increased TSH concentrations [fivefold]. Thiourea given with 0.1% vitamin A after initiation with NBHPA resulted in decreased serum concentrations of triiodothyronine and T4 [55% and 75%, respectively] and an increased TSH concentration [13-fold]. Thyroid weight gain was greater with the combined treatment. Thyroid hyperplasias and neoplasias were induced in both groups; however, the combination of thiourea and vitamin A induced more cell proliferation, as measured by bromodeoxyuridine incorporation (Takegawa *et al.*, 1997).

Mature (450–500 g) and immature (50–80 g, 21–23 days of age) male Sprague-Dawley rats were given an intraperitoneal dose of 0.6 mg/kg bw of [^{14}C]thiourea. The immature, but not the mature rats were tolerant to the toxic pulmonary effects of this treatment (Hollinger *et al.*, 1976). Vascular permeability, as determined by Evans blue dye injected into a femoral vein, increased with the age of male Sprague-Dawley rats that received an intraperitoneal dose of 10 mg/kg bw thiourea 2 h before sacrifice. The increased vascular permeability concorded with increased concentrations of histamine in lung and plasma (Giri *et al.*, 1991a).

The lethal intraperitoneal dose of thiourea in male Sprague-Dawley rats was 10 mg/kg bw, causing 100% mortality within 24 h. A non-lethal dose (0.5 mg/kg bw) given as pre-treatment provided complete protection against death for 8 days and partial protection for 24 days. The protection was correlated with histamine concentrations; that is, the histamine concentrations were low when the animals were protected (Giri *et al.*, 1991b).

In an assay for iodination with 2-methoxyphenol (guaiacol) in the presence of iodide and thiourea, thyroid peroxidase oxidized thiourea to formamidine disulfide. At neutral pH, formamidine then decomposed to cyanamide, which inhibited the function of thyroid peroxidase (Davidson *et al.*, 1979).

4.3   Reproductive and developmental effects

4.3.1   *Humans*

No data were available to the Working Group.

4.3.2   *Experimental systems*

Groups [size unspecified] of CF4 rats were given drinking-water containing 0.2% thiourea on days 1–14 of gestation, and the fetuses were examined on day 20. While the specific incidences of fetal effects were not provided, the authors noted that growth retardation and malformations of the nervous system and skeleton were present in the treated offspring (Kern *et al.*, 1980).

4.4   Effects on enzyme induction or inhibition and gene expression

4.4.1   *Humans*

No data were available to the Working Group.

4.4.2   *Experimental systems*

After initial treatment of male Fischer 344 rats with NBHPA at 2800 mg/kg bw, administration of 0.2% thiourea in the drinking-water for 10 weeks increased the activities of the cytochrome P450 isozymes CYP2E1 and CYP4A1 in the liver, while the activity of T4-UDP glucuronosyl transferase in the liver was similar to the control value (Takegawa *et al.*, 1997).

Thiourea at 10–100 mmol/L (optimum, 25 mmol/L) increased CYP2B1-catalysed oxidation of the tobacco-specific carcinogen 4-(nitrosomethylamino)-1-(3-pyridyl)-1-butanone (NNK) in a reconstituted cell-free system (Guo *et al.*, 1991).

4.5   Genetic and related effects

4.5.1   *Humans*

No data were available to the Working Group.

4.5.2   *Experimental systems* (see Table 1 for references)

   (*a*)   *DNA damage*

Thiourea did not induce differential survival in DNA repair-deficient strains of *Escherichia coli* or forward mutation to induce repair in the SOS chromotest. It produced differential cell killing in *E. coli uvrB/recA* cells without, but not with, metabolic activation. It did not induce mutation in *Salmonella typhimurium umu* and did not induce prophage in *E. coli* K12.

There is disagreement in the literature about the ability of thiourea to induce DNA single-strand breaks. Thiourea decreased the frequency of DNA strand breaks induced by X-rays or intercalating agents in mouse lymphoma cells, probably by altering chromatin structure (Pommier *et al.*, 1983). It did not induce unscheduled DNA synthesis in primary rat hepatocytes.

The reaction of [^{14}C]thiourea and hydrogen peroxide in the presence of calf thymus DNA produced formamidine sulfonate and cyanamide and gave rise to covalent binding of radiolabel to the DNA (Ziegler-Skylakakis *et al.*, 1998). This mechanism has not been observed *in vivo*.

   (*b*)   *Mutation and allied effects*

Thiourea was not mutagenic to *Salmonella typhimurium* or *E. coli* when tested without or with metabolic activation from liver microsomes from Aroclor-induced rats, mice or hamsters. It was weakly mutagenic in base-pair substitution and frameshift strains of *Salmonella* in the mouse host-mediated assay after intramuscular administration.

Thiourea was mutagenic in *Saccharomyces cerevisiae* and induced intrachromosomal recombination and petite mutations. It did not induce mutation or chromosomal malsegregation in *Aspergillus*.

Thiourea did not induce homologous or non-homologous recombination in cultured Chinese hamster cells.

There is disagreement in the literature about the ability of thiourea to induce mutation in mouse lymphoma L5178Y (*Tk* locus) or Chinese hamster V79 (*Hprt* locus) cells. Mutagenicity in Chinese hamster V79 cells was enhanced by depletion of intracellular glutathione.

Thiourea did not induce sister chromatid exchange in Chinese hamster V79 cells. It induced micronucleus formation in Syrian hamster embryo cells. There was weak induction of micronuclei in Chinese hamster V79 cells.

Thiourea transformed Syrian hamster embryo cells and Rauscher virus-infected rat embryo cells, and had weak transforming ability in a C3H10T1/2 cell line carrying bovine papillomavirus DNA.

Thiourea induced intrachromosomal recombination in transformed human lymphoblastoid cells.

Table 1. Genetic and related effects of thiourea

Test system	Result[a] Without exogenous metabolic system	Result[a] With exogenous metabolic system	Dose[b] (LED/HID)	Reference
Escherichia coli K12, prophage induction	NT	–	2000 µg/plate	Mamber et al. (1984)
Escherichia coli, SOS repair, forward mutation	–	–	38 000	Brams et al. (1987)
Escherichia coli, SOS repair, forward mutation	–	–	40 µg/tube	Kevekordes et al. (1999)
Escherichia coli pol A, differential toxicity (liquid suspension test)	NT	–	250	Rosenkranz & Poirier (1979)
Escherichia coli pol A, differential toxicity (liquid suspension test, other markers)	–	–	5000 µg/well	McCarroll et al. (1981)
Escherichia coli uvr/rec strains, differential toxicity	+	–	25 000	Hellmér & Bolcsfoldi (1992)
Salmonella typhimurium TA1535/pSK1002, umu test	–	–	1670	Nakamura et al. (1987)
Salmonella typhimurium TA100, TA1535, TA1537, TA1538, TA98, TA1536, reverse mutation	–	–	125 µg/plate	Simmon (1979a)
Salmonella typhimurium TA100, reverse mutation	–	–	150 µg/plate	Yamaguchi (1980)
Salmonella typhimurium TA100, TA1535, TA1537, TA1538, TA98, reverse mutation	–	–	333 µg/plate	Dunkel et al. (1984)
Salmonella typhimurium TA100, TA98, TA97, reverse mutation	–	–	1000 µg/plate	Brams et al. (1987)
Salmonella typhimurium TA100, TA1535, TA98, TA97, reverse mutation	–	–	10 000 µg/plate	Zeiger et al. (1988)
Salmonella typhimurium TA1535, TA1538, reverse mutation	–	–	250 µg/plate	Rosenkranz & Poirier (1979)
Escherichia coli RK, forward mutation	–	–	10 000	Hayes et al. (1984)
Escherichia coli WP2 uvrA, reverse mutation	–	–	333 µg/plate	Dunkel et al. (1984)
Aspergillus nidulans, mitotic malsegregation or forward mutation	–	NT	10 000	Crebelli et al. (1986)
Saccharomyces cerevisiae D3, mitotic recombination	–	–	50 000	Simmon (1979b)
Saccharomyces cerevisiae, intrachromosomal recombination	+	NT	30 000	Schiestl (1989)
Saccharomyces cerevisiae, intrachromosomal recombination	+	NT	20 000	Schiestl et al. (1989)
Saccharomyces cerevisiae, intrachromosomal recombination in G$_2$-arrested cells	+	NT	50 000	Galli & Schiestl (1995)

Table 1 (contd)

Test system	Result[a] Without exogenous metabolic system	Result[a] With exogenous metabolic system	Dose[b] (LED/HID)	Reference
Saccharomyces cerevisiae, intrachromosomal recombination in G$_1$-arrested cells	+	NT	10 000	Galli & Schiestl (1996)
Saccharomyces cerevisiae, intrachromosomal recombination in S-phase arrested cells	+	+	10 000	Galli & Schiestl (1998)
Saccharomyces cerevisiae, petite mutation	+	NT	4000	Egilsson et al. (1979)
Saccharomyces cerevisiae D3, petite mutation	+	NT	500	Wilkie & Gooneskera (1980)
Saccharomyces cerevisiae, reverse mutation, *trp* locus	–	+	500	Morita et al. (1989)
Drosophila melanogaster, somatic recombination, *zest-white* locus	+		7.6 µg/mL feed	Batiste-Alentorn et al. (1991)
Drosophila melanogaster, somatic recombination, *w/w'* locus	(+)		38 µg/mL feed	Vogel & Nivard (1993)
Drosophila melanogaster, somatic recombination, *white-ivory* system	?		152 µg/mL feed	Batiste-Alentorn et al. (1994)
Drosophila melanogaster, somatic recombination, wing-spot system	?		76 µg/mL feed	Batiste-Alentorn et al. (1995)
Drosophila melanogaster, somatic recombination, *w/w'* locus	–		76 µg/mL feed	Rodriguez-Arnaiz (1997)
DNA single-strand breaks, primary rat hepatocytes *in vitro*	+	NT	2280	Sina et al. (1983)
DNA single-strand breaks, primary rat hepatocytes *in vitro*	–	NT	1250	Fautz et al. (1991)
Unscheduled DNA synthesis, primary rat hepatocytes *in vitro*	–	NT	1900	Lonati-Galligani et al. (1983)
Unscheduled DNA synthesis, primary rat hepatocytes *in vitro*	–	NT	10 000	Fautz et al. (1991)
Gene mutation, Chinese hamster V79 cells, *Hprt* locus *in vitro*	–	NT	7600	Bradley et al. (1982)
Gene mutation, Chinese hamster V79 cells, *Hprt* locus *in vitro*	+	+[c]	760	Ziegler-Skylakakis et al. (1985)
Recombination, Chinese hamster V79 cell sub-line Sp5 *in vitro*	–	NT	25	Helleday et al. (1998)
Gene mutation, mouse lymphoma L5178Y cells, *Tk* locus *in vitro*	–	–	5000	Mitchell et al. (1988)
Gene mutation, mouse lymphoma L5178Y cells, *Tk* locus *in vitro*	–	(+)	5000	Myhr & Caspary (1988)
Gene mutation, mouse lymphoma L5178Y cells, *Tk* locus *in vitro*	(+)	(+)	1370	Wangenheim & Bolcsfoldi (1988)
Sister chromatid exchange, Chinese hamster V79 cells *in vitro*	–	NT	7600	Bradley et al. (1982)

Table 1 (contd)

Test system	Result[a] Without exogenous metabolic system	With exogenous metabolic system	Dose[b] (LED/HID)	Reference
Micronucleus formation, Syrian hamster embryo cells *in vitro*	+	NT	NR	Fritzenschaf *et al.* (1993)
Micronucleus formation, Chinese hamster V79 cells *in vitro*	(+)	NT	760	Ziegler-Skylakakis *et al.* (1998)
Cell transformation, Syrian hamster embryo cells	+	NT	0.1[d]	Pienta *et al.* (1977)
Cell transformation, Rauscher virus-infected rat embryo cells	+	NT	100	Dunkel *et al.* (1981)
Cell transformation, bovine papilloma virus DNA-enhanced C3H10T1/2 cells	(+)	NT	20	Kowalski *et al.* (2000)
Recombination (*HPRT* reversion), transformed human lymphoblastoid GM6804 cells *in vitro*	+	NT	5	Aubrecht *et al.* (1995)
Host-mediated assay, *Salmonella typhimurium* TA1530, TA1538, reverse mutation in mice *in vivo*	(+)		125 im × 1	Simmon *et al.* (1979)

[a] +, positive; −, negative; (+), weak positive; NT, not tested; ?, inconclusive
[b] LED, lowest effective dose; HID, highest ineffective dose; in-vitro tests, μg/mL; in-vivo tests, mg/kg bw per day; NR, not reported; im, intramuscular
[c] Co-culture with rat hepatocytes
[d] Higher concentrations were inactive.

Thiourea was mutagenic in somatic cells of *Drosophila melanogaster*. It induced mitotic recombination at one locus but not others.

4.6   Mechanistic considerations

Thiourea belongs to a class of drugs used in the treatment of hyperthyroidism and acts by inhibiting thyroid peroxidase, which decreases thyroid hormone production and increases proliferation by increasing the secretion of TSH. This is the probable basis of its thyroid tumour-promoting activity in experimental animals; however, no definitive conclusion regarding the mechanism of carcinogenicity of thiourea can be drawn in view of the mixed results obtained in tests for genotoxicity. Thiourea can interfere with thyroid peroxidase-mediated iodination of thyroglobulin.

Thiourea was not mutagenic in bacteria, but mixed results were obtained in assays in mammalian cells. Thiourea induced chromosomal recombination and mammalian cell transformation. The compound has not been adequately tested for genotoxicity *in vivo*.

5.   Summary of Data Reported and Evaluation

5.1   Exposure data

Thiourea is used in many industrial applications, including as a chemical intermediate or catalyst, in metal processing and plating and in photoprocessing.

5.2   Human carcinogenicity data

No data were available to the Working Group.

5.3   Animal carcinogenicity data

Thiourea has not been tested in a conventional bioassay of carcinogenicity in rodents that would meet present-day standards. In four early studies involving several strains of mice, thyroid hyperplasia but not thyroid tumours was reported after oral administration of thiourea. In several studies in rats given thiourea orally, either a high incidence of thyroid follicular-cell adenomas and carcinomas or increased incidences of hepatocellular adenomas or tumours of the Zymbal or meibomian glands were reported. However, there were deficiencies in each of these studies and no correspondence between studies with respect to tumour site. In five initiation–promotion studies in rats, thiourea promoted thyroid follicular-cell tumours initiated by *N*-nitroso-bis(2-hydroxypropyl)amine.

5.4   Other relevant data

Thiourea is well absorbed and concentrates in the thyroid. It is readily excreted. It can cross the placental barrier. Thiourea acts by inhibiting thyroid peroxidase, resulting in decreased thyroid hormone production and increased proliferation due to an increase in the secretion of thyroid-stimulating hormone. This is the probable basis of the tumorigenic activity of thiourea for the thyroid in experimental animals.

No data were available on reproductive or developmental effects of thiourea in humans. One study in rats showed growth retardation and malformations of the skeleton and nervous system in the offspring of thiourea-treated animals.

Thiourea did not induce gene mutation in bacteria, but mixed results were obtained in assays in mammalian cells. It consistently induced chromosomal recombination in yeast and insects and induced mammalian cell transformation.

5.5   Evaluation

There is *inadequate evidence* in humans for the carcinogenicity of thiourea.
There is *limited evidence* in experimental animals for the carcinogenicity of thiourea.

Overall evaluation

Thiourea is *not classifiable as to its carcinogenicity to humans (Group 3).*

6.   References

Abdalla, M.A. & Al-Swaidan, H.M. (1989) Iodimetric determination of iodate, bromate, hypochlorite, ascorbic acid, and thiourea using flow-injection amperometry. *Analyst*, **114**, 583–586

Akintonwa, D.A. (1985) High-pressure liquid chromatography separation of phenobarbitone, thiourea, and thioacetamide of toxicological interest. *Ecotoxicol. environ. Saf.*, **10**, 145–149

American Conference of Governmental Industrial Hygienists (2000) *TLVs and Other Occupational Exposure Values — 2000 CD-ROM*, Cincinnati, OH

Anisimova, L.A., Yushchenko, I.A. & Toropova, V.F. (1997) Photometric determination of thiourea with the use of sodium nitroprusside. *J. anal. Chem.*, **52**, 1049–1050

AOAC International (1999) *Official Methods of Analysis of AOAC International*, 16th Ed., 5th rev., Gaithersburg, MD [Methods 948.18, 948.19, 948.20, 961.10] [CD-ROM]

Aubrecht, J., Rugo, R. & Schiestl, R.H. (1995) Carcinogens induce intrachromosomal recombination in human cells. *Carcinogenesis*, **16**, 2841–2846

Batiste-Alentorn, M., Xamena, N., Creus, A. & Marcos, R. (1991) Genotoxicity studies with the unstable *zeste-white* (*UZ*) system of *Drosophila melanogaster*: Results with ten carcinogenic compounds. *Environ. mol. Mutag.*, **18**, 120–125

Batiste-Alentorn, M., Xamena, N., Creus, A. & Marcos, R. (1994) Further studies with the somatic *white-ivory* system of *Drosophila melanogaster*: Genotoxicity testing of ten carcinogens. *Environ. mol. Mutag.*, **24**, 143–147

Batiste-Alentorn, M., Xamena, N., Creus, A. & Marcos, R. (1995) Genotoxic evaluation of ten carcinogens in the *Drosophila melanogaster* wing spot test. *Experientia*, **51**, 73–76

Berestetskii, V.I. & Tulyupa, F.M. (1989) [Potentiometric titration of sulfide, thiocyanate, and thiosulfate ions and thiourea using a carbon indicator electrode.] *Zh. anal. Khim.*, **44**, 328–332 (in Russian)

Bian, G. (1985) [Cathodic stripping voltammetric determination of thiourea in cancer patient urine and pesticide plant wastewater.] *Fenxi Huaxue*, **13**, 917–919 (in Chinese)

Bradley, M.O., Patterson, S. & Zwelling, L.A. (1982) Thiourea prevents cytotoxicity and mutagenicity, but not sister-chromatid exchanges in V79 cells treated with *cis*-diaminedichloroplatinum(II). *Mutat. Res.*, **96**, 67–74

Brams, A., Buchet, J.P., Crutzen-Fayt, M.C., De Meester, C., Lauwerys, R. & Léonard, A. (1987) A comparative study, with 40 chemicals, of the efficiency of the Salmonella assay and the SOS chromotest (kit procedure). *Toxicol. Lett.*, **38**, 123–133

Budavari, S., ed. (2000) *The Merck Index*, 12th Ed., Version 12:3, Whitehouse Station, NJ, Merck & Co. & Boca Raton, FL, Chapman & Hall/CRC [CD-ROM]

Budnikov, G.K., Kargina, O.Y. & Vedernikova, E.Y. (1992) [Voltammetric method for determining thiourea.] *Izobreteniya*, **44**, 143–144 (in Russian)

Casas, C.B. & Koppisch, E. (1952) The thyroid and adrenal glands of castrated C₃H mice treated with thiourea. *Endrocrinology*, **51**, 322–328

Chemezova, K.S. & Khlynova, N.M. (1992) [Method for determination of thiourea using anodic stripping voltammetry.] *Izobreteniya*, **29**, 174 (in Russian)

CIS Information Services (2000a) *Directory of World Chemical Producers (Version 2000.1)*, Dallas, TX [CD-ROM]

CIS Information Services (2000b) *Worldwide Bulk Drug Users Directory (Version 2000)*, Dallas, TX [CD-ROM]

Crebelli, R., Bellincampi, D., Conti, G., Conti, L., Morpurgo, G. & Carere, A. (1986) A comparative study on selected chemical carcinogens for chromosome malsegregation, mitotic crossing-over and forward mutation induction in *Aspergillus nidulans*. *Mutat. Res.*, **172**, 139–149

Dalton, J., Morris, H.P. & Durnik, C.S. (1948) Morphologic changes in the organs of female C3H mice after long-term ingestion of thiourea and thiouracil. *J. natl Cancer Inst.*, **9**, 201–223

Davidson, B., Soodak, M., Strout, H.V., Neary, J.T., Nadamura, C. & Maloof, F. (1979) Thiourea and cyanamide as inhibitors of thyroid peroxidase: The role of iodide. *Endocrinology*, **104**, 919–924

Deichmann, W.B., Keplinger, M., Sala, F. & Glass, E. (1967) Synergism among oral carcinogens. IV. The simultaneous feeding of four tumorigens to rats. *Toxicol. appl. Pharmacol.*, **11**, 88–103

Deutsche Forschungsgemeinschaft (2000) *List of MAK and BAT Values 2000* (Report No. 36), Weinheim, Wiley-VCH Verlag GmbH, p. 102

Duan, M., Huang, J. & Yong, F. (1998) [Determination of thiourea in Cu electrolyte by extraction-spectrophotometry.] *Diandu Yu Huanbao*, **18**, 26–27 (in Chinese)

Dunkel, V.C., Pienta, R.J., Sivak, A. & Traul, K.A. (1981) Comparative neoplastic trans-formation responses of Balb/3T3 cells, Syrian hamster embryo cells, and Rauscher murine leukemia virus-infected Fischer rat embryo cells to chemical carcinogens. *J. natl Cancer Inst.*, **67**, 1303–1315

Dunkel, V.C., Zeiger, E., Brusick, D., McCoy, E., McGregor, D., Mortelmans, K., Rosenkranz, H.S. & Simmon, V.F. (1984) Reproducibility of microbial mutagenicity assays. I. Tests with *Salmonella typhimurium* and *Escherichia coli* using a standardized protocol. *Environ. Mutag.*, **6** (Suppl. 2), 1–254

Egilsson, V., Evans, I.H. & Wilkie, D. (1979) Toxic and mutagenic effects of carcinogens on the mitochondria of *Saccharomyces cerevisiae*. *Mol. gen. Genet.*, **174**, 39–46

Fautz, R., Forster, R., Hechenberger, C.M.A., Hertner, T., von der Hude, W., Kaufmann, G., Madle, H., Madle, S., Miltenberger, H.G., Mueller, L., Pool-Zobel, B.L., Puri, E.C., Schmezer, P., Seeberg, A.H., Strobel, R., Suter, W. & Baumeister, M. (1991) Report of a comparative study of DNA damage and repair assays in primary rat hepatocytes with five coded chemicals. *Mutat. Res.*, **260**, 281–294

Fitzhugh, O.G. & Nelson, A.A. (1948) Liver tumors in rats fed thiourea or thioacetamide. *Science*, **108**, 626–628

Fritzenschaf, H., Kohlpoth, M., Rusche, B. & Schiffmann, D. (1993) Testing of known carcinogens and noncarcinogens in the Syrian hamster embryo (SHE) micronucleus test *in vitro*; correlations with in vivo micronucleus formation and cell transformation. *Mutat. Res.*, **319**, 47–53

Galli, A. & Schiestl, R.H. (1995) *Salmonella* test positive and negative carcinogens show different effects on intrachromosomal recombination in G_2 cell cycle arrested yeast cells. *Carcinogenesis*, **16**, 659–663

Galli, A. & Schiestl, R.H. (1996) Effects of *Salmonella* assay negative and positive carcinogens on intrachromosomal recombination in G_1-arrested yeast cells. *Mutat. Res.*, **370**, 209–221

Galli, A. & Schiestl, R.H. (1998) Effect of *Salmonella* assay negative and positive carcinogens on intrachromosomal recombination in S-phase arrested yeast cells. *Mutat. Res.*, **419**, 53–68

Giri, S.N., Hollinger, M.A. & Rice, S.A. (1991a) Effects of thiourea on pulmonary vascular permeability and on lung and plasma histamine levels in rats. *Toxicol. Lett.*, **57**, 283–290

Giri, S.N., Hollinger, M.A. & Rice, S.A. (1991b) Effects of thiourea tolerance on plasma histamine, and lung vascular permeability. *Arch. Toxicol.*, **65**, 603–605

Gorbman, A. (1947) Thyroidal and vascular changes in mice following chronic treatment with goitrogens and carcinogens. *Cancer Res.*, **7**, 746–758

Grigorova, B. & Wright, S.A. (1986) Simultaneous determination of thiourea and formamidine disulfide, using reversed-phase high-performance liquid chromatography and a UV detector. *J. Chromatogr.*, **368**, 444–449

Guo, Z., Smith, T.J., Ishizaki, H. & Yang, C.S. (1991) Metabolism of 4-(methylnitrosamino)-1-(3-pyridyl)-1-butanone (NNK) by cytochrome P450IIB1 in a reconstituted system. *Carcinogenesis*, **12**, 2277–2282

Hayes, S., Gordon, A., Sadowski, I. & Hayes, C. (1984) RK bacterial test for independently measuring chemical toxicity and mutagenicity: Short-term forward selection assay. *Mutat. Res.*, **130**, 97–106

He, Z., Yuan, D., Luo, Q., Yu, X. & Zeng, Y. (1994) [Studies on thiourea and its derivatives by chemiluminescence analysis.] *Fenxi Ceshi Xuebao*, **13**, 33–36 (in Chinese)

He, Z., Wu, F., Meng, H., Ling, L., Yuan, L., Luo, Q. & Zeng, Y. (1999) Chemiluminescence determination of thiourea using tris(2,2′-bipyridyl)ruthenium(II)-KMnO4 system. *Anal. Sci.*, **15**, 381–383

Helleday, T., Arnaudeau, C. & Jenssen, D. (1998) Effects of carcinogenic agents upon different mechanisms for intragenic recombination in mammalian cells. *Carcinogenesis*, **19**, 973–978

Hellmér, L. & Bolcsfoldi, G. (1992) An evaluation of the *E. coli* K-12 *uvrB/recA* DNA repair host-mediated assay. I. In vitro sensitivity of the bacteria to 61 compounds. *Mutat. Res.*, **272**, 145-160

Hida, Y., Kikuchi, S. & Yanagishita, A. (1999) [Method for analysis of thiourea in plating solutions.] *Jpn. Kokai Tokkyo Koho*, Japanese Patent JP 01123668 (in Japanese)

Hollinger, M.A., Giri, S.N., Alley, M., Budd, E.R. & Hwang, F. (1974) Tissue distribution and binding of radioactivity from ^{14}C-thiourea in the rat. *Drug Metab. Disposition*, **2**, 521–525

Hollinger, M.A., Giri, S.N. & Budd, E. (1976) A pharmacodynamic study of [^{14}C]-thiourea toxicity in mature, immature, tolerant and nontolerant rats. *Toxicol. appl. Pharmacol.*, **37**, 545–556

Huang, F., Li, Z. & Jiang, H. (1997) [Analysis and control of thiourea content in ammonium-containing zinc plating bath.] *Cailiao Baohu*, **30**, 23–25 (in Chinese)

IARC (1974) *IARC Monographs on the Evaluation of Carcinogenic Risks of Chemicals to Man*, Vol. 7, *Some Anti-thyroid and Related Substances, Nitrofurans and Industrial Chemicals*, Lyon, IARCPress, pp. 95–109

IARC (1987) *IARC Monographs on the Evaluation of Carcinogenic Risks to Humans*, Suppl. 7, *Overall Evaluations of Carcinogenicity: An Updating of* IARC Monographs *Volumes 1 to 42*, Lyon, IARCPress, p. 72

Instituto Nacional de Farmacia e do Medicamento (2000) Lisbon

Kato, M., Hayashibe, Y., Taketani, M. & Sayama, Y. (1998) [Quantitative determination of thiourea in copper electrolysis solution by precipitation separation-flow analysis]. *Jpn. Kokai Tokkyo Koho*, Japanese Patent JP 10153592 (in Japanese)

Kern, M., Tatar-Kiss, Z., Kertai, P. & Foldes, I. (1980) Teratogenic effect of 2′-thiourea in the rat. *Acta morphol. acad. sci. hung.*, **18**, 259–267

Kevekordes, S., Mersch-Sundermann, V., Burghaus, C.M., Spielberger, J., Schmeiser, H.H., Arlt, V.M. & Dunkelberg, H. (1999) SOS induction of selected naturally occurring substances in *Escherichia coli* (SOS chromotest). *Mutat. Res.*, **445**, 81–91

Kiryushov, V.N. (1992) [Titrimetric method for determination of thiourea in ammoniacal cadmium- and zinc-plating baths.] *Zavod. Lab.*, **58**, 19–20 (in Russian)

Kiryushov, V.N., Vinokurova, O.B. & Rodin, V.V. (1986) [Rapid titrimetric method for determination of thiourea in solutions of a gold-extracting plant.] *Zavod. Lab.*, **52**, 18–19 (in Russian)

Komljenovic, J. & Radic, N. (1991) Potentiometric determination of thiourea by using ion-selective electrode with silver iodide-based membrane hydrophobized with PTFE. *Acta pharm. jugosl.*, **41**, 41–46

Kowalski, L.A., Laitinen, A.M., Mortazavi-Asl, B., Wee, R.K.-H., Erb, H.E., Assi, K.P. & Madden, Z. (2000) In vitro determination of carcinogenicity of sixty-four compounds using a bovine papillomavirus DNA-carrying C3H/10T1/2 cell line. *Environ. mol. Mutag.*, **35**, 300–311

Lebedev, A.E., Sokolov, E.M., Astakhov, R.K., Belen'ky, A.B. & Krasikov, B.S. (1992) [Determination of thiourea and glue in copper electrorefining solutions.] *Tsvetn. Met.*, **10**, 16–19 (in Russian)

Lee, J.-W., Mho, S.-I., Pyun, C.H. & Yeo, I.-H. (1994) Flow injective determination of thiourea by amperometry. *Bull. Korean chem. Soc.*, **15**, 1038–1042

Lide, D.R. & Milne, G.W.A. (1996) *Properties of Organic Compounds*, Version 5.0, Boca Raton, FL, CRC Press [CD-ROM]

Lonati-Galligani, M., Lohman, P.H.M. & Berends, F. (1983) The validity of the autoradiographic method for detecting DNA repair synthesis in rat hepatocytes in primary culture. *Mutat. Res.*, **113**, 145–160

Mamber, S.W., Bryson, V. & Katz, S.E. (1984) Evaluation of the *Escherichia coli* K12 inductest for detection of potential chemical carcinogens. *Mutat. Res.*, **130**, 141–151

Mandrou, B., Brun, S. & Kingkate, A. (1977a) [Determination of thiourea in fruits.] *Ann. Falsif. Expert. chim.*, **70**, 223–232 (in French)

Mandrou, B., Brun, S. & Kingkate, A. (1977b) Quantitative determination of thiourea in citrus fruits. *J. Assoc. off. anal. Chem.*, **60**, 699–671

McCarroll, N.E., Piper, C.E. & Keech, B.H. (1981) An *E. coli* microsuspension assay for the detection of DNA damage induced by direct-acting agents and promutagens. *Environ. Mutag.*, **3**, 429–444

Mertschenk, B. & Beck, F. (1995) Thiourea and thiourea derivatives. In: Elvers, B., Hawkins, S. & Russey, W., eds, *Ullmann's Encyclopedia of Industrial Chemistry*, Vol. A26, 5th rev. Ed., New York, VCH Publishers, pp. 803–815

Ministry of Health (2000) *Drugs*, Rome, Department of Drugs Assessment and Monitoring

Mitchell, A.D., Rudd, C.J. & Caspary, W.J. (1988) Evaluation of the L5178Y mouse lymphoma cell mutagenesis assay: Intralaboratory results for sixty-three coded chemicals tested at SRI International. *Environ. mol. Mutag.*, **12** (Suppl. 13), 37–101

Mitsumori, K., Onodera, H., Takahashi, M., Shimo, T., Yasuhara, K., Takegawa, K., Takahashi, M. & Hayashi, Y. (1996) Promoting effect of large amounts of vitamin A on cell proliferation of thyroid proliferative lesions induced by simultaneous treatment with thiourea. *Cancer Lett.*, **103**, 19–31

Morita, T., Iwamoto, Y., Shimizu, T., Masuzawa, T. & Yanagihara, Y. (1989) Mutagenicity tests with a permeable mutant of yeast on carcinogens showing false-negative in the *Salmonella* assay. *Chem. pharm. Bull.*, **37**, 407–409

Myhr, B.C. & Caspary, W.J. (1988) Evaluation of the L5178Y mouse lymphoma cell mutagenesis assay: Intralaboratory results for sixty-three coded chemicals tested at Litton Bionetics, Inc. *Environ. mol. Mutag.*, **12** (Suppl. 13), 103–194

Nakamura, S., Oda, Y., Shimada, T., Oki, I. & Sugimoto, K. (1987) SOS-inducing activity of chemical carcinogens and mutagens in *Salmonella typhimurium* TA1535/pSK1002: Examination with 151 chemicals. *Mutat. Res.*, **192**, 239–246

National Institute for Occupational Safety and Health (2000) *National Occupational Exposure Survey 1981–83*, Cincinnati, OH, Department of Health and Human Services, Public Health Service

Oesterle, D. & Deml, E. (1988) Lack of initiating and promoting activity of thiourea in rat liver foci bioassay. *Cancer Lett.*, **41**, 245–249

Onodera, H., Mitsumori, K., Takahashi, M., Shimo, T., Yasuhara, K., Kitaura, K., Takahashi, M. & Hayashi, Y. (1994) Thyroid proliferative lesions induced by anti-thyroid drugs in rats are not always accompanied by sustained increases in serum TSH. *J. toxicol. Sci.*, **19**, 227–234

Paynter, O.E., Burin, G.J., Jaeger, R.B. & Gregorio C.A. (1988) Goitrogens and thyroid follicular cell neoplasia: Evidence for a threshold process. *Regul. Toxicol. Pharmacol.*, **8**, 102–119

Pérez-Ruiz, T., Martínez-Lozano, C., Tomás, V. & Casajús, R. (1995) Flow injection fluorimetric determination of thiourea. *Talanta*, **42**, 391–394

Pienta, R.J., Poiley, J.A. & Lebherz, W.B., III (1977) Morphological transformation of early passage golden Syrian hamster embryo cells derived from cryopreserved primary cultures as a reliable in vitro bioassay for identifying diverse carcinogens. *Int. J. Cancer*, **19**, 642–655

Pommier, Y., Zwelling, L.A., Mattern, M.R., Erickson, L.C., Kerrigan, D., Schwartz, R. & Kohn, K.W. (1983) Effects of dimethyl sulfoxide and thiourea upon intercalator-induced DNA single-strand breaks in mouse leukemia (L1210) cells. *Cancer Res.*, **43**, 5718–5724

Purves, H.D. & Griesbach, W.E. (1947) Studies on experimental goitre. VIII: Thyroid tumours in rats treated with thiourea. *Br. J. exp. Pathol.*, **28**, 46–53

Radomski, J.L., Deichmann, W.B., MacDonald, W.E. & Glass, E.M. (1965) Synergism among oral carcinogens. I. Results of the simultaneous feeding of four tumorigens to rats. *Toxicol. appl. Pharmacol.*, **7**, 652–656

Raffaelli, A., Pucci, S., Lazzaroni, R. & Salvadori, P. (1997) Rapid determination of thiourea in wastewater by atmospheric pressure chemical ionization tandem mass spectrometry using selected-reaction monitoring. *Rapid Commun. mass Spectrom.*, **11**, 259–264

Rodriguez-Arnaiz, R. (1997) Genotoxic activation of hydrazine, two dialkylhydrazines, thiourea and ethylene thiourea in the somatic *w/w+* assay of *Drosophila melanogaster*. *Mutat. Res.*, **395**, 229–242

Rosenkranz, H.S. & Poirier, L.A. (1979) Evaluation of the mutagenicity and DNA-modifying activity of carcinogens and noncarcinogens in microbial systems. *J. natl Cancer Inst.*, **62**, 873–892

Rosin, A. & Ungar, H. (1957) Malignant tumors in the eyelids and the auricular region of thiourea-treated rats. *Cancer Res.*, **17**, 302–305

Sadtler Research Laboratories (1980) *Sadtler Standard Spectra, 1980 Cumulative Alphabetical Index*, Philadelphia, PA, p. 1482

Sastry, C.S.P., Satyanarayana, P., Rao, A.R.M., Singh, N.R.P. & Hemalatha, K. (1988) Spectrophotometric determination of some thiourea and thiol derivatives. *Acta cienc. indica chem.*, **14**, 227–230

Savela A., Vuorela R. & Kauppinen T. (1999) *ASA 1997* (Katsauksia 140), Helsinki, Finnish Institute of Occupational Health, p. 31 (in Finnish)

Schiestl, R.H. (1989) Nonmutagenic carcinogens induce intrachromosomal recombination in yeast. *Nature*, **337**, 285–288

Schiestl, R.H., Gietz, R.D., Mehta, R.D. & Hastings, P.J. (1989) Carcinogens induce intrachromosomal recombination in yeast. *Carcinogenesis*, **10**, 1445–1455

Shao, C. (1995) [Oscillopolarographic determination of microamounts of thiourea in copper electrolyte.] *Lihua Jianyan Huaxue Fence*, **31**, 151–152 (in Chinese)

Shepard, T.H., II (1963) Metabolism of thiourea S^{35} by the fetal thyroid of the rat. *Endocrinology*, **72**, 223–230

Shimo, T., Mitsumori, K., Onodera, H., Yasuhara, K., Takahashi, M., Takahashi, M., Ueno, Y. & Hayashi, Y. (1994a) Time course observation of thyroid proliferative lesions and serum TSH levels in rats treated with thiourea after DHPN initiation. *Cancer Lett.*, **85**, 141–149

Shimo, T., Mitsumori, K., Onodera, H., Yasuhara, K., Kitaura, K., Takahashi, M., Kanno, J. & Hayashi, Y. (1994b) Synergistic effects of phenobarbital and thiourea on proliferative lesions in the rat liver. *Cancer Lett.*, **81**, 45–52

Simmon, V.F. (1979a) In vitro mutagenicity assays of chemical carcinogens and related compounds with *Salmonella typhimurium*. *J. natl Cancer Inst.*, **62**, 893–899

Simmon, V.F. (1979b) In vitro assays for recombinogenic activity of chemical carcinogens and related compounds with *Saccharomyces cerevisiae* D3. *J. natl Cancer Inst.*, **62**, 901–909

Simmon, V.F., Rosenkranz, H.S., Zeiger, E. & Poirier, L.A. (1979) Mutagenic activity of chemical carcinogens and related compounds in the intraperitoneal host-mediated assay. *J. natl Cancer Inst.*, **62**, 911–918

Sina, J.F., Bean, C.L., Dysart, G.R., Taylor, V.I. & Bradley, M.O. (1983) Evaluation of the alkaline elution/rat hepatocyte assay as a predictor of carcinogenic/mutagenic potential. *Mutat. Res.*, **113**, 357–391

Slanina, P., Ullberg, S. & Hammarström, L. (1973) Distribution and placental transfer of ^{14}C-thiourea and ^{14}C-thiouracil in mice studied by whole-body autoradiography. *Acta pharmacol. toxicol.*, **32**, 358–368

Spector, A. & Shideman, F.E. (1959) Metabolism of thiopyrimidine derivatives: Thiamylal, thiopental and thiouracil. *Biochem. Pharmacol.*, **2**, 182–196

Takegawa, K., Mitsumori, K., Onodera, H., Mutai, M., Kitaura, K., Takahashi, M., Uneyama, C., Yasuhara, K., Takahashi, M., Yanai, T., Masegi, T. & Hayashi, Y. (1997) UDP-GT involvement in the enhancement of cell proliferation in thyroid follicular cell proliferative lesions in rats treated with thiourea and vitamin A. *Arch. Toxicol.*, **71**, 661–667

Toyoda, M., Ogawa, S., Ito, Y. & Iwaida, M. (1979) Gas–liquid chromatographic determination of thiourea in citrus peels. *J. Assoc. off. anal. Chem.*, **62**, 1146–1149

Ungar, H. & Rosin, A. (1960) The histogenesis of thiourea-induced carcinoma of the auditory duct sebaceous (Zymbal's) glands in rats. *Arch. De Vecchi Anat. pat.*, **31**, 419–430

Vazquez-Lopez, E. (1949) The effects of thiourea on the development of spontaneous tumours in mice. *Br. J. Cancer*, **3**, 401–414

Vogel, E.W. & Nivard, M.J.M. (1993) Performance of 181 chemicals in a Drosophila assay predominantly monitoring interchromosomal mitotic recombination. *Mutagenesis*, **8**, 57–81

Wang, X. (1996a) [Determination of thiourea in electrodeless bath for coating of tin.] *Diandu Yu Huanbao*, **16**, 21–22 (in Chinese)

Wang, X. (1996b) [Spectrophotometric determination of thiourea in low-cyanide zinc plating bath.] *Diandu Yu Tushi*, **15**, 34–36 (in Chinese)

Wangenheim, J. & Bolcsfoldi, G. (1988) Mouse lymphoma L5178Y thymidine kinase locus assay of 50 compounds. *Mutagenesis*, **3**, 193–205

Wilkie, D. & Gooneskera, S. (1980) The yeast mitochondrial system in carcinogen testing. *Chem. Ind.*, **21**, 847–850

Williams, R.H. & Kay, G.A. (1947) Thiouracils and thioureas: Comparisons of the absorption, distribution, destruction and excretion. *Arch. intern. Med.*, **80**, 37–52

Winkler, A.W., Man, E.B. & Danowski, T.S. (1947) Minimum dosage of thiourea, given together with iodine medication, necessary for the production and maintenance of a remission in hyperthyroidism. *J. clin. Invest.*, **26**, 446–452

Xu, J. & Tang, X. (1998) [Simultaneous determination of thiourea dioxide and thiourea by UV spectrophotometry.] *Shiyou Huagong*, **27**, 761–762 (in Chinese)

Xu, J., Liu, Y. & Cen, C. (1987) [Determination of thiourea in wastewater from pharmaceutical factories.] *Zhongguo Huanjing Kexue*, **7**, 61–64 (in Chinese)

Yamaguchi, T. (1980) Mutagenicity of isothiocyanates, isocyanates and thioureas in *Salmonella typhimurium*. *Agric. Biol. Chem.*, **44**, 3017–3018

Yao, S.Z., He, F.J. & Nie, L.H. (1992) Piezoelectric determination of traces of thiourea. *Anal. chim. Acta*, **268**, 311–314

Zeiger, E., Anderson, B., Haworth, S., Lawlor, T. & Mortelmans, K. (1988) *Salmonella* mutagenicity tests. IV. Results from the testing of 300 chemicals. *Environ. mol. Mutag.*, **11** (Suppl. 12), 1–158

Zejnilovic, R.M. & Jovanovic, S.I. (1986) Potentiometric determination of thiourea with ion selective electrode. *J. Serb. chem. Soc.*, **51**, 569–571

Zhou, L., Cai, H. & Li, Y. (1990) [Atomic absorption spectrometric determination of thiourea.] *Lihua Jianyan Huaxue Fence*, **26**, 293–295 (in Chinese)

Ziegler-Skylakakis, K., Rossberger, S. & Andrae, U. (1985) Thiourea induces DNA repair synthesis in primary rat hepatocyte cultures and gene mutations in V79 Chinese hamster cells. *Arch. Toxicol.*, **58**, 5–9

Ziegler-Skylakakis, K., Nill, S., Pan, J.F. & Andrae, U. (1998) S-Oxygenation of thiourea results in the formation of genotoxic products. *Environ. mol. Mutag.*, **31**, 362–373

SUMMARY OF FINAL EVALUATIONS

Agent	Degree of evidence of carcinogenicity		Overall evaluation of carcinogenicity to humans
	Human	Animal	
Amitrole	I	S	3*
Chlordane/heptachlor	I	S	2B
2,4-Diaminoanisole	I	S	2B
N,N'-Diethylthiourea	I (ND)	L	3
Doxylamine succinate	I	L	3
Ethylenethiourea	I	S	3*
Griseofulvin	I	S	2B
Hexachlorobenzene	I	S	2B
Kojic acid	I (ND)	L	3
Methimazole	I	L	3
Methylthiouracil	I	S	2B
Phenobarbital	I	S	2B
Propylthiouracil	I	S	2B
Spironolactone	I	L	3
Sulfamethazine	I (ND)	S	3*
Sulfamethoxazole	I	L	3
Thiouracil	I	S	2B
Thiourea	I (ND)	L	3
Toxaphene	I	S	2B

S, sufficient evidence of carcinogenicity; L, limited evidence of carcinogenicity; I, inadequate evidence of carcinogenicity; ND, no data; group 2B, possibly carcinogenic to humans; group 3, not classifiable as to its carcinogenicity to humans; for definitions of criteria for degrees of evidence and groups, see preamble, pp. 23–27.
* Overall evaluation downgraded on the basis of mechanistic data

SUPPLEMENTARY CORRIGENDA TO VOLUMES 1–78

Volume 78

p. 172, first paragraph, last line: *replace* ^{222}Ra *by* ^{224}Ra.

p. 173, last paragraph, third line from below: *before last word* and, *insert* lymphoblastic and second line from below: *replace* dysplastic *by* lymphocytic.

p. 208, first paragraph, line 14: *replace* fibroblastic spindle-cell sarcoma *by* fibroblastic osteosarcoma.

CUMULATIVE CROSS INDEX TO *IARC MONOGRAPHS ON THE EVALUATION OF CARCINOGENIC RISKS TO HUMANS*

The volume, page and year of publication are given. References to corrigenda are given in parentheses.

A

A-α-C	*40*, 245 (1986); *Suppl. 7*, 56 (1987)
Acetaldehyde	*36*, 101 (1985) (*corr. 42*, 263); *Suppl. 7*, 77 (1987); *71*, 319 (1999)
Acetaldehyde formylmethylhydrazone (*see* Gyromitrin)	
Acetamide	*7*, 197 (1974); *Suppl. 7*, 56, 389 (1987); *71*, 1211 (1999)
Acetaminophen (*see* Paracetamol)	
Aciclovir	*76*, 47 (2000)
Acridine orange	*16*, 145 (1978); *Suppl. 7*, 56 (1987)
Acriflavinium chloride	*13*, 31 (1977); *Suppl. 7*, 56 (1987)
Acrolein	*19*, 479 (1979); *36*, 133 (1985); *Suppl. 7*, 78 (1987); *63*, 337 (1995) (*corr. 65*, 549)
Acrylamide	*39*, 41 (1986); *Suppl. 7*, 56 (1987); *60*, 389 (1994)
Acrylic acid	*19*, 47 (1979); *Suppl. 7*, 56 (1987); *71*, 1223 (1999)
Acrylic fibres	*19*, 86 (1979); *Suppl. 7*, 56 (1987)
Acrylonitrile	*19*, 73 (1979); *Suppl. 7*, 79 (1987); *71*, 43 (1999)
Acrylonitrile-butadiene-styrene copolymers	*19*, 91 (1979); *Suppl. 7*, 56 (1987)
Actinolite (*see* Asbestos)	
Actinomycin D (*see also* Actinomycins)	*Suppl. 7*, 80 (1987)
Actinomycins	*10*, 29 (1976) (*corr. 42*, 255)
Adriamycin	*10*, 43 (1976); *Suppl. 7*, 82 (1987)
AF-2	*31*, 47 (1983); *Suppl. 7*, 56 (1987)
Aflatoxins	*1*, 145 (1972) (*corr. 42*, 251); *10*, 51 (1976); *Suppl. 7*, 83 (1987); *56*, 245 (1993)
Aflatoxin B₁ (*see* Aflatoxins)	
Aflatoxin B₂ (*see* Aflatoxins)	
Aflatoxin G₁ (*see* Aflatoxins)	
Aflatoxin G₂ (*see* Aflatoxins)	
Aflatoxin M₁ (*see* Aflatoxins)	
Agaritine	*31*, 63 (1983); *Suppl. 7*, 56 (1987)
Alcohol drinking	*44* (1988)
Aldicarb	*53*, 93 (1991)
Aldrin	*5*, 25 (1974); *Suppl. 7*, 88 (1987)

Allyl chloride   *36*, 39 (1985); *Suppl. 7*, 56 (1987);
                                                     71, 1231 (1999)

Allyl isothiocyanate   *36*, 55 (1985); *Suppl. 7*, 56 (1987);
                                                     73, 37 (1999)

Allyl isovalerate   *36*, 69 (1985); *Suppl. 7*, 56 (1987);
                                                     71, 1241 (1999)

Aluminium production   *34*, 37 (1984); *Suppl. 7*, 89 (1987)
Amaranth   *8*, 41 (1975); *Suppl. 7*, 56 (1987)
5-Aminoacenaphthene   *16*, 243 (1978); *Suppl. 7*, 56 (1987)
2-Aminoanthraquinone   *27*, 191 (1982); *Suppl. 7*, 56 (1987)
para-Aminoazobenzene   *8*, 53 (1975); *Suppl. 7*, 56, 390
                                                     (1987)

ortho-Aminoazotoluene   *8*, 61 (1975) (*corr. 42*, 254);
                                                     Suppl. 7, 56 (1987)

para-Aminobenzoic acid   *16*, 249 (1978); *Suppl. 7*, 56 (1987)
4-Aminobiphenyl   *1*, 74 (1972) (*corr. 42*, 251);
                                                     Suppl. 7, 91 (1987)

2-Amino-3,4-dimethylimidazo[4,5-*f*]quinoline (*see* MeIQ)
2-Amino-3,8-dimethylimidazo[4,5-*f*]quinoxaline (*see* MeIQx)
3-Amino-1,4-dimethyl-5*H*-pyrido[4,3-*b*]indole (*see* Trp-P-1)
2-Aminodipyrido[1,2-*a*:3′,2′-*d*]imidazole (*see* Glu-P-2)
1-Amino-2-methylanthraquinone   *27*, 199 (1982); *Suppl. 7*, 57 (1987)
2-Amino-3-methylimidazo[4,5-*f*]quinoline (*see* IQ)
2-Amino-6-methyldipyrido[1,2-*a*:3′,2′-*d*]imidazole (*see* Glu-P-1)
2-Amino-1-methyl-6-phenylimidazo[4,5-*b*]pyridine (*see* PhIP)
2-Amino-3-methyl-9*H*-pyrido[2,3-*b*]indole (*see* MeA-α-C)
3-Amino-1-methyl-5*H*-pyrido[4,3-*b*]indole (*see* Trp-P-2)
2-Amino-5-(5-nitro-2-furyl)-1,3,4-thiadiazole   *7*, 143 (1974); *Suppl. 7*, 57 (1987)
2-Amino-4-nitrophenol   *57*, 167 (1993)
2-Amino-5-nitrophenol   *57*, 177 (1993)
4-Amino-2-nitrophenol   *16*, 43 (1978); *Suppl. 7*, 57 (1987)
2-Amino-5-nitrothiazole   *31*, 71 (1983); *Suppl. 7*, 57 (1987)
2-Amino-9*H*-pyrido[2,3-*b*]indole (*see* A-α-C)
11-Aminoundecanoic acid   *39*, 239 (1986); *Suppl. 7*, 57 (1987)
Amitrole   *7*, 31 (1974); *41*, 293 (1986) (*corr.*
                                                     52, 513; *Suppl. 7*, 92 (1987);
                                                     79, 381 (2001)

Ammonium potassium selenide (*see* Selenium and selenium compounds)
Amorphous silica (*see also* Silica)   *42*, 39 (1987); *Suppl. 7*, 341 (1987);
                                                     68, 41 (1997)

Amosite (*see* Asbestos)
Ampicillin   *50*, 153 (1990)
Amsacrine   *76*, 317 (2000)
Anabolic steroids (*see* Androgenic (anabolic) steroids)
Anaesthetics, volatile   *11*, 285 (1976); *Suppl. 7*, 93 (1987)
Analgesic mixtures containing phenacetin (*see also* Phenacetin)   *Suppl. 7*, 310 (1987)
Androgenic (anabolic) steroids   *Suppl. 7*, 96 (1987)
Angelicin and some synthetic derivatives (*see also* Angelicins)   *40*, 291 (1986)
Angelicin plus ultraviolet radiation (*see also* Angelicin and some   *Suppl. 7*, 57 (1987)
   synthetic derivatives)
Angelicins   *Suppl. 7*, 57 (1987)
Aniline   *4*, 27 (1974) (*corr. 42*, 252);
                                                     27, 39 (1982); *Suppl. 7*, 99 (1987)

Benz[*a*]anthracene	*3*, 45 (1973); *32*, 135 (1983); *Suppl. 7*, 58 (1987)
Benzene	*7*, 203 (1974) (*corr. 42*, 254); *29*, 93, 391 (1982); *Suppl. 7*, 120 (1987)
Benzidine	*1*, 80 (1972); *29*, 149, 391 (1982); *Suppl. 7*, 123 (1987)
Benzidine-based dyes	*Suppl. 7*, 125 (1987)
Benzo[*b*]fluoranthene	*3*, 69 (1973); *32*, 147 (1983); *Suppl. 7*, 58 (1987)
Benzo[*j*]fluoranthene	*3*, 82 (1973); *32*, 155 (1983); *Suppl. 7*, 58 (1987)
Benzo[*k*]fluoranthene	*32*, 163 (1983); *Suppl. 7*, 58 (1987)
Benzo[*ghi*]fluoranthene	*32*, 171 (1983); *Suppl. 7*, 58 (1987)
Benzo[*a*]fluorene	*32*, 177 (1983); *Suppl. 7*, 58 (1987)
Benzo[*b*]fluorene	*32*, 183 (1983); *Suppl. 7*, 58 (1987)
Benzo[*c*]fluorene	*32*, 189 (1983); *Suppl. 7*, 58 (1987)
Benzofuran	*63*, 431 (1995)
Benzo[*ghi*]perylene	*32*, 195 (1983); *Suppl. 7*, 58 (1987)
Benzo[*c*]phenanthrene	*32*, 205 (1983); *Suppl. 7*, 58 (1987)
Benzo[*a*]pyrene	*3*, 91 (1973); *32*, 211 (1983) (*corr. 68*, 477); *Suppl. 7*, 58 (1987)
Benzo[*e*]pyrene	*3*, 137 (1973); *32*, 225 (1983); *Suppl. 7*, 58 (1987)
1,4-Benzoquinone (see *para*-Quinone)	
1,4-Benzoquinone dioxime	*29*, 185 (1982); *Suppl. 7*, 58 (1987); *71*, 1251 (1999)
Benzotrichloride (*see also* α-Chlorinated toluenes and benzoyl chloride)	*29*, 73 (1982); *Suppl. 7*, 148 (1987); *71*, 453 (1999)
Benzoyl chloride (*see also* α-Chlorinated toluenes and benzoyl chloride)	*29*, 83 (1982) (*corr. 42*, 261); *Suppl. 7*, 126 (1987); *71*, 453 (1999)
Benzoyl peroxide	*36*, 267 (1985); *Suppl. 7*, 58 (1987); *71*, 345 (1999)
Benzyl acetate	*40*, 109 (1986); *Suppl. 7*, 58 (1987); *71*, 1255 (1999)
Benzyl chloride (*see also* α-Chlorinated toluenes and benzoyl chloride)	*11*, 217 (1976) (*corr. 42*, 256); *29*, 49 (1982); *Suppl. 7*, 148 (1987); *71*, 453 (1999)
Benzyl violet 4B	*16*, 153 (1978); *Suppl. 7*, 58 (1987)
Bertrandite (*see* Beryllium and beryllium compounds)	
Beryllium and beryllium compounds	*1*, 17 (1972); *23*, 143 (1980) (*corr. 42*, 260); *Suppl. 7*, 127 (1987); *58*, 41 (1993)

Beryllium acetate (*see* Beryllium and beryllium compounds)
Beryllium acetate, basic (*see* Beryllium and beryllium compounds)
Beryllium-aluminium alloy (*see* Beryllium and beryllium compounds)
Beryllium carbonate (*see* Beryllium and beryllium compounds)
Beryllium chloride (*see* Beryllium and beryllium compounds)
Beryllium-copper alloy (*see* Beryllium and beryllium compounds)
Beryllium-copper-cobalt alloy (*see* Beryllium and beryllium compounds)
Beryllium fluoride (*see* Beryllium and beryllium compounds)
Beryllium hydroxide (*see* Beryllium and beryllium compounds)
Beryllium-nickel alloy (*see* Beryllium and beryllium compounds)
Beryllium oxide (*see* Beryllium and beryllium compounds)

C

Cabinet-making (*see* Furniture and cabinet-making)
Cadmium acetate (*see* Cadmium and cadmium compounds)
Cadmium and cadmium compounds   *2*, 74 (1973); *11*, 39 (1976)
(corr. 42, 255); *Suppl. 7*, 139
(1987); *58*, 119 (1993)

Cadmium chloride (*see* Cadmium and cadmium compounds)
Cadmium oxide (*see* Cadmium and cadmium compounds)
Cadmium sulfate (*see* Cadmium and cadmium compounds)
Cadmium sulfide (*see* Cadmium and cadmium compounds)
Caffeic acid   *56*, 115 (1993)
Caffeine   *51*, 291 (1991)
Calcium arsenate (*see* Arsenic and arsenic compounds)
Calcium chromate (see Chromium and chromium compounds)
Calcium cyclamate (*see* Cyclamates)
Calcium saccharin (*see* Saccharin)
Cantharidin   *10*, 79 (1976); *Suppl. 7*, 59 (1987)
Caprolactam   *19*, 115 (1979) *(corr. 42*, 258);
39, 247 (1986) *(corr. 42*, 264);
Suppl. 7, 59, 390 (1987); *71*, 383
(1999)

Captafol   *53*, 353 (1991)
Captan   *30*, 295 (1983); *Suppl. 7*, 59 (1987)
Carbaryl   *12*, 37 (1976); *Suppl. 7*, 59 (1987)
Carbazole   *32*, 239 (1983); *Suppl. 7*, 59
(1987); *71*, 1319 (1999)
3-Carbethoxypsoralen   *40*, 317 (1986); *Suppl. 7*, 59 (1987)
Carbon black   *3*, 22 (1973); *33*, 35 (1984);
Suppl. 7, 142 (1987); *65*, 149
(1996)
Carbon tetrachloride   *1*, 53 (1972); *20*, 371 (1979);
Suppl. 7, 143 (1987); *71*, 401
(1999)
Carmoisine   *8*, 83 (1975); *Suppl. 7*, 59 (1987)
Carpentry and joinery   *25*, 139 (1981); *Suppl. 7*, 378
(1987)
Carrageenan   *10*, 181 (1976) *(corr. 42*, 255); *31*,
79 (1983); *Suppl. 7*, 59 (1987)
Catechol   *15*, 155 (1977); *Suppl. 7*, 59
(1987); *71*, 433 (1999)
CCNU (*see* 1-(2-Chloroethyl)-3-cyclohexyl-1-nitrosourea)
Ceramic fibres (see Man-made mineral fibres)
Chemotherapy, combined, including alkylating agents (*see* MOPP and
     other combined chemotherapy including alkylating agents)
Chloral   *63*, 245 (1995)
Chloral hydrate   *63*, 245 (1995)
Chlorambucil   *9*, 125 (1975); *26*, 115 (1981);
Suppl. 7, 144 (1987)
Chloramphenicol   *10*, 85 (1976); *Suppl. 7*, 145
(1987); *50*, 169 (1990)
Chlordane (*see also* Chlordane/Heptachlor)   *20*, 45 (1979) *(corr. 42*, 258)
Chlordane and Heptachlor   *Suppl. 7*, 146 (1987); *53*, 115
(1991); *79*, 411 (2001)

D

Dacarbazine	*26*, 203 (1981); *Suppl. 7*, 184 (1987)
Dantron	*50*, 265 (1990) (*corr. 59*, 257)
D&C Red No. 9	*8*, 107 (1975); *Suppl. 7*, 61 (1987); *57*, 203 (1993)
Dapsone	*24*, 59 (1980); *Suppl. 7*, 185 (1987)
Daunomycin	*10*, 145 (1976); *Suppl. 7*, 61 (1987)
DDD (*see* DDT)	
DDE (*see* DDT)	
DDT	*5*, 83 (1974) (*corr. 42*, 253); *Suppl. 7*, 186 (1987); *53*, 179 (1991)
Decabromodiphenyl oxide	*48*, 73 (1990); *71*, 1365 (1999)
Deltamethrin	*53*, 251 (1991)
Deoxynivalenol (*see* Toxins derived from *Fusarium graminearum*, *F. culmorum* and *F. crookwellense*)	
Diacetylaminoazotoluene	*8*, 113 (1975); *Suppl. 7*, 61 (1987)
N,N'-Diacetylbenzidine	*16*, 293 (1978); *Suppl. 7*, 61 (1987)
Diallate	*12*, 69 (1976); *30*, 235 (1983); *Suppl. 7*, 61 (1987)
2,4-Diaminoanisole and its salts	*16*, 51 (1978); *27*, 103 (1982); *Suppl. 7*, 61 (1987); *79*, 619 (2001)
4,4'-Diaminodiphenyl ether	*16*, 301 (1978); *29*, 203 (1982); *Suppl. 7*, 61 (1987)
1,2-Diamino-4-nitrobenzene	*16*, 63 (1978); *Suppl. 7*, 61 (1987)
1,4-Diamino-2-nitrobenzene	*16*, 73 (1978); *Suppl. 7*, 61 (1987); *57*, 185 (1993)
2,6-Diamino-3-(phenylazo)pyridine (*see* Phenazopyridine hydrochloride)	
2,4-Diaminotoluene (*see also* Toluene diisocyanates)	*16*, 83 (1978); *Suppl. 7*, 61 (1987)
2,5-Diaminotoluene (*see also* Toluene diisocyanates)	*16*, 97 (1978); *Suppl. 7*, 61 (1987)
ortho-Dianisidine (*see* 3,3'-Dimethoxybenzidine)	
Diatomaceous earth, uncalcined (*see* Amorphous silica)	
Diazepam	*13*, 57 (1977); *Suppl. 7*, 189 (1987); *66*, 37 (1996)
Diazomethane	*7*, 223 (1974); *Suppl. 7*, 61 (1987)
Dibenz[*a,h*]acridine	*3*, 247 (1973); *32*, 277 (1983); *Suppl. 7*, 61 (1987)
Dibenz[*a,j*]acridine	*3*, 254 (1973); *32*, 283 (1983); *Suppl. 7*, 61 (1987)
Dibenz[*a,c*]anthracene	*32*, 289 (1983) (*corr. 42*, 262); *Suppl. 7*, 61 (1987)
Dibenz[*a,h*]anthracene	*3*, 178 (1973) (*corr. 43*, 261); *32*, 299 (1983); *Suppl. 7*, 61 (1987)
Dibenz[*a,j*]anthracene	*32*, 309 (1983); *Suppl. 7*, 61 (1987)
7*H*-Dibenzo[*c,g*]carbazole	*3*, 260 (1973); *32*, 315 (1983); *Suppl. 7*, 61 (1987)
Dibenzodioxins, chlorinated (other than TCDD) (*see* Chlorinated dibenzodioxins (other than TCDD))	
Dibenzo[*a,e*]fluoranthene	*32*, 321 (1983); *Suppl. 7*, 61 (1987)
Dibenzo[*h,rst*]pentaphene	*3*, 197 (1973); *Suppl. 7*, 62 (1987)
Dibenzo[*a,e*]pyrene	*3*, 201 (1973); *32*, 327 (1983); *Suppl. 7*, 62 (1987)
Dibenzo[*a,h*]pyrene	*3*, 207 (1973); *32*, 331 (1983); *Suppl. 7*, 62 (1987)

Di(2-ethylhexyl) phthalate	*29*, 269 (1982) (*corr. 42*, 261); *Suppl. 7*, 62 (1987); *77*, 41 (2000)
1,2-Diethylhydrazine	*4*, 153 (1974); *Suppl. 7*, 62 (1987); *71*, 1401 (1999)
Diethylstilboestrol	*6*, 55 (1974); *21*, 173 (1979) (*corr. 42*, 259); *Suppl. 7*, 273 (1987)
Diethylstilboestrol dipropionate (*see* Diethylstilboestrol)	
Diethyl sulfate	*4*, 277 (1974); *Suppl. 7*, 198 (1987); *54*, 213 (1992); *71*, 1405 (1999)
N,N′-Diethylthiourea	*79*, 649 (2001)
Diglycidyl resorcinol ether	*11*, 125 (1976); *36*, 181 (1985); *Suppl. 7*, 62 (1987); *71*, 1417 (1999)
Dihydrosafrole	*1*, 170 (1972); *10*, 233 (1976) *Suppl. 7*, 62 (1987)
1,8-Dihydroxyanthraquinone (*see* Dantron)	
Dihydroxybenzenes (*see* Catechol; Hydroquinone; Resorcinol)	
Dihydroxymethylfuratrizine	*24*, 77 (1980); *Suppl. 7*, 62 (1987)
Diisopropyl sulfate	*54*, 229 (1992); *71*, 1421 (1999)
Dimethisterone (*see also* Progestins; Sequential oral contraceptives)	*6*, 167 (1974); *21*, 377 (1979))
Dimethoxane	*15*, 177 (1977); *Suppl. 7*, 62 (1987)
3,3′-Dimethoxybenzidine	*4*, 41 (1974); *Suppl. 7*, 198 (1987)
3,3′-Dimethoxybenzidine-4,4′-diisocyanate	*39*, 279 (1986); *Suppl. 7*, 62 (1987)
para-Dimethylaminoazobenzene	*8*, 125 (1975); *Suppl. 7*, 62 (1987)
para-Dimethylaminoazobenzenediazo sodium sulfonate	*8*, 147 (1975); *Suppl. 7*, 62 (1987)
trans-2-[(Dimethylamino)methylimino]-5-[2-(5-nitro-2-furyl)-vinyl]-1,3,4-oxadiazole	*7*, 147 (1974) (*corr. 42*, 253); *Suppl. 7*, 62 (1987)
4,4′-Dimethylangelicin plus ultraviolet radiation (*see also* Angelicin and some synthetic derivatives)	*Suppl. 7*, 57 (1987)
4,5′-Dimethylangelicin plus ultraviolet radiation (*see also* Angelicin and some synthetic derivatives)	*Suppl. 7*, 57 (1987)
2,6-Dimethylaniline	*57*, 323 (1993)
N,N-Dimethylaniline	*57*, 337 (1993)
Dimethylarsinic acid (*see* Arsenic and arsenic compounds)	
3,3′-Dimethylbenzidine	*1*, 87 (1972); *Suppl. 7*, 62 (1987)
Dimethylcarbamoyl chloride	*12*, 77 (1976); *Suppl. 7*, 199 (1987); *71*, 531 (1999)
Dimethylformamide	*47*, 171 (1989); *71*, 545 (1999)
1,1-Dimethylhydrazine	*4*, 137 (1974); *Suppl. 7*, 62 (1987); *71*, 1425 (1999)
1,2-Dimethylhydrazine	*4*, 145 (1974) (*corr. 42*, 253); *Suppl. 7*, 62 (1987); *71*, 947 (1999)
Dimethyl hydrogen phosphite	*48*, 85 (1990); *71*, 1437 (1999)
1,4-Dimethylphenanthrene	*32*, 349 (1983); *Suppl. 7*, 62 (1987)
Dimethyl sulfate	*4*, 271 (1974); *Suppl. 7*, 200 (1987); *71*, 575 (1999)
3,7-Dinitrofluoranthene	*46*, 189 (1989); *65*, 297 (1996)
3,9-Dinitrofluoranthene	*46*, 195 (1989); *65*, 297 (1996)
1,3-Dinitropyrene	*46*, 201 (1989)
1,6-Dinitropyrene	*46*, 215 (1989)
1,8-Dinitropyrene	*33*, 171 (1984); *Suppl. 7*, 63 (1987); *46*, 231 (1989)

Ethylene dibromide	*15*, 195 (1977); *Suppl. 7*, 204 (1987); *71*, 641 (1999)
Ethylene oxide	*11*, 157 (1976); *36*, 189 (1985) (*corr. 42*, 263); *Suppl. 7*, 205 (1987); *60*, 73 (1994)
Ethylene sulfide	*11*, 257 (1976); *Suppl. 7*, 63 (1987)
Ethylenethiourea	*7*, 45 (1974); *Suppl. 7*, 207 (1987); *79*, 659 (2001)
2-Ethylhexyl acrylate	*60*, 475 (1994)
Ethyl methanesulfonate	*7*, 245 (1974); *Suppl. 7*, 63 (1987)
N-Ethyl-*N*-nitrosourea	*1*, 135 (1972); *17*, 191 (1978); *Suppl. 7*, 63 (1987)
Ethyl selenac (*see also* Selenium and selenium compounds)	*12*, 107 (1976); *Suppl. 7*, 63 (1987)
Ethyl tellurac	*12*, 115 (1976); *Suppl. 7*, 63 (1987)
Ethynodiol diacetate	*6*, 173 (1974); *21*, 387 (1979); *Suppl. 7*, 292 (1987); *72*, 49 (1999)
Etoposide	*76*, 177 (2000)
Eugenol	*36*, 75 (1985); *Suppl. 7*, 63 (1987)
Evans blue	*8*, 151 (1975); *Suppl. 7*, 63 (1987)

F

Fast Green FCF	*16*, 187 (1978); *Suppl. 7*, 63 (1987)
Fenvalerate	*53*, 309 (1991)
Ferbam	*12*, 121 (1976) (*corr. 42*, 256); *Suppl. 7*, 63 (1987)
Ferric oxide	*1*, 29 (1972); *Suppl. 7*, 216 (1987)
Ferrochromium (*see* Chromium and chromium compounds)	
Fluometuron	*30*, 245 (1983); *Suppl. 7*, 63 (1987)
Fluoranthene	*32*, 355 (1983); *Suppl. 7*, 63 (1987)
Fluorene	*32*, 365 (1983); *Suppl. 7*, 63 (1987)
Fluorescent lighting (exposure to) (*see* Ultraviolet radiation)	
Fluorides (inorganic, used in drinking-water)	*27*, 237 (1982); *Suppl. 7*, 208 (1987)
5-Fluorouracil	*26*, 217 (1981); *Suppl. 7*, 210 (1987)
Fluorspar (*see* Fluorides)	
Fluosilicic acid (*see* Fluorides)	
Fluroxene (*see* Anaesthetics, volatile)	
Foreign bodies	*74* (1999)
Formaldehyde	*29*, 345 (1982); *Suppl. 7*, 211 (1987); *62*, 217 (1995) (*corr. 65*, 549; *corr. 66*, 485)
2-(2-Formylhydrazino)-4-(5-nitro-2-furyl)thiazole	*7*, 151 (1974) (*corr. 42*, 253); *Suppl. 7*, 63 (1987)
Frusemide (*see* Furosemide)	
Fuel oils (heating oils)	*45*, 239 (1989) (*corr. 47*, 505)
Fumonisin B$_1$ (*see* Toxins derived from *Fusarium moniliforme*)	
Fumonisin B$_2$ (*see* Toxins derived from *Fusarium moniliforme*)	
Furan	*63*, 393 (1995)
Furazolidone	*31*, 141 (1983); *Suppl. 7*, 63 (1987)
Furfural	*63*, 409 (1995)

G

H

HC Yellow No. 4   *57*, 159 (1993)
Heating oils (*see* Fuel oils)
Helicobacter pylori (infection with)   *61*, 177 (1994)
Hepatitis B virus   *59*, 45 (1994)
Hepatitis C virus   *59*, 165 (1994)
Hepatitis D virus   *59*, 223 (1994)
Heptachlor (*see also* Chlordane/Heptachlor)   *5*, 173 (1974); *20*, 129 (1979)
Hexachlorobenzene   *20*, 155 (1979); *Suppl. 7*, 219
                                                          (1987); *79*, 493 (2001)
Hexachlorobutadiene   *20*, 179 (1979); *Suppl. 7*, 64 (1987);
                                                          73, 277 (1999)
Hexachlorocyclohexanes   *5*, 47 (1974); *20*, 195 (1979)
                                                          (*corr. 42*, 258); *Suppl. 7*, 220
                                                          (1987)
Hexachlorocyclohexane, technical-grade (*see* Hexachlorocyclohexanes)
Hexachloroethane   *20*, 467 (1979); *Suppl. 7*, 64 (1987);
                                                          73, 295 (1999)
Hexachlorophene   *20*, 241 (1979); *Suppl. 7*, 64 (1987)
Hexamethylphosphoramide   *15*, 211 (1977); *Suppl. 7*, 64
                                                          (1987); *71*, 1465 (1999)
Hexoestrol (*see also* Nonsteroidal oestrogens)   *Suppl. 7*, 279 (1987)
Hormonal contraceptives, progestogens only   *72*, 339 (1999)
Human herpesvirus 8   *70*, 375 (1997)
Human immunodeficiency viruses   *67*, 31 (1996)
Human papillomaviruses   *64* (1995) (*corr. 66*, 485)
Human T-cell lymphotropic viruses   *67*, 261 (1996)
Hycanthone mesylate   *13*, 91 (1977); *Suppl. 7*, 64 (1987)
Hydralazine   *24*, 85 (1980); *Suppl. 7*, 222 (1987)
Hydrazine   *4*, 127 (1974); *Suppl. 7*, 223
                                                          (1987); *71*, 991 (1999)
Hydrochloric acid   *54*, 189 (1992)
Hydrochlorothiazide   *50*, 293 (1990)
Hydrogen peroxide   *36*, 285 (1985); *Suppl. 7*, 64
                                                          (1987); *71*, 671 (1999)
Hydroquinone   *15*, 155 (1977); *Suppl. 7*, 64
                                                          (1987); *71*, 691 (1999)
4-Hydroxyazobenzene   *8*, 157 (1975); *Suppl. 7*, 64 (1987)
17α-Hydroxyprogesterone caproate (*see also* Progestins) *21*, 399 (1979) (*corr. 42*, 259)
8-Hydroxyquinoline   *13*, 101 (1977); *Suppl. 7*, 64 (1987)
8-Hydroxysenkirkine   *10*, 265 (1976); *Suppl. 7*, 64 (1987)
Hydroxyurea   *76*, 347 (2000)
Hypochlorite salts   *52*, 159 (1991)

I

Implants, surgical   *74*, 1999
Indeno[1,2,3-*cd*]pyrene   *3*, 229 (1973); *32*, 373 (1983);
                                                          Suppl. 7, 64 (1987)
Inorganic acids (*see* Sulfuric acid and other strong inorganic acids,
       occupational exposures to mists and vapours from)
Insecticides, occupational exposures in spraying and application of   *53*, 45 (1991)
Ionizing radiation (*see* Neutrons, γ- and X-radiation)

Lead chloride (*see* Lead and lead compounds)
Lead chromate (*see* Chromium and chromium compounds)
Lead chromate oxide (*see* Chromium and chromium compounds)
Lead naphthenate (*see* Lead and lead compounds)
Lead nitrate (*see* Lead and lead compounds)
Lead oxide (*see* Lead and lead compounds)
Lead phosphate (*see* Lead and lead compounds)
Lead subacetate (*see* Lead and lead compounds)
Lead tetroxide (*see* Lead and lead compounds)

Leather goods manufacture	*25*, 279 (1981); *Suppl. 7*, 235 (1987)
Leather industries	*25*, 199 (1981); *Suppl. 7*, 232 (1987)
Leather tanning and processing	*25*, 201 (1981); *Suppl. 7*, 236 (1987)
Ledate (*see also* Lead and lead compounds)	*12*, 131 (1976)
Levonorgestrel	*72*, 49 (1999)
Light Green SF	*16*, 209 (1978); *Suppl. 7*, 65 (1987)
d-Limonene	*56*, 135 (1993); *73*, 307 (1999)

Lindane (*see* Hexachlorocyclohexanes)
Liver flukes (*see Clonorchis sinensis, Opisthorchis felineus* and *Opisthorchis viverrini*)

Lumber and sawmill industries (including logging)	*25*, 49 (1981); *Suppl. 7*, 383 (1987)
Luteoskyrin	*10*, 163 (1976); *Suppl. 7*, 65 (1987)
Lynoestrenol	*21*, 407 (1979); *Suppl. 7*, 293 (1987); *72*, 49 (1999)

M

Magenta	*4*, 57 (1974) (*corr. 42*, 252); *Suppl. 7*, 238 (1987); *57*, 215 (1993)
Magenta, manufacture of (*see also* Magenta)	*Suppl. 7*, 238 (1987); *57*, 215 (1993)
Malathion	*30*, 103 (1983); *Suppl. 7*, 65 (1987)
Maleic hydrazide	*4*, 173 (1974) (*corr. 42*, 253); *Suppl. 7*, 65 (1987)
Malonaldehyde	*36*, 163 (1985); *Suppl. 7*, 65 (1987); *71*, 1037 (1999)

Malondialdehyde (*see* Malonaldehyde)

Maneb	*12*, 137 (1976); *Suppl. 7*, 65 (1987)
Man-made mineral fibres	*43*, 39 (1988)
Mannomustine	*9*, 157 (1975); *Suppl. 7*, 65 (1987)
Mate	*51*, 273 (1991)
MCPA (*see also* Chlorophenoxy herbicides; Chlorophenoxy herbicides, occupational exposures to)	*30*, 255 (1983)
MeA-α-C	*40*, 253 (1986); *Suppl. 7*, 65 (1987)
Medphalan	*9*, 168 (1975); *Suppl. 7*, 65 (1987)
Medroxyprogesterone acetate	*6*, 157 (1974); *21*, 417 (1979) (*corr. 42*, 259); *Suppl. 7*, 289 (1987); *72*, 339 (1999)
Megestrol acetate	*Suppl. 7*, 293 (1987); *72*, 49 (1999)

6-Nitrobenzo[a]pyrene	*33*, 187 (1984); *Suppl. 7*, 67 (1987); *46*, 255 (1989)
4-Nitrobiphenyl	*4*, 113 (1974); *Suppl. 7*, 67 (1987)
6-Nitrochrysene	*33*, 195 (1984); *Suppl. 7*, 67 (1987); *46*, 267 (1989)
Nitrofen (technical-grade)	*30*, 271 (1983); *Suppl. 7*, 67 (1987)
3-Nitrofluoranthene	*33*, 201 (1984); *Suppl. 7*, 67 (1987)
2-Nitrofluorene	*46*, 277 (1989)
Nitrofural	*7*, 171 (1974); *Suppl. 7*, 67 (1987); *50*, 195 (1990)
5-Nitro-2-furaldehyde semicarbazone (*see* Nitrofural)	
Nitrofurantoin	*50*, 211 (1990)
Nitrofurazone (*see* Nitrofural)	
1-[(5-Nitrofurfurylidene)amino]-2-imidazolidinone	*7*, 181 (1974); *Suppl. 7*, 67 (1987)
N-[4-(5-Nitro-2-furyl)-2-thiazolyl]acetamide	*1*, 181 (1972); *7*, 185 (1974); *Suppl. 7*, 67 (1987)
Nitrogen mustard	*9*, 193 (1975); *Suppl. 7*, 269 (1987)
Nitrogen mustard N-oxide	*9*, 209 (1975); *Suppl. 7*, 67 (1987)
Nitromethane	*77*, 487 (2000)
1-Nitronaphthalene	*46*, 291 (1989)
2-Nitronaphthalene	*46*, 303 (1989)
3-Nitroperylene	*46*, 313 (1989)
2-Nitro-*para*-phenylenediamine (*see* 1,4-Diamino-2-nitrobenzene)	
2-Nitropropane	*29*, 331 (1982); *Suppl. 7*, 67 (1987); *71*, 1079 (1999)
1-Nitropyrene	*33*, 209 (1984); *Suppl. 7*, 67 (1987); *46*, 321 (1989)
2-Nitropyrene	*46*, 359 (1989)
4-Nitropyrene	*46*, 367 (1989)
N-Nitrosatable drugs	*24*, 297 (1980) (*corr. 42*, 260)
N-Nitrosatable pesticides	*30*, 359 (1983)
N'-Nitrosoanabasine	*37*, 225 (1985); *Suppl. 7*, 67 (1987)
N'-Nitrosoanatabine	*37*, 233 (1985); *Suppl. 7*, 67 (1987)
N-Nitrosodi-*n*-butylamine	*4*, 197 (1974); *17*, 51 (1978); *Suppl. 7*, 67 (1987)
N-Nitrosodiethanolamine	*17*, 77 (1978); *Suppl. 7*, 67 (1987); *77*, 403 (2000)
N-Nitrosodiethylamine	*1*, 107 (1972) (*corr. 42*, 251); *17*, 83 (1978) (*corr. 42*, 257); *Suppl. 7*, 67 (1987)
N-Nitrosodimethylamine	*1*, 95 (1972); *17*, 125 (1978) (*corr. 42*, 257); *Suppl. 7*, 67 (1987)
N-Nitrosodiphenylamine	*27*, 213 (1982); *Suppl. 7*, 67 (1987)
para-Nitrosodiphenylamine	*27*, 227 (1982) (*corr. 42*, 261); *Suppl. 7*, 68 (1987)
N-Nitrosodi-*n*-propylamine	*17*, 177 (1978); *Suppl. 7*, 68 (1987)
N-Nitroso-N-ethylurea (*see* N-Ethyl-N-nitrosourea)	
N-Nitrosofolic acid	*17*, 217 (1978); *Suppl. 7*, 68 (1987)
N-Nitrosoguvacine	*37*, 263 (1985); *Suppl. 7*, 68 (1987)
N-Nitrosoguvacoline	*37*, 263 (1985); *Suppl. 7*, 68 (1987)
N-Nitrosohydroxyproline	*17*, 304 (1978); *Suppl. 7*, 68 (1987)
3-(N-Nitrosomethylamino)propionaldehyde	*37*, 263 (1985); *Suppl. 7*, 68 (1987)
3-(N-Nitrosomethylamino)propionitrile	*37*, 263 (1985); *Suppl. 7*, 68 (1987)
4-(N-Nitrosomethylamino)-4-(3-pyridyl)-1-butanal	*37*, 205 (1985); *Suppl. 7*, 68 (1987)

Phenacetin	*13*, 141 (1977); *24*, 135 (1980); *Suppl. 7*, 310 (1987)
Phenanthrene	*32*, 419 (1983); *Suppl. 7*, 69 (1987)
Phenazopyridine hydrochloride	*8*, 117 (1975); *24*, 163 (1980) (*corr. 42*, 260); *Suppl. 7*, 312 (1987)
Phenelzine sulfate	*24*, 175 (1980); *Suppl. 7*, 312 (1987)
Phenicarbazide	*12*, 177 (1976); *Suppl. 7*, 70 (1987)
Phenobarbital and its sodium salt	*13*, 157 (1977); *Suppl. 7*, 313 (1987); *79*, 161 (2001)
Phenol	*47*, 263 (1989) (*corr. 50*, 385); *71*, 749 (1999)
Phenolphthalein	*76*, 387 (2000)
Phenoxyacetic acid herbicides (*see* Chlorophenoxy herbicides)	
Phenoxybenzamine hydrochloride	*9*, 223 (1975); *24*, 185 (1980); *Suppl. 7*, 70 (1987)
Phenylbutazone	*13*, 183 (1977); *Suppl. 7*, 316 (1987)
meta-Phenylenediamine	*16*, 111 (1978); *Suppl. 7*, 70 (1987)
para-Phenylenediamine	*16*, 125 (1978); *Suppl. 7*, 70 (1987)
Phenyl glycidyl ether (*see also* Glycidyl ethers)	*71*, 1525 (1999)
N-Phenyl-2-naphthylamine	*16*, 325 (1978) (*corr. 42*, 257); *Suppl. 7*, 318 (1987)
ortho-Phenylphenol	*30*, 329 (1983); *Suppl. 7*, 70 (1987); *73*, 451 (1999)
Phenytoin	*13*, 201 (1977); *Suppl. 7*, 319 (1987); *66*, 175 (1996)
Phillipsite (*see* Zeolites)	
PhIP	*56*, 229 (1993)
Pickled vegetables	*56*, 83 (1993)
Picloram	*53*, 481 (1991)
Piperazine oestrone sulfate (*see* Conjugated oestrogens)	
Piperonyl butoxide	*30*, 183 (1983); *Suppl. 7*, 70 (1987)
Pitches, coal-tar (*see* Coal-tar pitches)	
Polyacrylic acid	*19*, 62 (1979); *Suppl. 7*, 70 (1987)
Polybrominated biphenyls	*18*, 107 (1978); *41*, 261 (1986); *Suppl. 7*, 321 (1987)
Polychlorinated biphenyls	*7*, 261 (1974); *18*, 43 (1978) (*corr. 42*, 258); *Suppl. 7*, 322 (1987)
Polychlorinated camphenes (*see* Toxaphene)	
Polychlorinated dibenzo-*para*-dioxins (other than 2,3,7,8-tetrachlorodibenzodioxin)	*69*, 33 (1997)
Polychlorinated dibenzofurans	*69*, 345 (1997)
Polychlorophenols and their sodium salts	*71*, 769 (1999)
Polychloroprene	*19*, 141 (1979); *Suppl. 7*, 70 (1987)
Polyethylene (*see also* Implants, surgical)	*19*, 164 (1979); *Suppl. 7*, 70 (1987)
Poly(glycolic acid) (*see* Implants, surgical)	
Polymethylene polyphenyl isocyanate (*see also* 4,4′-Methylenediphenyl diisocyanate)	*19*, 314 (1979); *Suppl. 7*, 70 (1987)
Polymethyl methacrylate (*see also* Implants, surgical)	*19*, 195 (1979); *Suppl. 7*, 70 (1987)
Polyoestradiol phosphate (*see* Oestradiol-17β)	
Polypropylene (*see also* Implants, surgical)	*19*, 218 (1979); *Suppl. 7*, 70 (1987)

Polystyrene (*see also* Implants, surgical)	*19*, 245 (1979); *Suppl. 7*, 70 (1987)
Polytetrafluoroethylene (*see also* Implants, surgical)	*19*, 288 (1979); *Suppl. 7*, 70 (1987)
Polyurethane foams (*see also* Implants, surgical)	*19*, 320 (1979); *Suppl. 7*, 70 (1987)
Polyvinyl acetate (*see also* Implants, surgical)	*19*, 346 (1979); *Suppl. 7*, 70 (1987)
Polyvinyl alcohol (*see also* Implants, surgical)	*19*, 351 (1979); *Suppl. 7*, 70 (1987)
Polyvinyl chloride (*see also* Implants, surgical)	*7*, 306 (1974); *19*, 402 (1979); *Suppl. 7*, *70* (1987)
Polyvinyl pyrrolidone	*19*, 463 (1979); *Suppl. 7*, 70 (1987); *71*, 1181 (1999)
Ponceau MX	*8*, 189 (1975); *Suppl. 7*, 70 (1987)
Ponceau 3R	*8*, 199 (1975); *Suppl. 7*, 70 (1987)
Ponceau SX	*8*, 207 (1975); *Suppl. 7*, 70 (1987)
Post-menopausal oestrogen therapy	*Suppl. 7*, 280 (1987); *72*, 399 (1999)
Post-menopausal oestrogen-progestogen therapy	*Suppl. 7*, 308 (1987); *72*, 531 (1999)
Potassium arsenate (*see* Arsenic and arsenic compounds)	
Potassium arsenite (*see* Arsenic and arsenic compounds)	
Potassium bis(2-hydroxyethyl)dithiocarbamate	*12*, 183 (1976); *Suppl. 7*, 70 (1987)
Potassium bromate	*40*, 207 (1986); *Suppl. 7*, 70 (1987); *73*, 481 (1999)
Potassium chromate (*see* Chromium and chromium compounds)	
Potassium dichromate (*see* Chromium and chromium compounds)	
Prazepam	*66*, 143 (1996)
Prednimustine	*50*, 115 (1990)
Prednisone	*26*, 293 (1981); *Suppl. 7*, 326 (1987)
Printing processes and printing inks	*65*, 33 (1996)
Procarbazine hydrochloride	*26*, 311 (1981); *Suppl. 7*, 327 (1987)
Proflavine salts	*24*, 195 (1980); *Suppl. 7*, 70 (1987)
Progesterone (*see also* Progestins; Combined oral contraceptives)	*6*, 135 (1974); *21*, 491 (1979) (*corr. 42*, 259)
Progestins (*see* Progestogens)	
Progestogens	*Suppl. 7*, 289 (1987); *72*, 49, 339, 531 (1999)
Pronetalol hydrochloride	*13*, 227 (1977) (*corr. 42*, 256); *Suppl. 7*, 70 (1987)
1,3-Propane sultone	*4*, 253 (1974) (*corr. 42*, 253); *Suppl. 7*, 70 (1987); *71*, 1095 (1999)
Propham	*12*, 189 (1976); *Suppl. 7*, 70 (1987)
β-Propiolactone	*4*, 259 (1974) (*corr. 42*, 253); *Suppl. 7*, 70 (1987); *71*, 1103 (1999)
n-Propyl carbamate	*12*, 201 (1976); *Suppl. 7*, 70 (1987)
Propylene	*19*, 213 (1979); *Suppl. 7*, 71 (1987); *60*, 161 (1994)
Propyleneimine (*see* 2-Methylaziridine)	
Propylene oxide	*11*, 191 (1976); *36*, 227 (1985) (*corr. 42*, 263); *Suppl. 7*, 328 (1987); *60*, 181 (1994)
Propylthiouracil	*7*, 67 (1974); *Suppl. 7*, 329 (1987); *79*, 91 (2001)

Sawmill industry (including logging) (*see* Lumber and
    sawmill industry (including logging))

Scarlet Red   *8*, 217 (1975); *Suppl. 7*, 71 (1987)

Schistosoma haematobium (infection with)   *61*, 45 (1994)

Schistosoma japonicum (infection with)   *61*, 45 (1994)

Schistosoma mansoni (infection with)   *61*, 45 (1994)

Selenium and selenium compounds   *9*, 245 (1975) (*corr. 42*, 255);
    Suppl. 7, 71 (1987)

Selenium dioxide (*see* Selenium and selenium compounds)

Selenium oxide (*see* Selenium and selenium compounds)

Semicarbazide hydrochloride   *12*, 209 (1976) (*corr. 42*, 256);
    Suppl. 7, 71 (1987)

Senecio jacobaea L. (*see also* Pyrrolizidine alkaloids)   *10*, 333 (1976)

Senecio longilobus (*see also* Pyrrolizidine alkaloids)   *10*, 334 (1976)

Seneciphylline   *10*, 319, 335 (1976); *Suppl. 7*, 71
    (1987)

Senkirkine   *10*, 327 (1976); *31*, 231 (1983);
    Suppl. 7, 71 (1987)

Sepiolite   *42*, 175 (1987); *Suppl. 7*, 71
    (1987); *68*, 267 (1997)

Sequential oral contraceptives (*see also* Oestrogens, progestins   *Suppl. 7*, 296 (1987)
    and combinations)

Shale-oils   *35*, 161 (1985); *Suppl. 7*, 339
    (1987)

Shikimic acid (*see also* Bracken fern)   *40*, 55 (1986); *Suppl. 7*, 71 (1987)

Shoe manufacture and repair (*see* Boot and shoe manufacture
    and repair)

Silica (*see also* Amorphous silica; Crystalline silica)   *42*, 39 (1987)

Silicone (*see* Implants, surgical)

Simazine   *53*, 495 (1991); *73*, 625 (1999)

Slagwool (*see* Man-made mineral fibres)

Sodium arsenate (*see* Arsenic and arsenic compounds)

Sodium arsenite (*see* Arsenic and arsenic compounds)

Sodium cacodylate (*see* Arsenic and arsenic compounds)

Sodium chlorite   *52*, 145 (1991)

Sodium chromate (*see* Chromium and chromium compounds)

Sodium cyclamate (*see* Cyclamates)

Sodium dichromate (*see* Chromium and chromium compounds)

Sodium diethyldithiocarbamate   *12*, 217 (1976); *Suppl. 7*, 71 (1987)

Sodium equilin sulfate (*see* Conjugated oestrogens)

Sodium fluoride (*see* Fluorides)

Sodium monofluorophosphate (*see* Fluorides)

Sodium oestrone sulfate (*see* Conjugated oestrogens)

Sodium *ortho*-phenylphenate (*see also ortho*-Phenylphenol)   *30*, 329 (1983); *Suppl. 7*, 71, 392
    (1987); *73*, 451 (1999)

Sodium saccharin (*see* Saccharin)

Sodium selenate (*see* Selenium and selenium compounds)

Sodium selenite (*see* Selenium and selenium compounds)

Sodium silicofluoride (*see* Fluorides)

Solar radiation   *55* (1992)

Soots   *3*, 22 (1973); *35*, 219 (1985);
    Suppl. 7, 343 (1987)

Spironolactone   *24*, 259 (1980); *Suppl. 7*, 344
    (1987); *79*, 317 (2001)

TCDD (*see* 2,3,7,8-Tetrachlorodibenzo-*para*-dioxin)	
TDE (*see* DDT)	
Tea	*51*, 207 (1991)
Temazepam	*66*, 161 (1996)
Teniposide	*76*, 259 (2000)
Terpene polychlorinates	*5*, 219 (1974); *Suppl. 7*, 72 (1987)
Testosterone (*see also* Androgenic (anabolic) steroids)	*6*, 209 (1974); *21*, 519 (1979)
Testosterone oenanthate (*see* Testosterone)	
Testosterone propionate (*see* Testosterone)	
2,2′,5,5′-Tetrachlorobenzidine	*27*, 141 (1982); *Suppl. 7*, 72 (1987)
2,3,7,8-Tetrachlorodibenzo-*para*-dioxin	*15*, 41 (1977); *Suppl. 7*, 350 (1987); *69*, 33 (1997)
1,1,1,2-Tetrachloroethane	*41*, 87 (1986); *Suppl. 7*, 72 (1987); *71*, 1133 (1999)
1,1,2,2-Tetrachloroethane	*20*, 477 (1979); *Suppl. 7*, 354 (1987); *71*, 817 (1999)
Tetrachloroethylene	*20*, 491 (1979); *Suppl. 7*, 355 (1987); *63*, 159 (1995) (*corr. 65*, 549)
2,3,4,6-Tetrachlorophenol (*see* Chlorophenols; Chlorophenols, occupational exposures to; Polychlorophenols and their sodium salts)	
Tetrachlorvinphos	*30*, 197 (1983); *Suppl. 7*, 72 (1987)
Tetraethyllead (*see* Lead and lead compounds)	
Tetrafluoroethylene	*19*, 285 (1979); *Suppl. 7*, 72 (1987); *71*, 1143 (1999)
Tetrakis(hydroxymethyl)phosphonium salts	*48*, 95 (1990); *71*, 1529 (1999)
Tetramethyllead (*see* Lead and lead compounds)	
Tetranitromethane	*65*, 437 (1996)
Textile manufacturing industry, exposures in	*48*, 215 (1990) (*corr. 51*, 483)
Theobromine	*51*, 421 (1991)
Theophylline	*51*, 391 (1991)
Thioacetamide	*7*, 77 (1974); *Suppl. 7*, 72 (1987)
4,4′-Thiodianiline	*16*, 343 (1978); *27*, 147 (1982); *Suppl. 7*, 72 (1987)
Thiotepa	*9*, 85 (1975); *Suppl. 7*, 368 (1987); *50*, 123 (1990)
Thiouracil	*7*, 85 (1974); *Suppl. 7*, 72 (1987); *79*, 127 (2001)
Thiourea	*7*, 95 (1974); *Suppl. 7*, 72 (1987); *79*, 703 (2001)
Thiram	*12*, 225 (1976); *Suppl. 7*, 72 (1987); *53*, 403 (1991)
Titanium (*see* Implants, surgical)	
Titanium dioxide	*47*, 307 (1989)
Tobacco habits other than smoking (*see* Tobacco products, smokeless)	
Tobacco products, smokeless	*37* (1985) (*corr. 42*, 263; *52*, 513); *Suppl. 7*, 357 (1987)
Tobacco smoke	*38* (1986) (*corr. 42*, 263); *Suppl. 7*, 359 (1987)
Tobacco smoking (*see* Tobacco smoke)	
ortho-Tolidine (*see* 3,3′-Dimethylbenzidine)	
2,4-Toluene diisocyanate (*see also* Toluene diisocyanates)	*19*, 303 (1979); *39*, 287 (1986)
2,6-Toluene diisocyanate (*see also* Toluene diisocyanates)	*19*, 303 (1979); *39*, 289 (1986)
Toluene	*47*, 79 (1989); *71*, 829 (1999)

List of IARC Monographs on the Evaluation of Carcinogenic Risks to Humans*

---

*Certain older volumes, marked out-of-print, are still available directly from IARCPress. Further, high-quality photo-copies of all out-of-print volumes may be purchased from University Microfilms International, 300 North Zeeb Road, Ann Arbor, MI 48106-1346, USA (Tel.: 313-761-4700, 800-521-0600).

All IARC publications are available directly from
IARCPress, 150 Cours Albert Thomas, F-69372 Lyon cedex 08, France
(Fax: +33 4 72 73 83 02; E-mail: press@iarc.fr).

IARC Monographs and Technical Reports are also available from the
World Health Organization Distribution and Sales, CH-1211 Geneva 27
(Fax: +41 22 791 4857; E-mail: publications@who.int)
and from WHO Sales Agents worldwide.

IARC Scientific Publications, IARC Handbooks and IARC CancerBases are also available from
Oxford University Press, Walton Street, Oxford, UK OX2 6DP (Fax: +44 1865 267782).

IARC Monographs are also available in an electronic edition,
both on-line by internet and on CD-ROM, from GMA Industries, Inc.,
20 Ridgely Avenue, Suite 301, Annapolis, Maryland, USA
(Fax: +01 410 267 6602; internet: https//www.gmai.com/Order_Form.htm)